Woelfel's
DENTAL ANATOMY
Its Relevance to Dentistry

SEVENTH EDITION

Woelfel's
DENTAL ANATOMY
Its Relevance to Dentistry

SEVENTH EDITION

Rickne C. Scheid, D.D.S., M.Ed.
Associate Professor
Section of Primary Care, Dental Hygiene;
and Restorative and Prosthetic Dentistry
The Ohio State University College of Dentistry
Columbus, Ohio

 Wolters Kluwer | Lippincott Williams & Wilkins
Health

Philadelphia • Baltimore • New York • London
Buenos Aires • Hong Kong • Sydney • Tokyo

Executive Edtior: John Goucher
Managing Editor: Kevin C. Dietz
Marketing Manager: Hilary Henderson
Production Editor: Gina Aiello
Compositor: Maryland Composition
Printer: Quebecor World-Dubuque

351 West Camden Street
Baltimore, Maryland 21201-2436 USA

530 Walnut Street
Philadelphia, Pennsylvania 19106 USA

The publisher is not responsible (as a matter of product liability, negligence, or otherwise) for any injury resulting from any material contained herein. This publication contains information relating to general principles of medical care, which should not be construed as specific instructions for individual patients. Manufacturers' product information and package inserts should be reviewed for current information, including contraindications, dosages, and precautions.

Printed in the United States of America.

Library of Congress Cataloging-in-Publication Data
Scheid, Rickne C.
  Woelfel's dental anatomy : its relevance to dentistry / Rickne C. Scheid. — 7th ed.
    p. ; cm.
  Rev. ed. of: Dental anatomy / Julian B. Woelfel, Rickne C. Scheid.
6th ed. ©2002.
  Includes bibliographical references and index.
  ISBN-13: 978-0-7817-6860-3
  ISBN-10: 0-7817-6860-8
1. Teeth—Anatomy. 2. Mouth—Anatomy. I. Woelfel, Julian B. Dental anatomy. II. Title. III. Title: Dental anatomy.
  [DNLM: 1. Tooth—anatomy & histology—Outlines. 2. Jaw—anatomy & histology—Outlines. 3. Mouth—anatomy & histology—Outlines. WU 18.2 S318w 2007]
QM311.W64 2007
611'.314—dc22   2006101078

The publishers have made every effort to trace the copyright holders for borrowed material. If they have inadvertently overlooked any, they will be pleased to make the necessary arrangements at the first opportunity.

To purchase additional copies of this book call our customer service department at **(800) 638-3030** or fax orders to **(301) 824-7390**. International customers should call **(301) 714-2324**.

2 3 4 5 6 7 8 9 10

Julian B. Woelfel, D.D.S.

Professor Emeritus Woelfel, known primarily for his expertise on complete dentures, research, and occlusion, taught clinical dentistry for 40 years in the College of Dentistry, The Ohio State University, Columbus, Ohio. He served as an Army prosthodontist for 2 years, conducted clinical research for the American Dental Association at the National Bureau of Standards in Washington, D.C. for 2 years, and was a visiting professor in Japan, Taiwan, England, and Brazil. Dr. Woelfel has lectured in 18 foreign countries. He has published 75 scientific articles, four editions of *Dental Anatomy*, and chapters in five books. He holds patents on two inventions that are used in Europe and the United States for accurately recording jaw relations. In addition to his love for students and teaching, he conducted a part-time private practice limited to partial and complete dentures for 33 years. One of his proudest accomplishments is this textbook. In 1967, he was the first recipient of the International Association of Dental Research Award for Research in Prosthodontics, and became a Life Member of the Nihon University Dental Alumni Association. In 1972, the New York Prosthodontic Society selected him for the Jerome and Dorothy Schweitzer Award for Outstanding and Continuing Research in Prosthodontics. In 1992, the Ohio Dental Association chose Dr. Woelfel for the prestigious Callahan Award, and in 2004, he was the recipient of the Distinguished Alumni Award of the College of Dentistry at The Ohio State University. He is a Life Member of several professional societies including Sigma Xi, the International Association for Dental Research, the American Prosthodontic Society, and the ADA, FDI, FICD, and FACD.

Rickne C. Scheid, D.D.S., M.Ed.

Dr. Rickne Scheid received his D.D.S. in 1972 at The Ohio State University and was inducted into the dental honorary fraternity, Omicron Kappa Upsilon. After serving in the U.S. Navy Dental Corps, he went into part-time practice and has taught at his alma mater since 1974. His appointments at the College of Dentistry have been in the Department of Operative Dentistry, the Division of Dental Hygiene, and currently, he holds a dual appointment in the Section of Restorative and Prosthetic Dentistry and the Section of Primary Care in Dental Hygiene. While teaching, he received his Masters in Education with honors in 1980. He has authored or coauthored nearly 50 scientific papers and abstracts. Throughout his teaching career, he has developed and directed 12 different courses, including directing the dental anatomy course, which is presented each year to 130 dental and dental hygiene students. Further, he helped develop and annually codirects over 184 hours of continuing education, including a review course for dental hygienists returning to practice, a dental anatomy review course for dentists and dental auxiliaries, and an expanded functions course for dental auxiliaries. He was inducted into the dental hygiene honorary, Sigma Phi Alpha, in 1989, and has received numerous dental and dental hygiene student teaching awards as well as the peer-evaluated Postle Teaching Award in 1996.

Preface to the Seventh Edition

Woelfel's Dental Anatomy: Its Relevance to Dentistry is primarily intended as a study guide for dental students, dental hygiene students, dental assistants, and dental laboratory technicians in the study of tooth morphology and related structures. The text is designed to help the reader appreciate the relationship of teeth to one another and to the bones, muscles, nerves, and vessels closely associated with the teeth and face. This text also includes considerable emphasis on the application of dental morphology to the practice of dentistry. The book is organized to be used by instructors of dental anatomy courses as a teaching manual during lectures, discussion periods, and laboratory sessions, and in early clinical experiences. It is also useful as a reference in a dental office.

HOW THE BOOK IS ORGANIZED:

Chapter 1 begins with a very brief overview of the teeth: just enough to help the reader appreciate the relationship of the teeth to the head and neck anatomy presented in the remaining sections of this chapter. Topics include the bones of the skull and associated bony landmarks, the temporomandibular joints, the chewing muscles, and the nerves, blood supply, and lymph drainage associated with the oral cavity. **Chapter 2** includes the location and description of *normal* oral structures observed during a head and neck cancer screening examination in the dental office, followed in **Chapter 3** by a more detailed description of general terminology of normal tooth morphology and ideal tooth and occlusal relationships. **Chapters 4 through 7** include detailed descriptions of each type of adult tooth, with drawings, photographs, and charts designed to illustrate the normal characteristics of each tooth type. These chapters also help the reader appreciate the variation that can occur between the same type of teeth in different mouths. The roots of the adult teeth are discussed in more detail in **Chapter 8** (relative to periodontics) and **Chapter 9** (relative to endodontics). **Chapter 10** includes the discussion of deciduous or primary teeth, along with eruption patterns occurring throughout the time when mixed dentition is present. **Chapter 11** provides a contemporary overview of occlusion. Here, the authors describe the relationship of the jaws and teeth during various normal and abnormal relationships, including a discussion of treatment modalities used to correct malocclusion or temporomandibular joint dysfunction. Next, in **Chapter 12**, there is an extensive discussion of many commonly encountered dental anomalies. The importance of dental anatomy and terminology related to operative and restorative dentistry is presented in **Chapter 13**. **Chapter 14** includes helpful techniques for learners to draw, sketch, and carve teeth, and **Chapter 15** includes the importance of tooth morphology within the field of forensic dentistry.

Each chapter includes methods designed to help you, the reader, master the content and put it to practice immediately.

- **Topic list:** Each *chapter* begins with a list of topics that are presented within that chapter. The topics are presented in the same order as the section outline headings within that chapter.
- **Learning objectives:** In each section, important learning objectives are presented to help you appreciate what you can expect to learn as you read. You can refer to the objectives to ensure that you are mastering the appropriate knowledge and skills.
- **New terms:** As each new term is encountered for the first time, it is highlighted in bold print and is defined within the text at that time, often with references to figures or diagrams to improve understanding. The bold print is helpful when using the text as a reference for understanding terms that can be found within the text's index.
- **Index (instead of a glossary):** The extensive index has been used instead of a glossary since many terms in dentistry are best appreciated by referring to illustrations or photographs for a complete understanding. In most cases, the first page where a term is referenced in the index is the page where you can find the term (in bold) and can refer to the suggested illustrations for the best learning.
- **Pronunciations:** New terms that may be difficult to pronounce have phonetic suggestions placed within brackets [like this] immediately after the word is first encountered.

- **Learning questions with answers:** Many chapters or sections end with a series of learning questions to test the learner's mastery of the objectives. These questions, in many cases, cover topics similar to those included on past dental and dental hygiene national examinations. For the convenience of quick and convenient feedback, the answers are presented immediately following the questions (but upside down). Available for instructors who use this edition is a CD that includes a bank of additional test items.
- **Learning exercises:** Practically every chapter provides the reader with a series of learning exercises. These exercises are presented within the body of each chapter at intervals where the authors feel an active learning experience would be helpful for you to understand and/or apply the topic. These exercises may suggest that you examine extracted teeth or tooth models, or skulls (or skull models), or perform specific self- or partner examinations. More advanced exercises (as in Chapter 14) provide methods for drawing, sketching, and carving teeth from wax, helping you to become intimately familiar with tooth shape and terminology.
- **Tables:** Throughout the text, the authors have placed numerous tables to help summarize the many facts presented within the text. These tables are helpful when reviewing the highlights of content found within each section.
- **Illustrations and drawings:** For complete understanding and clinical application of each topic, the authors have included a variety of photographs, illustrations, and original drawings selected and designed to illustrate key points and improve learning. A number of new illustrations and summary charts have been added to this edition, and many of the new illustrations are in color. Since a picture is worth a thousand words, it is critical that you refer to figures whenever they are referenced within the text in order to maximize your learning. Many figures are designed, so you can cover up the names of structures and test yourself. In some instances, important additional information is presented or clarified in the illustration legends. New in this edition is a CD for instructors containing all of the illustrations and drawings in the text that can be used when lecturing.
- **Appendix of comparative dental anatomy:** The text's unique appendix is designed to help the learner visualize the many tooth similarities and differences that are often difficult to understand with words alone. Each **adult tooth** class is referenced on two appendix pages. The first page includes characteristics (each labeled with a different letter) that are *common* to all teeth within that class. The second page is devoted to the *differences* (each identified with a letter) between the types of teeth within each class, and differences between teeth in each arch. Two additional appendix pages are included that illustrate the unique characteristics of anterior and posterior **primary teeth.** The layout on these pages makes it easy to compare the differences between teeth because various views of each tooth type are lined up on the same page next to other teeth in that class. As each tooth characteristic is described within the chapters on tooth morphology (Chapters 4–7 and 10), reference is frequently made to the illustrated representation of that characteristic on an appendix page as follows: the word "Appendix" is followed by the page number and letter denoting items being discussed (for example, "**Appendix 1a**" refers you to the Appendix, page 1, item "a"). Appendix pages are printed on heavier, perforated paper to permit removal and placement in a separate loose-leaf notebook. When used in this fashion, these pages provide you with increased *convenience* (since fewer page turns are required when referencing tooth characteristics within each chapter), *easier learning* (since the complex terminology used to describe each characteristic is best learned by visualizing that characteristic and comparing it to other similar teeth), and a separate *study guide* (since all labeled characteristics for each type of tooth are described on the back of each appendix page).
- For learning the morphology of individual teeth, the best learning resource is a collection of as many intact **extracted teeth** as you are able to acquire. A dentist, if presented with a quart jar of bleach, will remember his or her own student days and will probably be glad to put extracted teeth in the jar. Do not expect these teeth to be clean or sorted out; sorting is your job. While handling these teeth, **it is critical that the guidelines for infection control be followed:**

    GUIDELINES FOR STERILIZING EXTRACTED TEETH: Using protective gloves and a mask, tooth specimens should be scraped clean with a knife. Soaking for several hours in hydrogen peroxide before scraping is helpful. After scraping to remove hard deposits and soft tissue, tooth specimens should be further cleansed by soaking for 20 minutes in 4 ounces of household bleach containing 2 tablespoons of Calgon (a water softener). Teeth can then be placed in water (in a beaker covered with tin foil) to be autoclaved for 40 minutes at 121°C and 15 psi (Pantera E, Schuster G. J Dent Ed 1990;54[5]:284). Once prepared, teeth should be kept moist, either by soaking in water or, as suggested by Dr. Kim Loos, D.D.S., soaked in 25% glycerin and 75% water (parentsplace.com, Feb. 28, 2001).

As you begin learning the characteristics that differentiate each type of tooth as described in Chapters 4 through 7, you need to be aware of the considerable variation in tooth morphology that can occur from one patient to the next. You must keep in mind that relative tooth sizes and characteristics cited within the text do *not* apply to *all* patients' teeth, but are based on average sizes or particular morphology occurring with the greatest frequency. This text is unique in providing you with both **original and reviewed research** findings based on the study of thousands of teeth, casts, and mouths. The data from these studies are presented throughout the text in *brackets* [like this] and provide a scientific basis for understanding the frequency and extent to which differences from the norm occur. For example, the text states that "a mesial marginal groove is a distinguishing characteristic of the maxillary first premolar [but this occurred in only 97% of the 600 premolars checked, which means that, on the average, 3% may not have this groove], whereas the maxillary second premolar is not nearly as likely to have this groove [but 37% do have it]."

As you read the description of tooth morphology, not only identify each structure visually, but also use a dental explorer on an actual tooth or model to "feel" the contours being described since you will eventually be required to evaluate, reproduce, and/or clean the surfaces of these tooth contours with specific dental instruments. As you become familiar with the many similarities and differences of tooth morphology, you can later apply this information during patient treatment, evaluation, and education.

Hopefully, you will spend some time thinking about and comprehending the concepts as you read. After all, you are learning the "foreign" language of dental anatomy that you will be using for the rest of your professional lives. Have fun looking at teeth as though you were a tooth detective. Take notes, sketch different views of each tooth, and take advantage of all learning exercises, references to figures, and the appendix. Ask questions until your curiosity is satisfied. Most importantly, the authors hope this book will stimulate your interest and involvement in the wonderful and fascinating field of dentistry and that you will consider it to be a worthwhile addition to your library even after your formal education is complete.

Rickne C. Scheid

Comments or suggestions may be submitted to Dr. Scheid on e-mail (scheid.2@osu.edu).

Contents

Color plates follow page 256.

Introduction to the Seventh Edition and Acknowledgments

During my first year teaching at The Ohio State University College of Dentistry in 1974, I was fortunate to be assigned to teach in a laboratory for dental anatomy where I worked with and was mentored by, Dr. Julian Woelfel. He asked me to contribute the chapter on Operative Dentistry in the third edition in 1984. Little did I realize that in 1994, I would be selected by him to coauthor the fifth edition of a text on the very topic I began teaching in 1974: dental anatomy. During the preparation for the fifth and sixth editions, Julian permitted me great latitude in reorganizing the text to reflect my teaching style since I use this text as I teach over 135 dental and dental hygiene students each year. During this major reorganization, I was careful to maintain the unique aspects that he had incorporated into previous editions. This includes the results of his personal, science-based research, which formed the basis for many of the conclusions presented within this text: on everything from the average mandibular hinge opening to the frequency of Carabelli cusp formation and the comparative sizes of deciduous and permanent (or secondary) teeth. Now, in the seventh edition, Dr. Wolefel entrusted me to take over the text. In this edition, I was able to fine-tune the text to make it even more learner-friendly, adding more summary charts and more illustrations, including many color photographs and a CD for instructors.

I would like to express my appreciation to all of the contributors to this and previous editions of this book. Obviously, my thanks goes to Dr. Woelfel for selecting me to take over the new edition and teaching me to be meticulous, and for his many contributions to previous editions; to his wife, Marcile, who has helped tremendously in typing and editing previous editions; and to Dr. Gabriela Weiss (who proofed many pages and provided many test items for the CD), Dr. Lewis Claman (who organized and updated Chapter 8), Dr. John Nusstein (who organized and updated Chapter 9), Dr. Robert Rashid (who organized and updated Chapter 13), and Dr. Daniel Jolly (who completely rewrote Chapter 15). I would also like to recognize Ms. Dorothy Permar, who conceived and wrote the first edition in 1974, and Dr. Theodore Berg, Jr., Dr. Al Reader, and Ms. Connie Sylvester, who contributed to previous editions.

Rickne C. Scheid, D.D.S. M.Ed.

Structures That Form the Foundation for Tooth Function

1

Topics covered within the seven sections of this chapter include the following:

I. Naming teeth based on location within the normal, complete human dentition
   A. Complete primary dentition
   B. Complete permanent dentition
II. Bones of the human skull (with emphasis on the sphenoid, temporal, maxillae, and mandible bones)
   A. Bones of the neurocranium
   B. Bones of the face (visceral apparatus)
III. The temporomandibular joint
   A. Anatomy of the temporomandibular joint
   B. Ligaments that support the joint and limit joint movement
   C. Development of the temporomandibular joint
IV. Muscles of chewing (mastication)
   A. Muscles involved in mastication (chewing)
   B. Other muscles affecting mandibular movement

C. Other factors affecting tooth position or movement
   D. Summary of muscles that move and control the mandible
V. Nerves of the oral cavity (with emphasis on cranial nerves V, VII, IX, and XII)
   A. Trigeminal nerve (fifth cranial nerve)
   B. Facial nerve (seventh cranial nerve)
   C. Glossopharyngeal nerve (ninth cranial nerve)
   D. Hypoglossal nerve (12th cranial nerve)
   E. Summary of nerve supply to the tongue, salivary glands, facial skin, and facial muscles
VI. Vessels associated with the oral cavity (arteries, veins, and lymphatic system)
   A. Arteries
   B. Veins
   C. Lymph
VII. Structures visible on a panoramic radiograph

This chapter introduces the reader to the structures that form the foundation for tooth function: gross anatomy of the bones, muscles, nerves, blood supply, and lymph drainage of the head and neck. Emphasis is placed on the importance of these structures as they relate to the functioning of the jaws and teeth. Initially, however, the reader must master a few basic terms related to teeth.

SECTION I.	NAMING TEETH BASED ON LOCATION WITHIN THE NORMAL, COMPLETE HUMAN DENTITION

OBJECTIVES

This section is designed to prepare the learner to perform the following:
- Based on location in the normal, complete primary dentition, name all 20 teeth by dentition, arch, quadrant, class, and type.
- Based on location in the normal, complete permanent dentition, name all 32 teeth by dentition, arch, quadrant, class, and type.

Prior to a discussion of the structures that support the teeth, it is necessary to familiarize yourself with a brief description of the names of teeth based on their location in the human skull and mouth. This overview is necessary to appreciate and understand the full description of the bones, nerves, and blood vessels presented in this chapter, as well as the description of oral landmarks described in Chapter 2. A more in-depth description of all teeth begins in Chapter 3.

In general, each human tooth has a clinical **crown**, the portion of the tooth projecting beyond the gum line, and a clinical **root**, the portion hidden below the gum line. All of the teeth in the mouth together are referred to as the **dentition** [den TISH un]. Humans have two dentitions throughout life: one during childhood, called the **primary dentition**, and one that will hopefully last throughout adulthood, called the **secondary** (also known as **permanent**) **dentition**. The teeth in the upper jawbones (called the maxillae [mak SIL ee]) collectively form an arch shape known as the **maxillary** [MAK sei lair ee] **arch**, and those teeth in the lower jawbone (called the mandible) collectively form the **mandibular** [man DIB yoo ler] **arch**. Each arch can further be divided into the left and right halves (also known as left and right **quadrants** since each quadrant contains one-fourth of all teeth in that dentition).

A.   COMPLETE PRIMARY DENTITION

The *complete* primary dentition is normally present in a child from the ages of about 2 to 6 years. There are 20 teeth in the entire primary dentition (shown in *Fig. 1-1*): 10 in the maxillary arch and 10 in the mandibular arch. This dentition is also called the **deciduous** [de SIDJ oo us] **dentition**, referring to the fact that all of these teeth are eventually shed by age 12 or 13, being replaced sequentially by teeth of the permanent dentition. The complete primary dentition has five teeth in each quadrant. The primary teeth in each quadrant are further divided into three **classes**: incisors [in SI zerz], canines, and molars. Based on location, starting on either side of the midline between the right and left quadrants, the two front teeth in each quadrant of the primary dentition are **incisors** (I), followed by one **canine** (C), then two **molars** (M). Using these abbreviations for the classes of teeth, followed by a ratio composed of a top number representing the number of teeth in each upper quadrant and the bottom number representing the number of teeth in each lower quadrant, a formula can be used to represent the teeth in the human primary dentition as follows:

$$I\frac{2}{2}\ C\frac{1}{1}\ M\frac{2}{2} = 5 \text{ upper and 5 lower teeth on either side; 20 teeth in all}$$

The classes of primary teeth containing more than one tooth per quadrant (incisors and molars) are subdivided into **types** within each class. Each type can also be identified by its location within the complete quadrant. The primary incisor closest to the midline separating the right and left quadrants is called a **central incisor**; the incisor next to or lateral to the central incisor is called a **lateral incisor**. Next in each quadrant is a canine, followed by two molars: a **first molar** behind the canine and then a **second molar**.

LEARNING EXERCISE

Using either models of the complete primary dentition or Figure 1-1 while covering up the labels, identify each primary tooth based on its location in the arch. To identify each tooth accurately, include the dentition (primary); arch (maxillary or mandibular); quadrant (right or left); class (incisor, canine, or molar); type of incisor (central or lateral); and type of molar (first or second).

B.   COMPLETE PERMANENT DENTITION

The complete permanent (or secondary) dentition is present in the adult. It is composed of 32 teeth: 16 in the maxillary arch and 16 in the mandibular arch (shown in *Fig. 1-2*). The permanent dentition has eight teeth in each quadrant, which are divided into four **classes**: incisors, canines, **premolars** (PM; a new class for permanent teeth), and molars. Based on location, the two permanent front teeth in each quadrant are

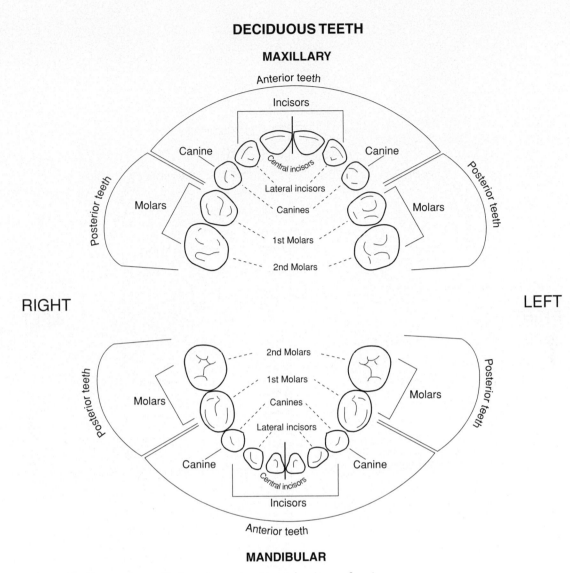

FIGURE 1-1. Maxillary and mandibular primary dentition (chewing surfaces).

incisors (I), followed by one *canine* (C), then two *premolars* (PM), and finally three *molars* (M). The dental formula for the human permanent dentition is:

$$I\frac{2}{2}\ C\frac{1}{1}\ PM\frac{2}{2}\ M\frac{3}{3} = 8 \text{ upper and } 8 \text{ lower teeth on either side, } 32 \text{ teeth in all}$$

The classes of permanent teeth containing more than one tooth per quadrant (namely, incisors, premolars, and molars) are subdivided into **types** within each class. Each type can also be identified by location within the quadrant. As in the primary dentition, the permanent incisor closest to the midline between the right and left quadrants is called a **central incisor**; the incisor next to or lateral to the central incisor is called a **lateral incisor**. Next in the arch is a **canine**, followed by a **first premolar**, then a **second premolar**. Continuing around toward the back in each quadrant are three molars: a **first molar**, a **second molar**, and finally a **third molar** (sometimes referred to as a wisdom tooth).

As noted by comparing the formulas for deciduous and permanent teeth, differences exist. Although central and lateral incisors and canines are similarly positioned in both dentitions, permanent dentitions have a new category of teeth called premolars, which are located between canines and molars. Premolars are positioned in the spaces left where the primary molars were located earlier in life. Behind the premolars, there are three instead of two molars.

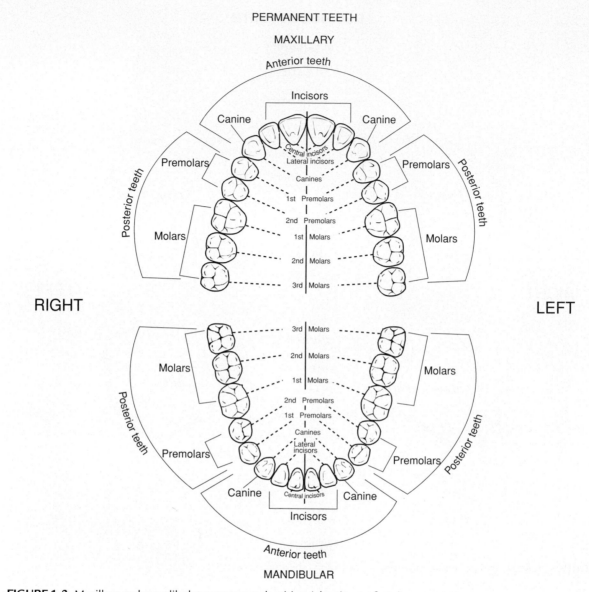

FIGURE 1-2. Maxillary and mandibular permanent dentition (chewing surfaces).

Two other terms are used to categorize or distinguish groups of teeth by their location: anterior and posterior teeth. **Anterior teeth** are those teeth in the front of the mouth, specifically, the incisors and the canines. **Posterior teeth** are those in the back of the mouth, specifically, the premolars and the molars.

It is interesting to note that animal dentition can be represented by the same type of formula as described above. Look at the formulas for animals in *Table 1-1* and note that cows have no upper incisors or upper canines. They have three upper and three lower premolars on each side. Did you know that dogs have twice as many premolars as humans if you include uppers and lowers, as well as the right and left sides?

LEARNING EXERCISE

Using either models of the complete permanent dentition or Figure 1-2 while covering up the labels, identify each permanent tooth based on its location in the arch. To identify each tooth accurately, include the dentition

Table 1-1	SOME DENTAL FORMULAE (ORDER OF TEETH PER QUADRANT) AND INTERESTING FACTS ABOUT TEETH IN ANIMALS[33–35]				
Humans, Old World monkeys, and apes	$1\frac{2}{2}\,c\frac{1}{1}\,p\frac{2}{2}$	$M\frac{3}{3}$	Porcupines and beavers	$1\frac{1}{1}\,c\frac{0}{0}\,p\frac{1}{1}$	$M\frac{3}{3}$
New World monkeys	$1\frac{2}{2}\,c\frac{1}{1}\,p\frac{3}{3}$	$M\frac{3}{3}$	Bears and pandas	$1\frac{3}{3}\,c\frac{1}{1}\,p\frac{4}{4}$	$M\frac{2}{3}$
Dogs, wolves, and foxes	$1\frac{3}{3}\,c\frac{1}{1}\,p\frac{4}{4}$	$M\frac{2}{3}$	Squirrels	$1\frac{1}{1}\,c\frac{0}{0}\,p\frac{2}{1}$	$M\frac{3}{3}$
Cats	$1\frac{3}{3}\,c\frac{1}{1}\,p\frac{3}{2}$	$M\frac{1}{1}$	Rabbit‡	$1\frac{2}{1}\,c\frac{0}{0}\,p\frac{3}{2}$	$M\frac{3}{3}$
Cows	$1\frac{0}{3}\,c\frac{0}{1}\,p\frac{3}{3}$	$M\frac{3}{3}$	Mice and rats	$1\frac{1}{1}\,c\frac{0}{0}\,p\frac{0}{0}$	$M\frac{3}{3}$
Horses and zebra*	$1\frac{3}{3}\,c\frac{1}{1}\,p\frac{4}{4}$	$M\frac{3}{3}$	Moles	$1\frac{3}{3}\,c\frac{1}{1}\,p\frac{4}{4}$	$M\frac{3}{3}$
Walruses	$1\frac{1}{0}\,c\frac{1}{1}\,p\frac{3}{3}$	$M\frac{0}{0}$	Vampire bats	$1\frac{1}{2}\,c\frac{1}{1}\,p\frac{2}{3}$	$M\frac{0}{0}$
Elephants	$1\frac{1}{0}\,c\frac{0}{0}\,Dm\dagger\frac{3}{3}$	$M\frac{3}{3}$	Shrews	$1\frac{3}{1}\,c\frac{1}{1}\,p\frac{3}{1}$	$M\frac{3}{3}$

* Pigs and hippopotami have the same formula, except that they have two or three upper and two or three lower incisors.

† Elephants have deciduous molars but no premolars. An elephant's skull is larger than necessary to house its brain. The size is needed to provide mechanical support for the tusks (one-third of their length is embedded in the skull) and the enormous molars. Each molar weighs about 9 pounds and is nearly a foot long mesiodistally on the occlusal surface. Tusks (the central incisors) can be as long as $11\frac{1}{2}$ feet and weigh 440 pounds.[42]

‡ Guinea pigs have the same formula, except that they have only one maxillary incisor.

The beaver has four strong curved incisors. They have very hard, bright orange enamel on the labial surface and much softer exposed dentin on the lingual surface. As the dentin wears off, this leaves very sharp cutting edges of enamel. The incisors continue to grow throughout life. The posterior teeth have flat, rough edges on the occlusal surface, and they stop growing at 2 years of age. There is a large diastema immediately posterior to the incisors, and flaps of skin fold inward and meet behind the incisors to seal off the back part of the mouth during gnawing. Therefore, splinters are kept out. The flaps of skin relax for eating and drinking.

The shrew has two hooked cusps on the upper first incisor. Its deciduous dentition is shed in utero. The shrew's 1- to $1\frac{1}{2}$-year life span is limited by the wear on their molars. Death occurs by starvation once the molars wear out. Also, their small body can store only enough food for 1-2 hours, so they must feed almost continually. Their diet consists of small invertebrates, woodlice, and fruit.

The vampire bat has large canines, but its highly specialized upper incisors, which are V-shaped and razor-edged, are what remove a piece of the victim's skin. The bat's saliva contains an anticoagulant, and its tongue rolls up in a tube to suck or lap the exuding blood.

Some vertebrates do not have any teeth (complete anodontia) but have descended from ancestors that possessed teeth. Birds have beaks but depend on a gizzard to do the grinding that molars would usually perform. Turtles have heavy law coverings, which are thin edged in the incisor region and wide posteriorly for crushing. The duck-billed platypus has its early-life teeth replaced by keratinous plates, which it uses to crush aquatic insects, crustaceans, and molluscs. The whalebone whale and anteaters also have no teeth, but their diets do not require mastication.

(permanent); arch (maxillary or mandibular); quadrant (right or left); class (incisor, canine, premolar, or molar); type of incisor (central or lateral); type of premolar (first or second); and type of molar (first, second, or third).

LEARNING QUESTIONS

Select the one best answer.

1. How many teeth are present in one quadrant of a complete adult (permanent) dentition?
    a. 5
    b. 8
    c. 10
    d. 20
    e. 32

2. What class of teeth is present in the permanent dentition that is NOT present in the primary dentition?
   a. incisors
   b. canines
   c. premolars
   d. molars

3. In a permanent dentition, the fifth tooth from the midline is a:
   a. canine
   b. premolar
   c. molar
   d. incisor

4. Posterior teeth in the permanent dentition include which of the following?
   a. premolars only
   b. molars only
   c. premolars and molars only
   d. canines, premolars, and molars

5. What permanent tooth erupts into the space previously held by the primary second molar?
   a. first molar
   b. second molar
   c. first premolar
   d. second premolar

ANSWERS: 1-b, 2-c, 3-b, 4-c, 5-d

SECTION II.   BONES OF THE HUMAN SKULL

OBJECTIVES

This section is designed to prepare the learner to perform the following:
- Describe and identify each bone seen on an intact human skull.
- Describe and identify each bony structure highlighted in bold in this chapter. Emphasis is placed on structures of the mandible, maxillae, temporal, and sphenoid bones.
- Describe and identify the location of the attachment of chewing muscles and ligaments attached to the mandible.
- Describe and identify the foramen of the nerves and arteries that supply the teeth and oral cavity.

LEARNING EXERCISE

To obtain a clear understanding of the bones of the skull and their relationship to one another and to the teeth, it is best to have a skull at hand to examine while reading this chapter. If you touch and trace each bone with your fingers as you read, you are not apt to forget its characteristics.

There are 206 distinct bones in our skeleton, 28 of which are in the skull if we count the malleus, stapes, and incus bones of each ear. The skull bones can be divided into two parts: the **neurocranium** [NOOR o CRAY ne um] surrounding the brain and the **facial** (or visceral) **apparatus** (making up the face).

When studying bones (and teeth), there are many descriptive terms that must be learned. Terms with similar definitions are grouped here to facilitate learning. Since anatomy terms are often similar to common familiar words, the new terms are compared to familiar words whenever possible.

BUMPS—(CONVEXITIES) ON BONES AND/OR TEETH

crest: a projecting ridge along a bone
eminence: a prominence or elevation of bone
process: a projection or outgrowth from a larger bone structure
protuberance [pro TU ber ahns]: a prominence or swelling (of bone)
ridge: linear, narrow, elevated portion of bone or tooth
tubercle [TOO ber k'l]: a small rounded projection on a bone or tooth

DEPRESSIONS—(CONCAVITIES) IN BONES AND/OR TEETH

alveolus [al VEE o lus] (plural: **alveoli** [al VEE o lie]): small hollow space or socket where the tooth root fits within the jaw bones
cavity: a hollow place within the body of bone (or within a tooth)
fissure [FISH er]: a cleft or groove (crack) between parts
fossa [FOS ah] (plural: **fossae** [FOS ee]): a small hollow or depressed area
fovea [FO ve ah]: small pit or depression
groove: linear depression or furrow
sinus: hollow, air-filled cavity or space within skull bones, or a channel for venous blood

OPENINGS—(HOLES) IN BONES AND/OR TEETH

aperture: an opening; compare a camera lens aperture
foramen [fo RA men] (plural: **foramina** [fo RAM i nah]): a small hole through bone or tooth for passage of nerves and vessels
foramen ovale [o VAL ee]: an oval or egg-shaped foramen (which is bigger than the round [rotundum] foramen)
foramen rotundum: a round foramen; recall the Capitol's rotundum or dome is round when viewed from above
meatus [me A tus]: a natural passage or opening in the body

RELATIVE LOCATION—FIGURE 1-3 WILL BE HELPFUL IN UNDERSTANDING TERMS WITH AN ASTERISK (*).

***anterior:** toward the front of the body
buccal [BUCK al]: related to or near the cheek; the buccal nerve innervates the cheek; the buccinator muscle is within the cheek; the buccal surface of a tooth is the side toward the cheek (also called *facial* side because it is toward the face that we see)
cervix: of the neck or neck-like; compare a *cervic*al vertebrae in the neck
external: toward the outside of the body; seen from the outside
***facial:** toward the face; seen when viewing the face side
***inferior** or the prefix **infra:** located below or beneath; lower than
***medial:** the surface toward, or closest to, the midline (medial) plane of the body; do not confuse medial with mesial, which will be described later
***median plane:** a longitudinal plane that divides the body into relatively equal right and left halves
***midsagittal plane** [SAJ i t'l]: same as median plane
***posterior:** toward the rear of the mouth or body
retro (prefix): back or behind
sub (prefix): under or beneath; compare to infra
superficial: closer to the surface
***superior** or the prefix **supra:** located above or over; higher or upper

GENERAL TERMS RELATED TO BONES

acoustic [ah KOOS tik]: referring to sounds or hearing; near the ear
cervical [SER vi kal]: related to the neck; like cervical vertebrae
condyle [KON dile]: an articular prominence of a bone resembling a knuckle

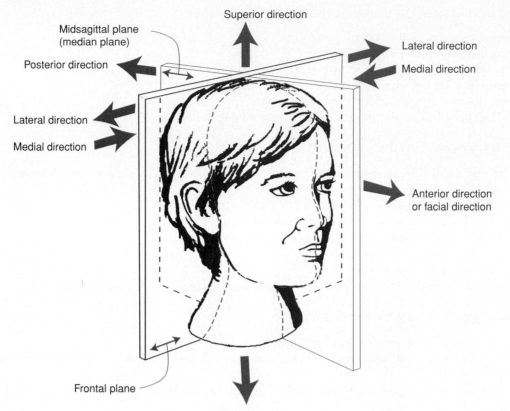

FIGURE 1-3. Planes of the head and directions used to identify relative location of structures or surfaces of the head.

coronoid: where the crown fits or the shape of a crown (compare coronation); for example, the coronoid process of the mandible is shaped like the point of a coronation crown; or a coronoid suture is where the crown fits

dura: hard, not soft (compare durable)

glenoid [GLE noyd]: socket-like

labial [LAY bee al]: related to the lips; toward the lips

lacrimal [LAK ri mal] (also spelled lachrymal): referring to the tears (compare lacrimosa)

lamina: a thin layer (compare laminated wood)

lingula [LING gyoo la]: tongue-shaped structure (compare lingual)

malar [MAY lar]: referring to the cheek or cheek bone (not to be confused with molar)

meatus [mee A tus]: a pathway or opening

palpebral [PAL pe bral]: referring to the eyelid

piriform [PEER i form]: pear shaped

septum: a partition (compare separate)

suture [SOO chur] **line:** the line of union of adjoining bones of the skull

symphysis [SIM fi sis]: fibrocartilaginous joint where opposed bony surfaces are joined (a suture line may not be evident)

trochlea [TROK lee ah]: pulley shaped

A. BONES OF THE NEUROCRANIUM

The **neurocranium** is the portion of the skull that supports, encloses, and protects the brain. It is made up of replacement bone (that is, there is a cartilaginous precursor or model for these bones). Other names for this type of bone are cartilage bone and endochondral bone. The eight bones of the neurocranium are

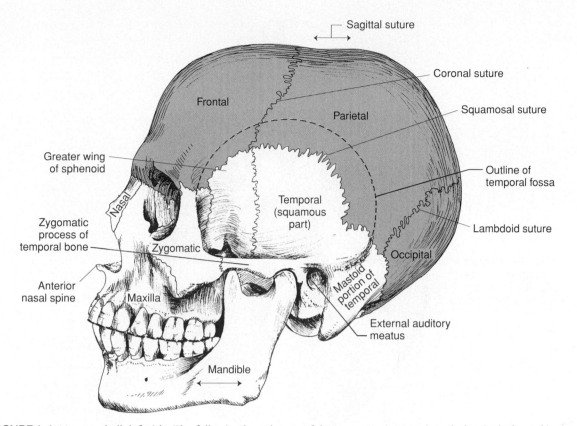

FIGURE 1-4. Human skull, left side. The following large bones of the neurocranium are in red: the single **frontal** bone forms the anterior superior portion, the **parietal** bones form the lateral and superior surfaces, and the **occipital** bone forms the posterior inferior portion. Note the outline of the shallow **temporal fossa**, which includes portions of temporal, parietal, sphenoid, and frontal bones.

four single bones (sphenoid, occipital, ethmoid, and frontal) and two paired bones (one on each side): temporal and parietal.

The following description of structures on each bone will focus on the location of key muscle and ligament attachments and the passageway (foramen and spaces) for the major cranial nerve branches to the mouth or oral cavity (especially the trigeminal, facial, glossopharyngeal, and hypoglossal nerves). The learner should become familiar with these bony structures in order to understand fully how the muscles move the jaw in each direction and where to apply local anesthetic along the path of a nerve, as described in subsequent sections of this chapter.

1. FRONTAL BONE

This single, large midline bone forms the "forehead" and eyebrow region (*Fig. 1-4*). A small portion of this bone in the temporal fossa region (outlined in *Fig. 1-4*) serves as part of the attachment for the superior end of the temporalis muscle.

2. PARIETAL BONES

These large, paired bones protect the brain laterally and posteriorly (*Fig. 1-4*). Like the frontal bone, part of this bone is located within the temporal fossa, which is where the superior end of the temporalis muscle attaches.

3. OCCIPITAL BONE

This bone provides the articulating surface between the skull and vertebral column at the **occipital condyle** [ahk SIP eh tal KON dile] (seen on the inferior surface in *Fig. 1-5*). The large **foramen**

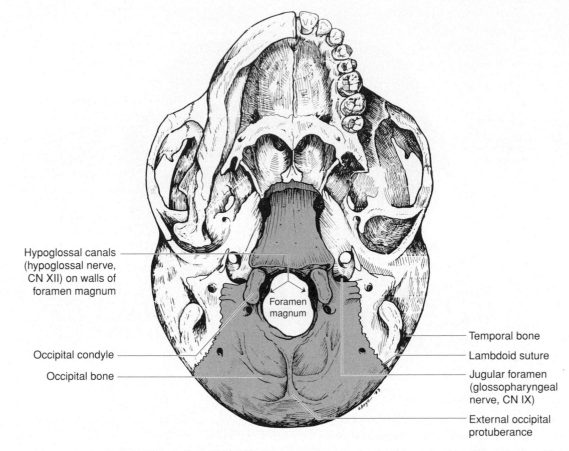

Hypoglossal canals
(hypoglossal nerve,
CN XII) on walls of
foramen magnum

Foramen
magnum

Temporal bone

Lambdoid suture

Occipital condyle

Jugular foramen
(glossopharyngeal
nerve, CN IX)

Occipital bone

External occipital
protuberance

FIGURE 1-5. Human skull: inferior surface with half of the mandible removed on the right side of the drawing. The **occipital** bone is highlighted in red. Note the location of the hypoglossal canals (in the lateral walls of the foramen magnum) and the jugular foramen just adjacent to the occipital bone.

magnum serves as the passageway for the spinal cord. On the lateral walls of the foramen magnum are the right and left **hypoglossal canals**, which are the passageways of the hypoglossal nerves (cranial nerve XII). Lateral to the foramen magnum (between the occipital and temporal bones) is the large **jugular** [JUG you lar] **foramen** (*Fig.1-5*), the passageway of the glossopharyngeal nerve (cranial nerve IX).

4.   SUTURE LINES BETWEEN BONES OF THE CRANIUM

Suture lines of the neurocranium are lines of fibrous connective tissue that join two bones of the skull immovably together, best seen in Figure 1-4. **Coronal sutures** are located between the frontal and two parietal bones. (*Hint:* This location is where a crown might fit during a *corona*tion.) **Squamosal** [skwa MO sal] **sutures** are located between the temporal and parietal bones. (Squamous refers to the fish-scale shape that this portion of the temporal bone resembles.) The **sagittal suture** (best seen on the top of the skull) joins the right and left parietal bones on the top midline of the skull, parallel to the sagittal plane of the skull. The **lambdoid** [LAM doid] **suture** joins the occipital bone with the parietal bones. Its shape from the posterior view resembles an upside-down "V" and can be compared to the shape of the Greek letter lambda (λ).

5.   SPHENOID BONE

This single, irregularly shaped, midline bone cradles the base of the brain and pituitary gland and forms the posterior part of the orbit (eye socket). The important pituitary gland is located within a depression called the **hypophysial fossa** or **sella turcica** (meaning Turkish chair or saddle) (*Fig. 1-6*).

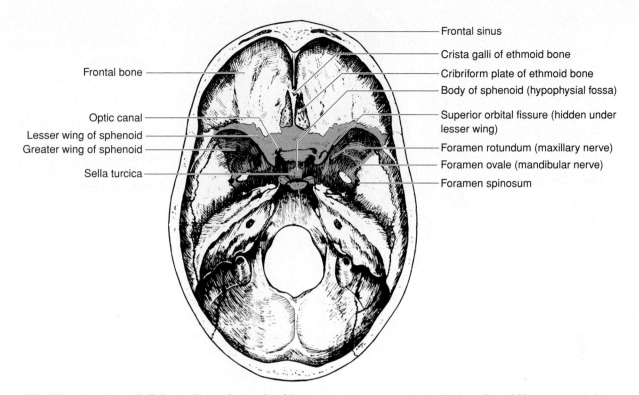

Frontal bone

Optic canal
Lesser wing of sphenoid
Greater wing of sphenoid

Sella turcica

Frontal sinus
Crista galli of ethmoid bone
Cribriform plate of ethmoid bone
Body of sphenoid (hypophysial fossa)
Superior orbital fissure (hidden under lesser wing)
Foramen rotundum (maxillary nerve)
Foramen ovale (mandibular nerve)
Foramen spinosum

FIGURE 1-6. Human skull: bones lining the inside of the neurocranium, superior view. The **sphenoid bone** is shaded in this figure. Also, notice the portion of the midline **ethmoid bone** that is visible in the anterior brain-case.

The complex shape of the sphenoid bone can only be appreciated by looking at it from several different views (best seen in Figs. 1-6 and 1-7 where it is shaded). The **sphenoid** [SFE noid] **bone** is important to dental professionals because it has processes that serve as part of the attachment for three of the four pairs of major chewing muscles. The sphenoid bone also has foramina (holes) that are the passageway for the nerve branches of the fifth cranial nerve (trigeminal) that supply all teeth and many surrounding structures.

The midline body of the sphenoid bone has processes or wings projecting laterally. The **lesser wings** are located superior to a fissure in the posterior surface of the eye socket, and can only be seen internally in Figure 1-6. The **greater wings** are also seen internally in Figure 1-6 but are best viewed externally in Figure 1-4. They extend superiorly from the body, posterior to the upper jaw bones, and medial to the lower jaw bone and cheek bones. The external surface of the greater wing (along with part of the temporal, frontal, and parietal bones) is part of the **temporal fossa** where the temporalis muscle attaches to the neurocranium. The fissure internally between the greater and lesser wing is called the **superior orbital fissure**, which is the passageway of the ophthalmic nerve (one branch of the trigeminal nerve). This fissure is labeled internally in Figure 1-6 and externally posterior to the eye socket in Figure 1-12.

The sphenoid bone also has two processes that project downward from the base of the skull just adjacent to the posterior surface of the maxillae (upper jaw bones). These are called **pterygoid** [TER i goid] **processes** and are best seen in the lateral view of Figure 1-8. (*Hint:* To remember the name of this process, note that it has a scalloped border somewhat like the wings of a *ptero*dactyl flying dinosaur.) Each pterygoid process contains a fossa about the size of the end of your little finger called the **pterygoid fossa** (*Fig. 1-7*). This fossa is where one end of a major chewing muscle, the medial pterygoid muscle, attaches. The pterygoid fossa is bounded laterally by a lateral plate of bone known as the **lateral pterygoid plate** (or lamina) and medially by a medial plate of bone (**medial pterygoid plate**) seen in Figure 1-7. The medial plate has a hook-like projection just posterior and medial to the third molars and behind the palate, called the **pterygoid hamulus** (Figs. 1-7 and 1-8). The space just lateral to and posterior to the lateral plate and inferior to the temporal bone is called the

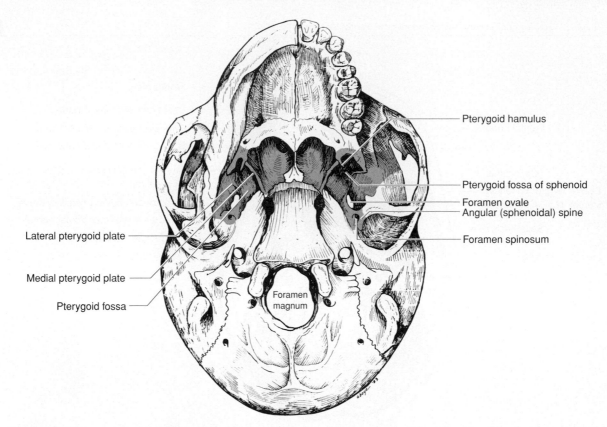

FIGURE 1-7. Human skull: inferior surface with half of the mandible removed on the right side of the drawing to permit easier viewing of the **sphenoid bone**, which is shaded. Notice the relative location of the **pterygoid plates and fossa** just posterior to the bones of the hard palate.

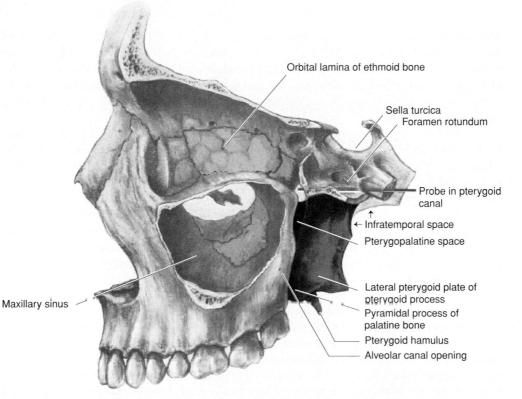

FIGURE 1-8. Part of human skull, lateral view, with the lateral wall of the left maxilla removed, exposing the large **maxillary sinus**. Note the lateral surface of the **lateral pterygoid plate** of the sphenoid bone (*shaded red*) just behind the maxilla. The **pterygoid hamulus** of the medial pterygoid plate is also visible and is just posterior (and slightly medial) to the third molars. (Reproduced by permission from Clemente CD, ed. Gray's anatomy of the human body. 30th ed. Philadelphia: Lea & Febiger, 1985:166.)

infratemporal space (*Fig. 1-8*), and it is filled with muscles, ligaments, vessels, and nerves, which will be described later. The lateral surface of the lateral pterygoid plate visible in Figure 1-8 is where one end of the lateral pterygoid muscle attaches.

Two pairs of foramina in this bone are important to dental professionals. Individually, these are known as the foramen rotundum and the foramen ovale. The oval, more posterior **foramen ovale** is the skull opening for the passage of the mandibular nerve (part of the trigeminal nerve), a major nerve to the mandibular teeth and jaw, and the chewing muscles. The foramen ovale is best seen internally in Figure 1-6 and externally in Figure 1-7. Pass a pipe cleaner through this foramen and appreciate that it drops inferiorly through the infratemporal space toward the mandible. It can be identified easily by its proximity to the much smaller foramen known as the **foramen spinosum** [spy NO sum]. Just posterior to the foramen ovale and spinosum on the inferior surface is a sharp, bony prominence called the **sphenoidal** [SFE noid al] **spine** (or **angular** spine) (*Fig 1-7*). This spine is the superior attachment of the *spheno*mandibular ligament, which extends inferiorly from the spine toward the medial surface of the lower jaw (mandible).

The rounder, more medial and anterior **foramen rotundum** [ro TUN dum] (seen only internally in *Fig. 1-6*) is the opening for the passage of another part of the trigeminal nerve called the maxillary nerve. If you are able to pass a pipe cleaner from the brain case through this foramen, it will be somewhat hidden in a space between the pterygoid process and upper jaw bone (maxilla). This space between the pterygoid process and the posterior wall of the maxillae (which is covered in part by vertical projections of the palatine bones) is known as the **pterygopalatine** [TER i go PAL eh tine] **space** labeled in Figure 1-8. The maxillary nerve that exits the skull through the foramen rotundum proceeds through this pterygopalatine space as it gives off branches to the upper jaw (maxillae) and teeth.

6. ETHMOID BONE

This single, hollow, sinus-filled bone is located on the midline beneath the anterior part of the brain, balloons out between the eye sockets, and extends inferiorly to form a thin plate of bone that helps separate the halves of the nasal cavities. The most superior aspect of this bone is visible within the brain case at the midline as the sieve-like **cribriform** [KRIB ri form] **plate** (*Fig. 1-6*) surrounding the triangular projection called the **crista galli** [KRIS ta GAL li, meaning rooster comb]. The cribriform plate is full of holes providing the passage from the nasal cavity for the fibers of the olfactory nerve (the nerve for smell). Inferior to the cribriform plate, the ethmoid bone spreads out to form part of the medial aspect of each orbit (orbital lamina of the ethmoid bone is visible in *Fig. 1-8*). It also has scrolled processes extending into the nasal cavity similar in appearance to the inferior nasal concha described later in this section. Finally, a vertical midline plate of the ethmoid bone extends downward into the nasal cavity to form (along with the separate single vomer bone) the **nasal septum** (*Fig. 1-12*), which separates the right and left nasal cavities.

7. TEMPORAL BONES

The **temporal bones** are a pair of complex bones that form part of the sides and base of the skull (best seen laterally in *Fig. 1-9* where one is shaded). The **temporal fossa** (outlined in *Fig. 1-9*) is a large, very shallow depression in the temple region formed by the lateral (**squamous** or fish-scale–shaped) part of the temporal bone, along with a portion of the sphenoid (greater wing) and the adjacent portions of the parietal and frontal bones. The temporal fossa is where the superior end of another major chewing muscle (the temporalis) attaches.

The paired temporal bones are especially important to dental professionals since each has a **mandibular fossa** (one is labeled on the right side of *Fig. 1-10*). The mandibular fossae (right and left) are located on the inferior aspect of the temporal bones. It is within these fossae that the lower jaw (or mandible) articulates with and moves against the temporal bones on the base of the neurocranium. This jaw joint (actually a joint on each side) is called the **temporomandibular joint** (commonly abbreviated TMJ) where the temporal bone and mandible articulate. Each mandibular fossa can be divided into two parts by the **petrotympanic fissure** (*Fig. 1-10*). The anterior two-thirds (anterior to the petrotympanic fissure) is the important functional part called the **articular** (or **glenoid**) **fossa**. Each articular fossa has a ridge of bone forming its anterior border, which is called the **articular eminence**.

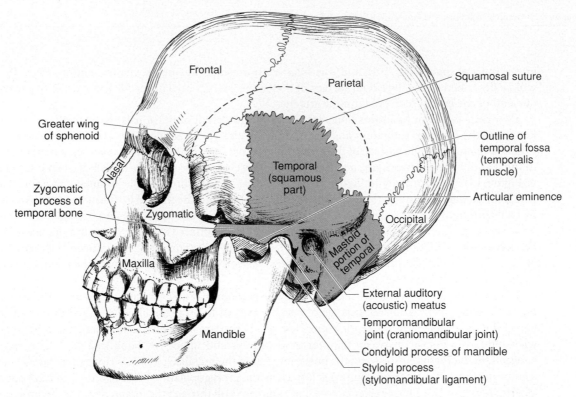

FIGURE 1-9. Human skull, left side. The lateral surface of the left **temporal bone** is shaded red. Note its squamous part, as well as its processes: mastoid, styloid, and zygomatic.

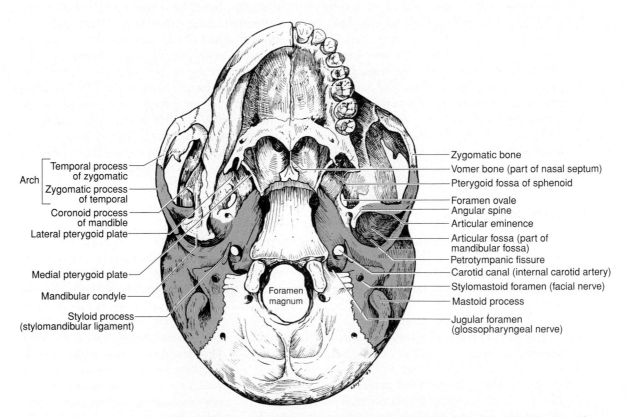

FIGURE 1-10. Human skull: inferior surface, with half of the mandible removed on the right side of the drawing. The right and left **temporal** bones are shaded red. Note the zygomatic process forming part of the zygomatic arch and the mandibular fossa and articular eminence. The small portion of the midline **vomer bone** is seen separating the right and left halves of the nasal passageways.

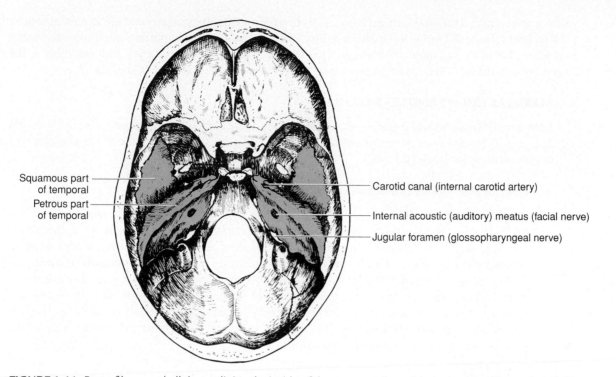

Squamous part of temporal

Petrous part of temporal

Carotid canal (internal carotid artery)

Internal acoustic (auditory) meatus (facial nerve)

Jugular foramen (glossopharyngeal nerve)

FIGURE 1-11. Part of human skull: bones lining the inside of the neurocranium with the **temporal bones** in red. The thick **petrous portion** of these bones contains the very small bones of the inner ear (incus, stapes, and malleus). Important nerves and vessels pass through the foramen labeled on this diagram. (Reproduced by permission from Clemente CD, ed. Gray's anatomy of the human body. 30th ed. Philadelphia: Lea & Febiger, 1985:166.)

Each temporal bone has several processes. The zygomatic [zy go MAT ik] process (*Fig. 1-9*) is the finger of bone anterior to the mandibular fossa that joins with another bone, the zygomatic, to form an arch called the zygomatic arch (sometimes referred to as the cheekbone). This arch shape of bones, seen from beneath in Figure 1-10, is the attachment of one end of the large muscle of mastication, the masseter. The prominent **mastoid process** (*Fig. 1-9*), seen inferiorly and posteriorly to the mandibular fossa, is the attachment for one end of a major neck muscle, the sternocleidomastoid muscle. You can feel the bump of the mastoid process behind the ear lobe. The **styloid process** (*Fig. 1-9*), shaped like a small skinny pencil (or stylus), is the attachment for one end of a ligament (stylomandibular ligament) that extends to the lower jaw.

Several paired foramina are of importance on this bone. Laterally, the **external acoustic meatus** [a KOO stik me A tus] is the opening into the ear canal (*Fig. 1-9*). Note the proximity of the TMJ to the ear canal opening. On the inferior surface, the **stylomastoid foramen** (*Fig. 1-10*) is located between the styloid and mastoid processes, and is where the facial nerve (cranial nerve VII) exits the temporal bone and passes into the infratemporal space. Internally, this nerve exits the brain case by entering the **internal acoustic meatus** (*Fig. 1-11*) of the temporal bone. This portion of the temporal bone is called the **petrous portion**, and it is within this bone that the auditory canal contains the minute bones of hearing known as the malleus, incus, and stapes. The **carotid canal** is the passageway of the internal carotid artery into the brain case, and the **jugular foramen** (between the temporal and occipital bones) is where the glossopharyngeal nerve (cranial nerve IX) passes out of the brain case (Figs. 1-10 and 1-11).

B. BONES OF THE FACE (VISCERAL APPARATUS)

The form of facial bones gives us our appearance. They function in both respiration and digestion and are made up of dermal or intramembranous bone, the type that is not preceded by cartilage. The facial bones are located anterior and inferior to the forehead and make up the major anterior part of the skull. There are 14 facial bones. Two single bones are the mandible (lower jaw) and the vomer. Six paired bones are the palatine, zygomatic, nasal, and lacrimal bones, as well as the maxillae (upper jaw) and inferior nasal concha [KONG kee] (also called turbinates). The mandible and maxillae are most important when considering the foundation for teeth and tooth function, so they will be discussed in more detail. The mandible is the largest bone in the face. Each maxilla (right and left) is the second largest bone in the face.

1. MAXILLAE (RIGHT AND LEFT MAXILLA)

Each maxilla [mak SILL a] (right or left) consists of one large, hollow, central mass called the *body* and four projecting *processes* or extensions of bone. It is best seen shaded in Figure 1-12. The plural of maxilla is maxillae [mak SILL ee].

a. Body of the Maxilla (structures seen in *Fig. 1-12*)

The *body* of the maxilla is shaped like a four-sided, hollow pyramid with the base oriented vertically next to the nasal cavity and the apex or peak extending laterally into part of the cheekbone (or zygomatic bone). Part of the maxilla forms the floor of the orbit of the eye where an **infraorbital fissure** is located. This fissure disappears anteriorly to become the **infraorbital canal** (not visible in *Fig. 1-12*). Important branches of the fifth cranial nerve and vessels enter this fissure and canal and give off branches within the canal, which supply some of the maxillary teeth and surrounding tissue. The infraorbital nerves and vessels exit the infraorbital canal on to the face through the **infraorbital foramen**. This foramen is on the anterior surface of the body of the maxilla, inferior to the eye and just superior to the canine fossa.

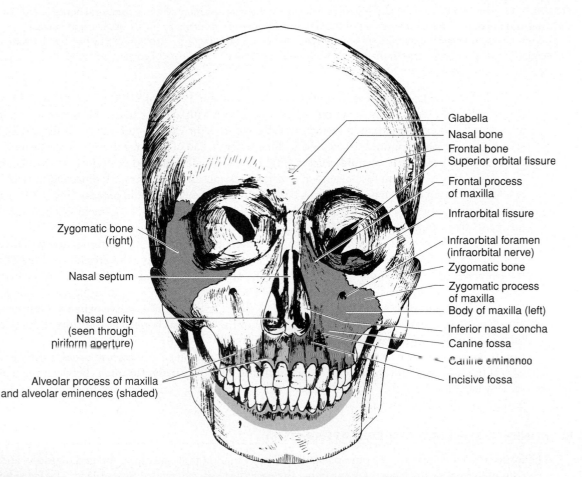

Glabella
Nasal bone
Frontal bone
Superior orbital fissure
Frontal process of maxilla
Infraorbital fissure
Infraorbital foramen (infraorbital nerve)
Zygomatic bone
Zygomatic process of maxilla
Body of maxilla (left)
Inferior nasal concha
Canine fossa
Canine eminence
Incisive fossa

Zygomatic bone (right)
Nasal septum
Nasal cavity (seen through piriform aperture)
Alveolar process of maxilla and alveolar eminences (shaded)

FIGURE 1-12. Human skull, frontal aspect. The left **maxilla** (on the right side of the drawing) and the right **zygomatic bone** (on the left side of the drawing) are shaded red. Also, the facial surface of the arch-shaped **alveolar process of the left maxilla** (process that surrounds the tooth roots) and the **alveolar process of the entire mandible** are shaded red.

b. Bony Processes on Each Maxilla

There are four processes extending out from the body of the maxillae. The first three described below are best viewed in Figure 1-12.

(1) Frontal (or Nasofrontal) Process

The **frontal (nasofrontal) process** derives its name from the fact that its medial edge joins with the nasal bone, extending superiorly to also articulate with the frontal bone. The medial or nasal surface forms part of the lateral wall of the nasal cavity and half of the opening of the nasal cavity (called the **piriform aperture** because of its pear shape).

(2) Zygomatic Process

The **zygomatic process** forms part of the anterior or facial surface of each maxilla. It extends laterally to join with the maxillary process of the zygomatic bone.

(3) Alveolar Process

The **alveolar** [al VEE o lar] **processes** of the right and left maxillae (and also of the mandible, described later) extend to form an arch shape of bone that surrounds the roots of the dental arch of teeth (seen shaded on the right maxilla and the entire lower jaw or mandible in *Fig. 1-12* and identified in cross section in *Fig. 1-13*). The roots of the teeth are embedded in individual **alveoli** (tooth sockets) only visible in the jaw bones if the teeth were recently extracted. The shape of each alveolus or thin bony socket naturally corresponds closely with the shape of the roots of the tooth it surrounds. **Alveolar eminences** are raised ridges of bone ex-

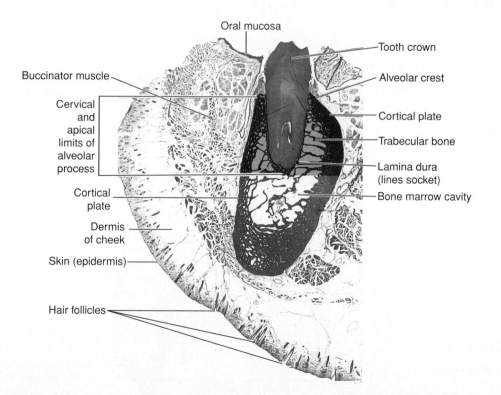

FIGURE 1-13. A buccolingual cross section [about 30 μm thick] of a human mandible and a molar. To the left of the mandible is the soft facial tissue of the cheek. Note the extent of the **alveolar process** (shaded red)—only the part of the mandible that surrounds the tooth root. The thick **cortical plate** surrounds the entire facial (left) and medial (right, inner) surfaces of the mandible, while the very thin **lamina dura** layer of bone lines the socket that surrounds the tooth root. A **periodontal ligament** (averaging only about twice as thick as this page [0.2 mm]) extends between the lamina dura and outer layer of tooth root, and supports the tooth within its socket. Note that much of this mandible has the texture of a sponge with many hollow spaces (bone marrow cavities), allowing nerves and blood vessels, after entering the bone through foramen, to pass through this spongy bone on their way to each tooth and adjacent bony structures. [Tooth enamel was destroyed by the decalcification of the specimen with nitric acid preparatory to embedding and sectioning.] For further information on the histology of these structures, refer to references 10, 23, and 37–41.

ternally overlying prominent tooth root convexities. The alveolar eminence over the canine tooth on each side is called the **canine eminence**. Anterior to the canine eminence is a shallow fossa over the root of the maxillary lateral incisor called the **incisive** [in SI siv] **fossa**. Posterior to the canine eminence is a fossa over the roots of maxillary premolars named the **canine fossa**.

The alveolar process is made up of several bony layers (seen in cross section of the mandible in *Fig. 1-13*). Supporting bone is made up of the thickened inner (lingual) and outer (facial) dense **cortical plate** with less dense **trabecular** [trah BEK u lar] **bone** sandwiched in between. Trabecular bone is composed of many plate-like bone partitions that separate the irregularly shaped marrow spaces located within this bone. Synonyms for trabecular bone include cancellous or spongy bone. Small nerve branches and vessels pass through this spongy bone to supply each tooth. The **lamina dura** is the much thinner, compact bony layer that lines the wall of each tooth socket (or alveolus). Synonyms for lamina dura include alveolar bony socket, alveolar bone, true alveolar bone, alveolar bone proper, and cribriform plate of the alveolar process. The only space between the outer layer of tooth root (which is covered with cementum) and this alveolar bone is occupied by a **periodontal ligament** that suspends each tooth within its alveolus by attaching the circumference of each tooth root to the surrounding lamina dura. The periodontal ligament is very thin [between 0.12 and 0.33 mm thick] and is composed of thousands of fibers.

(4) Palatine Process of the Maxilla
Refer to Figure 1-14 while reading about the palatine process. Each **palatine** [PAL a tine] **process** is a thin, bony shelf of each maxilla that projects horizontally. The right and left

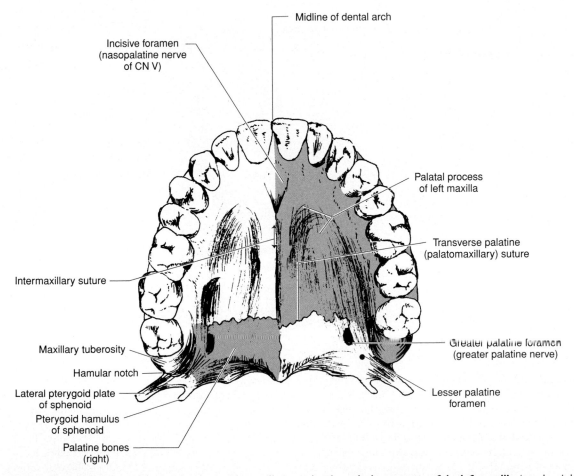

Midline of dental arch

Incisive foramen
(nasopalatine nerve
of CN V)

Palatal process
of left maxilla

Transverse palatine
(palatomaxillary) suture

Intermaxillary suture

Maxillary tuberosity

Greater palatine foramen
(greater palatine nerve)

Hamular notch

Lateral pterygoid plate
of sphenoid

Lesser palatine
foramen

Pterygoid hamulus
of sphenoid

Palatine bones
(right)

FIGURE 1-14. Inferior view of the hard palate with maxillary teeth. The **palatine process of the left maxilla** (on the right side of the drawing) and the **horizontal process of the right palatine bone** (on the left side of the drawing) are shaded. Note the important foramen where nerves and vessels can pass through to supply the palatal tissue.

processes join to form the anterior part of the **hard palate**. This hard palate forms the roof of the oral cavity and the floor of the nasal passageway. The anteroposterior line of fusion between the right and left palatine processes of the maxillae and the horizontal plates of the palatine bones is the **intermaxillary** (or midpalatine) **suture**. It is located on the midline running posteriorly from the incisive foramen. The **incisive foramen** is a centrally located hole at the most anterior part of this suture, just posterior to the central incisors. It transmits branches of the artery and nasopalatine nerve that supply adjacent palatal soft tissue. The most posterior part of the maxillary alveolar process is a bulge of bone called the **maxillary tuberosity**. A notch that separates the maxillary tuberosity of each maxilla from the adjacent pterygoid process of the sphenoid bone is called the **hamular notch**. Recall that the **pterygoid hamulus**, the hook-like projection of the medial plate of the pterygoid process, is located just posterior to the hamular notch. This may be felt in the mouth with your tongue (or clean fingers) just posterior to the hard palate and slightly medial to the maxillary tuberosity.

An embryonic **premaxilla** cannot normally be distinguished in the adult skull. It is the anterior part of the maxillary bone, which contains the incisors. When visible, a suture line separates the premaxilla from the palatine processes of the two maxillae.

c. Maxillary Sinus or Antrum

Sinuses are hollow spaces within bones and are found within the sphenoid, frontal, and ethmoid bones, as well as within each maxilla. The **maxillary sinus**, located within the body of each maxilla, functions to (a) lighten the skull, (b) give resonance to the voice, (c) warm the air we breathe, and (d) moisten the nasal cavity. [The average size of each maxillary sinus in an adult is about 25 mm from side to side, 30 mm from front to back, and 30 mm high, with an average capacity of 15 mL (range: 9.5–20 mL),[1] or about 1 tablespoon.]

Refer to Figure 1-15 while reading about the maxillary sinus. This large, four-sided, pyramid-shaped cavity is located within the body of each maxilla. One wall forms the sinus cavity floor. It extends inferiorly onto the superior portion of the maxillary alveolar process, where many projections of the ends (apices) of the molar roots, and sometimes premolar roots, are found. The most intimate relationship between the teeth and maxillary sinus is seen in Figure 1-16. Only very thin bone lies between the floor of the sinus and the ends (apices) of the roots of the maxillary molars. In rare cases, no bone separates the root apices from the sinus. There is always soft tissue, made up of the periodontal ligament on the tooth root and the mucous membrane lining the sinus cavity, between the root and the space of the cavity. Sometimes when a dentist extracts a molar and the root breaks off, he or she is unjustly accused of pushing the root into the sinus. It may have been located in the maxillary sinus prior to the extraction. The other three walls of the pyramid-shaped sinus are toward the orbit of the eye, toward the face, and posteriorly and laterally, next to the infratemporal space.

The maxillary sinus is a significant structure because of the close relationship it has to the teeth. The nerves to the maxillary teeth (posterior superior alveolar nerves) enter the maxilla and sinus through very small **foramina** located posterior and superior to the third molar, and through the **alveolar** [al VEE o lar] **canals** (*Fig. 1-15*). They pass just beneath the membrane lining of the sinus or through bony canals within the walls of the sinus. An infection in either the sinus or these teeth can spread to the other. Pain caused by a maxillary sinus infection can be mistaken for pain originating in any one or all of the molars or premolars on that side. Unfortunately, healthy teeth are sometimes extracted in a futile attempt to alleviate pain that was caused by a chronic maxillary sinus infection.

The maxillary sinus is lined with specialized cells (ciliated columnar epithelium) similar to those found in the respiratory tract. The mucous film it secretes moves spirally and upward (against gravity) across the membrane to the *opening* of the sinus located on the anterosuperior wall (*Fig. 1-15*), where it drains into the nasal cavity. If humans walked on all fours with the head forward like many animals, this opening for drainage would be on the floor of the sinus, not near the roof, and humans would have fewer sinus problems. Many people can get pain relief by placing their head in a prone position for several minutes to permit more rapid drainage of the maxillary sinuses.

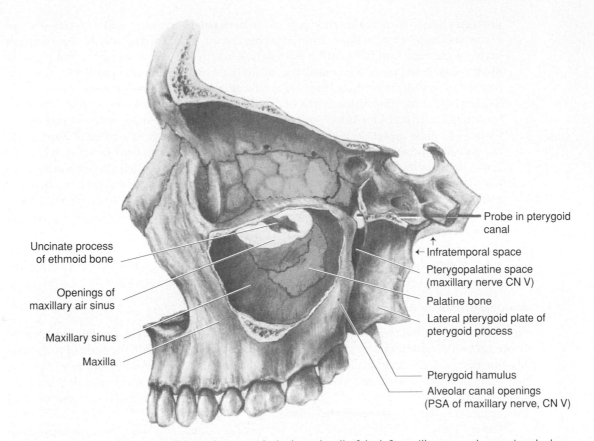

FIGURE 1-15. Part of human skull, lateral view, with the lateral wall of the left maxilla removed, exposing the large **maxillary sinus**. Note that the floor of this sinus is in proximity to the maxillary posterior teeth but does not extend forward as far as the maxillary anterior teeth. The **opening** of this sinus (into the nasal chamber) is located superiorly on the medial wall of the sinus. A portion of the palatine bone identified on the sinus wall is the vertical process of the **palatine bone** located adjacent to the posterior surface of each maxilla. Also, note the part of the midline **ethmoid bone** that balloons out between the right and left maxillary sinuses to form part of their medial walls. (Reproduced by permission from Clemente CD, ed. Gray's anatomy of the human body. 30th ed. Philadelphia: Lea & Febiger, 1985:166.)

2. MANDIBLE

The single horseshoe-shaped **mandible** [MAN de b'l], seen anteriorly in Figure 1-17, is the largest and strongest bone of the face. Generally speaking, it is bilaterally symmetrical. It bears the mandibular teeth and is attached only by ligaments and muscles to the relatively immovable bones of the neurocranium. The mandible is the only bone of the skull that can move. The other bones of the skull move only when the whole head is moved, and then they move in unison. The temporomandibular joints between the mandible and the temporal bones are movable articulations, the only visible movable articulations in the head.

The mandible has three parts: one horizontal *body* and two vertical **rami** [RAY mee] (singular, **ramus** [RAY mus]) (see *Fig. 1-17*). The landmarks of the mandible will be discussed according to their location: external surface of the body, then ramus, then the internal surface.

a. Body: External Surface

As with the maxillae, an **alveolar** [al VEE o lar] **process** surrounds the tooth roots (shaded in *Fig. 1-12*), and **alveolar eminences** are visible as vertical elevations over tooth roots on the facial surface. The prominent elevations overlying the roots of the canines are called the **canine eminences**.

The bulky, curved, horizontal body and the flattened vertical ramus join at the angle of the mandible on either side. The **angle** of the mandible is located where the inferior border of the body

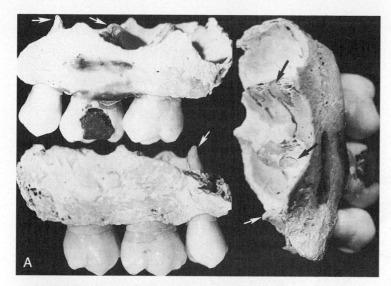

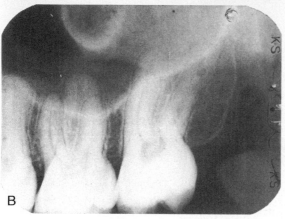

FIGURE 1-16. A. Three views of part of the left **alveolar process** of the maxilla surrounding the roots of the maxillary first and second molar and second premolar. Note the root tips (apices) shown by arrows extending out of the maxilla into what would have been the floor of the **maxillary sinus** space in an intact skull. **B.** Radiograph of the maxillary molar region showing the roots of the first molar several millimeters deep into the maxillary sinus (dark area surrounded by white border). Parts of the roots of the second molar are also within the sinus cavity. The root tip of the second premolar root is in the sinus as well. This is a common relationship.

joins the posterior border of the ramus (*Fig. 1-18*). The roughened portion of the lateral surface near the angle of the mandible is where the inferior end of the powerful masseter muscle attaches. The posterior border of the ramus is also the location of the attachment of the stylo*mandibular* ligament (whose other end attaches to the styloid process of the temporal bone).

The **symphysis** [SIM fi sis] is the line of fusion of the right and left sides at the midline where the two halves of the mandible fuse (join together) during the first year after birth. It is therefore usually not visible. Near the symphysis, two mental tubercles and one mental protuberance make up the human chin (*Fig. 1-17*). No other mammal has a chin. Two **mental tubercles** lie on either side of the midline near the inferior border of the mandible. The **mental protuberance** is centered on the midline between the two mental tubercles but is about 10 mm superior. The protuberance and the tubercles are more prominent on men than on women.

An **external oblique** [ob LEEK] **ridge** (*Fig. 1-18*) extends from the canine region to the anterior border of the ramus. The nearly horizontal ledge of bone in the molar region between the external oblique ridge and alveolar process is named the **buccal shelf**. This is the proximity of the buccal (or buccinator) nerve in the cheek.

The **mental foramen** is located near the root end (apex) of the second premolar (*Fig. 1-18*). On dental radiographs (x-rays), this foramen appears as a small dark circle next to the premolar root and must be distinguished from a periapical abscess (infection destroying bone near the root apex), which may appear very similar to the normal mental foramen. The nerves and vessels (inferior alveolar) that traverse the mandibular canal within the mandible divide while within the mandible, and a branch (mental branch) exits through this mental foramen in an outward,

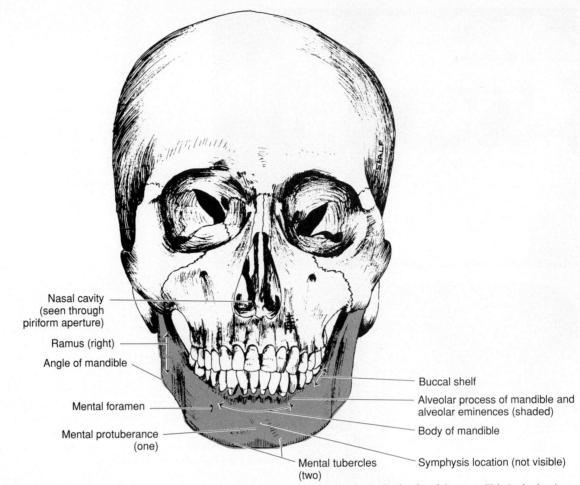

Nasal cavity
(seen through
piriform aperture)

Ramus (right)

Angle of mandible

Mental foramen

Mental protuberance
(one)

Mental tubercles
(two)

Buccal shelf

Alveolar process of mandible and
alveolar eminences (shaded)

Body of mandible

Symphysis location (not visible)

FIGURE 1-17. Human skull, frontal aspect. The **mandible** is shaded red. The bulky **body** of the mandible is the horizontal portion including the alveolar process that surrounds the mandibular teeth, and the two vertical processes extending to the base of the neurocranium (to the temporal bones) are called the rami (single is **ramus**).

upward, and posterior direction. Place a flexible probe carefully into this canal of your skull model to confirm this direction. The mental foramen is located at practically the same level on most humans: 13–15 mm superior to the inferior border of the mandible. [In a study of 40 skulls,[2] the mental foramen was found most often to be directly under the second premolar (42.5% of the time) or between the apices of the first and second premolars (40%). Infrequently, it was located distal to the apex of the second premolar (17.5%) and was never found under the apex of the first premolar.]

b. Ramus: Lateral Surfaces

Refer to Figure 1-18 while reading about this surface. There are two processes on the superior end of each ramus. The **coronoid** [KOR o noyd] **process** is the more pointed, anterior process on the upper border. The second more rounded and posterior process of the ramus is the **condyloid** [KON di loyd] **process** (also called the **mandibular condyle**). This process is composed of a bulky condyle head and a narrow neck that attaches the head to the ramus. The **sigmoid notch** (also called the mandibular or semilunar notch) is located between the coronoid process and the condyloid process. A portion of one of the important chewing muscles, the lateral pterygoid, attaches to the front of the neck of the condyloid process in a depression called the **pterygoid fovea** (*Fig. 1-19*). As stated earlier when discussing the temporal bone, the head of the mandibular condyle fits into and functions beneath the articular (glenoid) fossa of the temporal bone.

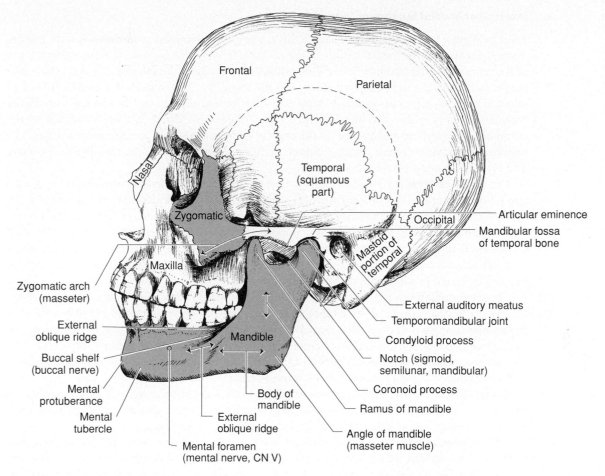

FIGURE 1-18. Human skull, left side. The lateral view of the **mandible** is shaded red, as well as the left **zygomatic** bone (of the cheek). In this view, the vertical ramus and its two processes (**condylar** and **coronoid processes**) are evident. Also, the zygoma bone, the zygomatic process of the temporal bone, and the zygomatic process of the maxilla form the **zygomatic arch**.

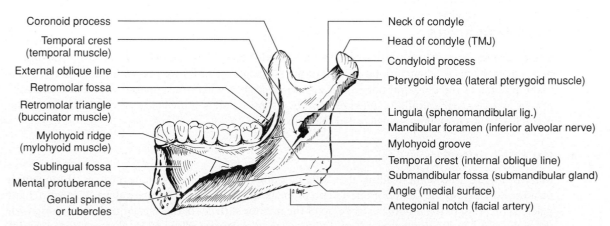

FIGURE 1-19. Mandible, medial surface. Notice the important **mandibular foramen**, as well as ridges, fossa, and processes.

c. Internal or Medial Surface of Mandible

Refer to Figure 1-19 while reading about this surface. The **mandibular foramen** is a prominent opening located on the medial surface of the ramus inferior to the sigmoid notch near the center of the ramus. It is the entrance into the mandibular canal where the inferior alveolar vessels and nerves pass from the infratemporal space into the mandible. The mandibular **lingula** [LING gu lah] is a tongue-shaped projection of bone just anterior and slightly superior to the mandibular foramen. This is where the inferior end of the spheno*mandibular* ligament attaches to the mandible. The superior end attaches to the angular (sphenoidal) spine on the sphenoid bone. The **mylohyoid groove** is a small groove running inferior and anterior from the mandibular foramen. The mylohyoid nerve rests in this groove.

The **temporal crest** is a ridge extending from the tip of the coronoid process onto the medial surface of the ramus and terminating near the third molar. The tendon from the fibers of the wide, flat, fan-shaped temporalis muscle attaches here. The inferior one-fourth of the temporal crest is called the **internal oblique line**. It is most important as a radiographic, rather than an anatomic, landmark. It appears on radiographs as a short, curved line somewhat inferior to the image of the external oblique line. The internal oblique line *is not synonymous with the mylohyoid ridge*, as incorrectly stated in some radiographic textbooks.

The **retromolar fossa** is a roughened shallow fossa distal to the last molar and bounded medially by the lowest portion of the temporal crest and laterally by the external oblique ridge. The **retromolar triangle** is in the lowest most anterior, and only horizontal, portion of the retromolar fossa. A **buccinator** [BUCK sin a tor] **crest** is a barely discernible ridge of bone that divides the smaller retromolar triangle from the rest of the larger retromolar fossa. The most posterior fibers of the buccinator (a pouch-shaped cheek muscle) muscle attach here.

Genial [JEE ne al] and mental **spines** or tubercles are located on either side of the midline on the internal surface of the mandible. Two large muscles (the genioglossus and the geniohyoid) attach to these spines and the elevated and roughened bone near them.

The **mylohyoid ridge** extends downward and forward from the molar region to the genial tubercles. The mylohyoid muscle, which forms part of the floor of the mouth, attaches from the mylohyoid ridge on the right medial side of the mandible to the ridge on the left medial side (somewhat like a hammock). A very broad, shallow **sublingual** [sub LING gwal] **fossa** is found just superior to the mylohyoid ridge and lateral to the genial tubercles on each side. The sublingual salivary gland rests in this fossa. A shallow **submandibular fossa** is found just inferior to the mylohyoid ridge in the premolar and molar regions. This is where the large submandibular salivary gland rests. On the inferior border of the mandible, a notch (called the antegonial notch) is located anterior to the angle of the mandible and is the passageway for the facial arteries and veins. You may be able to feel a pulse in this location of your own lower jaw.

3. ZYGOMATIC BONES

The **zygomatic bone** (one on each side of the face, shaded on the left side in *Fig. 1-18*) forms the prominence of each cheek. The temporal process of the zygomatic bone forms an arch along with the zygomatic process of the temporal bone. This **zygomatic arch** is where the superior end of the masseter muscle attaches to the skull. As stated previously, its lower end is connected to the lateral angle of the mandible. This cheek bone is also called the malar bone.

4. PALATINE BONES

Refer to Figure 1-20 while reading about the **palatine bone**. The horizontal processes of the paired palatine bones form the posterior one-fourth of the bony shelf called the **hard palate**. The entire hard palate (bony roof of the mouth) is made up of the inferior surfaces of these palatine bones, along with the right and left palatine processes of the maxillae. A **palatomaxillary** [PAL ah toe MAK si ler ee] **(transverse palatine) suture**, at right angles to the intermaxillary suture, is the junction between the palatine processes of the maxillae and the horizontal processes of the palatine bones.

The superior surfaces of the hard palate form the floor of the nasal cavity. The shape of the palate and the shape of the maxillary arch vary in length, breadth, and height. The hard palate blends

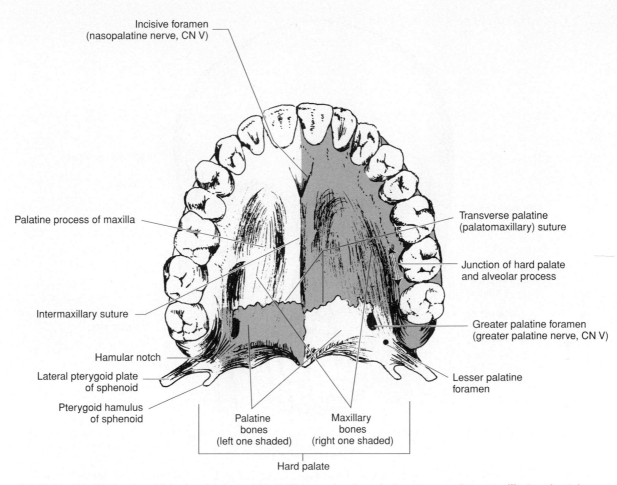

FIGURE 1-20. Inferior view of the hard palate with maxillary teeth. The **palatine process of one maxilla** (on the right side of the drawing) and the **horizontal process of one palatine bone** (on the left side of the drawing) are shaded. Note the **junction of the hard palate and alveolar process**, the location of the passage of the nerve that enters the palatal tissue through the **greater palatine foramen** in the palatine bones, which is distributed anteriorly, providing the sense of feeling to the palatal tissue (mucosa) medial to the posterior teeth.

smoothly with the palatal portion of the maxillary alveolar process. Part or all of the palatine processes are absent in a person who was born with a cleft palate.

The **greater palatine** [PAL ah tine] **foramina** (*Fig. 1-20*) are located posteriorly on each side near the angle where the right and left palatine bones meet the alveolar processes of the hard palate. They transmit the descending palatine vessels and greater (anterior) palatine nerves to the palate. The **lesser palatine foramina** are located on the palatine bone just behind and lateral to the greater palatine foramen. They transmit the middle and posterior palatine nerves.

The palatine bones also have vertical processes that are practically hidden from view on the intact skull. These vertical processes lie against the posterior wall of each maxilla (seen forming part of the posterior wall of the maxillary sinus in *Fig. 1-15*). These vertical processes are separated from the pterygoid process of the sphenoid bone by a space called the **pterygopalatine** [TER i go PAL ah tine] **space**, mentioned earlier when discussing the maxillae. Recall that this space is an important passageway of the maxillary nerve branches of cranial nerve V exiting from the cranium via the foramen rotundum on their way to the maxillary teeth and surrounding structures.

5. VOMER BONE

The **vomer bone** (*Figs. 1-10 and 1-21*) is a midline bone that, along with the vertical projection of the ethmoid bone, forms the **nasal septum**. This septum separates the right and left halves of the nasal cavity. A deviated septum may limit breathing and require surgery.

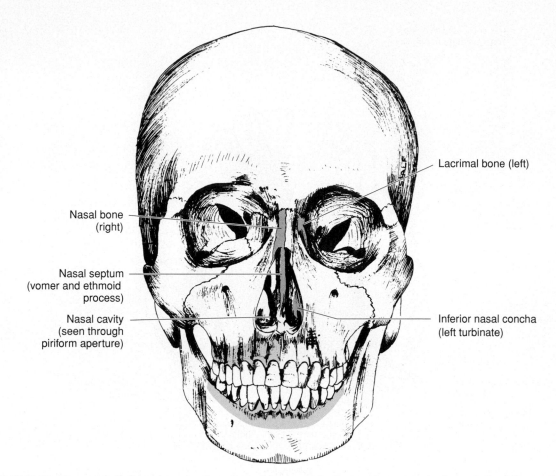

FIGURE 1-21. Human skull, frontal aspect. Several small bones of the face and nose are shaded red: the right **nasal** bone (on the left side of the diagram), the left **lacrimal** bone (on the medial surface of the eye socket), the left **inferior nasal concha** or **turbinate** bone (on the side of the nasal passageway), and the midline **nasal septum**, which is made up of two bones: the **vomer** bone and superiorly by the midline plate of the **ethmoid** bone.

6. NASAL BONES

The two **nasal bones** form the bony bridge of the nose (*Fig. 1-21*).

7. LACRIMAL BONES

The **lacrimal** [LAK ri mal] **bones** (also spelled lachrymal), small rectangular bones at the medial corner of each orbit, contain a depression for tear glands (*Fig. 1-21*).

8. INFERIOR TURBINATES OR CONCHAE

The **inferior nasal conchae** [CONG kee] or singular concha [KONG kah] (or **turbinates**) are scrolled bones (like the cross section scroll shape of a conch shell) in the nasal cavity forming part of the maxillary sinus wall. These are best seen through the opening to the nasal cavity (piriform aperture) (*Fig. 1-21*). Along with other scrolled processes of the ethmoid bone, they increase the area of mucous membrane inside the nasal cavity to warm and moisten air that we breathe.

9. HYOID BONE

The **hyoid** [HI oid] **bone** (see *Fig. 1-38*) is not really a bone of the skull but floats alone above the laryngeal prominence of the thyroid cartilage (known to many as the Adam's apple or voice box). All of the bones of the skull, except the mandible, are firmly attached to one another by irregular sutures.

The hyoid bone is not connected to the bones of the skull except via soft tissue. Muscles extend in a superior direction (suprahyoid muscles) from the hyoid bone to the mandible (e.g., the geniohyoid) and in an inferior direction (infrahyoid muscles) from the hyoid to the **sternum** (breastbone) and **clavicle** (collar bone). Like the bones of the neurocranium, the hyoid bone has a cartilaginous model precursor.

LEARNING QUESTIONS

Select the one best answer.

1. Which of the following bones does not form part of the temporal fossa?
    a. parietal
    b. frontal
    c. sphenoid
    d. temporal
    e. occipital

2. The mental foramen is located where?
    a. on the external surface of the mandible
    b. on the internal surface of the mandible
    c. on the palatal surface of the maxilla
    d. on the external surface of the maxillae
    e. on the sphenoid bone

3. What space does the maxillary nerve pass through immediately after exiting the foramen rotundum?
    a. nasopalatine canal
    b. mandibular canal
    c. maxillary sinus
    d. infraorbital canal
    e. pterygopalatine space

4. What bony process of the maxilla surrounds tooth roots?
    a. nasofrontal process
    b. frontal process
    c. alveolar process
    d. zygomatic process
    e. palatine process

5. Which structure is not located on the sphenoid bone?
    a. foramen ovale
    b. foramen rotundum
    c. greater wing
    d. pterygoid process
    e. articular fossa

6. Which teeth are most likely to have the roots in proximity with the maxillary sinus?
    a. maxillary molars and premolars
    b. maxillary canines
    c. maxillary incisors
    d. mandibular posterior teeth

7. The suture line joining the two parietal bones is called the:
    a. squamosal suture
    b. coronoid suture
    c. sagittal suture
    d. intermaxillary suture
    e. lambdoid suture

ANSWERS: 1-e, 2-a, 3-e, 4-c, 5-e, 6-a, 7-c

LEARNING EXERCISES

Each of the following bony landmarks can be seen or felt underneath the soft tissue on the face or in the mouth and could be used to describe the location of abnormalities during a clinical examination. First, describe the location; then, identify each of the following landmarks on an actual skull (or figures within this text). Use the referenced figures to confirm that you have correctly located each landmark.

- canine eminence of the mandible and maxillae—Figure 1-12

- mental protuberance—Figure 1-17

- maxillary tuberosity—Figure 1-14

- external auditory meatus—Figure 1-4

Each of the following landmarks is the attachment of a major muscle or ligament of importance to the dental professional. First, describe the location; then, identify each of the following landmarks on an actual skull (or figures within this text). Use the referenced figures to confirm that you have correctly described the location of the attachment on the skull. When possible, also feel or point to the landmark's location on your own head, or within your mouth.

- Angle of the mandible, lateral surface (**masseter muscle**)—Figure 1-18

- Zygomatic arch (**masseter muscle**)—Figure 1-18

- Angle of the mandible, medial surface (**medial pterygoid muscle**)—Figure 1-19

- Medial surface of the lateral pterygoid plate and adjacent pterygoid fossa of the sphenoid bone (**medial pterygoid muscle**)—Figure 1-7

- Temporal fossa (**temporalis muscle**)—Figure 1-4

- Coronoid process and temporal crest of mandible (**temporalis muscle**)—Figure 1-19

- Lateral surface of the lateral pterygoid plate of the sphenoid bone (**lateral pterygoid muscle**)—Figure 1-8

- Pterygoid fovea: anterior neck of mandibular condyle (**lateral pterygoid muscle**)—Figure 1-19

- Angular spine of the sphenoid (**sphenomandibular ligament**)—Figure 1-7

- Lingula of the mandible (**sphenomandibular ligament**)—Figure 1-19

- Styloid process of the temporal bone (**stylomandibular ligament**)—Figure 1-9

- Mastoid process of the temporal bone (**sternocleidomastoid muscle**)—Figure 1-9

- Mylohyoid ridge of the mandible (**mylohyoid muscle**)—Figure 1-19

- Genial spines of the mandible (**some suprahyoid muscles**)—Figure 1-19

Each of the following foramen or spaces is the passageway for nerves and blood vessels of importance to the dental professional. First, describe the location; then, identify each of the following foramina or spaces on an actual skull (or figures within this text). Use the referenced figures to confirm that you have correctly located the foramen, canal, or space on the skull.

- foramina rotundum in the sphenoid bone (for the **maxillary division of trigeminal nerve**)—Figure 1-6

- pterygopalatine space (for the **maxillary division of trigeminal nerve**)—Figure 1-8

- foramina ovale in the sphenoid bone (for the **mandibular division of trigeminal nerve**)—Figures 1-6 and 1-7

- mandibular foramina in the mandible (for the **inferior alveolar nerve**)—Figure 1-19

- mental foramina in the mandible (for the **mental nerve**)—Figure 1-18

- greater palatine foramina in the palatine bones (for the **greater palatine nerve**)—Figure 1-20

- incisive foramen in the maxillary bones (for the **nasopalatine nerve**)—Figure 1-20

- infraorbital foramina in the maxillae (for the **infraorbital nerve**)—Figure 1-12

SECTION III.   THE TEMPOROMANDIBULAR JOINT

OBJECTIVES

The objectives for this section are to prepare the reader to perform the following:
- Describe and locate (on a skull) the articulating parts of the temporomandibular joint (TMJ).
- Describe the location and functions of the articular disc.
- Palpate the lateral and posterior surfaces of the condyle of the mandible during movement of the jaws.
- On a skull, describe and locate the attachments of the ligaments of the temporomandibular joint.

A joint, or articulation, is a connection between two separate parts of the skeleton. The **temporomandibular joint** is the articulation between the mandible and the two temporal bones. The mandibular articulation with the skull on each side may also correctly be termed the **craniomandibular articulation** since it is the articulation between the movable mandible and the stationary cranium or skull.[3] It is a bilateral articulation: the right and left sides work as a unit. It is the only visible free-moving articulation in the head; all others are sutures and are immovable.[4] The coordinated movements of the right and left joints are complex and usually controlled by reflexes. Within some limit or range, the great adaptability of the joints permits the freedom of movement of the mandible required during speech and mastication (chewing). One can learn, however, to move the mandible voluntarily into specific, well-defined positions or pathways.[5-9] Both the maxillae and mandible support teeth whose shape and position greatly influence the most closed portions of mandibular movements.[3] Proper functioning of the temporomandibular joints has a profound effect on the occlusal contacts of teeth, which involve nearly all phases of dentistry.

A.   ANATOMY OF THE TEMPOROMANDIBULAR JOINT

There are three articulating parts to each temporomandibular joint: the mandibular condyle, the articular fossa with its adjacent eminence (or tubercle) of the temporal bone, and the articular disc interposed between the bony parts (Figs. 1-22 and 1-23). These parts are enclosed by a fibrous connective tissue capsule.[1,4,7]

1.   MANDIBULAR CONDYLE

The **mandibular condyle** [KON dile] is about the size and shape of a large date pit with the greater dimension mediolaterally (*Fig. 1-23*). From the side, it looks like a round knob (*Fig. 1-22*). From the posterior (or anterior) aspect, it is wide mediolaterally with a narrow neck. The upper surface of the

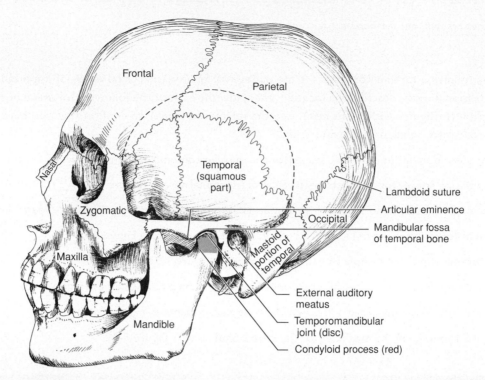

FIGURE 1-22. Human skull, left side. This lateral view shows the articulation of the bones of the **temporomandibular joint**, namely, the temporal bones and the mandible. The head of the condyle of the mandible is shaded red, and the red line on the inferior border of the zygomatic process of the temporal bone (zygomatic process) clearly outlines the concave **mandibular** (with its **articular**) **fossa**, and the convex **articular eminence** just anterior to it. For the mandibular to move forward, the condyles move the mandible down over the articular eminence, so the mandible is depressed and the mouth opens.

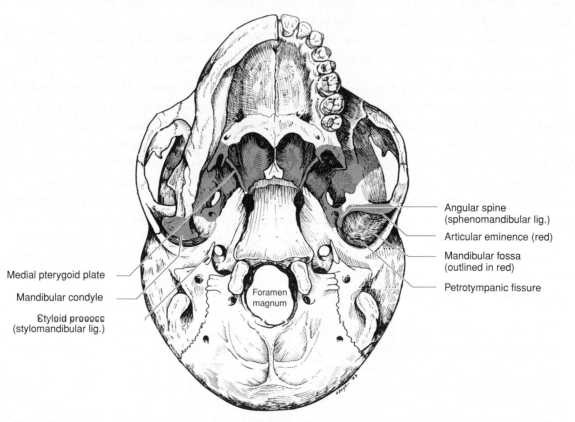

FIGURE 1-23. Human skull: inferior surface with half of the mandible removed on the right side of the drawing. Parts of the mandible and temporal bone that make up the **temporomandibular joint** are highlighted in red. On the left side, the **condylar process** of the mandible is shaded red, and on the right side with the mandible removed, the **mandibular** (and **articular**) **fossa** of the temporal bone is outlined in red, with the thicker anterior portion being the **articular eminence**. The sphenoid bone is also red.

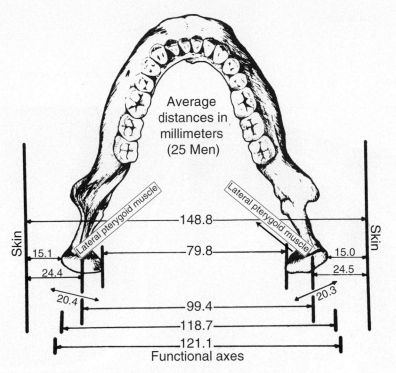

FIGURE 1-24. Depth (beneath the skin) of the landmarks of the head of the mandibular condyle and relative **direction of the right lateral pterygoid muscle** fibers (*red arrow*) from its insertion on the neck of the condyle toward its origin (not seen, but on the lateral surface of the lateral plate the sphenoid bone). [To obtain these measurements, metal markers were placed on the skin and some teeth on 25 men prior to taking submental vertex cephalometric radiographs for analysis, tracing, and measuring. The location of the center of rotational opening of the mandible (the hinge axis) was found to pass through or near the center of the heads of the condyles. The functional axes were determined from pantographic recordings. Resultant articular settings were found to be wider than the outer poles of the condyles. This means that lateral and protrusive excursions are controlled by ligaments and muscles, rather than by bone, as previously reported. This research was conducted by Drs. Woelfel and Igarashi and supported by the Ohio State University College of Dentistry and Nihon University School of Dentistry in Tokyo.]

mandibular condyle is strongly convex anteroposteriorly, and mildly convex mediolaterally. [Note the width of the condyle and its depth beneath the skin in *Fig. 1-24*. It is a large solid structure, about 10 mm thick anteroposteriorly and 20.4 mm wide mediolaterally. Although the average depth of the outer surface of the condyle is 15 mm beneath the skin, it is readily palpated, and its movements are visible (seemingly just beneath the skin) when eating. Research by Drs. Woelfel and Igarashi on 25 men found the average depth of the outer surface of the mandibular condyle on each side to be 15.0 mm; the range was 10.3–21.4 mm beneath skin.]

Carefully examine the photomicrograph of a human temporomandibular joint seen in Figure 1-25. The condyle is in the position it would occupy when the teeth come together as tightly and as comfortably as possible (maximum intercuspation), about 1 mm anterior to its most retruded position. The functioning regions are covered with fibrous connective tissue. The fibrous layers of the joint and the disc are avascular (devoid of blood vessels and nerves),[10] indicating that considerable force occurs on these surfaces of the joint. This fibrous, avascular type of connective tissue is adapted to resist pressure. It is particularly thick on the superior and anterior surfaces of the condyle over the region where most function occurs when the condyle is forward from its resting position, as when we bite our front teeth or incisors together (seen as the shaded structure in *Fig. 1-25*). Notice on the photomicrograph that this same type of fibrous covering also lines the posterior articulating surfaces of the articular eminence and adjacent fossa, as well as the center portion of the disc.

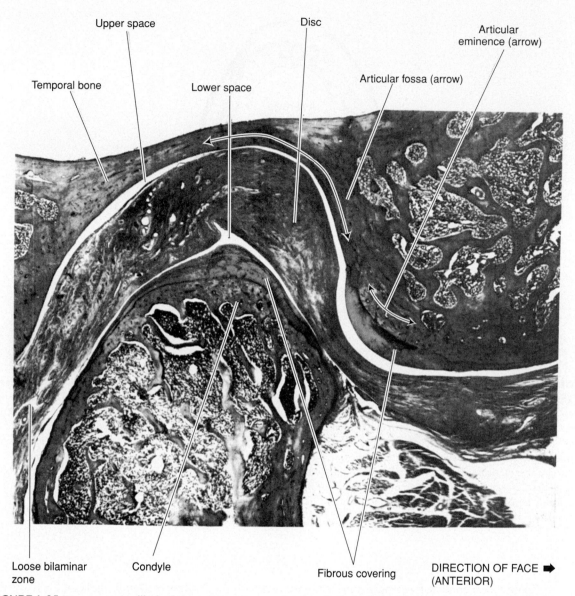

Upper space | Disc | Articular eminence (arrow)

Temporal bone | Lower space | Articular fossa (arrow)

Loose bilaminar zone | Condyle | Fibrous covering | DIRECTION OF FACE ➡ (ANTERIOR)

FIGURE 1-25. Temporomandibular joint, photomicrograph of the lateral aspect. The anterior of the skull (the face) is toward the right of the picture. The white area across the top is the space of the brain case. Notice the thicker **fibrous covering** (highlighted in red) and underlying compact bone on the **functional** part of the posterior inferior articular eminence and superior anterior part of the mandibular condyle. Also, notice the arrows indicating the contours of the concave articular fossa, and convex articular eminence, of the temporal bone. [This specimen was removed in a block of tissue, fixed in formalin, demineralized, embedded in celloidin, sectioned at a thickness of about 25 mm, and stained with hematoxylin and eosin.] (Courtesy of Professor Rudy Melfi.)

2. ARTICULAR FOSSA (NONFUNCTIONING PORTION) AND ARTICULAR EMINENCE (FUNCTIONING PORTION)

Study the right side of Figure 1-23 where half of the mandible has been removed, exposing the maxillary teeth, tuberosity, and articular fossa and eminence. The **articular** (glenoid) **fossa** is the anterior three-fourths of the larger **mandibular fossa**, and is anterior to the petrotympanic fissure. It is considered to be a nonfunctioning portion of the joint because, when the teeth are in *tight* occlusion, there is no tight contact among the head of the condyle, the disc, and the concave part of the articular fossa. [The fossa is about 23 mm mediolaterally and extends 15 mm posteriorly from the eminence. The intracapsular surface area is two to three times greater than on the very mobile mandibular condyle. The anterior part of the capsule that surrounds the entire mandibular fossa and articular eminence attaches 10 mm in front of the crest of the articulating eminence.[11]]

The **articular eminence** or transverse bony ridge is located just anterior and inferior to the articular fossa (*Fig. 1-22*). As stated earlier, its posterior surface is padded or lined by a thickened layer of fibrous connective tissue, more than the rest of the articular fossa, indicating that this is the functional portion of the joint when we are chewing food with the mandible in a protruded and/or lateral position. The thickest functional part of this lining is on the posterior inferior portion of the articular eminence (*Fig. 1-25*). This is where the anterior superior portion of the mandibular condyle rubs against it, but only indirectly since the articular disc is normally interposed between the two functioning bony elements.

3. ARTICULAR DISC

Examine a skull with the posterior teeth fitting together (in tight occlusion) and study how the mandibular condyle fits loosely into the articular fossa. The disc is not present in a prepared dry skull because the disc is not bone. There should be a visible space between the mandibular condyle and the articular fossa that in life was occupied by the disc.

The disc (*Figs. 1-25* and *1-26*) is a tough oval pad of dense fibrous connective tissue acting as a shock absorber between the mandibular condyle and the articular fossa and articular eminence. The disc surfaces are very smooth. It is thinner in the center than around the edges. Its periphery is thinner anteriorly and laterally but thicker medially and posteriorly. Rarely, it may become perforated. The center of the disc has no blood supply[10]; however, it is richly supplied elsewhere.

The *upper* contour of the disc is both concave and convex anteroposteriorly to conform to the shape of the articular eminence and fossa. In other words, it is concave anteriorly to conform to the convex articular eminence, and it is convex posteriorly, conforming to the concave shape of the articular fossa that it loosely rests against. The *lower* surface of the disc is concave anterior to posterior, thus adapting to the upper surface of the convex mandibular condyle.

The disc forms one natural wedge anterior to the condyle head and a second wedge posterior to the condyle. The lining of the capsule surrounding the disc produces **synovial** [si NO vee al] **fluid** that lubricates the joint. Because of the extremely slippery surfaces and the peripheral thickening of the disc, the disc moves harmoniously with the condyle. Also, the mandible and right and left discs move forward together because the lateral pterygoid muscle that pulls the jaw forward is attached

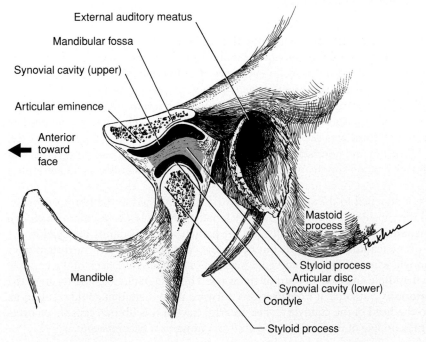

External auditory meatus
Mandibular fossa
Synovial cavity (upper)
Articular eminence
Anterior toward face
Mandible
Mastoid process
Styloid process
Articular disc
Synovial cavity (lower)
Condyle
Styloid process

FIGURE 1-26.
Temporomandibular joint, sagittal section. The anterior surface of the skull (face) is to the left. The sectioned temporal bone (with mandibular fossa and articular eminence) forms the superior part of the joint, and the sectioned head of the condyle forms the inferior part. The **articular disc** is shaded red. The **upper and lower synovial cavities** surround the disc. (Reproduced by permission from Clemente CD, ed. Gray's anatomy of the human body. 30th ed. Philadelphia: Lea & Febiger, 1985:340.)

Table 1-2	PREVALENCE OF CREPITUS DURING MAXIMUM OPENING*				
	NONE (%)	BOTH SIDES (%)	RIGHT SIDE (%)	LEFT SIDE (%)	ONE SIDE (R OR L) (%)
594 Dental hygiene students	52.0	13.3	18.2	16.8	35.0
505 Dental students	72.0	4.2	15.9	7.9	23.8
Percentage of all 1099 students	61.2	9.1	17.1	12.7	29.8

* Determinations by Dr. Woelfel, 1970–1986. More than 20% of these professional students had or were undergoing orthodontic treatment.

to the pterygoid fovea on the neck of the condyle as well as to the disc. When the thicker peripheral portions become flattened or the center of the disc thickens, the disc fails to move synchronously with the condyle, resulting in a popping or grating noise (**crepitus**), which is quite an annoying yet a fairly common occurrence. The frequency of this occurrence is presented in *Table 1-2*. With an elastic posterior attachment, the disc moves with the head of the condyle during function but only about half as far.

The articular disc has many functions.[11,12] It divides the space between the head of the condyle and the articulating fossa into upper and lower spaces (synovial cavities seen in *Fig. 1-26*), which permits complex functional movements of the mandible.[12] Because the anterior and posterior portions of the disc contain some specialized nerve fibers called **proprioceptive** [PRO pri o SEP tiv] **fibers**, which help unconsciously to determine the position of the mandible, the disc helps regulate movements of the condyle. It stabilizes the condyle by filling the space between incongruous articulating surfaces of the convex condyle and concave-convex articular fossa and articular eminence.[12] The disc cushions the loading of the joint at the point of contact (like a shock absorber). The cushioning and lubrication reduce physical wear and strain on joint surfaces.

B. LIGAMENTS THAT SUPPORT THE JOINT AND LIMIT JOINT MOVEMENT

Ligaments are slightly elastic bands of tissue. They do *not* move the joint; muscles move the joint. They do support and confine the movement of the mandible to protect muscles from being stretched beyond their capabilities.

1. FIBROUS CAPSULE (CAPSULAR LIGAMENT)

The **fibrous (or articular) capsule** is a fibrous tube of tissue that encloses the joint, best seen in Figures 1-27 and 1-28. It is fairly thin, except laterally, where the thicker **lateral** (formerly temporomandibular) **ligament** is located.[13] The upper border of the capsule is attached to the temporal bone around the circumference of the articular fossa and the articular eminence. The lower border is attached around the neck of the condyloid process, thus enclosing the condyle and completing the tube.

The internal surface of the fibrous capsule is lined with a **synovial membrane** that covers the bones to the borderline of their articulating surfaces and part of the mandibular neck. This thin membrane secretes a fluid, **synovia**, which lubricates the joint. This fluid is three times more slippery than ice. The synovial fluid both lubricates and nourishes the fibrous covering of the articulating surfaces and center of the disc, which lack a blood supply. In a normal joint space, there is only a small amount of fluid (one or two drops).

The articular disc is not attached to the skull, but anteriorly it is attached to the fibrous capsule. Posteriorly, the disc and the capsule are connected by a thick pad of loose elastic vascular connective tissue called the **bilaminar zone** (*Fig. 1-25*). Laterally and medially, the disc is tightly attached to the lateral and medial sides of the mandibular condyle but not to the capsule. Therefore, the disc follows the movement of the condyle when the lateral pterygoid muscles (attached to the neck of the condyle and the discs) move the mandible and disc forward or sideways. This design of attachments gives the disc freedom to move anteriorly but limits it from excessive forward movement that could result in its displacement anterior to the head of the condyle.[14] The anterior part of this fibrous capsule restricts posterior movement of the condyle of the mandible on wide openings as it becomes taut.

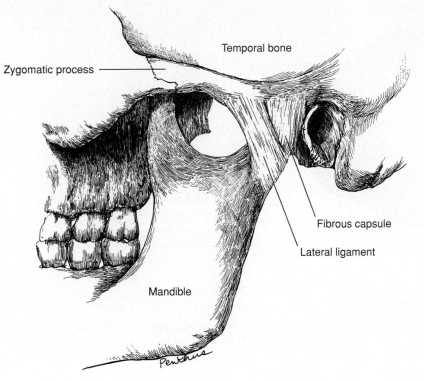

FIGURE 1-27. **Fibrous capsule** of the temporomandibular joint, lateral aspect, enclosing the joint, and the thickened outer **lateral ligament**. (Reproduced by permission from Clemente CD, ed. Gray's anatomy of the human body. 30th ed. Philadelphia: Lea & Febiger, 1985:339.)

2. LATERAL LIGAMENT (FORMERLY TMJ LIGAMENT)

The outer layer of the fibrous capsule is a thicker layer of fibrous tissue that is reinforced by accessory ligaments, which strengthen it. The **lateral ligament** of this joint is the strong reinforcement of the anterior lateral wall of the capsule (*Fig. 1-27*). It attaches to the zygomatic arch, then narrows as it drops obliquely down and backward to the lateral and posterior neck of the condyle. It keeps the condyle close to the fossa and helps to prevent lateral and posterior displacement of the mandible. It has no counterpart medially, and seemingly none is needed, since the right and left temporomandibular articulations work together as a unit. The lateral ligament on the opposite side, by failing to stretch, prevents excess medial displacement on the side moving medially.

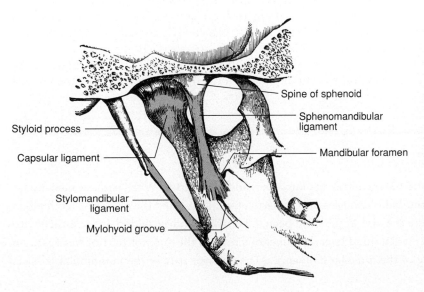

FIGURE 1-28. **Ligaments of the temporomandibular joint** limit mandibular movement. The **fibrous capsule (capsular ligament)** surrounds the joint, the **stylomandibular ligament** connects the styloid process of the temporal bone to the posterior surface of the mandible near the angle, and the **sphenomandibular (or spinomandibular) ligament** connects the spine of the sphenoid bone with the medial surface of the mandible near the lingula (tongue-like process) adjacent to the mandibular foramen. (Reproduced by permission from Clemente CD, ed. Gray's anatomy of the human body. 30th ed. Philadelphia: Lea & Febiger, 1985:339.)

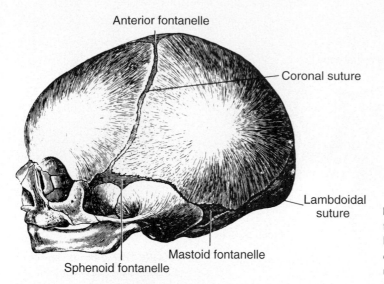

Anterior fontanelle

Coronal suture

Lambdoidal suture

Mastoid fontanelle

Sphenoid fontanelle

FIGURE 1-29. Skull at birth showing fontanelles (membrane-covered openings between bones). Notice that the mandibular condyle is barely higher than the crest of the mandibular ridge.

3. STYLOMANDIBULAR LIGAMENT

The **stylomandibular** [STY lo man DIB yoo lar] **ligament** is posterior to the joint but also gives support to the mandible (*Fig. 1-28*). It is relaxed when the mouth is closed but becomes tense on extreme protrusion of the mandible.[13] It is attached above to the styloid process of the temporal bone and below to the posterior border and angle of the mandible.

4. SPHENOMANDIBULAR LIGAMENT

The **sphenomandibular** [SFE no man DIB yoo lar] **ligament** is medial to the joint (*Fig. 1-28*). It gives some support to the mandible and may help limit maximum opening of the jaw. It is attached above to the angular (sphenoidal) spine of the sphenoid bone. Then it spreads out like a fan and attaches on the lingula of the mandible near the mandibular foramen.

C. DEVELOPMENT OF THE TEMPOROMANDIBULAR JOINT

In infants, the articular fossa, the articular eminence, and the condyle are rather flat. This flatness allows for a wide range of sliding motions in the temporomandibular joint. Also, this joint is at about the same level as the occlusal plane at birth with relatively no ramus height (*Fig. 1-29*). During growth, the articular fossa deepens, the articular eminence becomes prominent, the condyle becomes rounded, and the shape of the disc changes to conform to the change in shape of the fossa and condyle. There is also a downward lengthening of the ramus. The condyle contains cartilage beneath its surface, and the condyloid process and ramus lengthen until a person is 20–25 years old. This is one way the mandible grows in depth. As a result of growth in the condyle area, the body of the mandible is lowered from the skull, and the occlusal plane is located about 1 inch below the level of the condyles in an adult.

LEARNING EXERCISE

Study a skull and see how the mandibular condyle fits into the mandibular fossa. When you examine the fit, notice the space between the mandibular condyles and the articular fossae when the posterior teeth are in tight occlusion. This space is where the disc would have been in life. The condyle, with the disc attached to the neck of the condylar process medially and laterally, functions toward the anterior part of this fossa on the posterior and inferior surface of the articular eminence. (The anterior part of the mandibular fossa is called the articular fossa.)

On yourself, palpate the temporomandibular joint and feel the movement of the mandibular condyle. First, put your index fingers immediately in front of either ear opening and open and close your mouth. Notice that when you open and close the mandible just a little, you feel little movement of the condyles, whereas when you open the mandible wide, you feel more movement. This happens because during minimal opening the condyles only rotate within the articular fossa, but when we open wide, the entire mandible moves bodily (translates) forward and downward as the condyles are pulled forward over the articular eminence. Next, move your jaw to the right and left sides. You are feeling the movement of the outer pole (surface) of each mandibular condyle. Finally, place your little finger gently inside either ear opening, then open and close your mouth and pull your jaw back or posteriorly. You are feeling the upper and posterior portion of the mandibular condyle, especially when you close or retrude (pull back) your mandible.

LEARNING QUESTIONS

Select the one best answer.

1. What two structures articulate with the disc in the temporomandibular joint?
    a. the coronoid process of the mandible and the mandibular fossa of the temporal bone
    b. the condyloid process of the mandible and the mandibular fossa of the temporal bone
    c. the coronoid process of the mandible and the mandibular fossa of the sphenoid bone
    d. the condyloid process of the mandible and the mandibular fossa of the sphenoid bone
    e. the condyloid process of the mandible and the mandibular fossa of the maxillae

2. The ligament that limits the amount of movement of the mandible and attaches from the inferior surface of the neurocranium to the lingula of the mandible is the:
    a. lateral (TMJ) ligament
    b. stylomandibular ligament
    c. sphenomandibular ligament
    d. sternocleidomastoid ligament

3. Where on the temporal bone does the mandible function?
    a. in the anterior three-quarters of the mandibular fossa called the articular fossa
    b. in the posterior quarter of the mandibular fossa called the articular fossa
    c. on the posterior inferior portion of the articular eminence
    d. on the anterior inferior position of the articular eminence

ANSWERS: 1-b, 2-c, 3-c

SECTION IV. MUSCLES OF CHEWING (MASTICATION)

OBJECTIVES

The objectives for this section are to prepare the reader to perform the following:
- Identify the four pairs of major muscles of mastication.
- Describe and identify the origin and insertion of each of these muscles of mastication on a skull and be able to palpate each (if possible) on yourself or a partner.
- Describe and demonstrate the function of each of these muscles.
- List other factors that contribute to the position of teeth and movement of the mandible.
- Describe the location and list the functions of the groups of muscles that contribute to facial expression.

The following general terms relate to muscles and will be helpful to know as you read this section:

anguli [ANG gu li]: triangular area or angle of a structure

depressor: acts to depress or make lower

insertion of the muscles of mastication: place of attachment of muscles to the bone that moves, like muscle attachment on the movable mandible

labial [LAY bee al]: related to, or toward, the lips; like the labial surface of a tooth

levator [le VA tor]: acts to raise (cf. elevator)

lingual [LIN gwal]: related to the tongue; for example, the lingual nerve innervates the tongue; the lingual muscle is within the tongue; and the lingual surface of a tooth is the side toward the tongue

mental: referring to the chin; the mental foramen is the hole in the mandible where the mental nerve passes out of the mandible to the chin; the mentalis muscle inserts into the chin[1]

orbicularis [or BIK u lar is]: round; compare an orbit

origin (of muscles of mastication): are the source, beginning or fixed proximal end attachment of a muscle as compared to its insertion, which is a muscle's more movable attachment or distal end[1]

oris: referring to the edge of the mouth; compare oral

procerus [pro SE rus]: long and slender

The muscles of the body contribute 40–50% of the total body weight.[15] Muscles produce the desired action by pulling or by shortening, never by pushing or by lengthening. **Skeletal** or **voluntary muscles** are made up of specialized cells that contract. Skeletal muscles are very active metabolically and therefore require a rich blood supply.[15] There are two other kinds of muscles, **cardiac and smooth (involuntary) muscles**, which we are unable to control or direct.

Muscle cells are small (10–40 microns [μm] in diameter), elongated contractile fibers, each enclosed in a delicate envelope of loose connective tissue. Many individual parallel muscle fibers make up a bundle, and various numbers of bundles comprise a muscle. The longest muscle fibers are 300 mm (11.4 inches) long. Each contractile bundle of cells can contract about 57% of its fully stretched length.[16] The all-or-none law states that any single muscle *fiber* always contracts to its fullest extent.[11] When a weak effort or contraction is required of the whole muscle, then only a few fibers contract (each to the fullest extent). Many fibers contracting produce greater power as needed. No single muscle acts alone to produce a movement or to maintain posture. Many muscles must work in perfect coordination to produce a steady, well-directed motion of a body part.

When a muscle becomes shorter as it moves a structure, the movement is called an **isotonic contraction**. When a muscle maintains its length as it contracts to stabilize a part, this movement is called **isometric contraction**. As you close your jaw until all teeth contact, the closing muscles work isotonically because they become shorter as the mandible moves superiorly. If you maintain contact of all of your teeth but squeeze them together hard, these same muscles are contracting isometrically because they cannot shorten any more once your teeth are together.

A few or more individual muscles fibers of all of our voluntary muscles are continually or alternately contracting during consciousness. This minimal amount of contraction needed to maintain posture is called muscle **tone** or **tonus**, and the muscles involved are named "antigravity" muscles. As you read this, the muscles of mastication are probably in a state of minimal tonic contraction or balance with each other, with the neck muscles, and with gravity, enabling a comfortable, restful position for your mandible with the teeth apart. This normal resting jaw position varies slightly according to whether you are sitting, lying on your back, or standing up, and depending on how tense or stressed you are. When you fall asleep at your desk, antigravity muscles relax and, as you may have seen on others, the mouth drops open. Hopefully, this brief discussion will whet your appetite for seeking further knowledge. The list of references at the end of this chapter offers several choices.

A. MUSCLES INVOLVED IN MASTICATION (CHEWING)

Muscles of mastication move the mandible. They include four pairs of muscles (right and left): masseter, temporalis, medial pterygoid, and lateral pterygoid muscles. These muscles have the major control over the movements of the mandible. Each of these muscles has one end identified as its origin and the other end identified as its insertion. The **origin end** of each of the muscles of mastication is the source, beginning, or

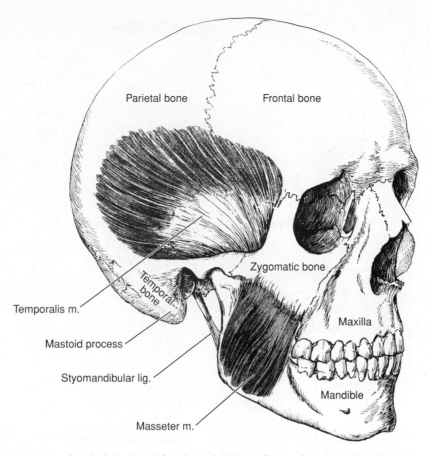

FIGURE 1-30. Masseter muscle (*shaded red*) and fan-shaped **temporalis muscle**. (Reproduced by permission from Clemente CD, ed. Gray's anatomy of the human body. 30th ed. Philadelphia: Lea & Febiger, 1985:450.)

fixed proximal attachment located, in this case, on the bones of the neurocranium, which are relatively immovable. The **insertion end** is the attachment on the movable bone that for each of these muscles is attached to, and moves, the mandible.

There are five different ways the mandible moves. We can **elevate** it (closing the mouth), **depress** it (opening the mouth), **retrude** it (retracting or pulling back the mandible), **protrude** it (protracting or moving the mandible anteriorly), and move it into **lateral excursions** (moving the mandible sideways, as in chewing).

1. MASSETER MUSCLE

The **masseter** [ma SEE ter] **muscle** (*Fig. 1-30*) is the largest, most superficial, bulky, and powerful of the muscles of mastication. It is four-sided in shape. [Its average volume on 25 males is $30.4 \pm 4.1 \text{ cm}^3$, which is 2.6 times larger than the medial pterygoid muscle (second largest one at $11.5 \pm 2.1 \text{ cm}^3$).[17]]

Origin: The masseter arises from the inferior and medial surfaces of the zygomatic bone, the zygomatic process of the maxillae, and the temporal process of zygomatic bone (collectively known as the zygomatic arch seen in *Fig. 1-31*). From here it extends inferiorly and posteriorly toward its insertion.

Insertion: The masseter inserts on the inferior lateral surface of the ramus and angle of the mandible (*Fig. 1-31*).

Action: It **elevates** the mandible (closes the mouth) and applies great power in crushing food.[6,8,9]

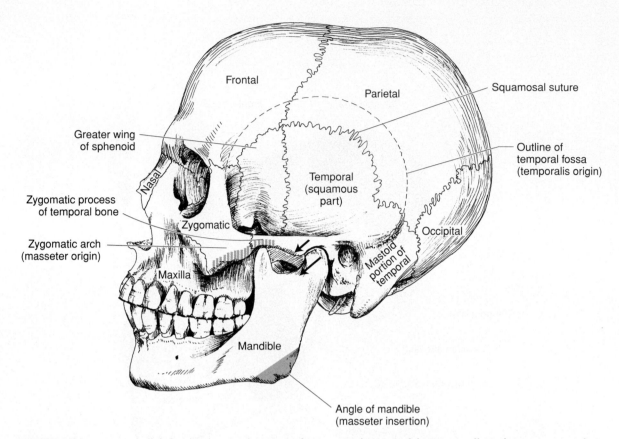

FIGURE 1-31. Human skull, left side, showing location of some **attachments of the temporalis and masseter muscles** (*shaded red*). This lateral view shows the origin of the fan-shaped temporalis muscle (within the shallow temporal fossa outlined with a *red dotted line*) and the origin of the masseter (on the zygomatic arch), as well as the insertion of the masseter muscle (lateral surface of the angle of the mandible). The red arrows indicate the slope of the posterior surface of the articular eminence and the subsequent downward (opening) movement of the mandible when it is pulled forward by both lateral pterygoid muscles.

LEARNING EXERCISE

As you clench your teeth several times, feel the contraction of the masseter by placing a finger on the outside of your cheek posterior to the third molar region. The muscle will produce a noticeable bulge beneath your finger each time. The part felt just inferior to the cheek bone (anterior to the ear) is the origin, and the bulge felt over the angle of the mandible is the insertion.

2. TEMPORALIS MUSCLE

The **temporalis** [tem po RA lis] **muscle** is a fan-shaped, large but flat muscle with both vertical anterior (and middle) fibers and more horizontal posterior vertical fibers. Vertical and horizontal fibers are shaded in *Figure 1-32*.

Origin: The temporalis arises from the entire temporal fossa (*Fig. 1-31*) (composed of the squamous part of temporal bones and the greater wing of the sphenoid bones and the adjacent portions of the frontal and parietal bones). From here, its **anterior** (and middle) fibers are directed vertically downward while its **posterior** fibers are directed more horizontally, mostly anteriorly and somewhat inferiorly, passing medial to the zygomatic arch.

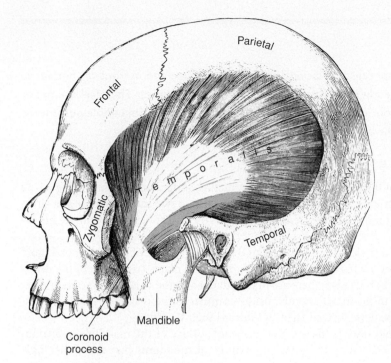

FIGURE 1-32. Temporalis muscle: some vertical (anterior) and horizontal (posterior) fibers are shaded red. The zygomatic process of the temporal bone and temporal process of the zygomatic bone have been removed. When studying this drawing, you should understand why the contraction of the anterior, vertically oriented fibers of the temporal muscle act to close the jaw, while contraction of the posteriorly positioned, horizontally oriented fibers act to pull the jaw back or to retract (retrude) the mandible. (Reproduced by permission from Clemente CD, ed. Gray's anatomy of the human body. 30th ed. Philadelphia: Lea & Febiger, 1985:449.)

Insertion: The temporalis inserts on the coronoid process of the mandible, the medial surface of the anterior border of the ramus, and the temporal crest of the mandible (*Fig. 1-33*) via one common tendon.

Action: The **anterior** (and middle) vertical fibers contract to act to **elevate** the mandible (close the jaw) especially when great power is not required, and the **posterior** horizontal fibers **retrude** or pull the mandible posteriorly.[6,8,9] This muscle can position the mandible slightly more anterior or posterior while also closing the teeth together.

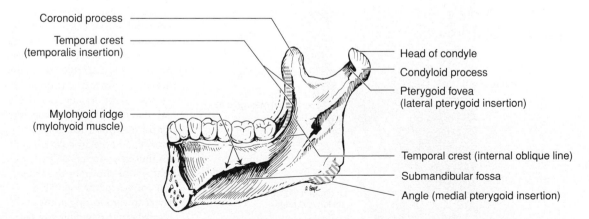

FIGURE 1-33. Mandible, medial surface, with the location of the **muscle insertions** of the temporalis, medial pterygoid, and lateral pterygoid muscles. The insertion of the **temporalis** muscle is located on the anterior medial ridge (temporal crest) of the mandibular ramus. The insertion of the **medial pterygoid** muscle is on the internal surface of the angle of the mandible. The insertion of the **lateral pterygoid** muscle is on the anterior surface of the neck of the condyle in the pterygoid fovea (as well as the articular disc, which is not shown).

LEARNING EXERCISE

Feel contraction of the origin of the temporalis by placing several fingers above and in front of your ear to feel the vertical fibers contract as you gently close your teeth together several times. Then feel the nearly horizontal fibers just above and behind your ears contract as you retrude or pull your mandible posteriorly. This may be more difficult to feel since the bulge is less evident.

3. MEDIAL PTERYGOID MUSCLE

The **medial pterygoid** [TER i goid] **muscle** is located on the medial surface of the ramus (*Figs. 1-34* and *1-35*). Along with the masseter located on the lateral surface, these two muscles serve as a sling, one on the medial side and one on the lateral side of the angle of the mandible, and result in similar actions.

Origin: The medial pterygoid muscle arises mainly from the medial surface of the lateral pterygoid plate and the pterygoid fossa between the medial and lateral pterygoid plates (right side of the drawing in *Fig. 1-37*) of the sphenoid bone. [Also, there are fibers attached to the palatine bone and posterior surface of the maxillae, and to the maxillary tuberosity.[3]] Similar to the masseter, the fibers pass from their origin inferiorly and posteriorly (but laterally) toward their insertion.

Insertion: The medial pterygoid muscle inserts on the *medial* surface of the mandible in a triangular region at the angle and on the superior adjacent portions of the ramus just above the angle (*Fig. 1-33*).

Action: It **elevates** the mandible (closes jaw) like the masseter and the anterior (and middle) fibers of the temporalis muscles. Although not as large or powerful, it is a synergist of (i.e., works together with) the larger masseter muscle in helping apply the power or great force on closures.

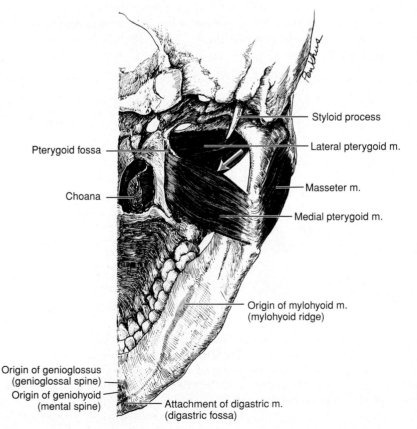

Pterygoid fossa

Choana

Styloid process

Lateral pterygoid m.

Masseter m.

Medial pterygoid m.

Origin of mylohyoid m.
(mylohyoid ridge)

Origin of genioglossus
(genioglossal spine)

Origin of geniohyoid
(mental spine)

Attachment of digastric m.
(digastric fossa)

FIGURE 1-34. The skull from the inferior view showing the **medial pterygoid** and **masseter muscles,** as well as the **lateral pterygoid** muscle. Note how the **medial pterygoid muscle** (*shaded red*) and **masseter** muscles form a sling that supports the mandible. Also, from this view, it is clear that the **lateral pterygoid** muscle has its origin (on the base of the cranium) more medial than its insertion (on the anterior portion of the neck of the condyle, and the articular disc). If this muscle contracts only on the right side as shown by the arrow, that condyle of the mandible moves toward its origin, thus bodily moving the mandible toward the left or opposite side. (Reproduced by permission from Clemente CD, ed. Gray's anatomy of the human body. 30th ed. Philadelphia: Lea & Febiger, 1985:452.)

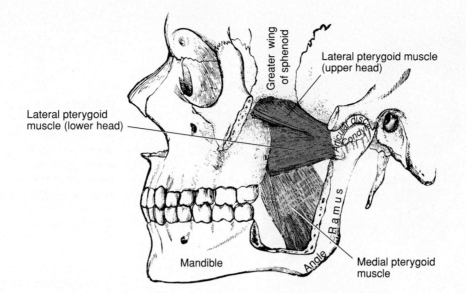

FIGURE 1-35. A lateral view of two heads of the **lateral pterygoid muscle** (*shaded red*) and the **medial pterygoid** muscle, with **the** zygomatic arch and the anterior part of the ramus removed. The **upper head of the lateral pterygoid** muscle has its origin on the infratemporal surface of the sphenoid bone, and the **lower head** has its origin on the lateral surface of the lateral pterygoid plate of the sphenoid bone (covered by the muscle in this drawing). The insertion of both heads of the lateral pterygoid muscle is on the fovea of the neck of the condyle of the mandible, and on the articular disc. Notice the horizontal orientation of the lateral pterygoid fibers in direct contrast to the vertical direction of the medial pterygoid fibers. Simultaneous contraction of both lateral pterygoid muscles pulls the condyle (and disc) forward, which causes the mandible to protrude and the mouth to open. Contraction of the **medial pterygoid** muscle in harmony with the masseter elevates the mandible (closes the mouth). (Reproduced by permission from Clemente CD, ed. Gray's anatomy of the human body. 30th ed. Philadelphia: Lea & Febiger, 1985:451.)

LEARNING EXERCISE

Attempt to palpate the insertion of the medial pterygoid muscle in your mouth by bending the head forward to relax the skin on the neck, and placing the forefinger medial to the internal angle of the mandible while gently pressing upward and outward. When the teeth are squeezed together, you should feel the bulge of this muscle.

4. LATERAL PTERYGOID MUSCLE

The **lateral pterygoid muscle**, unlike the other three pairs of muscles where most fibers are oriented primarily vertically, has its fibers aligned mostly horizontally (*Fig. 1-35*). The lateral pterygoid muscle is a short, thick, somewhat conical muscle located deep in the infratemporal fossa (inferior to the temporal bone and posterior to the maxillae) and is the prime mover of the mandible except for closing the jaw.

Origin: The lateral pterygoid muscle arises from two heads, both located on the sphenoid bone. The smaller superior head is attached to the infratemporal surface of the greater wing of the sphenoid bone (*Fig. 1-35*); the larger inferior head is attached to the adjacent lateral surface of the lateral pterygoid plate on the sphenoid bone (*Figs. 1-35* and *1-36*). Fibers pass posteriorly and laterally in a horizontal direction toward their insertion. When viewed from below, the direction of these fibers, from their insertion on the anterior surfaces of the heads of the mandibular condyles, is represented by the arrow in *Figure 1-37*.

Insertion: The lateral pterygoid muscle inserts on the depression on the front of the neck of the condyloid process called the pterygoid fovea (*Fig. 1-33*) and into the anterior margin of the articular disc. Minor forward contractions of the upper head pulling the disc forward work in concert with the

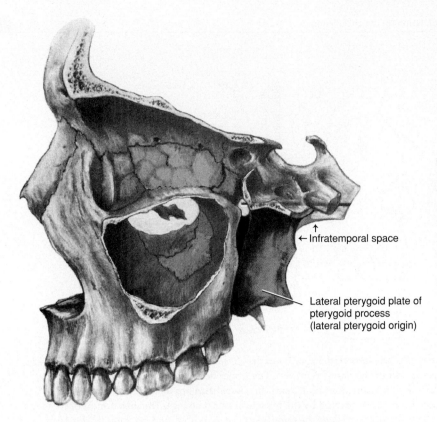

FIGURE 1-36. Part of human skull, lateral view, with the lateral wall of the maxilla removed to expose the maxillary sinus. Posterior to the maxilla, note the location of the **origin** of the two heads of the **lateral pterygoid muscle**: the lateral surface of the **lateral pterygoid plate** (*shaded red*) just posterior to the maxilla and the **infratemporal** surface (superior to the infratemporal space) on the base of the cranium. (Reproduced by permission from Clemente CD, ed. Gray's anatomy of the human body. 30th ed. Philadelphia: Lea & Febiger, 1985:166.)

← Infratemporal space

Lateral pterygoid plate of pterygoid process (lateral pterygoid origin)

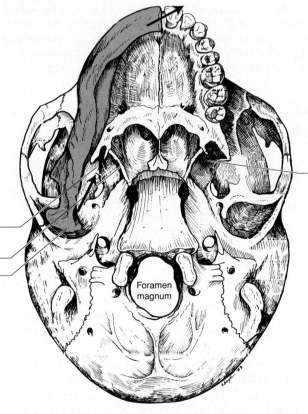

Pterygoid fossa of sphenoid (medial pterygoid origin)

Lateral pterygoid plate (lateral pterygoid origin)

Medial pterygoid plate

Mandibular condyle

Foramen magnum

FIGURE 1-37. Human skull, inferior surface, showing the location of the origin and insertion of the lateral pterygoid muscle and the origin of the medial pterygoid muscle in the pterygoid fossa. Only half of the mandible (*shaded red*) is shown, on the left side of the drawing. As you study this drawing, notice the arrow that connects the insertion of the lateral pterygoid muscle (on the **anterior neck of the condyle of the mandible**) with its origin (on the **lateral surface of the lateral pterygoid plate** denoted by a red line). When only this one lateral pterygoid muscle contracts and pulls the insertion end toward its origin, the mandible moves medially, toward the opposite side, as shown by the second arrow near the anterior part of the mandible. The location of the origin of the medial pterygoid muscle is shown on the right side of the drawing in the **pterygoid fossa**.

stretching of the elastic band of tissues behind the disc (retrodiscal tissues) and permit the disc to accompany the mandible as it moves forward, preventing posterior displacement of the disc.[14]

Actions: When *both lateral pterygoids* contract simultaneously, the action is:

- to **protrude** the mandible. No other muscle or groups of muscles are capable of doing this but can only assist in this action as stabilizers or by controlling the degree of jaw opening during the protrusion.[5,6,8,9,18]
- to **depress** the mandible. They do this by pulling the articular discs and the condyles forward and down onto the articular eminences, which moves the mandible inferiorly and helps rotate it, thereby opening the mouth (illustrated by arrows in Figure 1-31 that show the incline of the articular eminence and the same downward direction that condyles take when pulled forward under the bump of the eminence). The lateral pterygoids are assisted somewhat in this task by groups of muscles in the neck attached from the mandible to the hyoid bone (called the suprahyoid muscles), and from the hyoid bone to the clavicle and sternum called the infrahyoid muscles.

When *only one lateral pterygoid* contracts, it pulls the condyle on that side medialward and anteriorly, moving the body of the mandible and its teeth *toward the opposite side* (since the origin of the lateral pterygoid muscle is medial to its insertion as seen by the arrow in Figure 1-37). For example, contraction of the right lateral pterygoid muscle draws the right condyle medially (to the left) and forward, causing the mandible to move toward the left side (into **left lateral excursion**).[8] Conversely, the contraction of the left lateral pterygoid muscle causes the mandible to move to the right side (**right lateral excursion**).[8] No other muscle is capable of moving the mandible sideways, although synergistic (in harmony with) unilateral contraction of the posterior fibers of the temporalis muscle occurs on the side toward which the jaw moves.[8]

LEARNING EXERCISE

Viewing the inferior surface of a skull with a movable mandible, imagine elastic bands attached from the location of the origins to the insertions of the lateral pterygoid muscles, right and left side. Since the origin on the base of the skull stays stationary, but the mandible at the insertion can move, confirm that the mandible moves anterior and inferior if both elastic bands were contracted (shortened). Next, see what would happen if only one band was shortened (contracted). If only the right side is shortened, the right condyle moves medially (to the left), closer to its origin on the lateral pterygoid plate, so the body of the mandible and its teeth also move toward the left side. Practice this until you understand why the jaw moves the way it does when one lateral pterygoid muscle works. Next, attempt to palpate the origin of the lateral pterygoid muscle in your mouth. Slip a clean little finger into your mouth along the lateral surface of the maxillary alveolar process. Then gently move the finger posteriorly and medially, around to the posterior surface of the maxilla, and superiorly toward the lateral surface of the lateral pterygoid plate where the lateral pterygoid muscle attaches. Moving the mandible toward the side you are palpating will give your finger more room to reach the muscle. This palpation may be slightly uncomfortable.

B. OTHER MUSCLES AFFECTING MANDIBULAR MOVEMENT

Other muscles affecting mandibular movement include the suprahyoid and infrahyoid group of muscles. The **suprahyoid** [SOO prah HI oid] **muscle group** extends superiorly from the superior surface of the hyoid bone to the mandible, whereas the **infrahyoid muscle group** extends inferiorly from the inferior surface of the hyoid bone to the clavicle (collarbone) and sternum (breast bone) (*Fig. 1-38*). The inferior hyoid muscles must stabilize the hyoid bone in order for the suprahyoid muscles to move the mandible. These muscle groups act together with both lateral pterygoid muscles to help depress the mandible (open the mouth) and act with the posterior (horizontal) fibers of the temporalis muscles to retrude (pull back) the mandible.

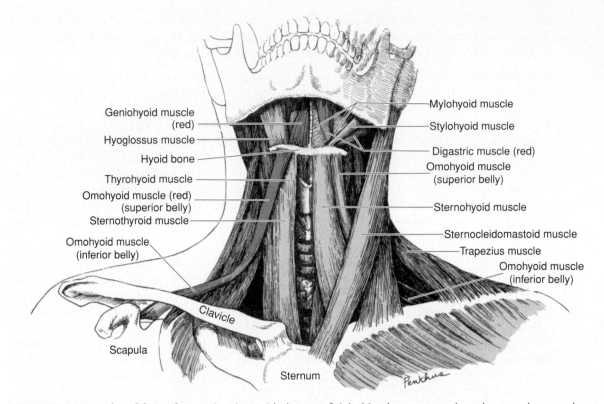

FIGURE 1-38. Muscles of the neck, anterior view, with the superficial, thin platysma muscle and some other muscles removed. Note the **hyoid bone** with a group muscles superior to the hyoid (called the **suprahyoid muscle group**) and another group of muscles inferior to the hyoid bone (called the **infrahyoid muscle group**). The suprahyoids generally attach the hyoid bone to the mandible, and include the **digastric** muscle and the **geniohyoid** muscle, shaded red on the right side of the drawing. The infrahyoids generally attach the hyoid bone to the clavicle (collar bone) and sternum (breast bone), and include the **omohyoid** muscle, shaded red on the left side of the drawing. When both muscle groups work together, they can help open and retrude the mandible. (Reproduced by permission from Clemente CD, ed. Gray's anatomy of the human body. 30th ed. Philadelphia: Lea & Febiger, 1985:451.)

The suprahyoid muscles include the **stylohyoid** [STY lo HI oid] muscles (which arise on the styloid process), **digastric** [di GAS trik] (the anterior bellies attach near the genial spines or tubercles), **mylohyoid** (arising from the mylohyoid ridges on each half of the medial surface of the mandible and found inferior to the floor of the mouth), and **geniohyoid** [JEE ni o HI oid] (arising from the genial tubercles). The infrahyoid muscles include the **omohyoid**, **sternohyoid**, **sternothyroid**, and **thyrohyoid**, and muscles that arise from the clavicle (collarbone), sternum (breastbone), and adjacent structures.

Another neck muscle, the **sternocleidomastoid**, attaches from the mastoid process of the temporal bone to the sternum breastbone) and clavicle (collar bone). This muscle does not move the mandible, but is palpated during a cancer screening exam since it is the location of cervical (neck) lymph nodes (*Fig. 1-38*).

C.   OTHER FACTORS AFFECTING TOOTH POSITION OR MOVEMENT

Other factors affecting relative tooth positions and movements include the ligaments, fascia, and, to a certain extent, the muscles of facial expression. The **ligaments**, including the capsular, temporomandibular, stylomandibular, and sphenomandibular ligaments (recall *Figs. 1-27* and *1-28*), provide some limits to protrusive, lateral, and opening movements of the mandible.

Fascia [FASH e ah] is also thought to limit movement of the mandible to some extent. Fascia is connective tissue that forms sheets or bands between anatomic structures. It attaches to bones and surrounds muscles, glands, vessels, nerves, and fat.

Some **muscles of facial expression** (especially in the lips and cheeks) and the tongue muscles are thought to influence development, position, and shape of the dental arches. The muscles of facial expression are shown in *Fig. 1-39* and include the following:

- **Orbicularis oris** [or BIK u LAR is O ris] is located within the lips around the opening of the mouth and acts to close or purse the lips (as around a straw or around a saliva ejector within the dental office).
- **Buccinator** [BUCK si na tor] attaches on the buccinator crest (posterior to the mandibular third molar) and adjacent soft tissue forming a pouch in the cheeks. When contracting, it pulls the cheek inward to keep food on the chewing surfaces of teeth during chewing.
- *Upper oral group* includes the **zygomaticus** [ZI go MAT i kus] **major and minor, levator labii** [LAB e e] **superioris**, and **levator anguli oris**. All contribute to raising the upper lip and/or angle, as in smiling. (The levator labii superioris alaeque [a LY kwe] nasi dilates the nostrils, as in contempt. The **risorius** [ri SO ri us] retracts [spreads] the angle of the mouth.)

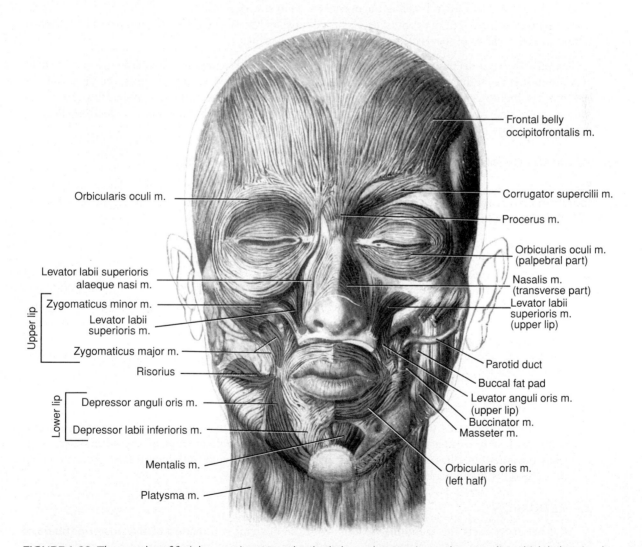

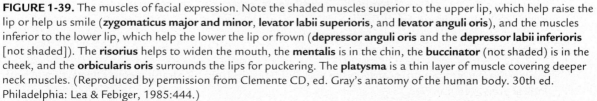

FIGURE 1-39. The muscles of facial expression. Note the shaded muscles superior to the upper lip, which help raise the lip or help us smile (**zygomaticus major and minor, levator labii superioris**, and **levator anguli oris**), and the muscles inferior to the lower lip, which help the lower the lip or frown (**depressor anguli oris** and the **depressor labii inferioris** [not shaded]). The **risorius** helps to widen the mouth, the **mentalis** is in the chin, the **buccinator** (not shaded) is in the cheek, and the **orbicularis oris** surrounds the lips for puckering. The **platysma** is a thin layer of muscle covering deeper neck muscles. (Reproduced by permission from Clemente CD, ed. Gray's anatomy of the human body. 30th ed. Philadelphia: Lea & Febiger, 1985:444.)

- *Lower oral group* (including the **depressor labii inferior** and **depressor anguli oris**) contracts to lower the lower lip or angle, as in a frown. The **mentalis** [men TA lis] is located in the chin and raises or protrudes the chin as in a pout.
- *Nose muscles* include the **nasalis** [na SA lis], which flares the nostrils; the **depressor septi nasi** (not shown in figure), which pulls the nares down, thereby constricting the opening of the nose (nares); and the **procerus** [pro SE rus] superior from the bridge of the nose, which lowers the medial eyebrow and wrinkles the nose.
- *Eye muscles* include the **orbicularis oculi** [or BIK u lar is AHK u li], which surrounds the eye and acts to squint the eye, and the **corrugator supercilii** [COR u gay tor su per SIL e e], which draws the medial end of the eyebrow down, as in a frown.
- *Ear muscles* include the **posterior, superior,** and **anterior auricular** [aw RIK u lar] muscles (not shown), which act to move the ears and/or scalp. Can you wiggle your ears by contracting these muscles? Give it a try.
- The broad **occipitofrontalis** [ahk SIP i toe fron TAL is] (or epicranial) muscle draws back the scalp, wrinkling the forehead and raising the eyebrows, as in surprise.
- The **platysma** [plah TIZ mah] muscle is a broad muscle that extends from the mouth to the anterior and lateral surfaces of the neck and contracts during a grimace.

The posterior and deep muscles of the neck, as well as the overlying fascia and skin, all have a slight postural influence on the physiologic resting position of the mandible. Other than this, the numerous facial muscles, including the buccinator, do *not* influence any movements of the mandible. However, a person's posture, state of mind, stress, health, and physical and mental fatigue each have a decided effect on the resting posture of the mandible at any given time.[19]

D. SUMMARY OF MUSCLES THAT MOVE AND CONTROL THE MANDIBLE

There are five specifically different ways that we can voluntarily move our mandible. There are limitless combinations of these movements that occur throughout any 24 hours. In review, here are the muscles that contribute to each movement:

1. ELEVATION

Elevation (elevates the mandible and closes the mouth) results from the bilateral contraction of three pairs of muscles. Right and left **temporalis** muscles (vertical fibers) bring the mandible upward into position for crushing food. The temporalis muscles are primarily the *positioning* muscles, as they elevate the mandible upward until it is in position to have the real force applied by the other two pairs of closing muscles. Right and left **masseter** muscles and right and left **medial pterygoid muscles** act together to apply the power for forceful jaw closures, as in crushing food, such as biting through a carrot.

2. DEPRESSION

Depression (depresses the mandible and opens the mouth) results primarily from the bilateral contraction of **both lateral pterygoid** muscles, assisted by **suprahyoid and infrahyoid** muscles, especially the anterior bellies of the digastric muscles and the omohyoid (infrahyoid) muscles, which help fix or hold the hyoid bone.

3. RETRUSION

Retrusion (retracts the mandible) results from the bilateral contraction of the **posterior fibers of the temporalis** muscles assisted by the **suprahyoids**, especially the **digastric** muscles (anterior and posterior bellies seen in *Fig. 1-38*).

4. PROTRUSION

Protrusion (or protraction, protrudes the mandible) results from the simultaneous contraction of **both lateral pterygoid** muscles.

5. LATERAL EXCURSION

Lateral excursion (moves sideways) results from the contraction of **one lateral pterygoid** muscle. (The mandible is moved bodily to the left by the contraction of the right lateral pterygoid muscle.)[8,20]

LEARNING QUESTIONS

Select the one best answer.

1. Which muscle has its origin in the pterygoid fossa?
    a. medial pterygoid muscle
    b. lateral pterygoid muscle
    c. masseter
    d. temporalis muscle

2. The masseter muscle elevates the mandible. Which other muscles are involved in elevating the mandible?
    a. temporalis (anterior fibers) and lateral pterygoid muscles
    b. lateral pterygoid muscles and medial pterygoid muscles
    c. temporalis (posterior and anterior fibers) and medial pterygoid muscles
    d. medial pterygoid muscles and temporalis (anterior fibers)
    e. lateral pterygoid muscles and temporalis (posterior fibers)

3. In which direction do the fibers of the lateral pterygoid muscles travel from their origin to their insertion?
    a. medial and posterior
    b. medial and anterior
    c. lateral and anterior
    d. lateral and posterior

4. Which of the following muscles of facial expression does not contribute to moving the lips?
    a. orbicularis oris
    b. risorius
    c. levator labii superioris
    d. depressor labii inferioris
    e. orbicularis oculi

5. Which of the following would you palpate anterior and 1–2 inches superior to the ear?
    a. masseter, the origin
    b. masseter, the insertion
    c. temporalis, posterior fibers
    d. temporalis, anterior fibers
    e. temporalis, the insertion

6. Which muscle, when contracting, moves the mandible to the right?
    a. the left medial pterygoid muscle
    b. the right medial pterygoid muscle
    c. the left temporalis muscle, horizontal fibers
    d. the right lateral pterygoid muscle
    e. the left lateral pterygoid muscle

ANSWERS: 1–a, 2–d, 3–d, 4–e, 5–d, 6–e

SECTION V. NERVES OF THE ORAL CAVITY

OBJECTIVES

The objectives for this section are to prepare the reader to perform the following:
- List the 12 cranial nerves and briefly describe their function.
- Describe in depth the important branches of the trigeminal nerve and trace the route of each important branch from the brain to the structures that they innervate in the oral cavity.
- Describe the pathway to the oral cavity of the facial nerve and identify the oral structure(s) it innervates (both motor and sensory).
- Describe the pathway to the oral cavity of the glossopharyngeal nerve and identify the oral structure(s) it innervates.
- Describe the pathway to the oral cavity of the hypoglossal nerve and identify the oral structure(s) it innervates.

There are three types of nerve fibers based on their function: afferent, efferent, and secretory. **Afferent** [AF er ent] (or **sensory**) fibers convey impulses (such as feeling, touch, pain, taste) from peripheral organs (like the skin or surface of the tongue) to the central nervous system. (*Hint:* Afferent: where "a" [as in *a*pproach] means sending impulses *toward* the brain [i.e., from an organ receiving sensory input], so the brain can "feel" it; therefore, these impulses are sensory, related to the senses of feeling, touch, pain, taste, etc.)

Efferent [EF er ent] (or **motor**) nerve fibers convey impulses from the central nervous system to the peripheral organs, such as to muscle fibers to initiate contraction. They supply the four pairs of muscles of mastication and other muscles in the region of the mouth. (*Hint:* Efferent: where "e" [as in *e*xit] means sending an impulse *from* the brain, often to a muscle, to have a bone move in the intended direction [or to increase force on that bone without movement]; therefore, these impulses are motor.)

Secretory fibers are specialized efferent nerve fibers that, upon stimulation, can send messages to glands, like the salivary and lacrimal glands to produce and secrete saliva or tears.

Table 1-3 lists the **12 cranial nerves** (indicated by Roman numerals I–XII) that are responsible for the following functions.[1,21–26]

A. TRIGEMINAL NERVE (FIFTH CRANIAL NERVE)

When discussing the function of the oral cavity, probably the most important nerve is the trigeminal. The trigeminal nerve or fifth cranial nerve is the largest of the cranial nerves and is the major sensory nerve of the face and scalp. It originates in the large semilunar or trigeminal ganglion, a group of nerve cell bodies located on the internal, superior surface of the temporal bone in a small depression within the cranium medial to the foramen ovale. The trigeminal nerve is divided into **three major divisions** (or three nerve branches). (*Hint:* "tri" in *tri*geminal refers to the nerve's three divisions.) **Division I** (**ophthalmic** [ahf THAL mik] **nerve**) and **Division II** (**maxillary nerve**) are only afferent (sensory). **Division III** (**the mandibular nerve**) is both afferent (sensory) and efferent (motor). Its efferent fibers supply the muscles of mastication. This is the only cranial nerve with sensory (feeling) innervation to the skin of the face, and the divisions or branches are distributed to the face as shown in *Figure 1-40*.

The maxillary and mandibular divisions of the trigeminal nerve also supply afferent or sensory neurons that provide the brain with information about the position of the teeth and jaws at all times. The interpretation of postural information by the brain (sense of position) is called **proprioception**. Proprioceptive nerve receptors are located in muscles and ligaments, including the ligaments around the teeth (called periodontal ligaments), and in the lateral aspects of the temporomandibular joints. The periodontal ligament around each tooth is well supplied with proprioceptive (sense of position) neurons from the maxillary and mandibular divisions of the trigeminal nerve. These branches continually send messages to the brain as to the relative position of the mandibular to maxillary teeth. This has a tremendous influence on relative jaw position, movement, and occlusion (the fitting together) of the teeth. Canines are reported to have the richest supply of proprioceptive nerve endings.

The temporomandibular joint also has proprioceptive neurons in the capsule and disc that are innervated by the auriculotemporal branch of the mandibular division of the trigeminal nerve. To a great extent,

Table 1-3	THE 12 CRANIAL NERVES	
NERVE #	CRANIAL NERVE	FUNCTION
I	Olfactory [ol FAK toe ree]	Smell
II	Optic	Sight
III	Oculomotor [AHK u lo MO tor]	Orbital muscles for eye movement
IV	Trochlear [TROK le ar]	Orbital muscles for eye movement
V	***Trigeminal [tri JEM i nal]**	**Motor: movement of the jaws and muscles of mastication**
		Sensory: sensation of feeling for the face, teeth, and periodontal ligaments, and anterior two-thirds of the tongue
VI	Abducent [ab DOO sent]	Orbital muscles for eye movement
VII	***Facial**	**Motor: to the muscles of facial expression, taste to anterior two-thirds of tongue**
		Secretory: to submandibular and sublingual glands
VIII	Auditory (acoustic)	Sense of hearing, position, and balance
IX	***Glossopharyngeal [GLOSS o feh rin JI al]**	**Secretory: secretory to parotid gland, pharyngeal movements**
		Sensory: feeling to pharynx and posterior one-third of tongue and taste to posterior one-third of tongue
X	Vagus [VAY gus]	Pharyngeal and laryngeal movements: digestive tract
XI	Spinal accessory	Neck movements: sternocleidomastoid and trapezius muscles
XII	***Hypoglossal**	**Motor: tongue movement (muscles)**

* **The asterisked nerves in bold** are most important when discussing the function of the oral cavity. A detailed discussion of these nerves will include the major branches to structures of the mouth, including teeth, periodontal ligaments and alveolar processes, gingiva (gums), the palate and floor of the mouth, and muscles of mastication, of facial expression, and of the tongue (both for muscular action and our sense of taste). Also, a pneumonic that may help you remember the cranial nerves (where the first letter of each word is the same as the first letter of each cranial nerve) is "On Old Olympus Towering Tops, A Finn and German Viewed Some Hops."

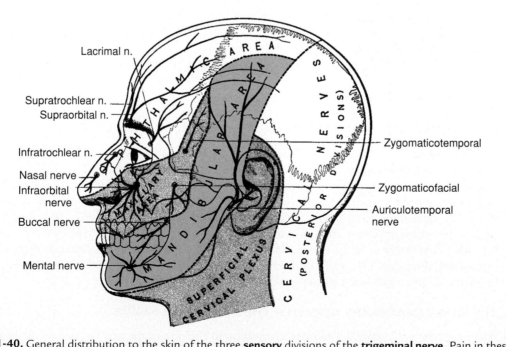

FIGURE 1-40. General distribution to the skin of the three **sensory** divisions of the **trigeminal nerve**. Pain in these areas is felt by impulses sent through the **ophthalmic**, **maxillary**, and **mandibular** branches (divisions) of this nerve. These three branches are distributed to the face as indicated in this drawing. (Reproduced by permission from Clemente CD, ed. Gray's anatomy of the human body. 30th ed. Philadelphia: Lea & Febiger, 1985:1164.)

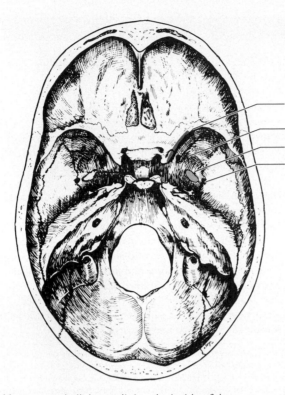

Superior orbital fissure
(beneath lesser wing)

Foramen rotundum (maxillary nerve)

Foramen ovale (mandibular nerve)

Foramen spinosum

FIGURE 1-41. Human skull: bones lining the inside of the neurocranium, superior view. Note the location of the three pairs of openings where the three branches of the **trigeminal nerve** leave the brain: the **superior orbital fissure** for the ophthalmic branch, the **foramen rotundum** for the maxillary branch, and the **foramen ovale** for the mandibular branch. The openings on the right side of the drawing are shaded red.

proprioceptive information, especially from the teeth, determines the subconscious but well-coordinated function of the two complex temporomandibular joints.[24,25] Otherwise, we could experience many unpleasant tooth interferences or frequent joint pain.

Each of the three divisions is divided into many branches. The branches of the maxillary nerve and the mandibular nerve are those that innervate the region of, and around, the oral cavity and will be discussed in the most depth in this section.

1. DIVISION I (OPHTHALMIC NERVE) OF THE TRIGEMINAL NERVE

The **ophthalmic** [of THAL mik] **nerve** is about 25 mm long and exits from the skull by way of the superior orbital fissure on the superior surface of the orbit (*Fig. 1-41*). It has three main branches: the smallest lacrimal nerve, the largest frontal nerve (which further divides into supraorbital and supratrochlear), and the nasociliary nerve (with its infratrochlear and nasal branches). The distribution of these sensory branches that supply the skin of the face is shown in Figure 1-40. The ophthalmic nerve and its branches supply sensory innervation (feeling) to the upper third of the face (i.e., the eyeball, the skin of the forehead, scalp, eyelid and nose, and part of the nasal mucosa and maxillary sinus) *The ophthalmic nerve does not supply the oral cavity.* (Hint: "Ophthalmic" is related to the eye; compare *ophthal*mologist, a physician who specializes in eyes.)

2. DIVISION II (MAXILLARY NERVE) OF THE TRIGEMINAL NERVE

The maxillary nerve provides sensory innervation to the skin of the middle third of the face, including the palate and maxillary teeth (*Fig. 1-40*). It exits the braincase of the skull through the **foramen rotundum** (*Fig. 1-41*). After passing through the foramen rotundum, the maxillary nerve passes into the **pterygopalatine space** and eventually splits into four branches: the pterygopalatine, posterior superior alveolar, infraorbital, and zygomatic nerves. These branches are best viewed in *Figure 1-42*.

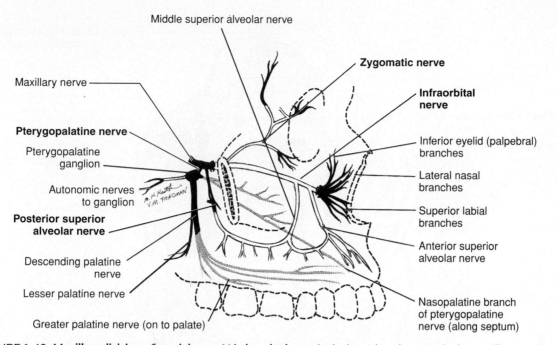

FIGURE 1-42. Maxillary division of cranial nerve V (trigeminal nerve): the branches that supply the maxillary teeth and surrounding structures. Note that the black portions are outside the maxillae, the white parts are within the maxillae and maxillary sinuses, and the red shaded parts pass through the nasal cavity to enter the palate. The major branches are in bold print. (Reproduced by permission from Brand RW, Isselhard DE. Anatomy of oral structures. 2nd ed. St. Louis: C.V. Mosby, 1998:221.)

a. First Branch of the Maxillary Nerve: Pterygopalatine Branch

The first branch of the maxillary nerve, the **pterygopalatine nerve**, splits off closest to the origin of the maxillary nerve, then passes through the pterygopalatine ganglion (*Fig. 1-42*). A branch of this nerve, called the **descending palatine nerve**, passes through the greater palatine foramen to become the **greater palatine nerve** as it enters the back of the palate (shaded red in *Fig. 1-42*). The greater palatine nerve spreads anteriorly to supply the mucosa (soft tissue covering) of the posterior portion of the hard palate and the palatal gingiva (gum tissue) next to the posterior teeth (molars and premolars) (*Fig. 1-43*). Just posterior to the greater palatine foramen, the **middle** and **posterior (lesser) palatine nerves** enter the palate through the lesser palatine foramina to spread posteriorly to supply the tonsils and mucosa of the soft palate.

Another long branch of the pterygopalatine nerve, the **nasopalatine nerve** (shaded red in *Fig. 1-42*) runs along the roof of the nasal cavity and diagonally down along the **nasal septum** to emerge onto the anterior palate through the **incisive foramen**. This branch innervates the soft tissue of the nasal septum and gingiva and palatal soft tissue lingual to the anterior teeth. The right and left nasopalatine nerves communicate with the greater palatine nerves to innervate the entire hard palate. Innervation of the entire palate is shown in Figure 1-43.

b. Second Branch of the Maxillary Nerve: Posterior Superior Alveolar Nerve

Just before the maxillary nerve branch enters the infraorbital fissure and canal on the floor of the orbit, it gives off its second branch, the **posterior superior alveolar (PSA) nerve**. This branch enters the **alveolar canals** on the infratemporal portion of the maxilla (*Fig. 1-44*). Once within the trabecular (spongy) bone of the maxilla and the maxillary sinus, its **dental branches** enter small openings in the tooth roots to supply the *maxillary molars* (except for one root, the mesiobuccal root of the maxillary first molars). It also innervates the supporting alveolar bone, periodontal ligaments, and facial gingiva next to the maxillary molars, the mucosa of part of the maxillary sinus, and cheek mucosa next to maxillary molars.

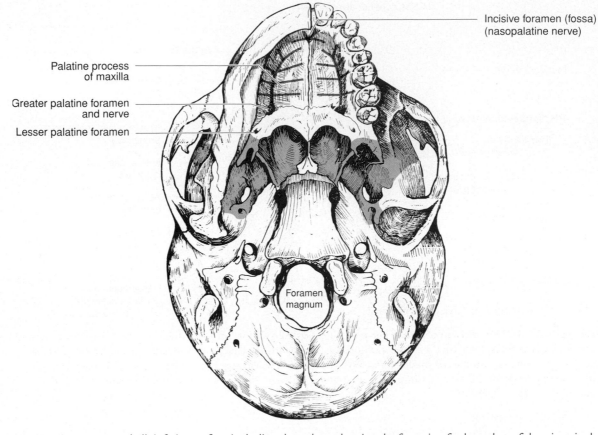

Palatine process
of maxilla

Greater palatine foramen
and nerve

Lesser palatine foramen

Incisive foramen (fossa)
(nasopalatine nerve)

Foramen
magnum

FIGURE 1-43. Human skull: inferior surface including the palate, showing the foramina for branches of the trigeminal nerve that innervates the mucosa of the palate: the **greater palatine foramen** (for the greater palatine nerve) and the **incisive foramen** (for the nasopalatine nerve). The red lines indicate the diagrammatic distribution of the branches of the greater palatine nerves as they spread out along the junction of the alveolar processes with the palatine processes of the maxillae to the tissues (mucosa) of the palate located between the posterior teeth. The **nasopalatine nerve** branches spread out to the mucosa between the anterior teeth.

c.   Third Branch of the Maxillary Nerve: Infraorbital Nerve

In the pterygopalatine space, a third branch splits off and passes through the inferior orbital fissure on the floor of the orbit and enters the infraorbital canal, where it becomes the **infraorbital nerve** (*Figs. 1-42* and *1-44*). While within this canal, the infraorbital nerve gives off two branches, the middle superior alveolar and the anterior superior alveolar nerves (shown in *Fig. 1-44*).

The **middle superior alveolar (MSA)** nerve passes forward along the lining of the maxillary sinus. It gives off small dental branches that enter premolars through their root openings (apical foramina) to supply the *maxillary premolars* (and the mesiobuccal root of the maxillary first molar), supporting alveolar bone, periodontal ligaments, and facial gingiva in the maxillary premolar region and part of the maxillary sinus. It is important to realize that the nerve supplying primary teeth is the same as that to the permanent teeth that replace them. Therefore, the nerve branch to the primary molars is the MSA, the same one that supplies their successors, the permanent premolars.

The second branch given off of the infraorbital nerve while in the infraorbital canal is the **anterior superior alveolar (ASA) nerve**. Its small dental branches supply the pulp, supporting alveolar bone, periodontal ligaments, and facial gingiva of the *maxillary anterior teeth* and part of the maxillary sinus. Comparison of descriptions of the superior alveolar nerves indicates a great lack of uniformity in their distribution. Sometimes, the middle superior alveolar nerve is missing, and the function is taken over by the anterior and posterior alveolar nerves.

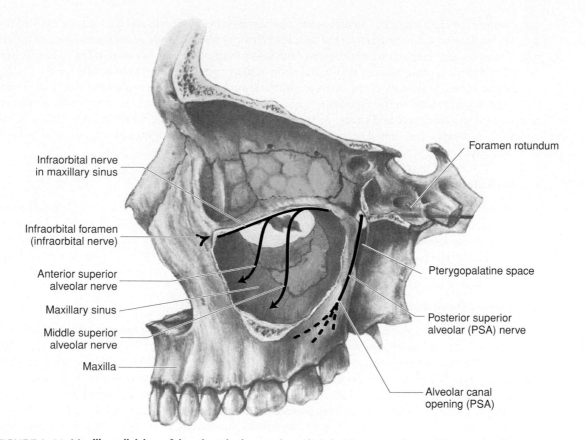

Infraorbital nerve
in maxillary sinus

Infraorbital foramen
(infraorbital nerve)

Anterior superior
alveolar nerve

Maxillary sinus

Middle superior
alveolar nerve

Maxilla

Foramen rotundum

Pterygopalatine space

Posterior superior
alveolar (PSA) nerve

Alveolar canal
opening (PSA)

FIGURE 1-44. Maxillary division of the trigeminal nerve: branches that innervate the maxillary teeth. The lateral wall of the left maxilla has been removed exposing the large maxillary sinus. One nerve branch (the posterior superior alveolar nerve) exits the **pterygopalatine space** and goes down the posterior surface of the maxilla before entering the maxilla through the **alveolar canals** on its way to most maxillary molar roots. Another branch, the infraorbital, passes from the pterygopalatine space to the **floor of the eye orbit** (which also forms the **roof of the maxillary sinus**) where it enters the infraorbital canal (not shown). Within the infraorbital canal, two branches split off to pass downward along the walls of the **maxillary sinus** and into the maxilla. The middle superior alveolar nerve passes through the spongy bone of the maxilla to the maxillary premolars (and one first molar root on each side), and the anterior superior alveolar passes to the roots of the maxillary anterior teeth. The infraorbital branch continues through the infraorbital canal to exit the maxilla through the **infraorbital foramen**, which provides feeling to the skin on the side of the nose, the anterior part of the cheek, and the upper lip on that side.

After exiting from the infraorbital foramen, the **infraorbital nerve** splits into its end (terminal) branches innervating the skin and mucosa of the side of the nose (**nasal nerve**), skin and mucosa of the lower eyelid (**palpebral** [PAL pe bral] **nerve**), skin and mucosa of the upper lip, facial gingiva of maxillary premolars, and facial gingiva of anterior teeth (**labial** [LAY bee al] **nerve**) (*Fig. 1-42*).

d. Fourth Branch of the Maxillary Nerve: Zygomatic Nerve

The **zygomatic nerve** arises in the pterygopalatine fossa, enters the orbit via the inferior orbital fissure, and then divides into the zygomaticotemporal and zygomaticofacial nerves (the upper and lower branches, respectively, of the zygomatic nerve in *Fig. 1-40*). It supplies the skin of the temporal region and part of the orbit.

3. DIVISION III (MANDIBULAR NERVE) OF THE TRIGEMINAL NERVE

The mandibular nerve is a mixed nerve; that is, it contains both afferent (sensory) and efferent (motor) fibers. It is the only efferent portion of the trigeminal nerve. These motor fibers of the mandibular nerve supply the eight muscles of mastication, plus the mylohyoid muscle and the anterior belly of the digastric muscle, which help to retract the mandible. Sensory fibers provide general sensations of touch, pain, pressure, and temperature to the skin of the lower third of the face (as seen in *Fig. 1-40*), as well as the floor of the mouth, anterior two-thirds of the tongue (not taste), and mandibular teeth.

The mandibular nerve exits the neurocranium through the **foramen ovale** (*Fig. 1-41*). It passes into a space just medial to the zygomatic arch and mandibular ramus, and inferior to the temporal bone, called the **infratemporal space**. As it passes inferiorly toward the mandibular foramen in the mandible, it divides into four sensory branches: the auriculotemporal, buccal, lingual, and inferior alveolar nerves.

a. Auriculotemporal Nerve

The first branch of the mandibular division, the **auriculotemporal** [aw RIK u lo TEM po ral] **nerve** (*Fig. 1-40*), comes off the main trunk immediately below the base of the skull, turning backward beneath the lateral pterygoid muscle to supply pain and proprioception fibers to the temporomandibular joint and sensation to the outer ear and the skin of the lateral aspect of the skull and cheek.

b. Buccal (Buccinator) Nerve

Another branch is the **buccal (buccinator** [BUCK sin a tor] **or long buccal) nerve** (*Fig. 1-45*), which comes off just below the foramen ovale and passes through the infratemporal space between the two heads of the lateral pterygoid muscles, then down and forward, emerging between the anterior border of the masseter and posterior border of the buccinator muscle. It innervates the buccal gingiva in the area of the mandibular molars, and sometimes the second premolars. The best place to anesthetize the buccinator nerve is inside the cheek by injecting or depositing the solution into the buccinator muscle near the mandibular molars (*Fig. 1-46*). This nerve also supplies the mucosa and skin of the cheek up to the corner of the mouth.

c. Lingual Nerve

The next branch of the mandibular nerve, given off about 15 mm below the foramen ovale, is the **lingual nerve** branch (*Figs. 1-45* and *1-46*), which goes to the tongue. It passes downward, medial to the ramus but lateral to the medial pterygoid muscle, to the posterior part of the mylohyoid ridge. It is located closely beneath the mucous membrane near the last molar. The lingual nerve provides general sensation (touch, pain, pressure, and temperature, but not taste) to the top (dorsal) and bottom (ventral) surfaces of the anterior two-thirds of the tongue and adjacent tissues. The adjacent tissues include the soft tissue (mucosa) on the floor of the mouth and inner surface of the mandible, and the lingual gum tissue (gingiva) of the entire mandible.

d. Inferior Alveolar Nerve

Finally, the **inferior alveolar nerve** (*Figs. 1-45* and *1-46*) comes off the mandibular nerve on the medial side of the lateral pterygoid muscle. This large nerve roughly parallels the direction of the lingual nerve to descend between the sphenomandibular ligament and ramus to the mandibular foramen, where it gives off the **mylohyoid nerve** just before it enters the mandible through the **mandibular foramen** (represented on the medial surface of the mandible in *Fig. 1-46*). The **mylohyoid nerve** (efferent) pierces the sphenomandibular ligament and travels forward in the mylohyoid groove to supply the mylohyoid muscle and the anterior belly of the digastric muscle.

Once the inferior alveolar nerve passes through the mandibular foramen, it is in the **mandibular canal** within the body of the mandible, where it gives off the dental branches that spread through trabecular (spongy) bone of the mandible, into the mandibular molar and premolar teeth through the openings into their root tips. It also innervates the periodontal ligaments and alveolar processes of these teeth. In the area of the premolars, the inferior alveolar nerve splits into its two terminal branches: the mental and incisive nerves.

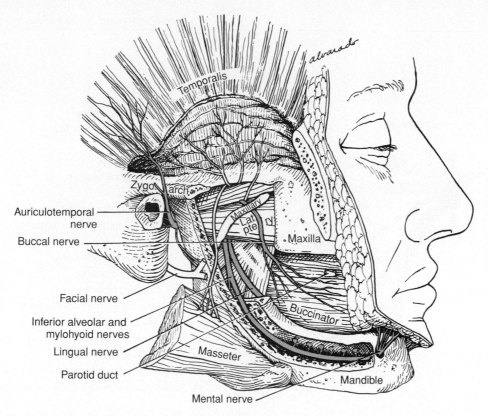

Labels on figure: Temporalis, alvarado, Zygo[matic] arch, Auriculotemporal nerve, Buccal nerve, Maxillary, Lat [pterygoid], Maxilla, Facial nerve, Inferior alveolar and mylohyoid nerves, Lingual nerve, Parotid duct, Buccinator, Masseter, Mandible, Mental nerve

FIGURE 1-45. Mandibular division of the trigeminal nerve branches. The external wall of the right mandible has been removed to expose the **inferior alveolar nerve** within the mandible, where it gives off the many small branches to each mandibular tooth. (From this view, the teeth are not visible.) Within the mandible near the premolar area, the inferior alveolar nerve splits into two end (terminal) branches. One branch, the **mental nerve**, exits through the mental foramen to innervate the skin of the chin and lip on that side, while the other branch is really a continuation of the inferior alveolar nerve anteriorly within the mandible where it is called the **incisive nerve** (not visible here). Also, note the other major branches of the mandibular division: the **lingual nerve**, which is in close proximity to the inferior alveolar nerve posteriorly, but then diverges anteriorly to enter the tongue, and the **buccal nerve**, which innervates the cheek and tissue next to mandibular molars. Other branches (not shaded) are motor branches of the mandibular nerve supplying the muscles of mastication. (One motor branch can be seen entering the masseter muscle.) (Reproduced by permission from Clemente CD, ed. Gray's anatomy of the human body. 30th ed. Philadelphia: Lea & Febiger, 1985:1166.)

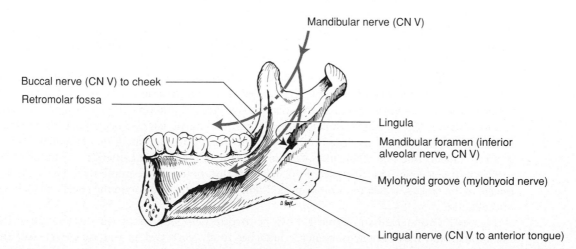

Labels on figure: Mandibular nerve (CN V), Buccal nerve (CN V) to cheek, Retromolar fossa, Lingula, Mandibular foramen (inferior alveolar nerve, CN V), Mylohyoid groove (mylohyoid nerve), Lingual nerve (CN V to anterior tongue)

FIGURE 1-46. Location of the branches of the **mandibular division of the trigeminal nerve** (*in red*) overlying the medial surface of the mandible. As the mandibular nerve passes through the infratemporal space, it gives off the **buccal nerve** to the cheek. Before entering the mandibular foramen, the mandibular nerve gives off a **lingual nerve** branch that passes to the tongue. The **inferior alveolar nerve** enters the **mandibular foramen** (and canal) where it and its terminal incisal branch give off branches through the spongy bone to all mandibular teeth.

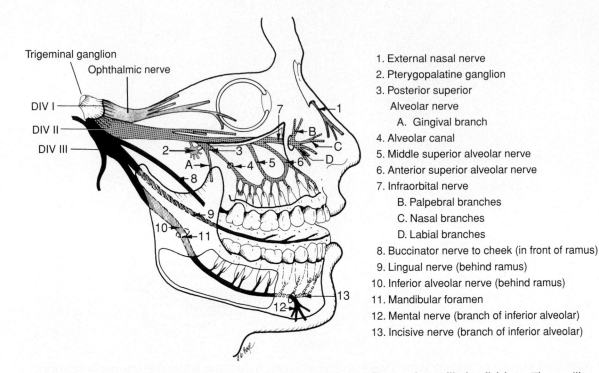

1. External nasal nerve
2. Pterygopalatine ganglion
3. Posterior superior
   Alveolar nerve
   A. Gingival branch
4. Alveolar canal
5. Middle superior alveolar nerve
6. Anterior superior alveolar nerve
7. Infraorbital nerve
   B. Palpebral branches
   C. Nasal branches
   D. Labial branches
8. Buccinator nerve to cheek (in front of ramus)
9. Lingual nerve (behind ramus)
10. Inferior alveolar nerve (behind ramus)
11. Mandibular foramen
12. Mental nerve (branch of inferior alveolar)
13. Incisive nerve (branch of inferior alveolar)

FIGURE 1-47. Trigeminal nerve distribution of the branches of the **maxillary and mandibular divisions**. The maxillary nerve and branches are shaded red; the mandibular nerve and branches are black. Note that the buccinator (long buccal) branch (labeled #8) of the mandibular division passes superficial to the ramus to enter the cheek, whereas the lingual nerve (labeled #9) and inferior alveolar nerve (labeled #10) pass medial to the ramus (denoted by the gray color) as they go to the tongue and mandible, respectively. Also, note that the infraorbital branch of the maxillary division gives off the middle superior alveolar and anterior superior alveolar branches while in the infraorbital canal on the floor of the eye orbit (roof of the maxillary sinus).

After splitting off the mandibular nerve, the **mental nerve** (*Fig. 1-45*) exits from the body of the mandible via the **mental foramen** and supplies the facial gingiva of the mandibular incisors, canines, and premolars and the mucosa and skin of the lower lip and chin on that side up to the midline. The **incisive nerve** (*Fig. 1-47*) branch can really be considered a continuation of the inferior alveolar nerve, continuing forward within the mandibular canal to supply the mandibular incisor and canine teeth, their periodontal ligaments, and surrounding alveolar process.

Note that if an anesthetic solution is deposited next to the opening of the mandibular foramen, it could *block* the passage of afferent nerve signals from *all* mandibular teeth on that side (by blocking the inferior alveolar and its terminal incisive branch) and on that side of the lower chin and lip area (because another terminal branch, the mental nerve, has also been blocked). Further, since the lingual nerve is in close proximity to the mandibular foramen, its fibers may also be blocked, causing that side of the floor of the mouth, lingual gingiva, and anterior two-thirds of the tongue to lose feeling. The only part of the mandible that would *not* be numb would be the tissue buccal to the molars, which requires some additional anesthetic solution in the cheek to block the buccal nerve.

Figures 1-47 and *1-48* and Table 1-4 can be used to help summarize the distribution of the mandibular and maxillary sensory nerve branches to all teeth and surrounding tissues of the mouth.

Other *efferent (motor) branches* of the mandibular nerve supply the muscles of mastication: the **masseteric nerve** to the masseter muscle, as well as to the temporomandibular joint, the **posterior and anterior temporal nerves** to the temporalis muscle, the **medial pterygoid nerve** to the medial pterygoid muscle, and the **lateral pterygoid nerve** to the lateral pterygoid muscle.

NERVES

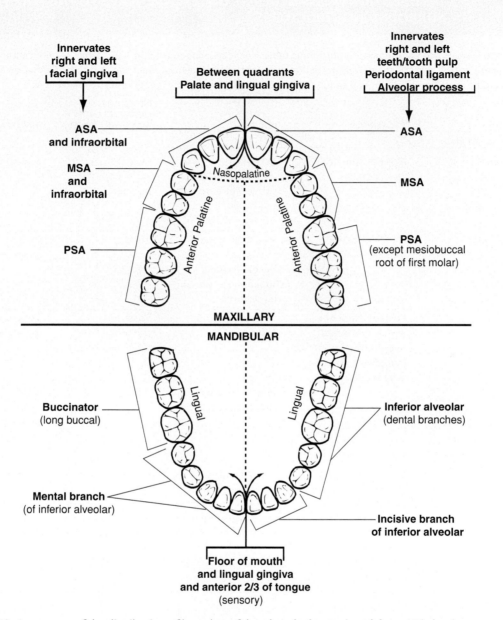

FIGURE 1-48. A summary of the distribution of branches of the **trigeminal nerve (cranial nerve V)** that innervate the tissues of the mouth. Nerves listed on the *left* side of the diagram supply **facial gingiva** on both the right *and* left side of the face; nerves listed on the *right* side of the diagram supply the **teeth, tooth pulps, periodontal ligaments, and alveolar processes** on both sides of the face. Mucosa medial to the teeth is innervated by the nerves listed in those areas.

B. FACIAL NERVE (SEVENTH CRANIAL NERVE)

The **facial nerve** is a mixed nerve (efferent and afferent). From the brain, the facial nerve enters the temporal bone through the **internal acoustic meatus** (*Fig. 1-49*) and exits from the skull between styloid and mastoid processes through the **stylomastoid foramen** (*Fig. 1-50*). It passes through the parotid gland. It then divides into two terminal branches: temporofacial (to the side of forehead) and cervicofacial (to the lower side of the face, orbicularis oris muscle, and chin).

Efferent [EF er ent] **fibers** innervate muscles of facial and visual expression of the face and the scalp. Other muscles supplied by the facial nerve include the posterior belly of the digastric muscle and

Table 1-4	DISTRIBUTION OF BRANCHES OF TRIGEMINAL NERVE TO THE TEETH AND SURROUNDING STRUCTURES

Carefully study this comprehensive but simple table. Then, covering one column at a time, see how many nerves you can recall. These are the nerves any dental student, dental hygiene student, or graduate of either profession should be most familiar with. You should also be able to determine the location of each nerve.

TEETH	TOOTH PULP	GINGIVA	PERIODONTAL LIGAMENT AND ALVEOLAR PROCESS	HARD PALATE
MAXILLARY ARCH				
Anteriors	Anterior superior alveolar n.	Palatal— Nasopalatine n. Labial—infraorbital and anterior superior alveolar n.	Anterior superior alveolar n.*	Nasopalatine n.
Premolars	Middle superior alveolar n.	Palatal—anterior palatine n. Buccal—middle superior alveolar and infraorbital n.	Middle superior alveolar n.*	Anterior palatine n.
Molars	Posterior superior alveolar n. except mesiobuccal root of first (supplied by middle superior alveolar n.)	Palatal—anterior palatine n.	Posterior superior alveolar n.*	Anterior palatine n.
		Buccal—Posterior superior alveolar n.		SOFT PALATE: middle and posterior palatine n.
MANDIBULAR ARCH AND FLOOR OF MOUTH				
Anteriors	Incisive branch of the inferior alveolar n.	Lingual—lingual n. Labial—mental n.	Incisive n.	Lingual n.
Premolars	Dental branch of inferior alveolar n.	Lingual—lingual n. Buccal—mental n.	Dental branch of inferior alveolar n.	Lingual n.
Molars	Dental branch of inferior alveolar n.	Lingual—lingual n.	Dental branch of inferior alveolar n.	Lingual n.
		Buccal—buccinator n. (long buccal n.)		

* Also supply the maxillary sinus.

stylohyoid muscle (*Fig. 1-38*); the platysma muscle (a broad, thin superficial muscle that covers much of the anterior part of the neck, seen in *Fig. 1-39*); and the stapedius muscle (in middle ear cavity). None of these muscles has any influence on moving the mandible. Efferent **secretory fibers** end in the pterygopalatine and submandibular ganglia and bring about secretions from two pairs of salivary glands: the sublingual glands located just under the mucosa in the floor of the mouth superior to the mylohyoid muscle and the submandibular glands located in the submandibular fossae on the medial surface of the mandible inferior to the mylohyoid muscle.

Afferent [AF er ent] **fibers** of the facial nerve come off superior to the stylomastoid foramen and course through the tympanic cavity inside of the petrous portion of the temporal bone, eventually coming out of the skull by way of the **petrotympanic** [PET ro tim PAN ik] **fissure**. These fibers of the facial nerve (**chorda tympani nerve**) join with the lingual nerve (branch of the mandibular division of the trigeminal nerve) and

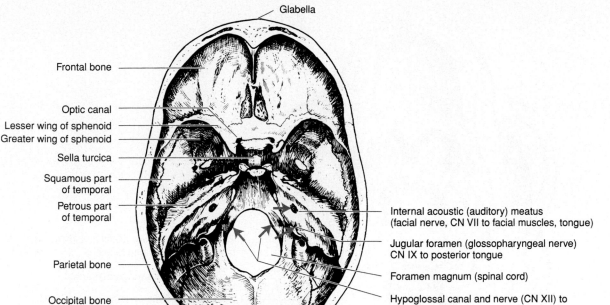

FIGURE 1-49. Foramen for **cranial nerves VII (facial), IX (glossopharyngeal)**, and **XII (hypoglossal)** as they exit the brain case through bones lining the inside of the neurocranium. Arrows indicate the location of the facial nerve as it passes through the **internal acoustic foramen**, the glossopharyngeal nerve as it passes through the **jugular foramen**, and the hypoglossal nerve as it passes through the **hypoglossal canals** (not visible but on the lateral walls of the foramen magnum).

supply the sense of taste to the anterior two-thirds of the tongue (the body and the tip of the tongue). There are approximately 8000–9000 taste buds in the young adult, more in children, and fewer with advancing age. Originally, four primary tastes were identified: sour (acid), sweet, salty, and bitter.[27] Some authors add alkaline and metallic to the taste senses. Others are currently citing a unique taste associated with monosodium glutamate (amino acids) called umami.[43] Early research on taste was interpreted by mapping the tongue for the quality of taste sensed in each area: the tip of the tongue is where one best distinguishes sweet, salty, or alkaline substances, and the sides of the tongue are most sensitive to sour (acidic) substances.[27] However, newer research has shown that cells within each taste bud may respond to multiple tastes, but the sense of taste in each area of the tongue is dependant upon the intensity of each taste. [An excellent discussion of taste is found in the chapter by Travers and Travers in the text edited by Cummings.]

C. GLOSSOPHARYNGEAL NERVE (NINTH CRANIAL NERVE)

The **glossopharyngeal** [GLOSS o feh rin JI al] **nerve** exits from the skull via the **jugular** [JUG yoo lar] **foramen** (*Figs. 1-49* and *1-50*). It then passes down and forward, medial to the styloid process, to enter the tongue. It is a mixed nerve (efferent and afferent) and supplies parts of the tongue and pharynx.

The glossopharyngeal nerves' **efferent** fibers innervate the stylopharyngeus muscle of the pharynx.

Secretory fibers innervate the parotid gland, effecting secretion. This gland is located in front of each ear lobe in the cheek tissues just inferior to the zygomatic arch. The **afferent** fibers of this nerve supply the sense of taste and general sensation to the posterior one-third of the tongue and general sensation to the mucosa of the pharynx and tonsils. (Bitter sensations are prominent on the dorsal [top] surface in the region of the circumvallate papillae on the posterior third of the tongue. Additional taste buds can be found in other structures in the back of the mouth [such as the pillars of the fauces, hard and soft palate, epiglottis, and pharynx].[27,28]) (*Hint:* Glossopharyngeal = glosso [tongue] + pharyngeal [pharynx or throat]).

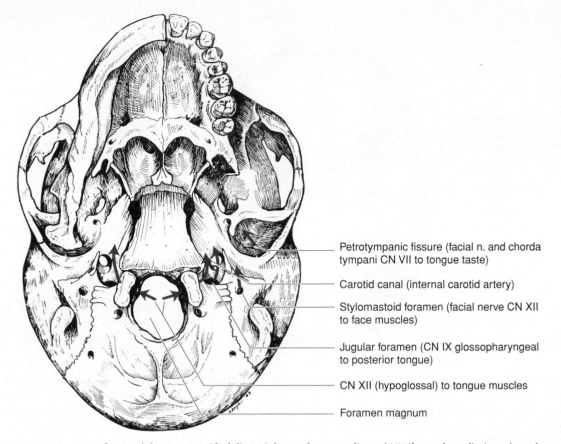

Petrotympanic fissure (facial n. and chorda tympani CN VII to tongue taste)

Carotid canal (internal carotid artery)

Stylomastoid foramen (facial nerve CN XII to face muscles)

Jugular foramen (CN IX glossopharyngeal to posterior tongue)

CN XII (hypoglossal) to tongue muscles

Foramen magnum

FIGURE 1-50. Foramen for **cranial nerves VII (facial), IX (glossopharyngeal)**, and **XII (hypoglossal)** viewed on the inferior surface of the neurocranium. One part of the facial nerve exits through the **stylomastoid foramen** and another small branch exits through the **petrotympanic fissure** where it joins up with the lingual branch of the trigeminal nerve to provide the anterior two-thirds of the tongue with feeling (trigeminal nerve neurons) and taste (facial nerve neurons). The glossopharyngeal nerves exit through the **jugular foramen**. The hypoglossal nerves exit through the **hypoglossal canals**. Also, note the **carotid canal** where the internal carotid *artery* enters the braincase.

D. HYPOGLOSSAL NERVE (TWELFTH CRANIAL NERVE)

The **hypoglossal nerve** exits from the skull through the **hypoglossal canals** just above the **occipital condyles** near the anterior border of the large **foramen magnum** (visible inside the walls of the foramen magnum [*Fig. 1-50*]). It descends steeply, entering the oral cavity at the posterior border of the mylohyoid muscle. This efferent nerve supplies the muscles that move the tongue. These are genioglossus, styloglossus, hyoglossus, longitudinal, vertical, and transverse. If this nerve becomes damaged from injury or tumor, the tongue will deviate noticeably toward the affected side. (*Hint:* Hypoglossal = hypo [beneath; like a *hypo*dermic needle] + glossal [tongue].)

E. SUMMARY OF NERVE SUPPLY TO THE TONGUE, SALIVARY GLANDS, FACIAL SKIN, AND FACIAL MUSCLES

AFFERENT FIBERS TO THE TONGUE

- Cranial nerve V, the lingual nerve (branch of division III or the mandibular branch), provides general sensation to the anterior two-thirds (body) of the tongue.
- Facial nerve (cranial nerve VII) provides taste sensation to anterior two-thirds (body) of tongue.
- Glossopharyngeal nerve (cranial nerve IX) is responsible for taste and general sensation in the posterior one-third (or root) of the tongue.

EFFERENT FIBERS TO THE TONGUE MUSCLES

- Hypoglossal nerve (cranial nerve XII) supplies motor fibers to the muscles of the tongue.

SECRETORY FIBERS TO SALIVARY GLANDS

- Glossopharyngeal nerve (cranial nerve IX) supplies the parotid salivary glands.
- Facial nerve (cranial nerve VII) supplies the submandibular and sublingual salivary glands.

AFFERENT FIBERS TO SKIN OF THE FACE

- Cranial nerve V supplies all sense of feeling to the skin of the face through branches of the ophthalmic division (upper face), maxillary division (middle face). and mandibular division (lower face).

EFFERENT MOTOR NERVES TO THE MAJOR MUSCLES OF MASTICATION

- Cranial nerve V, the motor branches of the mandibular division of cranial nerve V, supply the masseter (masseteric nerve), the temporalis (temporalis nerves), and the medial and lateral pterygoid (pterygoid nerve branches).

EFFERENT MOTOR NERVES TO MOST MUSCLES OF FACIAL EXPRESSION

- Facial nerve (cranial nerve VII) supplies most muscles of facial expression.

LEARNING EXERCISE

- Describe the pathway of the branches of the mandibular division of the fifth cranial nerves as they pass from the brain toward their target organs (especially the teeth and surrounding soft tissue). Name the location where branches split off of the main nerves and name the foramina through which each branch passes. Then, if it is possible on your study skull, take a pipe cleaner and carefully pass it through the foramina to show the passageway of these nerves. Think about where these nerves might be reached by an anesthetic syringe needle and what structures would be anesthetized if anesthetic deposited in that location blocked nerve impulses from all branches of that nerve that are farther away from the brain.

- Repeat the previous exercise for the branches of the maxillary division.

- Sketch the dorsal view of the tongue and label which nerves innervate the anterior two-thirds and posterior one-third for general sensation, taste, and movement (muscles).

- List all 12 cranial nerves in order and their functions.

- Review all words in bold that have phonetic spelling to confirm that your pronunciation is correct.

LEARNING QUESTIONS

Select the one best answer.

1. The branches of which nerve cause the masseter muscle fibers to contract, thus squeezing the teeth together?
    a. cranial nerve V: maxillary division
    b. cranial nerve V: mandibular division
    c. cranial nerve V: ophthalmic division
    d. facial nerve
    e. lingual nerve

2. Which of the following nerve branches does not need to be anesthetized in order to block the sensation of pain to the pulp and all surrounding bone and gingiva of tooth #27 prior to an extraction?
   a. buccal nerve
   b. mental nerve
   c. incisive nerve
   d. inferior alveolar nerve
   e. lingual nerve

3. Which two nerves branch off the infraorbital nerve while it is in the infraorbital canal?
   a. MSA and PSA
   b. ASA and MSA
   c. PSA and ASA
   d. MSA and nasopalatine
   e. nasopalatine and greater palatine

4. Anesthetizing nerve fibers of what nerve results in numbness in half of the anterior two-thirds of the tongue?
   a. hypoglossal nerve
   b. glossopharyngeal nerve
   c. lingual nerve branch of the trigeminal nerve
   d. lingual nerve branch of the facial nerve

5. The nerve branch of the trigeminal that provides pain sensation to the mandibular teeth exits the skull through what foramen?
   a. f. ovale
   b. f. rotundum
   c. mandibular f.
   d. mental f.
   e. infraorbital f.

ANSWERS: 1-b, 2-a, 3-b, 4-c, 5-a

SECTION VI.   VESSELS ASSOCIATED WITH THE ORAL CAVITY

OBJECTIVES

The objectives for this section are to prepare the reader to perform the following:
- Trace blood through the major blood vessels (arteries) from the heart to the teeth and back (through veins) to the heart.
- Describe the pathway (fossa, spaces, etc.) of the key arteries that supply the teeth and, where possible, feel the pulse.
- Trace the route of infection from teeth and associated oral structures through the lymph system.
- Palpate the location of lymph nodes associated with the spread of infection of the oral cavity.

Nerves and arteries tend to parallel one another, often passing through the same foramen and canals within bones after they meet. Arteries pass up toward the mouth from the heart and nerves come down to the mouth from the brain. Generally, arteries of the face and jaw run a more wiggly or corkscrew course than do veins.

A. ARTERIES

Refer to the pathway of blood from the heart to the teeth in *Figure 1-51*. Blood courses from the left ventricle of the heart through the aorta to the common carotid artery, which ascends in the neck and divides into the **external carotid** [kah ROT id] **artery** (*Fig. 1-52*), which gives off the maxillary branches supplying structures in the mouth, and the internal carotid artery (enters the skull through the carotid canal and does not supply the mouth). You can feel the pulse of the external carotid just in front of the sternocleidomastoid muscle as required during cardiopulmonary resuscitation training.

As the external carotid passes superiorly behind the angle of the mandible, it gives off two important branches to the mouth. First, the **lingual artery** (not seen on *Fig. 1-52*) comes off near the hyoid bone, then enters the tongue. As with the lingual nerve, this artery supplies the floor of the mouth, adjacent gingiva, and the sublingual gland.

Second, the **facial artery** (*Fig. 1-52*) comes off just superior or with the lingual artery. It then passes forward obliquely beneath the submandibular gland, then laterally around the lower border of the mandible. The facial artery and nerve pass together through a shallow notch on the inferior border of the mandible just anterior to the insertion of the masseter muscle. This notch is called the **antegonial notch** (*Fig. 1-19*). This is an important landmark to be aware of so that you will be able to stop the flow of blood to the face in an emergency. Try to find the facial artery at the antegonial notch with your finger or thumb. You may feel pulsations of the facial artery if you are in the correct spot. From here, the facial artery goes upward over the outer surface of the mandible to the face.

Now four branches of the facial artery will be described. The **ascending palatine artery** comes off at the highest point of the first bend of the facial artery before it passes onto the face and ascends to supply structures adjacent to the pharynx (the soft palate, the pharyngeal muscles, the mucosa of the pharynx, and the palatine tonsil). The **submental artery**, which converges with the mylohyoid nerve, supplies structures in the floor of the mouth (the mylohyoid muscle, anterior belly of the digastric muscle, and lymph nodes inferior to the mylohyoid muscle). After passing onto the face, the **inferior** and **superior labial arteries** (*Fig. 1-52*) surround and supply the lips and the orbicularis oris muscle. **Lateral nasal** and **angular arteries** are the terminal branches of the facial arteries.

There is considerable merging at the midline of the arteries from both sides of the face, rather than the more conventional system whereby an artery terminates with many small capillaries. This merging of small arteries from opposite sides is called an end-to-end anastomosis. One example is where the right and left superior and inferior labial arteries join at the midline. As one might guess, such an anastomosis can cause problems in arresting hemorrhage on the face.

The **maxillary artery** is probably the most important artery to the dentist and dental hygienist. It arises from the external carotid within the parotid gland (*Fig. 1-52*). The branches of this artery can be considered in *three parts* as shown in *Figure 1-53*. The branches of the mandibular and pterygopalatine (or first and third) parts are directly involved with the blood supply to the mandibular and maxillary teeth, respectively. The branches of the pterygoid (or middle) part provide blood to the four pairs of muscles of mastication (masseter, temporalis, medial, and lateral pterygoids). Study Figure 1-53 as you read about the following branches of each part of the maxillary artery. Also, notice the similarity between the names of the vessels and the names of the nerves that supply the same structures.

> ARTERIES TO MANDIBLE: The branch coming off of the *mandibular* (or first) *part* of the maxillary artery is the **inferior alveolar artery**, which, like the inferior alveolar nerve, enters the mandible through the mandibular foramen, supplying branches to the mandibular molars and premolars. It then divides into two branches: the **mental artery**, which exits from the mental foramen to the lower lip and chin, and the **incisive artery**, which continues forward within the mandible to supply the anterior teeth (similar to the path of nerves of the same name seen in the mandible in *Fig. 1-47*).

> ARTERIES TO MUSCLES: Branches coming off of the *pterygoid* (or second) *part* of the maxillary artery are not involved directly with the teeth but supply blood to the muscles of mastication (posterior and anterior deep temporalis, masseteric, and pterygoid and buccinator branches).

> ARTERIES TO MAXILLAE: Branches that come off of the *pterygopalatine* (or third) *part* of the maxillary artery supply the maxillary teeth and the periodontal ligaments. The

Pathway of Blood From Heart to Tooth and Back to Heart*

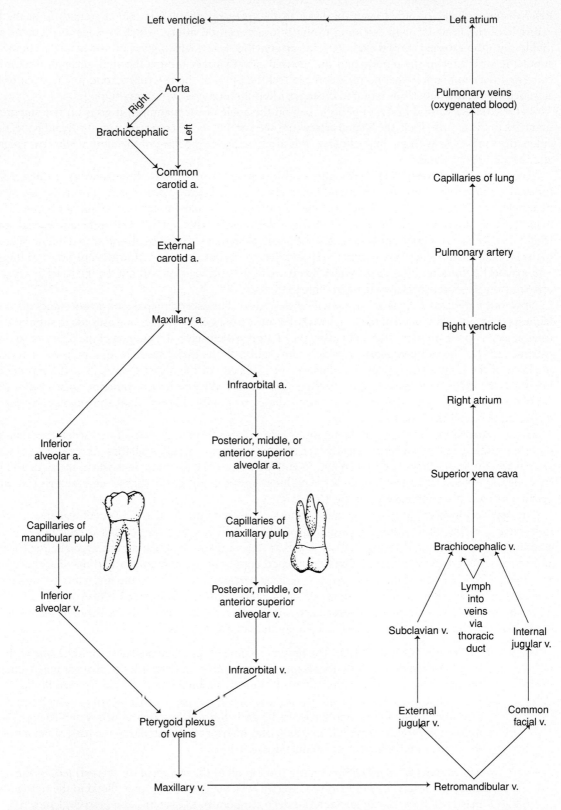

*Think in terms of a drop of blood making this round trip.

FIGURE 1-51. Pathway of blood from the heart to the teeth and back to the heart.

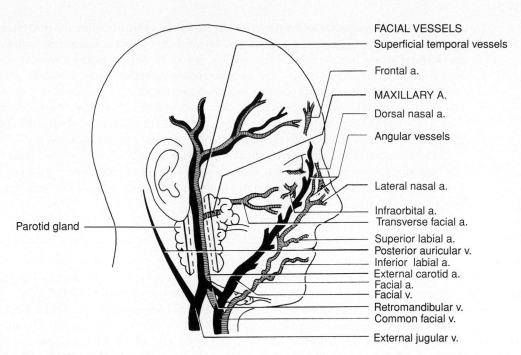

FACIAL VESSELS
Superficial temporal vessels
Frontal a.
MAXILLARY A.
Dorsal nasal a.
Angular vessels
Lateral nasal a.
Infraorbital a.
Transverse facial a.
Superior labial a.
Posterior auricular v.
Inferior labial a.
External carotid a.
Facial a.
Facial v.
Retromandibular v.
Common facial v.
External jugular v.

Parotid gland

FIGURE 1-52. Facial vessels. The parotid gland is split apart to show the **external carotid artery and vein**, with the **maxillary artery** coming off and passing deep to this gland. Arteries are shaded red; veins are black.

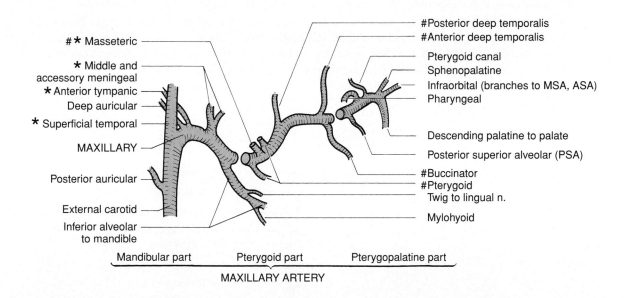

#★ Masseteric
★ Middle and accessory meningeal
★ Anterior tympanic
Deep auricular
★ Superficial temporal
MAXILLARY
Posterior auricular
External carotid
Inferior alveolar to mandible

#Posterior deep temporalis
#Anterior deep temporalis
Pterygoid canal
Sphenopalatine
Infraorbital (branches to MSA, ASA)
Pharyngeal
Descending palatine to palate
Posterior superior alveolar (PSA)
#Buccinator
#Pterygoid
Twig to lingual n.
Mylohyoid

Mandibular part | Pterygoid part | Pterygopalatine part

MAXILLARY ARTERY

FIGURE 1-53. Maxillary artery and the branches of its three major parts. The branches of the *mandibular part* supplies blood to the mandible and teeth, the *pterygoid part* supplies the muscles of mastication, and the *pterygopalatine part* supplies the maxillae and teeth. Vessels labeled with (*) are branches to the temporomandibular joint. Branches labeled with (#) supply blood to muscles of mastication.

posterior superior alveolar artery traverses the maxillary sinus, and, like the posterior superior alveolar nerve, supplies the maxillary molars. While within the infraorbital canal, the **infraorbital artery**, like the infraorbital nerve, gives off the **middle superior alveolar artery**, which supplies the premolars, and the **anterior superior alveolar** artery, which supplies the anterior teeth. The **descending palatine** branch of the maxillary artery supplies part of the nasal cavity before it emerges onto the palate through the greater palatine foramina (*Fig. 1-43*) like the nerves to supply the mucosa of the hard and soft palate and the lingual gingiva. Its terminal part ascends through the incisive canal into the nasal cavity.

The temporomandibular joint is supplied with oxygenated blood from five branches: the ascending pharyngeal (not visible in figure) and superficial temporal branches of the external carotid artery and by the anterior tympanic, masseteric, and middle meningeal branches of the maxillary artery (*Fig. 1-53*).

B. VEINS

Veins tend to be straighter than arteries.[29,30] In many instances, they travel almost the same course as arteries. There are no valves in any of the facial veins. Therefore, an infection in the face can go in either direction through veins. Drainage normally takes place through the veins shown in Figure 1-54.

The **pterygoid** [TER i goid] **plexus of veins** is a network of veins medial to the upper part of the ramus of the mandible between the temporal and lateral pterygoid muscles or between the lateral and medial pterygoids.[30] The pterygoid plexus collects blood from the upper part of the face, the lips and muscles around the mouth, the posterior part of the nasal cavity, the palate, the maxillary alveolar process, and teeth. The pterygoid plexus empties into the **maxillary vein**, which helps drain the plexus. The dense venous plexus surrounds the maxillary *artery* and helps protect it from becoming flattened when the masticatory muscles contract. During muscle contractions, however, blood is driven from the veins.[30]

The **inferior alveolar vein** (not visible in *Fig. 1-54*) drains the mandible and the mandibular teeth and also empties into the pterygoid plexus of veins. The **facial vein** is formed by the angular and lateral nasal veins. It receives blood from the superior and inferior labial veins and from the muscles of mastication. The course of the facial vein closely parallels that of the facial artery, but, of course, the blood flows in opposite directions. The **deep facial vein** connects the pterygoid plexus with the facial vein.

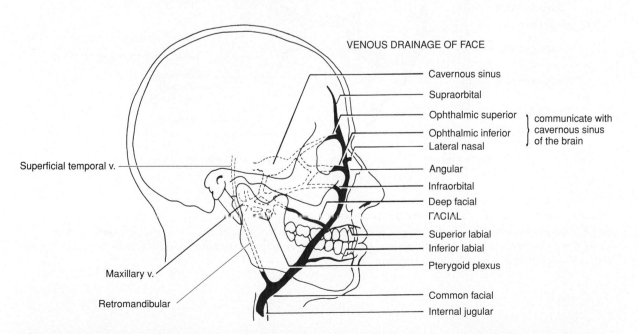

VENOUS DRAINAGE OF FACE

Cavernous sinus
Supraorbital
Ophthalmic superior ⎫
Ophthalmic inferior ⎬ communicate with cavernous sinus of the brain
Lateral nasal ⎭
Angular
Infraorbital
Deep facial
FACIAL
Superior labial
Inferior labial
Pterygoid plexus
Common facial
Internal jugular

Superficial temporal v.
Maxillary v.
Retromandibular

FIGURE 1-54. Venous drainage of the face. The dotted lines represent deeper (less superficial) vessels. Notice how many veins come together in the **pterygoid plexus** of veins, an area prone to bleeding if the anesthetic syringe cuts any vessel wall within this plexus.

The **lingual veins** (not visible on *Fig. 1-54*) drain the tongue and empty into either the common facial or internal jugular vein.

The **retromandibular vein** is formed by the union of the superficial temporal and maxillary veins within the parotid gland. It drains the regions supplied by the maxillary and superficial temporal arteries. It drains into the facial vein. The retromandibular and facial veins empty indirectly into the **internal jugular vein** via the **common facial vein**. Blood then passes into the brachiocephalic vein, to the superior vena cava, then through the heart and lungs to become oxygenated before being pumped back to the mouth (*Fig. 1-51*).

LEARNING EXERCISE

Draw the route of a drop of blood from the heart to both a maxillary and mandibular tooth and then back to the heart as shown in Figure 1-51. Name each vessel along the way. Try to visualize this interesting round trip, which takes place about every 10–15 seconds. Remember, the maxillary artery and its branches are probably the most important to the dentist or dental hygienist.

C. LYMPH

The lymph system is somewhat more complex[31] since it serves to collect tissue fluid that got outside the blood capillary bed and then to return this fluid to the vascular system. In the arterial side of a capillary bed, blood pressure exceeds osmotic pressure, so fluid escapes into the tissue spaces. On the venous side of each capillary bed, the blood pressure is lower, and the osmotic pressure becomes higher, forcing 90% of the tissue fluid back into the venous capillary bed.[32] The major bulk of the remaining 10% of the fluid is the lymph, which passes into the lumen of lymph capillaries, and is then collected in the nodes (shown in *Fig. 1-55*) and returned to the blood vascular system.

During times of infection, trauma, or cancerous growth, abnormal amounts of fluids escape (with specialized cells to fight infection, etc.) and result in swollen lymph glands. Since lymph nodes form chains that are then connected by lymph vessels, infection spreads predictably from the site of infection to a specific lymph node, which then drains to another until the lymph system empties back into the veins. The spread pattern is as follows. Refer to Figure 1-55 while reading.

Infection in the area of the chin and adjacent structures including the tip of the tongue and tissues surrounding the mandibular incisors—anterior floor of the mouth, lower lip, and adjacent gingiva (gum tissue)—all drain into the **submental nodes** just lingual to the mandibular symphysis area. When enlarged, these nodes can be palpated just posterior to the symphysis area of the mandible.

The **submandibular chain of nodes** is located over the surface of the mandibular salivary gland and can be palpated medial but anterior to the angle of the mandible, with the most prominent node in this chain located over the facial artery medial to the antegonial notch. The **submental nodes** drain into the submandibular nodes. Also, the submandibular nodes drain most other intraoral structures, including all maxillary and mandibular teeth, facial and palatal gingiva or gum tissue (except around the mandibular anteriors), posterior floor of the mouth, sides of the tongue anteriorly (but not the tip), cheek and side of the nose, and upper lip and lateral lower lip; the maxillary sinus drains into the **submandibular nodes**.

Parotid [pa ROT id] (or preauricular) **nodes**, located over the parotid gland in front of the ear, receive lymph from the area around the parotid gland, including the adjacent scalp, ear, prominence of the cheek, and eyelids. The parotid and submandibular nodes, as well as excess lymph resulting from a sore throat (inflamed tonsils and pharynx), drain into the **deep and superficial cervical chain of nodes**. These are located along the large sternocleidomastoid neck muscles. To cite an example of the spread of infection, if an infection like a pimple or aphthous ulcer formed on the lower lip, it would drain into the mental nodes, which would in turn drain into the submandibular nodes, which in turn, along with parotid nodes from the side of the face, would drain into the cervical nodes. An enlarged cervical node could be the result of the lower lip infection.

From here, the lymph returns via the venous drainage of the cardiovascular system. On the *left* side, drainage is through the **thoracic** [tho RAS ik] **duct**, which empties into veins at the junction of the **left subclavian** [sub CLAY vi an] and **internal jugular veins**, which ultimately form the **brachiocephalic**

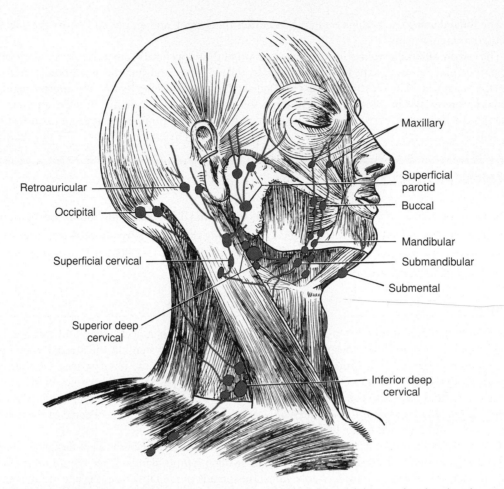

FIGURE 1-55. Lymph nodes of the head and neck. These areas should be palpated during a head and neck examination. (Reproduced by permission from Clemente CD, ed. Gray's anatomy of the human body. 30th ed. Philadelphia: Lea & Febiger, 1985:880.)

[BRAY ki o se FAL ik] **vein**. On the *right* side, lymph empties into the junction of the **right subclavian** and **internal jugular vein**.

LEARNING EXERCISE

• Describe the pathway by which an infection (or cancer cells) might spread from a maxillary tooth to the neck through the lymph system, then through the venous system.

• Describe the pathway by which an infection might spread from a mandibular tooth to the neck through the lymph system, then through the venous system.

LEARNING QUESTIONS

Select the one best answer.

1. Which node would first show enlargement from an infection of a mandibular incisor?
    a. submental
    b. submandibular

    c. parotid

    d. cervical

    e. preauricular

2. At what location would you palpate the cervical lymph node chain?

    a. around the sternocleidomastoid muscle

    b. near the symphysis of the mandible

    c. over the submandibular gland

    d. behind the ear

    e. over the parotid gland

3. Branches of what artery supply blood to the mandibular teeth?

    a. maxillary artery

    b. masseteric artery

    c. pterygoid artery

    d. pterygopalatine artery

    e. superficial temporal artery

4. Branches of what artery supply blood to the maxillary teeth?

    a. maxillary artery

    b. masseteric artery

    c. pterygoid artery

    d. pterygopalatine artery

    e. superficial temporal artery

ANSWERS: 1-a, 2-a, 3-a, 4-a

SECTION VII. STRUCTURES VISIBLE ON A PANORAMIC RADIOGRAPH

OBJECTIVE

The objective for this section is to prepare the reader to perform the following:
* Based on relative location and shape, identify key structures already discussed in this text as they appear on a panoramic radiograph.

Now that you have learned the location and shape of many bony structures within the head, it is possible to look at a radiograph and identify many of these structures based on their shape and location. In order to do this, you need to know that the denser structures in the head (especially the bones and teeth) will appear on the radiograph as the most white (or **radiopaque**). Further, the least dense structures in the head (like foramina passing through bones, sinuses, and nerve canals) will appear on the radiograph as darker structures (called **radiolucent**). Finally, a panoramic radiograph is taken by a device that rotates around the jaws, so that the operator can capture structures viewed from the right, front, and left in one film. It is as though you could take the horseshoe-shaped mandible with its teeth and rami and flatten it out, with its inner surface lying flat on a table and the outer (lateral) surfaces visible as one flat object.

LEARNING EXERCISE

With this simple background, and your knowledge of the shape and location of structures in the skull, study the radiograph in Figure 1-56 and see how many of the following structures you can identify without looking at the answers. MATCH the following lettered items with the corresponding number and arrow on the radiograph. Use the clues only if needed.

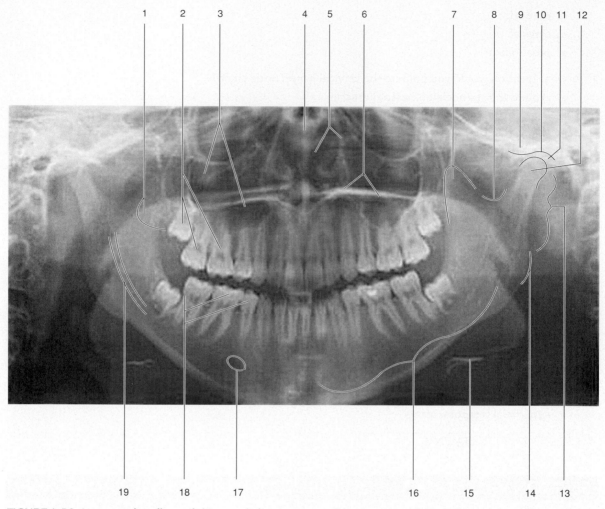

FIGURE 1-56. A panoramic radiograph (Panorex) showing many of the structures of the skull. Test your ability to identify these structure based on their shape and relative location by matching the letter of a description (A–S) with the number of each structure (1–19). (Radiograph courtesy of Dr. R. M. Jaynes, DDS, Assistant Professor at Ohio State University.)

A. **Mandibular teeth.** Note that each tooth has one or more roots embedded into the bony (opaque) alveolar processes. How many are there? Can you see the radiolucent, very thin (almost invisible) periodontal ligaments around each root?

B. **Maxillary teeth.** Note that each tooth has one or more roots embedded into the bony (opaque) alveolar processes. How many are there?

C. **Body of the mandible**

D. **Angle of the mandible**

(Clue: It is the inferior posterior corner of the horizontal body of the mandible where it joins the vertical ramus.)

E. **Ramus**

(Clue: It is the vertical part of the mandible.)

F. **Coronoid process**

(Clue: It is like the point of a king's crown.)

G. **Condylar process**

(Clue: It articulates within the concavity of the temporal bone called the mandibular [articular] fossa).

H. **Sigmoid notch**

(Clue: This notch is between the coronoid and condyloid processes.)

I. **Mandibular canal**

(Clue: It is a radiolucent canal with its mandibular foramen where the inferior alveolar nerve enters the mandible.)

J. **Mental foramen**

(Clue: It is a radiolucent circle near the ends of the premolar roots where the mental nerve branch of the inferior alveolar nerve splits off and exits the mandible to innervate the lower lip and chin on that side.)

K. **Maxillary tuberosity**

(Clue: It is the bump of bone behind the last maxillary molar.)

L. **Maxillary sinus.** Note its proximity to the roots of the maxillary molars and premolars.

M.**Hard palate** composed of the palatal processes of maxillae and PALATINE bones

N. **Mandibular (articular) fossa**

(Clue: It is the depression on the base of the cranium in the temporal bone where the condyle of the mandible fits.)

O. **Articular eminence**

(Clue: It is the opaque bump of temporal bone anterior to the mandibular fossa that deflects the condyles and the mandible downward [opening the mouth] as it moves forward.)

P. **Articular disc space**

(Clue: It is a radiolucency between the condyle and fossa.)

Q. **Nasal passageway** (also called **nasal fossa**)

(Clue: This hollow radiolucent space is located superior to the maxillary anterior teeth.)

R. **Nasal septum**: VOMER and vertical plate of ETHMOID bone

(Clue: The septum separates the right and left halves of the nasal passageways.)

S. **Hyoid bone**

(Clue: This bone appears to float below the mandible since the infra- and suprahyoid muscles attached to it are radiolucent and are not visible.)

ANSWERS: A–18 (there are 14 mandibular teeth; two premolars are missing). B–2 (there are 14 maxillary teeth; two premolars are missing), C–16, D–14, E–13, F–7, G–12, H–8, I–19, J–17, K–1, L–3, M–6, N–10, O–9, P–11, Q–5, R–4, S–15.

REFERENCES

1. Clemente CD, ed. Gray's anatomy of the human body. 30th ed. Philadelphia: Lea & Febiger, 1985.
2. Roman-Ruiz LA. The mental foramen: a study of its positional relationship to the lower incisor and premolar teeth [Master's Thesis]. Columbus, OH: Ohio State University, College of Dentistry, 1970.

3. Sicher H, DuBrul EL. Oral anatomy. 7th ed. St. Louis: C.V. Mosby, 1975:174–209.
4. Edwards LF, Gaughran GRL. Concise anatomy. 3rd ed. New York: McGraw-Hill, 1971.
5. Hickey JC, Allison ML, Woelfel JB, et al. Mandibular movements in three dimensions. J Prosthet Dent 1963;13:72–92.
6. Hickey JC, Woelfel JB, et al. Influence of occlusal schemes on the muscular activity of edentulous patients. J Prosthet Dent 1963;13:444–451.
7. Woelfel JB, Hickey JC, Rinear L. Electromyographic evidence supporting the mandibular hinge axis theory. J Prosthet Dent 1957;7:361–367.
8. Woelfel JB, Hickey JC, Stacy RW. Electromyographic analysis of jaw movements. J Prosthet Dent 1960;10:688–697.
9. Woelfel JB, Hickey JC, Allison ML. Effect of posterior tooth form on jaw and denture movement. J Prosthet Dent 1962;12:922–939.
10. Melfi RC. Permar's oral embryology and microscopic anatomy. 8th ed. Philadelphia: Lea & Febiger, 1988:247–257.
11. Sharry JJ. Complete denture prosthodontics. New York: McGraw-Hill, 1962:45–86.
12. Ricketts RM. Abnormal function of the temporomandibular joint. Am J Orthod 1955;41:425, 435–441.
13. Burch JG. Activity of the accessory ligaments of the temporomandibular joint. J Prosthet Dent 1970;24:621–628.
14. Turell J, Ruiz HG. Normal and abnormal findings in temporomandibular joints in autopsy specimens. J Craniomandib Disord Facial Oral Pain 1987;1:257–275.
15. Osborn JW, ed., with Armstrong WG, Speirs RL. Anatomy, biochemistry and physiology. Oxford: Blackwell Scientific Publications, 1982:324–343.
16. Haines RW. On muscles of full and of short action. J Anat 1934;69:20–24.
17. Gionhaku N, Lowe AA. Relationship between jaw muscle volume and craniofacial form. J Dent Res 1989;68:805–809.
18. Montgomery RL. Head and neck anatomy with clinical correlations. New York: McGraw-Hill, 1981:202–214.
19. Winter CM, Woelfel JB, Igarashi T. Five-year changes in the edentulous mandible as determined on oblique cephalometric radiographs. J Dent Res 1974;53(6):1455–1467.
20. Kraus B, Jordan R, Abrams L. Dental anatomy and occlusion. Baltimore: Williams & Wilkins, 1969:203–222.
21. Basmajian JV. Grant's medical method of anatomy. 9th ed. Baltimore: Williams & Wilkins, 1975.
22. Edwards LF, Gaughran GRL. Concise anatomy. 3rd ed. New York: McGraw-Hill, 1971.
23. Sicher H, DuBrul EL. Oral anatomy. 6th ed. St. Louis: C.V. Mosby, 1975:344–378.
24. Crum RJ, Loiselle RJ. Oral perception and proprioception. A review of the literature and its significance to prosthodontics. J Prosthet Dent 1972;28:215–230.
25. Jerge CR. Organization and function of the trigeminal mesencephalic nucleus. J Neurophysiol 1963;26:379–392.
26. Renner RP. An introduction to dental anatomy and esthetics. Chicago: Quintessence Publishing, 1985:162.
27. Jenkins GN. The physiology of the mouth. 3rd ed. Revised reprint. Oxford: Blackwell Scientific Publications, 1970:310–328.
28. Osborn JW, ed. Anatomy, biochemistry and physiology. Oxford: Blackwell Scientific Publications, 1982:542.
29. Edwards LF, Gaughran GRL. Concise anatomy. 3rd ed. New York: McGraw-Hill, 1971.
30. Sicher H, DuBrul EL. Oral anatomy. 7th ed. St. Louis: C.V. Mosby, 1980:351–376.
31. Montgomery RL. Head anatomy with clinical correlations. New York: McGraw-Hill, 1981:75–82.
32. Paff GH. Anatomy of the head and neck. Philadelphia: W.B. Saunders, 1973.
33. Osborn JR, ed. Dental anatomy and embryology. Oxford: Blackwell Scientific Publications, 1981:133.
34. Palmer RS. Elephants. World Book Encyclopedia 1979;6:178C.
35. Brant D. Beavers. World Book Encyclopedia 1979;2:147.
36. Melfi RC. Permar's oral embryology and microscopic anatomy. 8th ed. Philadelphia: Lea & Febiger, 1988.
37. Osborn JW, ed. Dental anatomy and embryology. Oxford: Blackwell Scientific Publications, 1981.
38. Montgomery RL. Head and neck anatomy with clinical correlations. New York: McGraw-Hill, 1981.
39. Brand W, Isselhard B. Anatomy of orofacial structures. 5th ed. St. Louis: C.V. Mosby, 1994.
40. Francis CC. Introduction to human anatomy. 6th ed. St. Louis: C.V. Mosby, 1973.
41. Osborn JW, ed. Anatomy, biochemistry and physiology. Oxford: Blackwell Scientific Publications, 1982.
42. Zoo Books: Elephants. Wildlife Education Ltd. San Diego: Frye & Smith, 1980:14.
43. Kawamura Y, Kare MR. Umami: a basic taste. New York: Marcel-Dekker, 1987.

GENERAL REFERENCES

Ash MM. Wheeler's dental anatomy, physiology and occlusion. 7th ed. Philadelphia: W.B. Saunders, 1993.
Clemente CD, ed. Gray's anatomy of the human body. 30th ed. Philadelphia: Lea & Febiger, 1994.

Clemente CD. Anatomy: a regional atlas of the human body. 4th ed. Baltimore: Williams & Wilkins, 1997.

Dorland's illustrated medical dictionary. 28th ed. Philadelphia: W.B. Saunders, 1985.

Fehrenbach MJ, Herring SW. Illustrated anatomy of the head and neck. Philadelphia: W.B. Saunders, 1996.

Reed GM, Sheppard VF. Basic structures of the head and neck. Philadelphia: W.B. Saunders, 1976.

Travers JB, Travers SP. Physiology of the oral cavity. In: Cummings CW, ed. Otolaryngology head and neck surgery, vol. 2, 4th ed. Philadelphia: Elsevier Mosby, 2005.

Web site: http://education.yahoo.com/reference/gray/—Bartleby.com edition of Gray's Anatomy of the Human Body side of the drawing in the **pterygoid fossa**.

Oral Examination: Normal Anatomy of the Oral Cavity

Topics covered within the two sections of this chapter include the following:

I. Extraoral examination: normal structures
    A. General appearance
    B. Head
    C. Skin and underlying muscles of mastication
    D. Eyes
    E. Temporomandibular joint
    F. Neck
    G. Lymph nodes
    H. Salivary glands (extraorally)
    I. Lips

II. Intraoral examination: normal structures (and landmarks for placing local anesthetic)
    A. Labial and buccal mucosa: vestibule and cheeks
    B. Palate: roof of the mouth
    C. Oropharynx: fauces, palatine arches, and tonsils
    D. Tongue
    E. Floor of the mouth
    F. Salivary glands (intraorally)
    G. Alveolar process
    H. Gingiva
    I. Teeth (count them)

OBJECTIVES

This chapter is designed to prepare the learner to perform the following:

- While systematically following all of the steps suggested for a thorough head and neck (cancer screening) examination, identify and describe all normal structures found during an extraoral and intraoral examination.
- Describe the location and palpate (examine by touching) the major muscles of mastication.
- Describe the location of the temporomandibular joint, and palpate the joint posteriorly and laterally to the condyles.
- Describe the location of the lymph nodes that drain the face and neck, and palpate these areas.
- Describe the location of the major salivary glands, and palpate these areas.
- Describe the location for injecting anesthetic in order to anesthetize the teeth and surrounding structures.

Anatomic Terms
The following general anatomic terms would be helpful to know before reading this chapter:

circumvallate [sir kum VAL ate]: circum (around), vallate (valley or trench)
filiform: shaped like a thread or filament
fornix: referring to a vault-like space
frenum [FREE num] (also frenulum; pl. frena): small fold of tissue that limits movement
fungiform [FUN ji form]: shaped like a fungi or mushroom
linea alba [LIN e a AL ba]: the white (alba) line (linea)
mastication [MAS ti KA shen]: chewing food
vestibule: entrance to the mouth; like an anteroom, known as a vestibule in an old house

During the periodic head and neck (cancer screening) examination, the dental professional should evaluate all oral and surrounding structures for evidence of pathology. This examination begins with an evaluation of the patient's general health and then includes an assessment of extraoral structures of the head and neck, followed by an intraoral examination that includes an evaluation of all structures from the lips to the throat.

The purpose of a complete and thorough extraoral and intraoral examination is to identify any areas of pathology that might require follow-up or treatment. The primary purpose of this section is to describe *normal* landmarks that can be identified within the mouth, so that deviations from normal can more easily be distinguished. It should also help the reader describe the location of *abnormal* lesions relative to the location of *normal* adjacent structures, which is necessary when following the progression of changes of a lesion, or when referring a patient for a lesion biopsy. A secondary purpose of this chapter is to highlight landmarks that are helpful when injecting local anesthetic for dental treatment.

The authors suggest performing an examination on a partner after studying the description and location of each normal landmark. Also, keep in mind that soft tissue structures cover the bones of the skull and are supplied by the nerves and blood vessels that were discussed in Chapter 1. As you study this material and examine the mouth, recall the underlying bones, nerves, and vessels.

SECTION I   EXTRAORAL EXAMINATION: NORMAL STRUCTURES

A. GENERAL APPEARANCE

The first thing to notice during an initial meeting with a patient is his or her general appearance. You can obtain clues regarding possible health problems that have not yet been diagnosed, and you can begin to predict how well the patient will tolerate dental treatment. Notice the posture, gait, breathing, and general well-being during your greeting.

B. HEAD

A close look at the head may reveal asymmetry of the head, or a discrepancy in the relationship of the upper and lower jaw bones. This could be important when determining how to treat problems with the bite (tooth occlusion) and to identify swelling that could be a sign of pathology or infection.

C. SKIN AND UNDERLYING MUSCLES OF MASTICATION

Observe the skin for any unusual lesions, and describe each lesion by location (relative to adjacent normal landmarks), size, and the person's knowledge of its history. The evaluator's knowledge of pathology will be helpful when distinguishing benign lesions from those requiring follow-up pathology consult and/or biopsy.

Muscles of the head and neck may be palpated to identify pain or tenderness that could be related to problems with the temporomandibular joint or an imbalance in the occlusion of the teeth (made worse when the person habitually clenches or squeezes the teeth together). For this reason, it is important to be able to locate and palpate these muscles where possible. Each muscle pair can be palpated bilaterally with the middle finger of each hand while using the index and fourth finger to palpate surrounding soft tissue. Palpate these muscles on a partner while using *Figure 2-1* as a guide.

- **Masseter:** Feel the body of the masseter by palpating the bulge over the lateral angle of the mandible when your partner clenches the jaws together. Move your finger down toward the angle of the mandible to feel the insertion, and move up toward the zygomatic arch (inferior border of the zygomatic bone and zygomatic process of the temporal bone) to feel the origin.
- **Medial pterygoid:** Feel the bulge when your partner clenches while palpating the medial surface of the angle of the mandible at the insertion. It may help to have your partner lean the head forward to relax the skin of the neck as you gently palpate upward and outward against the medial surface of the mandible near the angle, using the tips of your middle finger and forefinger. This may cause some discomfort.
- **Temporalis, anterior fibers:** Palpate the origin of the anterior (horizontal) fibers on the forehead just above a line between the eyebrow and superior border of the ear. Since these muscle fibers help close the mouth, see if you feel the bulge when your partner clenches the teeth.
- **Temporalis, posterior fibers:** Palpate the origin of the posterior (vertical) fibers of the temporalis just above and posterior to the superior border of the ear. Since these muscle fibers are involved in retruding the mandible, see if you can feel a bulge when your partner retrudes (pulls back) the mandible.

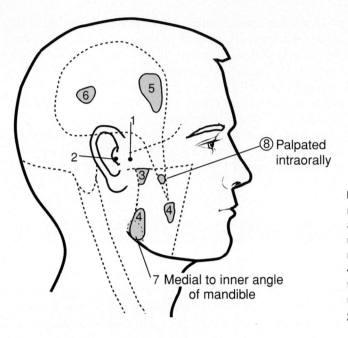

FIGURE 2-1. Sites for palpation of temporomandibular joint and muscles of mastication (origin and insertion locations). **1.** Lateral surface of mandibular condyle. **2.** Posterior surface of mandibular condyle. **3.** Masseter (origin). **4.** Masseter (insertion). **5.** Temporalis (anterior fibers that close mandible). **6.** Temporalis (posterior fibers that retract mandible). **7.** Medial pterygoid. **8.** Lateral pterygoid (palpated intraorally).

- **Lateral pterygoid** (intraoral palpation): The lateral pterygoid can only be palpated intraorally. Feel this muscle by placing your little finger in the vestibule behind the maxillary tuberosity. (Use a skull to see how to reach the lateral plate of the pterygoid process of the sphenoid bone.) With your partner's mouth slightly open and the mandible moved slightly toward the side being palpated, slide your little finger back toward the lateral pterygoid plate for the origin of the lateral pterygoid muscle. This may be uncomfortable to a patient even if the muscle is not sore. The anterior surface of the neck of the condyloid process is the location of part of the insertion of this muscle, but it cannot be palpated.

D. EYES

The normally white part of the eyes (**sclera**) should be white and clear, not bloodshot, and not yellow (a possible indication of jaundice from liver disease). The thin layer of tissue covering the eyeball and reflected onto the inner surfaces of the eyelids (called the **conjunctiva**) should appear healthy and not be severely inflamed (red) or irritated (a possible sign of allergy or disease). The **pupil** (dark center opening surrounded by the colored iris) should not be severely pinpoint or dilated, both of which may be signs of disease or drug use.

E. TEMPOROMANDIBULAR JOINT

Locate and palpate the lateral aspects of both mandibular condyles simultaneously by standing behind your partner and pressing your middle fingers over the skin just anterior to the external opening of the ear and inferior to the zygomatic arch while your partner opens wide and closes (*Fig. 2-2*, labeled #1). Feel the head of the condyle move as your partner opens and closes the mandible and moves the mandible from side to side. Movement of the condyles during minimal opening of the mandible cannot be felt as well as when the mandible is opened wide since the condyles and mandible only rotate around a line connecting the condyles (like a swing) during *minimal* opening, but the condyles and mandible move bodily (translate forward and downward over the articular eminences) when *opening wide*. Also, feel the condyles during lateral movement to see if you discern differences in movement on the right side versus the left side during movement to the right, then movement to the left. Sometimes you may feel a jerky movement accompanied by a clicking, popping, or grating sound. This is likely due to the head of the condyle slipping off, or wrinkling, the articular disc.

Palpate the posterior surface of the mandibular condyle by placing your little fingers into each external auditory meatus (ear canal openings) and press anteriorly forward (*Fig. 2-1*, labeled #2). Feel the posterior surface of the condyles as your partner opens, closes, and moves the mandible laterally from side to side.

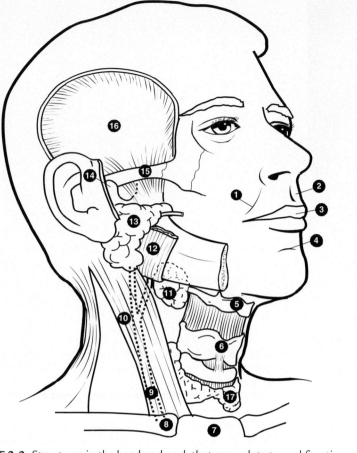

1. Nasolabial groove
2. Philtrum
3. Tubercle (upper lip)
4. Labiomental groove
5. Hyoid bone
6. Laryngeal prominence
   (Adam's apple)
7. Sternum
8. Clavicle
9. Carotid artery (dotted lines)
10. Sternocleidomastoid muscle
11. Submandibular gland
12. Masseter muscle
13. Parotid gland
14. Head of condyle
15. Zygomatic process
16. Temporalis muscle
17. Thyroid gland

FIGURE 2-2. Structures in the head and neck that may relate to oral function.

F. NECK

The neck should be evaluated for symmetry and to confirm that there are no lumps or bumps. The **thyroid gland** (a major gland that secretes the thyroid hormone, which is responsible for controlling much of the metabolism of the body) is located in the neck. It is just inferior to the voice box (**larynx** or **laryngeal prominence**), and is shaped somewhat like a butterfly with wings extending laterally on either side of the larynx (*Fig. 2-2*, labeled #17). This gland should be evaluated visually and palpated (as in *Fig. 2-3*) to ensure that there is no swelling (a possible goiter), which could be a sign of dysfunction of this gland and its output of thyroid hormone. Lymph nodes in the neck that are located around the sternocleidomastoid muscles are described next.

G. LYMPH NODES

The evaluation of lymph nodes during a dental exam is important since enlarged nodes may indicate infection from sites that drain into them, or may be an indicator of the spread of cancer. Healthy nodes are normally not palpable, but infection or malignancies may cause them to become enlarged. A node that becomes palpable due to an infection that drains into the node is more likely to be firm, tender, enlarged, and warm, and adjacent skin may be reddened. In this case, look for the site of infection based on your knowledge of the spread pattern within the nodes discussed in the previous chapter. Even after the infection is resolved, the nodes may remain enlarged but would be nontender and rubbery in consistency. If a node becomes enlarged due to the effect of a malignancy, it is more likely to feel firm and nontender, but it also feels like it is attached to the underlying tissue, so it is relatively immovable, and it will continue to get bigger.

Nodes, when enlarged, can be felt by passing the sensitive fleshy part of the fingertips over the location of each node location. Using Figure 1-55 as your guide, palpate the skin located over the *submental* nodes

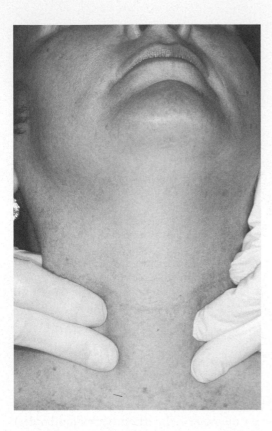

FIGURE 2-3. Palpation of the tissue in the neck surrounding the thyroid gland and laryngeal prominence, feeling for asymmetry or swelling.

(just inferior and posterior to the chin), the *submandibular* nodes (inside the angle of the mandible and over the submandibular glands), the *superficial parotid* and the *retroauricular* nodes (anterior and posterior to the ear, respectively), and the *cervical* nodes (surrounding the large sternocleidomastoid neck muscle, as demonstrated in *Fig. 2-4*).

H. SALIVARY GLANDS (EXTRAORALLY)

Two pairs of major salivary glands can be palpated extraorally: the submandibular glands and the parotid glands. The **submandibular glands** are located just medial to the inferior border of the mandible within the shallow submandibular fossae (Fig. 2-2). These glands produce almost two-thirds of our saliva, mostly the thinner (serous) type but also some thicker (mucous) types.[1] They are positioned just anterior to where

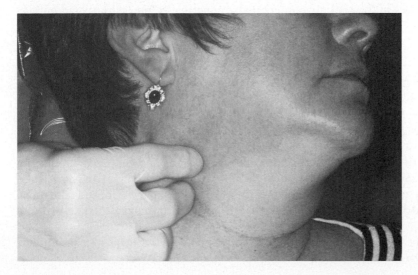

FIGURE 2-4. Palpation of tissue of the neck that surrounds the sternocleido-mastoid muscle in order to detect any enlarged cervical lymph nodes that are located around this muscle.

the facial artery passes over the inferior surface of the mandibular on its way from the neck to the face. Palpate this vessel on the inferior border of the mandible (you may feel its pulse) and move medially in order to locate the submandibular gland.

The large four-sided **parotid glands** are located just anterior and inferior to each ear lobe (lateral to the ramus and extending posteriorly to the sternocleidomastoid muscle, Fig. 2-2). They produce 23–33% or our saliva (the serous or thinner type).[1] These glands may become enlarged during mumps or a duct blockage.

I. LIPS

Use *Figure 2-5* as a guide while studying the lips. The lips are the two fleshy borders of the mouth (an upper and a lower) that join at the labial **commissure.** The upper lip is bounded by the cheeks (laterally) at the **nasolabial groove** and by the nose (superiorly). The nasolabial groove runs diagonally downward and laterally from the side of the nostrils toward an area near the commissure of the mouth. The lower lip is also bounded laterally by the cheeks, and bounded inferiorly by the chin at a horizontal groove called the **labiomental groove.** Recall that the underlying orbicularis oris muscle is the muscle within the lips surrounding the mouth opening that permits us to close our lips around a straw. The upper lip has a small rounded nodule of tissue in the center of the lowest part of the upper lip called the **tubercle,** and the skin superior to the tubercle has a depression running toward the center of the nose called the a **philtrum** [FIL trum].

The **vermilion border** (also margin or zone) is the red border of the lips, representing a transitional zone where the lips merge into the mucous membrane or **mucosa** [mu KO sah] (tissue lining the mouth). It is the area where females often place lipstick. It is bounded externally on the face by the **mucocutaneous** [MYOO ko kyoo TAY ne us] **junction,** the junction between the skin of the face and the vermilion border of the lips. The vermilion border is bounded internally in the mouth by the wet line where labial mucosa begins. A **wet line** (or wet–dry line) is the junction between the outer red portion (vermilion border), which is usually dry, and the inner smooth and moist mucosa. (See Color Plate #1.) The wet line is located about 10 mm back from the skin or mucocutaneous junction. The lips are redder in younger persons than

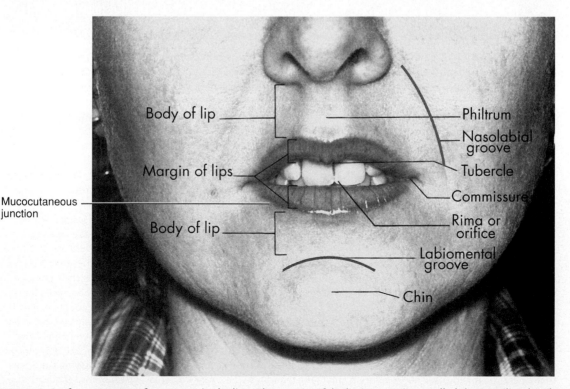

FIGURE 2-5. Surface anatomy of structures in the lips. The margin of the lip is sometimes called the vermilion border. The mucocutaneous junction is the junction of the skin of the face with the vermilion border.

in older persons. In some individuals, the lip color is reddish brown due to the presence of brown melanin pigment. The vermilion border and mucocutaneous junction are important in the head and neck examination because changes here may be caused by exposure to the sun and could lead to skin cancer.

| SECTION II | INTRAORAL EXAMINATION: NORMAL STRUCTURES (AND LANDMARKS FOR PLACING LOCAL ANESTHETIC) |

The **oral cavity** is bounded anteriorly by the lips, laterally by the cheeks, superiorly by the palate, and inferiorly by the floor of the mouth. The oral cavity can be divided into the outer **oral vestibule,** or space between the teeth (and supporting alveolar processes) and lips, and the **oral cavity proper,** the inner space bounded anteriorly and laterally by the teeth and alveolar processes.

Mucous membrane (mucosa) lines any body cavity opening up to where it joins the skin on the outside of the body. **Oral mucous membrane** lines the oral cavity. It is made up of two layers: outer stratified surface epithelium and underlying connective tissue. It resembles the skin on the outside of the body, except that it is moist. Some areas subjected to the most wear, such as the roof the mouth (over the hard palate) and the gingiva, are covered by a toughened outer tissue called a **keratin** [KER ah tin] **layer.** As wear occurs, this portion takes on a grayish appearance and is replaced by underlying cells. Other areas of the oral mucous membrane that are protected are more delicate in structure, such as the cheeks and floor of the mouth, and have no keratin layer. This lining mucosa is so thin that the blood vessels located in the underlying connective tissue may easily be seen, giving it a reddish or bluish color.

Many of the nerves that innervate the teeth and adjacent oral structures can be reached with the anesthetic syringe needle by penetrating the labial and buccal mucosa. The landmarks that are helpful for locating these injection sites will be described throughout this section.

TECHNIQUE FOR INJECTING LOCAL ANESTHETIC TO NUMB ORAL STRUCTURES: BACKGROUND

In order for you to "feel" pain, the tooth or surrounding tissue that is being stimulated must pass the message to the brain by way of the branches of the cranial nerves. When anesthetic is placed near a nerve and can spread (or infiltrate) though soft tissue or spongy bone to enter the nerve cells with sufficient concentration, it can reduce pain messages being sent back to the brain. Anesthetic, to be effective, must be placed at a location along the nerve between the tissues to be numbed and the brain. Therefore, it is important to recall the passageway of the nerves of the mouth to know where to apply the anesthetic in order to block the pain elicited in the tissues being treated (such as tooth pulps and tissues surrounding the teeth) to keep the message from reaching (and being "felt" by) the brain.

Recall that most nerves parallel arteries and veins. In order to avoid injecting local anesthetic into these vessels where it can produce an exaggerated negative effect on the entire body (systemic effect), an **aspirating syringe** is used. This type of syringe permits the operator to pull back on the stopper of the anesthetic cartridge and apply a negative pressure through the solution and needle. Therefore, if the needle tip is in a blood vessel, the negative pressure can aspirate (suck in) blood into the glass anesthetic cartridge where it is visible. When blood is observed, the operator can reposition the needle prior to injecting the anesthetic and aspirate again to ensure that the anesthetic will *not* enter the vessel where it would quickly reach the heart.

In order for the anesthetic to block the signal of *tooth* pain being sent along the nerve branches that pass from each tooth to the brain, a sufficient concentration of anesthetic must enter the nerve cells along their passageway from the tooth to the brain to block the nerve. In order to accomplish this, anesthetic may be applied as close as possible to a nerve before it enters the bone, or, if the bone is porous enough or thin enough, it may be applied outside of the bone where it can pass (infiltrate) through the bone directly to the dental nerve branches in the bone before they enter the tooth root. The maxillae bones are less dense than the mandible, permitting anesthetic to infiltrate more readily from adjacent soft tissue into bone and reach nerve branches that enter the tooth pulps. In the mandible, nerves supplying the pulps can be blocked more effectively by applying the anesthetic near the mandibular nerve before it enters the mandible (the inferior alveolar nerve) or into the mental foramen (which permits the solution to enter the mandible and block only the inferior alveolar nerve branches to the premolars [and possibly the anterior teeth], but not the molars).

A. LABIAL AND BUCCAL MUCOSA: VESTIBULE AND CHEEKS

The arch or vault-shaped space between the cheek or lips externally and the teeth and gingiva (gum tissue) of the maxilla or mandible internally is called a **vestibule** (maxillary or mandibular). The **buccal vestibule** is next to the posterior teeth (premolars and molars), whereas the **labial vestibule** is next to the anterior teeth. It is covered with dark pink-colored alveolar mucosa and is rich in blood vessels and minor salivary glands. The tip of your tongue (and a toothbrush) can easily reach into each vestibule to assist in cleaning the facial surfaces of the teeth, and while chewing, to lift food back between the upper and lower teeth. The **vestibular fornix** (see *Fig. 2-15*) is the lowest part of the vestibule next to the mandible or highest part next to the maxillae. The vestibular fornix next to the cheeks is where food may collect in patients with nerve damage to the cheek (as with unilateral loss of function of the facial nerve from Bell's palsy or from stroke).

INJECTIONS FOR THE POSTERIOR, MIDDLE, AND ANTERIOR SUPERIOR ALVEOLAR NERVES

Consider the nerves that can be blocked in order to anesthetize the teeth and surrounding tissues of the upper jaw. These are all branches of the maxillary division of the fifth cranial (trigeminal) nerve. In order to anesthetize the pulp of one or two teeth, or the soft tissue in a specified area, it is necessary to block the appropriate individual branches of the posterior superior alveolar (PSA), middle superior alveolar (MSA), or anterior superior alveolar (ASA) nerve branches that innervate these tissues.

If you want to anesthetize only the maxillary second or third molar and adjacent tissue, you can reach the **PSA** *(Fig. 2-6)* before it enters the **alveolar canals** *(Fig. 2-7)* by directing the anesthetic toward the posterior surface of the maxilla, just superior, distal, and slightly medial to the apex of the third molar. Entry to this site is through the mucosa at the height of the buccal vestibule (vestibular fornix) superior to the **maxillary tuberosity** *(Fig. 2-8)*. The cheek can be stretched slightly outward to permit an angle that is directed superiorly and medially. Specific dental branches of the PSA can also be blocked by depositing the anesthetic next to the maxilla as close to the apex of the tooth being anesthetized as possible, and the solution will infiltrate through the maxillary bone to block the dental branches to these molars. When using this technique to anesthetize a maxillary first molar, the anesthetic will not only reach the dental branches of the PSA that enter two of its roots, but also the MSA branches that enter the third root.

For all other maxillary teeth and adjacent facial gingiva, you need to block branches of the **MSA** or **ASA**. Since you cannot easily reach the MSA and ASA nerves as they pass from the brain though the base of the orbit and maxillary sinus, you deposit the solution in the soft tissue of the **vestibular fornix** adjacent to the maxillae, at a **level of the tooth root tips** of the teeth you want to get numb *(Figs. 2-9 and 2-10)*. The anesthetic can infiltrate through the soft tissue and bone to reach dental nerve branches of the ASA (supplying the pulps of anterior teeth, *Fig. 2-11*) or MSA (supplying the pulps of premolars and one root [mesiobuccal] of the maxillary first molar, *Fig. 2-12*) in order to block pain. The anesthetic placed to block the MSA nerve branches may also infiltrate through the bone to block some of the PSA nerve branches, thereby numbing the entire first molar.

End branches of the **infraorbital nerve** branches that supply the soft tissue facial to premolars and anterior teeth can be anesthetized using the infiltration technique described above. However, blocking all of the terminal branches of the infraorbital nerve may also be helpful. This nerve can be reached by applying the anesthetic near the opening of the **infraorbital foramen** *(Fig. 2-13)*. This foramen can be palpated with the forefinger just below the inferior border of the eye socket while the thumb is placed in the facial vestibule to raise the upper lip. The needle passes into tissue at the height (**fornix**) of the vestibule near the premolars (similar to the MSA injection), but the tip is moved parallel to the facial surface of the maxilla until reaching the level of the infraorbital foramen *(Fig. 2-14)*.

Refer to Figure 2-15 as a guide while studying the following structures. The labial frenum [FREE num] (plural: frena [FREE nah]) is the thin sheet of tissue that attaches the internal center of the lip (upper and lower) to the mucosa covering the maxillae or mandible near the central incisors. The buccal frenum loosely attaches the cheek to the mucosa of the jaw in the area of the premolars (maxillary and mandibular). These buccal frena may be seen by pulling the lower lip and cheek out and upward and the upper lip and cheek out and downward. Facial muscles move the buccal frena forward and backward and upward and downward during eating to help, along with the tongue, to place our food back over the chewing surfaces of our teeth while eating. Movement of these frena can dislodge complete dentures if the denture border is designed improperly.

The **buccal mucosa** lining of the inside of the cheeks is shiny, but in spots may be rough. Often there is a horizontal white line extending anteroposteriorly on each side at the level where the upper and lower teeth come together, called the **linea alba** [LIN e ah AL ba] buccalis. (*Hint:* "Linea" means line; "alba" means white.) It may extend from the commissural area to the third molar region at a level of the occlusal surfaces of the posterior teeth. (See Color Plate #2.) This area is often irritated by trauma from biting the cheek. Usually 4–6 mm posterior to the commissure, an elevation of mucous membrane called the **commissural papule** is commonly seen and may be palpated (*Fig. 2-15*).

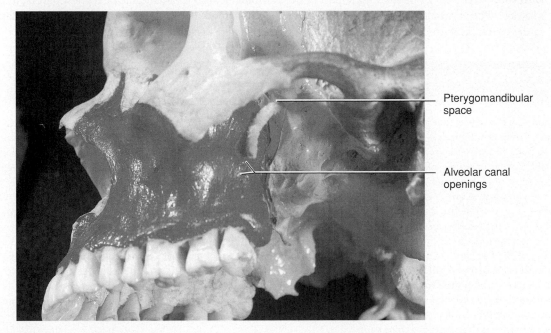

Pterygomandibular space

Alveolar canal openings

FIGURE 2-6. Human skull with shaded maxilla. A pipe cleaner, representing the **posterior superior alveolar nerve,** passes out of the pterygomandibular space superiorly, toward the alveolar canals on the posterior surface of the maxilla.

Alveolar canal openings

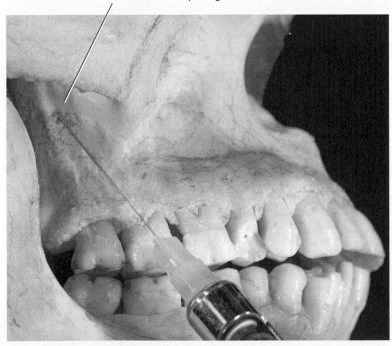

FIGURE 2-7. Anesthetic syringe needle aimed toward the alveolar canals where the **posterior superior alveolar nerve** would enter the maxilla on its way to the maxillary molar roots.

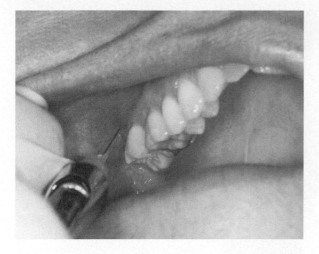

FIGURE 2-8. Penetration of the needle through the oral mucosa at the height of the maxillary vestibular fornix just posterior to the maxillary tuberosity is directed medially and superiorly toward the alveolar canals where the **posterior superior alveolar nerve** enters the maxilla. This injection location should reduce pain sensation to the maxillary molars (except the mesiobuccal root of the maxillary first molar) and adjacent facial soft tissue and gingiva.

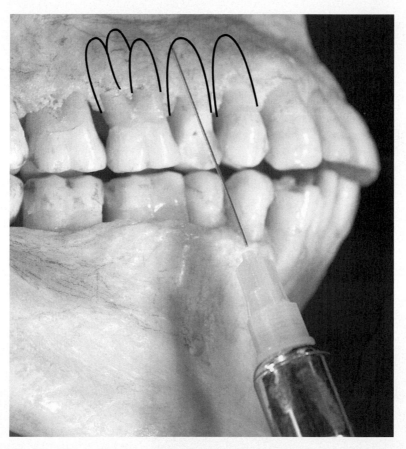

FIGURE 2-9. Human maxilla with maxillary first molar and premolar roots sketched on the maxilla. The anesthetic syringe needle is aimed parallel to the contour of the maxilla to reach the level of the root ends of the maxillary premolar or molar teeth to be anesthetized. The anesthetic can infiltrate through the maxilla to reduce pain sensation to these teeth (and adjacent facial soft tissue and gingiva) by simultaneously blocking the **middle superior alveolar nerve** and branches of the adjacent **posterior superior alveolar nerve.**

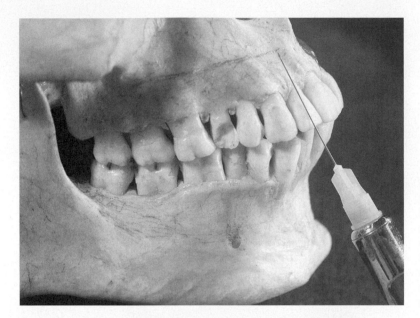

FIGURE 2-10. Human maxilla with a pencil line indicating the approximate level of the end of the maxillary tooth roots. The anesthetic syringe needle is aimed parallel to the contour of the maxilla to reach the level of the root ends of the maxillary anterior teeth in order to block the **anterior superior alveolar nerve.**

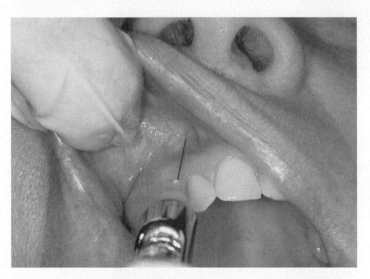

FIGURE 2-11. The anesthetic syringe needle penetrates through the oral mucosa at the height of the maxillary vestibular fornix adjacent to the maxillary lateral incisor until the needle tip reaches the estimated level of the root tip. This injection location should reduce sensation to the maxillary incisors by infiltrating through the maxilla to block the **anterior superior alveolar nerve.**

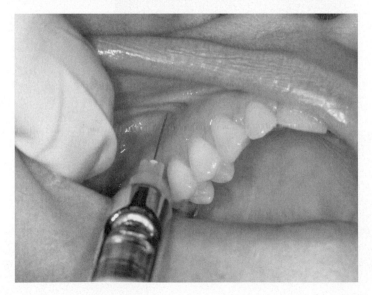

FIGURE 2-12. The anesthetic syringe needle penetrates through the oral mucosa at the height of the maxillary vestibular fornix (near the buccal frenum) adjacent to the maxillary premolars until the needle tip reaches the estimated level of the root tips. This injection location should reduce sensation to the maxillary premolars and adjacent first molar by infiltrating through the maxilla to block the **middle superior alveolar nerve** and the adjacent branches of the **posterior superior alveolar nerve.**

Infraorbital foramen

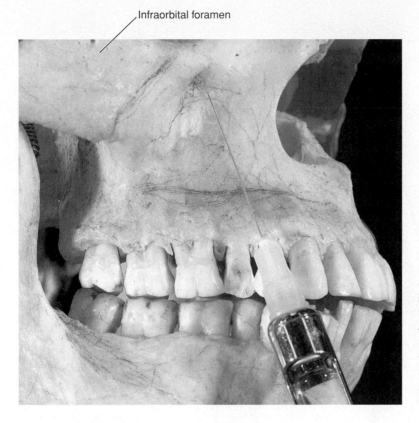

FIGURE 2-13. The anesthetic syringe needle is aimed parallel to the contour of the maxilla to reach the level of the **infraorbital nerve.** Anesthetic can block the infraorbital nerve where it exits the infraorbital foramen to reduce pain sensation in the tissues of the upper lip and facial gingiva (and part of the nose and lower eyelid) that are supplied by the infraorbital nerve branches.

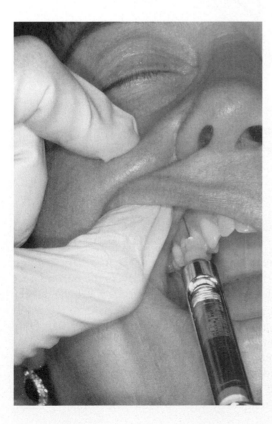

FIGURE 2-14. The anesthetic syringe needle penetrates through the oral mucosa at the height of the maxillary vestibular fornix adjacent to the maxillary canine or first premolar (similar in location and angulation to a middle superior alveolar or an anterior superior alveolar block), but the needle penetrates farther, beyond the level of the root tips, to the level of the **infraorbital nerve** (felt by palpating to find the depression of the infraorbital foramen and marking the level with the finger as in the photograph).

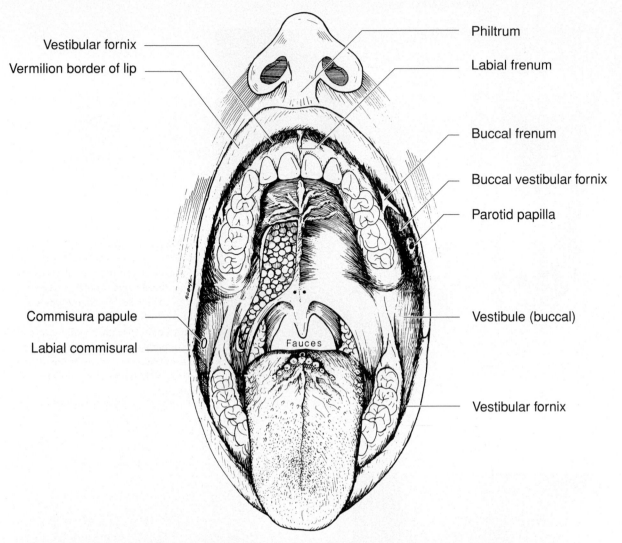

Vestibular fornix

Vermilion border of lip

Philtrum

Labial frenum

Buccal frenum

Buccal vestibular fornix

Parotid papilla

Commisura papule

Labial commisural

Fauces

Vestibule (buccal)

Vestibular fornix

FIGURE 2-15. Structures of the vestibule and adjacent cheek mucosa.

LONG BUCCAL INJECTION:

The **buccinator (long buccal)** nerve is a branch of the mandibular nerve that does not pass through the mandibular foramen, but is located in the soft tissue of the cheek. The anesthetic can be applied just beneath the buccal mucosa and just superior to the buccal shelf next to the mandibular molar requiring facial tissue numbness (*Figs. 2-16 and 2-17*).

The **parotid papilla** [pa ROT id pah PILL e] is a rounded flap of tissue next to the maxillary first and second molars at or just superior to the occlusal plane (Fig. 2-15). This papilla covers the **parotid duct (Stensen's duct)** opening. [In 1971 and 1972, Dr. Woelfel and Dr. Igarashi supervised 331 dental students as they recorded the position of the right and left parotid papilla on each other. Of 662 parotid papillae, 78% were located between the maxillary first and second molar or by the second molar. Only 22% were by the first molar. In height, 87% of these same papillae were located level with (34%) or above the level (53%) of the occlusal plane. Only 13% were found below the level of the occlusal plane. The widest variation in location among these dental students was in two men, one having his parotid papilla on each side 11 mm above the occlusal plane and the other man with his 8 mm below the level of the occlusal plane. In a similar study of 293 adult men and 114 adult women (258 white, 11 black,

9 Hispanic), the parotid papilla averaged 3.3 mm above the occlusal plane (right 3.0, left 3.5 mm)[2.]
Palpation of the cheeks (or lips) for lumps or bumps can be accomplished by pressing with the thumb
on one side against the forefinger on the other side (called bidigital palpation) as seen in *Figure 2-18*.

Fordyce's granules or spots are small, yellowish irregular areas and may be conspicuous in some persons. They are most commonly located on the buccal mucosa inside the cheeks posterior to the corner of
the mouth. (See Color Plate #2.) They are really the manifestation of intraoral sebaceous glands—glands
normally associated with hair follicles on the skin outside of the mouth. Their presence here may be the
result of fusion of the upper and lower parts of the cheek during embryonic development. Such glands have
also been found, however, on other parts of the oral mucosa.

B. THE PALATE: ROOF OF THE MOUTH

The **hard palate** is the firm anterior part of the roof of the mouth with mucosa over the underlying bone
(namely, the horizontal plates of the palatine bones and palatine processes of the maxillae). The **soft palate**
is the posterior movable part of the roof of the mouth without underlying bony support. The **vibrating line**
is the junction between the hard and soft palate (*Fig. 2-19*).

1.   HARD PALATE STRUCTURES

Refer to Figures 2-19 and 2-20 while studying the structures of the hard palate. The hard palate
is covered by keratinized, grayish red to coral pink tissue. The **incisive papilla** is the small
rounded elevation of tissue on the midline of the palate just behind (or lingual to) the central

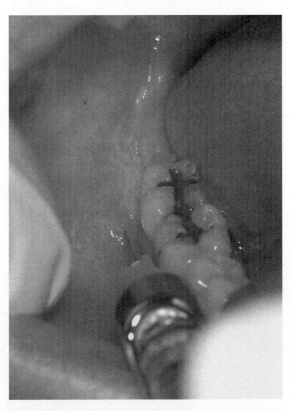

FIGURE 2-17. Anesthetic syringe used to block the
(long) **buccal nerve** by penetrating the mucosa into the
cheek just buccal to the maxillary molars. This anesthetic
should reduce pain sensation to the facial soft tissue and
gingiva of the mandibular molars.

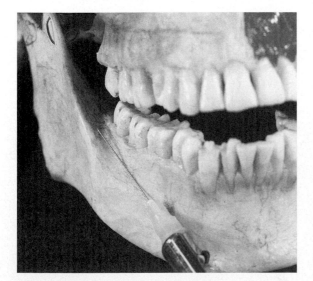

FIGURE 2-16. Location on the skull for blocking the end
branches of the (long) **buccal nerve** facial to the
mandibular molars and superior to the buccal shelf.

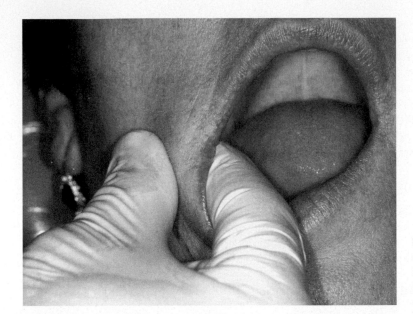

FIGURE 2-18. Bidigital palpation of the soft tissue of the cheeks, feeling for lumps or bumps by opposing the thumb on one side of the cheek and forefinger on the other.

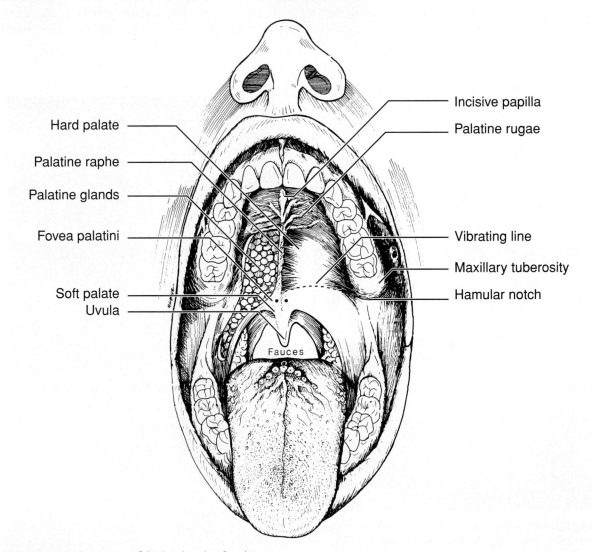

FIGURE 2-19. Structures of the hard and soft palate.

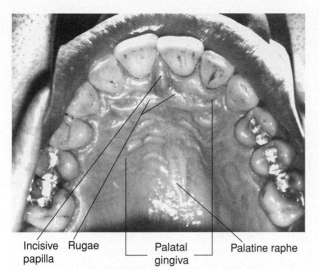

Incisive papilla · Rugae · Palatal gingiva · Palatine raphe

FIGURE 2-20. Structures of the hard palate. Note the prominent palatine rugae (ridges) and incisive papilla (anterior midline). The palatine raphe is not conspicuous in this subject. In some mouths, this raphe is more distinguishable as a ridge extending anteroposteriorly in the center of the hard palate. It is located over the intermaxillary suture line between the right and left maxillary palatine processes.

incisors. This papilla is located over the incisive foramen, where the nasopalatine nerve passes from the nasal cavity to innervate the anterior portion of the hard palate. It is the location for injecting anesthetic to numb palatal tissue in this area. [There is a relatively constant 8.5-mm distance from the facial surface of the maxillary central incisors and the center of the incisive papilla. On 326 casts measured by Dr. Woelfel, the average distance was 8.4 mm, with a range of 5.5 to 12 mm.]

NASOPALATINE NERVE INJECTION

In order to anesthetize the tissues of the palate, we need to block one or two nerves. The greater (anterior) palatine nerve innervates most of the palate (all tissue covering the hard palate, lingual to molars and premolars) and the nasopalatine nerve for tissue lingual to the anterior teeth. Recall that both of these nerve branches split off of the maxillary nerve while in the pterygopalatine space, then pass through the nasal passageways before entering the palatal tissue. The nasopalatine nerve passes from the pterygopalatine space along the nasal septum in the nasal cavity and into palatal mucosa through the incisive foramen (*Fig. 2-21*), which is located immediately under the bump of very firm tissue called the incisive papilla (*Fig. 2-22*). This papilla is located on the palate just lingual to the midline between the maxillary central incisors. Since this tissue is very firm, only a small amount of anesthetic can be applied into this tissue, and this injection can be most painful. Applying pressure over the injection site with the handle of a mirror or with the end of a cotton-tipped applicator for 15–20 seconds prior to injecting can minimize this discomfort.

The **palatine raphe** [RAY fee] is the slightly elevated centerline of firm tissue running from front to back (anteroposteriorly) in the hard palate (*Fig. 2-19*). The intermaxillary suture attachment between right and left maxillae is immediately beneath the surface along this line. The mucosa is firm over the raphe because it is firmly attached to the underlying bone without intervening fat or gland cells. The rest of the tissue on both sides of the raphe has fat or salivary gland tissue beneath the surface, so it is softer than over the palatine raphe. This spongy tissue at the junction of the hard palate and alveolar process next to premolars and molars is the location of the **greater palatine nerve.** There are more than 350 very small palatine glands in the posterior third of the hard palate.[3] They secrete thick but slippery saliva.

GREATER PALATINE NERVE INJECTION

The greater palatine nerve passes from the nasal cavity to palatal tissue through the greater palatine foramen located just lingual to the third molars at the junction of the most posterior part of the horizontal bone of the hard palate and the more vertical alveolar process surrounding the maxillary posterior teeth (*Fig. 2-23*). The anterior palatine nerve extends anteriorly toward the first premolar along the junction of the alveolar process and palate covered by tissue that is softer and more spongy than the tissue covering the midline of the hard palate.

When locating or palpating this location, care must be taken to avoid touching the soft plate (posterior to the underlying bones of the palate) since this may elicit a gag reflex causing the patient to vomit. A small amount of anesthetic may be placed into this spongy tissue resulting in numbness of tissues adjacent to and anterior to the injection site *(Fig. 2-24)*.

Note: It is also possible to reach the entire maxillary branch of the trigeminal nerve just after it exits the cranium through the foramen rotundum while it is still within the pterygopalatine space and anesthetize all of the maxillary branches (called a second division block). This location is more superior than the location of the PSA block already discussed. Anesthetic deposited in this location reduces pain to the structures supplied by the PSA, MSA, ASA, greater palatine, and nasopalatine nerves. Caution must be taken in this area because the pterygoid plexus of vessels is located here, and cutting a vessel wall could result in bleeding under the skin called a hematoma.

Palatine rugae [ROO ge] or [ROO je] are a series of palatal tissue elevations, or wrinkles, located just behind the maxillary anterior teeth. They form a pattern like branches on a tree, coming off of the common midline "trunk," the palatine raphe. [Among casts from 939 hygiene students, rugae trees had three, four, or five branches on each side in 87% of the students. The first main branch was aligned lingual to the canine in 72%. The rugae were well elevated in 85% of the students and flattened in only 14%. Rugae are more distinct in young persons than in other persons. However, a longitudinal study of 20 females and 21 males, from age 4 to 22 years, indicated a slight but steady growth in the length of rugae during this period (average: 1.4–2.3 mm). Rugae growth occurred earlier in females, but the males had more branches.[4]] Rugae function in two important ways: in tactilely sensing objects or food position and in aiding the tongue's proper placement for the production of certain speech sounds.[5] This part of the palate is often burned by eating pizza when it is too hot or becomes abraded from chewing too much popcorn.

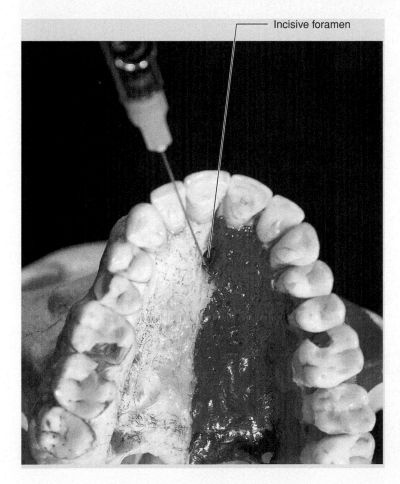

Incisive foramen

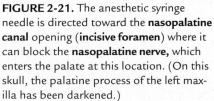

FIGURE 2-21. The anesthetic syringe needle is directed toward the **nasopalatine canal** opening (**incisive foramen**) where it can block the **nasopalatine nerve,** which enters the palate at this location. (On this skull, the palatine process of the left maxilla has been darkened.)

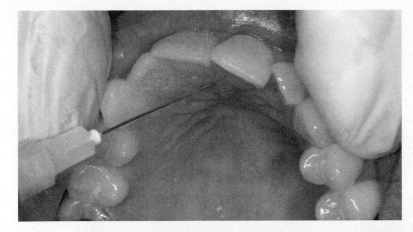

FIGURE 2-22. The anesthetic syringe needle is penetrating the very firm **incisive papilla** overlying the opening to the incisive foramen in order to block the **nasopalatine nerve.** This should reduce pain sensation to the palatal soft tissues lingual to the anterior teeth. Since this injection site is so sensitive (it has been known to bring tears to the eyes), it is recommended to place pressure over the incisive papilla with a mirror handle or cotton-tip applicator for a brief time prior to injecting with the needle.

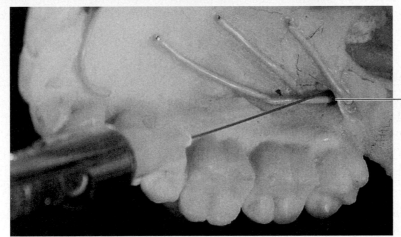

Greater palatine foramen

FIGURE 2-23. The anesthetic syringe needle is directed toward the **greater palatine foramen** opening where can block the **greater palatine nerve,** which enters the palate at this location. The wires represent the spread of branches of this nerve to half of the hard palate tissue located between the posterior teeth.

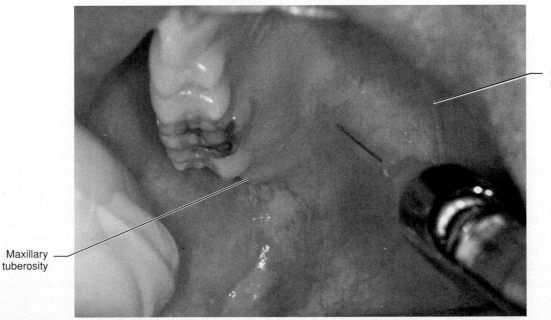

Palatine raphe

Maxillary tuberosity

FIGURE 2-24. The anesthetic syringe needle is penetrating the relatively spongy palatal mucosa near the junction of the vertical alveolar process and horizontal palatine processes near the third molars to reach the **greater palatine nerve.** This injection should reduce pain sensation on that side to the palatal soft tissues between the posterior teeth.

2. THE SOFT PALATE

The soft palate (*Fig. 2-19*) is located posterior to the hard palate beginning at the vibrating line. Along with the hard palate, it separates the mouth from the nasal passage. It is sometimes redder than the hard palate because of its slightly increased vascularity. Its anterior border extends between the right and left third molars. Unlike the hard palate, there is no bone beneath the surface of the soft palate. Say "ah, ah, ah" forcefully and see the soft palate move up and down or vibrate. The hinged place where you observe the beginning movement of the soft palate is the **vibrating line. Fovea palatini** [FO ve ah pal a TEEN ee] are a pair of pits in the soft palate located on either side of the midline, near but posterior to the vibrating line. They are openings of ducts of minor palatine mucous glands.[5] The **uvula** [YOU view la] is a small fleshy structure hanging from the center of the posterior border of the soft palate.

The soft palate functions during swallowing and speech. The **pharynx** [FAR inks] is the superior part of the digestive tube between the nose, mouth, and esophagus. During swallowing, the soft palate moves to close off the nasal pharynx from the oral pharynx to prevent regurgitation of food into the nasal cavity. The soft palate is raised to seal the oral cavity from the nasal cavity during blowing or when producing explosive consonants (like "b" and "p").

C. OROPHARYNX: FAUCES, PALATINE ARCHES, AND TONSILS

Refer to *Figure 2-25* while studying the fauces and surrounding structures. The **fauces** [FAW seez] is the posterior boundary of the oral cavity. It is the opening from the mouth into the oropharynx (throat) for air when breathing through the mouth and for food, since the oropharynx leads to the esophagus and stomach. The fauces is bounded inferiorly by the dorsum of the tongue, laterally by a palatal arch or pillars, and superiorly by the soft palate. Examine the fauces and palatine arches by having the patient open and say "ahhh . . . . ." You may have to gently push the tongue down with a tongue depressor. *Be careful:* Patients may gag.

Identify the anterior and posterior palatine pillars or arches that descend from the soft palate. The **anterior arch** is also named the **glossopalatine** [GLOSS o PAL a tine] arch, and the **posterior arch** is named the **pharyngopalatine** [fah RING go PAL a tine] arch, after the muscles beneath them. (*Hint:* The arch from the tongue [glosso] to the palate [*glosso*palatine anterior arch] is more anterior than the arch from the pharynx or throat behind it [*pharyngo*palatine posterior arch].) (See Color Plate #3.) The **palatine tonsils,** when present, are located between the anterior and posterior pillars. These tonsils may become enlarged and inflamed during infections of the respiratory system. Patients may have had these surgically removed.

Although not part of the oropharynx, there are several landmarks just posterior to the last molars that will be presented here. Immediately posterior to the *maxillary* last molar is a firm tissue bulge over bone of the alveolar ridge called the **maxillary tuberosity** (*Fig. 2-25*). This tuberosity is present even after all of the teeth have been lost, and is included in an impression of the upper arch when constructing a maxillary complete denture. A similar, less prominent, pear-shaped elevation of movable tissue distal to the *mandibular* last molar is the **retromolar pad.** (See Color Plate #3.) (*Hint:* "Retro" means behind, or distal, to the last molar). When a person has fully erupted third molars, the maxillary tuberosities and retromolar pads are small because teeth occupy these regions. The **pterygomandibular** [TER i go mand DIB you lar] **fold** is a fold of tissue that appears to connect the mandible and the maxilla. This is easy to see when the mouth is opened wide, as this action stretches this fold, extending from the **retromolar pad** on the mandible to the pterygoid process of the sphenoid bone just behind the **maxillary tuberosity.** This fold is an important landmark for the anesthetic syringe needle to enter when aiming toward the mandibular foramen, where the inferior alveolar nerve can best be anesthetized at a point just before entering the mandibular canal and going into the body of the mandible. The **retromylohyoid** [REH tro my lo HI oid] **curtain** is a curtain of mucous membrane along the medial, posterior portion of the mandible near the floor of the mouth, extending between the anterior pillar of the fauces and the pterygomandibular fold. An arrow points to the location of this curtain (but it is not visible) in Figure 2-25. It is an important limiting structure in forming the lingual flange (edge) of a mandibular complete denture.

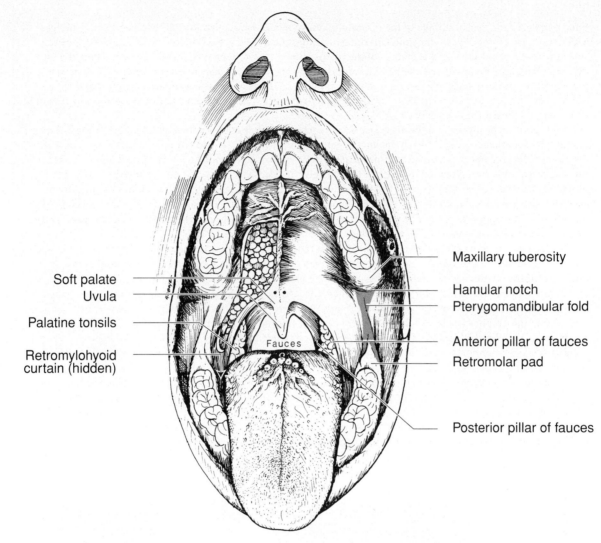

Soft palate
Uvula

Palatine tonsils

Retromylohyoid
curtain (hidden)

Fauces

Maxillary tuberosity

Hamular notch
Pterygomandibular fold

Anterior pillar of fauces
Retromolar pad

Posterior pillar of fauces

FIGURE 2-25. Structures surrounding the fauces (oropharynx).

INFERIOR ALVEOLAR INJECTION: ANESTHETIZING MANDIBULAR TEETH, SURROUNDING TISSUE, AND ADJACENT FLOOR OF THE MOUTH AND TONGUE

The nerves being blocked here are branches of the third division or mandibular branch of the fifth cranial (trigeminal) nerve. Since the bone of the mandible is more dense than in the maxillae, it is often more effective to anesthetize mandibular teeth by applying the anesthetic next to the inferior alveolar nerve before it enters the mandible, or, for premolars and anterior teeth, to apply anesthetic into the mandible at the opening of the mental foramen. To reduce pain for all structures supplied by the entire **inferior alveolar nerve,** the anesthetic is deposited next to the mandibular nerve before it enters the mandible (through the **mandibular foramen**). Recall that the mandibular foramen is located on the medial surface of the ramus of the mandible, a *little over halfway* from the anterior to the posterior border of the ramus (*Fig. 2-26*). On most adults, the foramen is also located superiorly inferiorly a small distance (on average about 5 mm or ¼–½ inch) superior to the level of the chewing surfaces of the posterior teeth. To reach this nerve through the oral mucosa, the injection site is often coincident with the level of the center of a shallow concavity that can be palpated with the finger or thumb on the anterior border of the ramus just superior to the buccal shelf (where the vertical ramus and horizontal alveolar processes join) (*Fig. 2-27*). In order to reach the mandibular foramen, the needle penetrates mucosa about ½ inch above the occlusal plane. (On an edentulous patient, use the landmark of the **retromolar pad** and inject just slightly superior to it.) At this level, enter into the mucosa through the **pterygomandibular fold** (Fig. 2-27) and continue parallel to the medial surface of the ramus until the mandible is touched. Recall that each ramus diverges wider as it goes posteriorly, so the handle of the syringe must be angled across the premolars on the opposite side in order to parallel the medial surface of the ramus (Fig. 2-28). If bone is touched before reaching the estimated depth of the foramen, or if the bone is not reached when you are well beyond the foramen, you need to pull back the needle, reangle the syringe, and try again. If bone is reached at the estimated location of the inferior alveolar nerve, pull back the needle slightly to avoid damaging the bone, then aspirate to ensure you are not in a vessel, and inject the anesthetic.

Anesthetic can be placed at intervals (reaspirating each time) while entering through the mucosa toward the mandibular foramen in order to reach the lingual nerve branch, which is next to the inferior alveolar nerve. Because the **lingual nerve** is located within the tissue adjacent to the mandibular nerve (Fig. 2-29), the anesthetic can infiltrate through tissue toward the lingual nerve and result in numbness to the anterior half of the tongue and adjacent lingual mucosa of the floor of the mouth on the side being injected. Blocking the inferior alveolar nerve *and* lingual nerve should reduce pain in all mandibular teeth and surrounding tissues and should numb half of the tongue and half of the lip on that side. The only area not numb would be the tissue just buccal to the molars, which is innervated by the **buccinator (long buccal)** nerve (described earlier).

If only tissue or teeth of mandibular premolars or anterior teeth needs to be anesthetized, the anesthetic solution can be applied at the location of the mental foramen (Fig. 2-30). At this location, the **mental nerve** branches off the inferior alveolar nerve and exits the mandible to spread anteriorly and innervate the lower lip and adjacent labial tissue. Just inside of this foramen, the inferior alveolar nerve continues forward within the mandible as **incisive branches** to innervate the pulps of anterior teeth. This foramen is normally palpable (and evident on radiographs) at a level between or near the root tips of the mandibular premolars. The injection enters mucosa at the depth (fornix) of the buccal vestibule extending to the level of the palpated foramen. Due to the posterior superior direction of this foramen and canal, it is best entered by directing the needle inferiorly and slightly from the distal (Fig. 2-30).

Note: It may also be possible to anesthetize only mandibular incisors by placing the anesthetic just labial to the alveolar bone facial to the root tips of the mandibular anterior teeth. Even though the mandibular bone is dense, this may be successful *if* the bone overlying these roots is quite thin. Using this technique may get the mandibular facial tissue and anterior and premolar teeth numb, but neither this mandibular facial infiltration technique nor the mental nerve block will affect the lingual tissue or tongue.

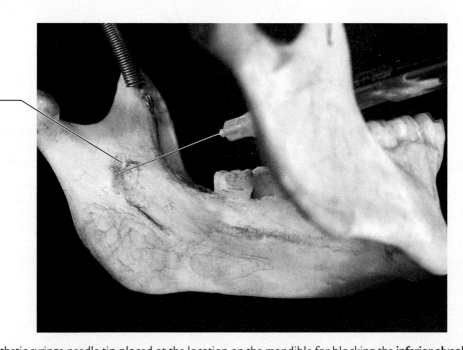

Mandibular foramen

FIGURE 2-26. Anesthetic syringe needle tip placed at the location on the mandible for blocking the **inferior alveolar nerve** before it enters the **mandibular foramen** and canal. Note the position of the mandibular foramen about halfway between the anterior and posterior border of the ramus, and the foramen location relative to the occlusal plane of the mandibular teeth (which is slightly superior to the plane by about 5 mm).

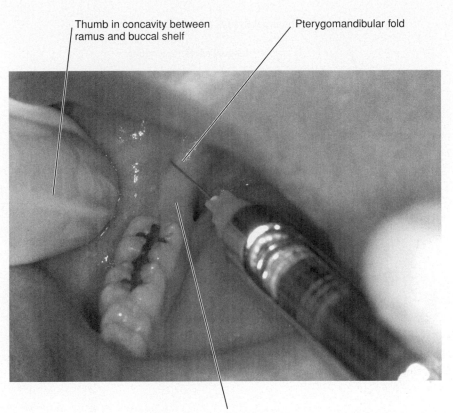

Thumb in concavity between ramus and buccal shelf

Pterygomandibular fold

Retromolar pad

FIGURE 2-27. Anesthetic syringe needle tip penetrating the oral mucosa at the location of the **pterygomandibular fold** just occlusal to the **retromolar pad.** By angling the syringe cartridge over the premolars on the opposite side, the needle can be directed toward the inferior alveolar nerve where it enters the mandible through the mandibular canal. For the average-size person, a long needle penetrates to about half of its total length in order to reach the ramus and foramen, but this depth may be deeper for a very large-boned person or less deep for a very small-boned person.

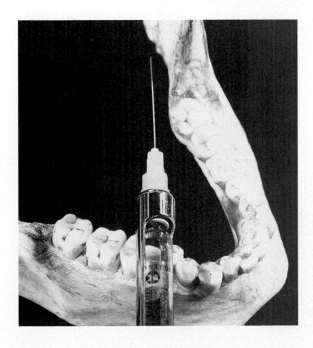

FIGURE 2-28. A superior view of the mandible and ramus showing the angulation required to reach the opening of the mandibular canal. The syringe cartridge must be directed over the premolars on the opposite side in order to parallel the internal surface of the ramus (which diverges considerably posteriorly).

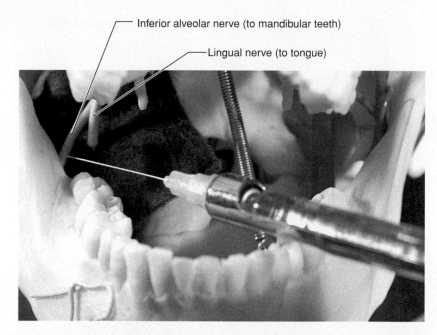

FIGURE 2-29. Two wires represent the inferior alveolar nerve (touched by the needle), and a cut portion of the lingual nerve branch, which goes to the tongue. Notice that the **lingual nerve** would be anesthetized if some anesthetic were applied prior to reaching the inferior alveolar nerve.

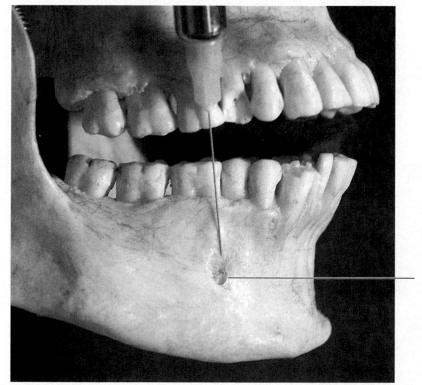

FIGURE 2-30. The syringe needle tip is located adjacent to the **mental foramen.** Note its location near the estimated root tips of the mandibular premolars. Applying anesthetic here can reduce pain to the soft tissue of the chin and lower lip on that side by blocking the **mental nerve,** which splits off the inferior alveolar nerve and exits the mandibular at this location. If enough concentration of anesthetic makes its way into the opening of the mental foramen, it can also reduce pain to premolar teeth (and possibly anterior teeth) and adjacent gingiva by blocking the **incisive branches** of the inferior alveolar nerve that supply these teeth. This injection would *not* numb the tongue.

D. TONGUE

The tongue is a broad, flat organ largely composed of muscle fibers and glands. It rests in the floor of the mouth within the curved body of the mandible. The tongue changes its shape with each functional movement. The anterior two-thirds is called the **body,** and the posterior one-third is the tongue **base** or **root.** (Recall that the body of the tongue is innervated for feeling by cranial nerve V or the trigeminal nerve and for taste by cranial nerve VII or the facial nerve. The base or root is innervated for taste and feeling by cranial nerve IX or the glossopharyngeal nerve.) Examine the tongue by wrapping it in a damp gauze square to grab its slippery surface and gently pulling it first to one side, then to the other. (The tongue muscles that may fight you in this endeavor are innervated by cranial nerve XII or the hypoglossal nerve.)

1. DORSUM OF THE TONGUE

Use Figure 2-31 as a guide for landmarks on the dorsum (top) of the tongue. However, most people are unable to stick their tongue as far forward as in this illustration. The **dorsum** (dorsal or superior surface) of the tongue is the principal organ of taste and is invaluable during speech, mastication, and deglutition (swallowing). The dorsum of the tongue is grayish-red and is rough. It is covered by two kinds of papillae. The fine hair-like **filiform papillae,** which are quite numerous, cover the anterior two-thirds of the dorsal surface of the tongue. They are arranged in

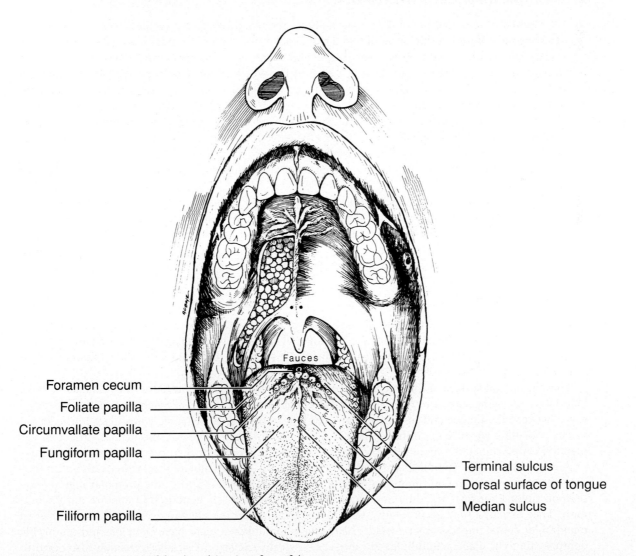

Fauces

Foramen cecum

Foliate papilla

Circumvallate papilla

Fungiform papilla

Filiform papilla

Terminal sulcus

Dorsal surface of tongue

Median sulcus

FIGURE 2-31. Structures of the dorsal (top) surface of the tongue.

lines somewhat parallel to the terminal sulcus.[3] The more sparse, scattered, and shorter **fungiform papillae** are easy to identify because of their round mushroom cap shape and deep red color. Fungiform papillae are most concentrated near the tip of the tongue.[3] (See Color Plate #4.)

Two other papillae types are also found near the junction of the posterior one-third of the tongue. The first are large, red, leaf-like projections actually located on the lateral surface of the tongue known as **foliate papillae** [FO li ate pah PILL e]. (See Color Plate #5.) They contain some taste buds. The **circumvallate** [ser kum VAL ate] **papillae** are 8–12 large, flat, mushroom-shaped papillae forming a V-shaped row on the dorsum near the posterior third of the tongue. (See Color Plate #4.) Their walls contain numerous taste buds. The **foramen cecum** [SEE kum] is a small circular opening immediately posterior to the center of the "V," formed by the circumvallate papilla. This foramen is the remnant of the thyroglossal duct from which the thyroid gland developed. The **terminal sulcus** is a shallow groove running laterally and forward on either side of the foramen cecum but posterior to the circumvallate papillae. It is usually necessary to hold the tongue quite firmly with gauze and pull it forward in order to see the circumvallate papillae and their neighboring structures because of their extremely posterior location. Posterior to the terminal sulcus, the smoother posterior one-third of the dorsum contains numerous mucous producing glands and lymph follicles (or nodules) referred to as the lingual tonsil (not visible on *Fig. 2-31*).

2. VENTRAL SURFACE OF THE TONGUE

The **ventral** or undersurface of the tongue is shiny, and blood vessels are visible. Refer to Figure 2-32. The **lingual frenum** is a thin sheet of tissue that attaches the center of the undersurface of the tongue to the floor of the mouth. Raise your tongue and watch how this tissue fold limits the amount of tongue movement. [Measurements on 333 casts by Dr. Woelfel indicated the frenum attachment to be 8.03 ± 1.5 mm below the gingival sulcus of the mandibular central incisors; range 5.4–11 mm. Assuming an average-length mandibular central incisor (8.8 mm), the lingual frenum attaches about 17 mm below the incisal edge of these teeth.] In a person who is tongue-tied, the lingual frenum is firmly attached perhaps only 3 or 4 mm below the gingival margins of the central incisors and may severely limit tongue movement. Further, as the tongue moves, this type of frenum could pull on the attached gingiva, contributing to periodontal problems. A simple surgical procedure corrects this type of situation.

Plica fimbriata [PLY kah fim bri AH tah] (fimbriated folds) are delicate fringes of mucous membrane on each side of the frenum on the ventral surface of the tongue. The free edge of this fold may have a series of fringe-like processes. These are very delicate and often difficult to see unless gently moved by the tongue blade or mirror. In some animals, these fringes of tissue serve to keep the teeth clean.

E. FLOOR OF THE MOUTH

Visually examine the floor of the mouth by having the patient raise the tongue. Also, feel for unusual lumps by palpating the floor of the mouth with the forefinger of one hand pressing against the floor and opposed outside of the mouth by the fingers of the other hand. This method of palpation is called bimanual palpation since it requires two hands (*Fig. 2-33*).

Like the ventral surface of the tongue, the tissues of the floor of the mouth are shiny, and some large blood vessels may be seen near the surface. The **alveolingual sulcus** (Fig. 2-32) is the broad, valley-shaped space between the tongue and mandibular alveolar bone. You can gently place your finger in this broad sulcus and press laterally to confirm whether there are any bony ridges on the medial surface of the mandible. A prominent bump in this area might be a relatively common occurrence: a mandibular torus.

A **mandibular torus** (plural tori) (*Fig. 2-34*) is a bulbous protuberance of bone beneath a thin mucous membrane covering on the medial side of the mandible often found in the premolar region (also seen on Color Plate #6). Mandibular tori are probably inherited as a genetic trait and are not uncommon. They usually cause no problems, but may be irritated during chewing of coarse foods or when mandibular dental impressions are made. After several or all lower teeth have been lost and removable dentures are to be made, mandibular tori must be surgically excised. [A similar torus may also occur in the middle of the palate and is called a **torus palatinus** or **palatine torus** (*Fig. 2-34*).] **Exostosis** [ek sos

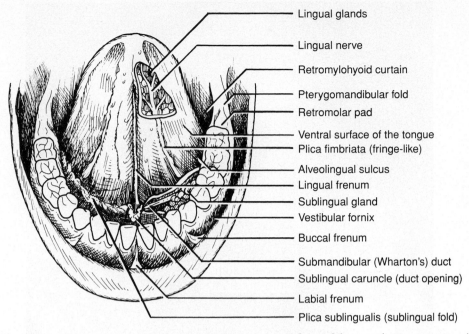

Lingual glands

Lingual nerve

Retromylohyoid curtain

Pterygomandibular fold

Retromolar pad

Ventral surface of the tongue

Plica fimbriata (fringe-like)

Alveolingual sulcus

Lingual frenum

Sublingual gland

Vestibular fornix

Buccal frenum

Submandibular (Wharton's) duct

Sublingual caruncle (duct opening)

Labial frenum

Plica sublingualis (sublingual fold)

FIGURE 2-32. Structures of the ventral (under) surface of the tongue and floor of the mouth. Some mucosa is dissected away on the right side of the tongue and floor of the mouth to reveal the sublingual salivary gland and the submandibular duct passing from the submandibular gland to the openings on the sublingual caruncles.

TOE sis, plural is exostoses] is the general term used to describe any hyperplastic bony growth projecting outward from the bone surface, such as a torus palatinus or mandibular torus, but can also be used to describe bony ridges that may form on the facial (cheek) surface of the alveolar processes of the mandible or maxillae.

F.   SALIVARY GLANDS (INTRAORALLY)

Refer to Figure 2-32 while studying these landmarks on the floor of the mouth. On the floor, the overlying sublingual folds, called the **plica sublingualis** [PLY ka sub ling GWAL is], extend anteriorly on each side of the floor of the mouth from the first molar region to the lingual frenum. Along these folds are many small openings of ducts from underlying **sublingual salivary glands** located in this region. These sublingual glands secrete purely mucous (ropy-type) saliva, producing only 5–8% of our saliva.[1]

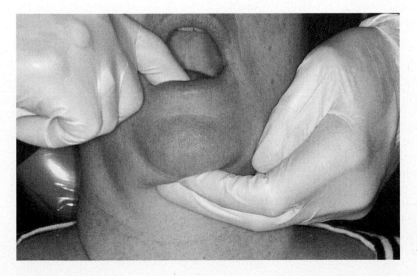

FIGURE 2-33. Bimanual palpation (using the opposing fingers of two hands) in order to feel for lumps or bumps (like a salivary duct blockage) within the floor of the mouth.

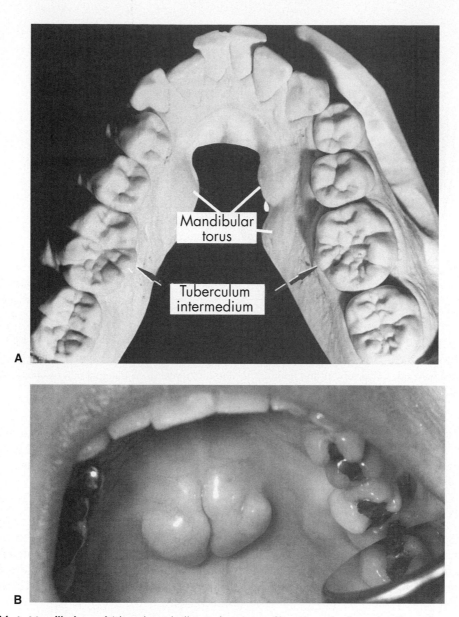

FIGURE 2-34. A. Mandibular tori (three large bulbous elevations of bone) on the lingual surface of a stone cast of the mandible. (Note: The mandibular first molars have six, instead of the usual five, cusps. The extra lingual cusp is called a tuberculum intermedium.) **B.** A maxillary **torus palatinus** or palatal torus.

In the center line at the junction between the right and left sublingual folds, on either side of the lingual frenum, is a pair of bulges called **sublingual caruncles** (see Color Plate #6), each with an opening from ducts of the mandibular salivary glands (**Wharton's ducts**). Wharton's ducts drain the large submandibular glands located posteriorly on either side in the submandibular fossae of the internal surface of the mandible. These glands produce about two-thirds of our saliva.[1] Their secretions are primarily serous (two-thirds serous cells, one-third mucous cells[6]). A person normally secretes over a pint of saliva during 24 hours (300 mL between meals, 300 mL while eating, and only 20 mL while sleeping), based on averages from 600 people.[1]

If you use bimanual palpation and gently move one finger in the floor of the mouth (opposing another outside of the mouth) from posterior to anterior over the sublingual folds and the underlying submandibular ducts, saliva may flow out of the caruncles of the glands. Saliva may even squirt out of the mouth through the openings in the caruncles when the patient opens wide (as when you yawn during a boring lecture) and the surrounding muscles apply pressure to the duct. It is possible for saliva to calcify within the ducts and block the flow of saliva. This could cause symptoms that get worse when eating since the saliva cannot make its way out of the ducts. This calcified blockage (called a sialolith [si AL o lith]) may be palpated, confirmed with a radiograph, and surgically removed.

G. ALVEOLAR PROCESS

The bone surrounding the roots of the teeth should be palpated for bony growths (exostosis) or lesions.

H. GINGIVA

The **periodontium** [per e o DON she um] is defined as the supporting tissues of the teeth, including surrounding alveolar bone (already discussed), the gingiva, the periodontal ligaments, and the outer layer of the tooth roots (covered with cementum). The **periodontal ligament** is a very thin ligament composed of many fibers that connects the outer layer of the tooth root (which is covered with cementum) with the thin layer of dense bone (lamina dura) lining each alveolus or tooth socket. The groups of fibers of the periodontal ligament represented in *Figure 2-35* are greatly enlarged. The entire thickness of the ligament would only be about twice as thick as this page. The **gingiva** is that part of the masticatory (keratinized) oral mucous membrane that covers the alveolar processes of the jaws and surrounds the portions of the teeth near where the root and crown join (cervical portion). It is firmly attached to the teeth and to the surrounding bone. The gingiva is the only visible part of the periodontium that is seen in the initial oral examination.

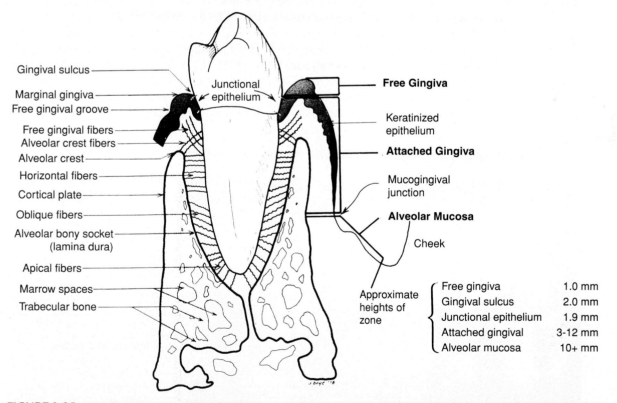

FIGURE 2-35. Periodontium including zones of gingiva and periodontal fiber groups. A mandibular left first premolar is suspended in its alveolus by the five groups of periodontal ligament fibers: apical, oblique, horizontal, alveolar crest, and free gingival fibers are visible. A sixth group, called transseptal fibers, not visible in this drawing, attaches from the cementum of one tooth to the cementum of the adjacent tooth at a level between the free gingival and alveolar crest fibers. The fibers of the periodontal ligament are much shorter than depicted here, averaging only 0.2 mm long (about as thick as two pages in this text).

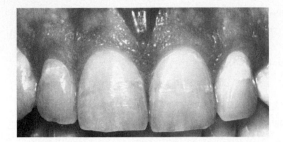

FIGURE 2-36. Healthy gingiva, close up. Note the ideal contours and stippled (orange peel) surface texture, usually most noticeable on the maxillary labial attached gingiva.

Healthy gingiva is stippled (that is, textured with many small depressions, like an orange peel, *Fig. 2-36*) and coral pink in persons with light skin pigmentation. (See Color Plate # 7.) In persons with dark coloring of the hair and skin and in those of Mediterranean origin, the gingiva may be brown or spotted with brown (**melanin pigmentation**). (See Color Plate #8.) This pigmentation may occur up to the mucogingival junction. It is a common occurrence in people with darkly colored and black skin, Asians, people from India, and people of Mediterranean origins (such as many Italians, Arabs, Yemenites, and Turks).

Healthy gingiva varies in appearance from individual to individual and in different areas of the same mouth. It is usually pink (or pigmented), with thin margins just covering or parallel to the junction of the tooth crown and root (cervical line or cementoenamel junction). Therefore, the shape of the margin around each tooth is like a parabolic arch (similar in shape to the St. Louis Arch). This repeated parabolic arch pattern around each tooth is evident in *Figure 2-36*.

Gingiva can be visually divided into zones as shown in *Figure 2-37*. The zone closest to the tooth crown is *un*attached gingiva, which includes the free gingiva and the interproximal papillae. **Free gingiva** (or marginal gingiva) is the tissue that is not attached to the tooth or alveolar bone. It surrounds each tooth to form a collar of tissue with a space or gingival sulcus (crevice) hidden between it and the tooth. Free gingiva extends from the **free gingival margin** (the edge of gingiva closest to the chewing or incising surfaces of the teeth) to the **free gingival groove** (visible in about one-third of adults) that separates free gingiva from attached gingiva. The **interdental (interproximal) papilla** [pah PILL ah] (plural is **papillae** [pa PILL ee]) is that part of the unattached gingiva between the teeth. A healthy papilla conforms to the space between two teeth (interproximal space), so it comes to a point near where the adjacent teeth contact. The papilla also has the hidden sulcus where dental floss can fit once it passes between the teeth.

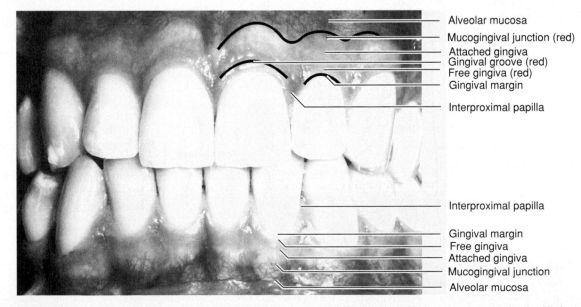

FIGURE 2-37. Clinical zones of the gingiva. Note that the interdental papillae should, but do not completely, fill the interproximal spaces between the mandibular incisors. The tissues are otherwise healthy. (Courtesy of Lewis J. Claman, D.D.S., M.S.)

Attached gingiva is a band or zone of gray to light or coral pink keratinized masticatory mucosa that is firmly bound to the underlying bone (*Fig. 2-37*). It extends between the free gingiva (at the free gingival groove if present) and the more movable alveolar mucosa. The amount or width of attached gingiva varies normally from 3 to 12 mm.

The **mucogingival line** (junction) (*Fig. 2-37*) is a scalloped junction between attached gingiva and the looser, redder alveolar mucosa. **Alveolar mucosa** is movable mucosa, dark pink to red, due to increased vascularity and more delicate nonkeratinized tissue just apical to the mucogingival line. It is more delicate and less firmly attached to the underlying bone than the attached gingiva and is more displaceable as well, because of the underlying vessels and connective tissue. Palpate these two types of tissues and you will feel the difference in firmness. This movable alveolar mucosa is found in three places: in the maxillary and mandibular *facial* vestibule and in the mandibular lingual aspects (alveolingual sulcus), but not on the palate, which has firm, attached keratinized tissue for almost the entire surface. Therefore, the mucogingival line is present on the *facial* aspects of the maxillary and mandibular gingiva but only on the *lingual* aspect of mandibular gingiva.

Keratinized gingiva is the general term used to describe both the free and attached gingiva. It is widest on the facial (vestibular) aspect of maxillary anterior teeth and the lingual aspect of mandibular molars. It is narrowest on the facial aspect of mandibular premolars.[7]

The **gingival sulcus** (*Figs. 2-35 and 2-38*) is not seen visually but can be evaluated with a periodontal probe, since it is actually a space (or potential space) between the tooth surface and the narrow unattached cervical collar of free gingiva. The gingival sulcus is lined with the sulcular epithelium. It extends from the free gingival margin to the junctional epithelium [averaging 0.69 mm in depth].[8] **Junctional** (or attached) **epithelium** (seen in cross section in *Fig. 2-35*) is a band of tissue at the most apical portion of the gingival sulcus that attaches the gingiva to the tooth. It is about 1 mm in width.[8] Then there is a 1- to 1.5-mm connective tissue attachment to the root above the osseous (bony) crest of bone. It is usually recommended that the margins of artificial crowns and inlays be kept 3 mm from this osseous crest.

Clinically, the healthy gingival sulcus ranges in probing depth from about 1 to 3 mm and should not bleed when correctly probed. The periodontal probe usually penetrates into the junctional epithelium, hence the difference between the depth determined through clinical probing and the depth seen on a microscopic cross section.[9] [In a survey by Dr. Woelfel, 267 dental hygiene students measured their gingival sulcus depth with a calibrated periodontal probe. The average gingival sulcus depths for mandibular first molars midbuccal were 1.5 ± 0.5 mm; midlingual: 1.7 = 0.6 mm; mesiolingual and distolingual: 2.5 ± 0.5 mm. These measurements indicate that the gingival sulcus is usually deeper interproximally. Similar measurements made on the mesiofacial aspect of mandibular canines (1.9 ± 0.8 mm), maxillary canines (1.8 mm), maxillary first premolars (1.9 ± 0.7 mm), and maxillary first molars (2.1 ± 0.7 mm) indicate sulci slightly deeper on posterior teeth than those on anterior teeth.] Sometimes, during the process of eruption of the mandibular last molar through the mucosa, a flap of tissue may remain over part of the chewing surface called an **operculum** (seen in Color Plate #9). This operculum can easily be irritated during chewing and become infected.

Note in Figure 2-35 that the periodontal ligament (between the bone and tooth root) is made up of four groups of tiny fibers with differing directions and attachments and different names. The **apical, oblique,**

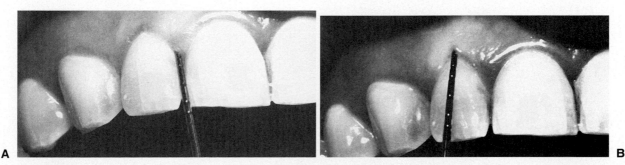

A   B

FIGURE 2-38. Periodontal probe in place in the gingival sulcus. **A.** Interproximal probing in sulcus bounded by interdental papilla. **B.** Facial probing in gingival sulcus bounded by free gingiva.

horizontal, and **alveolar crest fibers** connect different parts of the tooth root (cementum) to the lamina dura of the tooth socket. The oblique fibers provide the major support to the tooth during function. **Free gingival fibers** are directed from tooth root (cementum) into free gingiva. A sixth group, the **transseptal fibers,** are not seen on Figure 2-35 since they run directly from the root (cementum) of one tooth to the cementum of the adjacent tooth at a level between the free gingival and alveolar crest fibers.

I.   THE TEETH: COUNT THEM

An important part of the oral examination is to determine which teeth are erupted in the mouth, identify them by name or universal number, and determine which teeth are missing. When the number of teeth is fewer than expected for a patient, a careful history can confirm tooth loss by disease or accident, or teeth removed prior to orthodontic treatment. When history does not confirm such reasons for tooth loss, radiographs are recommended to rule out the possibility of unerupted teeth beneath the mucosa or surrounded by bone (impacted teeth) or to confirm that a tooth never formed. It is also possible for the patient to have extra (supernumerary) teeth or unexpected teeth (such as primary teeth in a 30 year old). These factors impact treatment planning decisions and should be documented.

The total number of teeth depends on the age of the individual and the stage of development of the teeth. As stated in the first section in this text, the complete **primary dentition** consists of 20 teeth. Children between 2½ and 5¾ years of age will usually have all 20 primary teeth present in the mouth. For the next 6 years, there is normally a mix of some primary and some permanent teeth (called **mixed dentition**) until about 12 years of age, when all primary teeth have been lost and only permanent teeth are present. At age 12, there would normally be 28 permanent teeth (all but the unerupted third molars). Eventually (by the late teens or early 20s), the complete **permanent** (or secondary) **dentition** consists of 32 teeth, including the four third molars that erupt (become visible) into the mouth.

LEARNING EXERCISE

Examine a partner (using infection control procedures) and identify each of the structures listed on this modified Head and Neck examination form. (The order of structures listed on this form is the same order as that encountered within the chapter, so it should be easy to follow the text as you perform the exam.) Use a tongue depressor or a mouth mirror to retract the lips and cheeks. A good light is needed, and a mouth mirror is useful for reflecting light into remote areas and for holding the tongue or cheek out of the way during your examination.

NORMAL STRUCTURES FOUND

DURING THE HEAD AND NECK EXAM

(Key: * = not found on all patients)

Extraoral Examination:

General Appearance: healthy walk and posture; normal breathing

Head: symmetrical (or not); jaw midline symmetrical (or not)

Skin: palpate underlying muscles: masseter (origin, insertion); temporalis (anterior and posterior origin); medial pterygoid (insertion)

Eyes: clear sclera; pupil not considerably dilated or constricted

Temporomandibular joint: palpate lateral surface of condyle during function; posterior surface of condyle (in internal auditory meatus)

Neck: palpate thyroid gland; submandibular salivary gland

Nodes: palpate for submental; submandibular; parotid (preauricular); postauricular; cervical (around sternocleidomastoid muscle)

Salivary glands: palpate parotid gland and submandibular gland (bimanual for sublingual [intraoral])

Lips: commissure; nasolabial fold; labiomental groove; tubercle; philtrum; vermilion zone; mucocutaneous junction; wet line

Intraoral Examination:

Mucosa: Labial: labial frenum; fornix
    Buccal: buccal frenum; commissural papule; *linea alba; parotid papilla from parotid gland (Stensen's duct: press along it for saliva); *Fordyce granules (orange-colored spots)

Palate: Hard palate: incisive papilla; palatine raphe; reggae; *torus palatinus; pterygoid hamulus
    Soft palate: vibrating line (say "ah"); fovea palatine; uvula

Tonsils/oropharynx: fauces; glossopalatine arch; pharyngopalatine arch; * palatine tonsils; pterygomandibular fold; retromylohyoid curtain

Tongue: Dorsum: filiform, fungiform and circumvallate papillae (way back); foramen cecum and terminal sulcus
    Lateral: foliate papillae
    Ventral: lingual frenum; plica fimbriata (may need to "separate" from tongue with mirror handle)

Floor of mouth: alveololingual sulcus; *mandibular torus, palpate bimanual: sublingual folds over sublingual glands; joining at sublingual caruncles with Wharton's ducts of submandibular gland (may squirt)

Salivary glands: Buccal mucosa: parotid papilla ("milk" Stensen's duct)
Floor of mouth: sublingual folds over submandibular glands with caruncle and opening to submandibular gland (may squirt)

Alveolar process: *exostosis (particularly on buccal aspect); maxillary tuberosity (*pterygoid hamulus behind*)

Gingiva: free gingival (has sulcus; would confirm with probe); *free gingival groove: interdental papilla; attached (keratinized) gingiva; mucogingival junction; retromolar pad (mandibular), *tissue overlapping last molar = operculum*

Teeth: count all erupted teeth; note retained primary teeth: *impacted (on radiographs), malformations, etc.

Occlusion (circle one): class I II III: evaluate first molar and canine relationships

LEARNING QUESTIONS

Test your newly acquired knowledge by matching the forty landmarks with their descriptions. Place the appropriate letter or letters on line on left.

_____ 1. Dorsum of tongue
2. Hard palate
3. Pharynx
_____ 4. Elevated midline of hard palate
_____ 5. Stensen's duct
6. Alveolar mucosa
7. Fordyce's spots
_____ 8. Melanin
_____ 9. Gingiva between teeth
10. Palatal tissue bump between teeth #8, 9
11. Vibrating line
12. Wharton's duct openings
_____ 13. Labial frenum
_____ 14. Ventral surface of tongue
15. Oral cavity
16. Retromolar pad
_____ 17. Maxillary tuberosity
_____ 18. Filiform papillae
19. Torus mandibularis
20. Attached gingiva
_____ 21. Fauces
_____ 22. Nasolabial groove
23. Labiomental groove
24. Sublingual gland
_____ 25. Submandibular gland
_____ 26. Plica sublingualis
27. Uvula
28. Plica fimbriata
_____ 29. Foliate papilla
_____ 30. Circumvallate papillae
31. Alveololingual sulcus
32. Palatine tonsils
_____ 33. Retromylohyoid curtain
_____ 34. Fungiform papillae
35. Alveolar mucosa
36. Fovea palatini
_____ 37. Parotid gland
_____ 38. Philtrum
39. Commissure
40. Exostosis

a. Mouth
b. Dark pigment on attached gingiva
c. Anteriorly in floor of mouth where the plica sublingualis meet
d. Underside of tongue
e. Hair-like papillae covering two-thirds of dorsum of tongue
f. Top side of tongue
g. Sebaceous glands on inside of cheek
h. Interdental papillae
i. Opens on inside of cheek near maxillary molars
j. Palatine raphe
k. Attaches lip to mucosa covering jaw (upper and lower)
l. Behind soft palate
m. Incisive papilla
n. Lines floor of vestibule
o. Firm, covered by gingiva, has rugae
p. Ridge of bone lingual to mandibular premolars
q. Elevation of tissue distal to mandibular last molar
r. Elevation of tissue distal to maxillary last molar
s. Junction of hard and soft palate
t. Tightly attached—pink color
u. Mucous salivary glands beneath anterior third of tongue
v. Large serous salivary gland beneath posterior third of tongue
w. At corners of mouth where lips join
x. Diagonal grooves from nostrils to corner of mouth
y. Horizontal depression below lower lip
z. Vertical depression on upper lip
aa. Opening from oral cavity to pharynx
bb. Serous salivary gland just in front of ear
cc. Loosely attached
dd. Fold in floor of mouth beneath tongue
ee. Slight fold on each side of ventral surface of tongue
ff. Hangs downward in center of soft palate
gg. On lateral surfaces of posterior third of tongue
hh. Space between mandibular teeth and tongue
ii. 8 to 12 circular papillae arranged in a "V" shape
jj. Pocket of mucous membrane between anterior pillar and pterygomandibular fold
kk. Located between anterior and posterior pillars in throat
ll. Bulbous protuberance on facial side of mandible in premolar region
mm. Sparse round mushroom-shaped papillae on dorsum of tongue
nn. Located just posterior to vibrating line

ANSWERS: 1-f, 2-o, 3-l, 4-j, 5-i, 6-n or cc, 7-g, 8-b, 9-h, 10-m, 11-s, 12-c, 13-k, 14-d, 15-a, 16-q, 17-r, 18-e, 19-p, 20-t, 21-aa, 22-x, 23-y, 24-u, 25-v, 26-dd, 27-ff, 28-ee, 29-gg, 30-ii, 31-hh, 32-kk, 33-jj, 34-mm, 35-n or cc, 36-nn, 37-bb, 38-z, 39-w, 40-ll

REFERENCES

1. Jenkins GN. The physiology of the mouth. 3rd ed. Revised reprint. Oxford: Blackwell Scientific, 1970:310–328.
2. Foley PF, Latta GH. A study of the position of the parotid papillae relative to the occlusal plane. J Prosthet Dent 1985;53:124–126.
3. Osborn JW, Armstrong WG, Speirs RL, eds. Anatomy, biochemistry and physiology. Oxford: Blackwell Scientific, 1982:535.
4. Simmons JD, Moore RN, Errickson LC. A longitudinal study of anteroposterior growth changes in the palatine rugae. J Dent Res 1987;66:1512–1515.
5. Renner RP. An introduction to dental anatomy and esthetics. Chicago: Quintessence Publishing, 1985.
6. Brand RW, Isselhard DE. Anatomy of orofacial structures. 5th ed. St. Louis: C.V. Mosby, 1994.
7. Lang N, Loe H. The relationship between the width of keratinized gingiva and gingival health. J Periodontol 1972;43:623.
8. Gargiulo A, Wentz F, Orban B. Dimensions and relationships of the dentogingival junction in humans. J Periodontol 1961;32:261.
9. Polson A, Caton J, Yeaple R, et al. Histological determination of probe tip penetration into gingival sulcus of humans using an electronic pressure-sensitive probe. J Clin Periodontol 1980;7:479.

GENERAL REFERENCES

Beck EW. Mosby's atlas of functional human anatomy. St. Louis: C.V. Mosby, 1982.

Clemente CD. Anatomy: a regional atlas of the human body. 4th ed. Baltimore: Williams & Wilkins,1997.

Clemente CD, ed. Gray's anatomy of the human body. 30th ed. Philadelphia: Lea & Febiger, 1985.

DuBrul EL. Sicher and DuBrul's oral anatomy. St. Louis: C.V. Mosby, 1988.

Dunn MJ, Shapiro CZ. Dental anatomy/head and neck anatomy. Baltimore: Williams & Wilkins, 1975.

Montgomery RL. Head and neck anatomy with clinical correlations. New York: McGraw-Hill, 1981:236–240.

Web site: http://education.yahoo.com/reference/gray/

3 Basic Terminology for Understanding Tooth Morphology

Prior to reading this chapter, be sure to master the terms used to identify teeth in Chapter 1, Section I.

The background terminology and concepts presented in this chapter are divided into seven sections as follows:

I. Tooth identification systems: Universal, Palmer, and International Numbering Systems
II. Terminology used to describe the parts of a tooth
    A. Four tissues of a tooth
    B. *Anatomic* versus *clinical* crown and root
III. Terminology used to define tooth surfaces
    A. Terms that identify outer surfaces (toward the cheeks or lips) of anterior versus posterior teeth
    B. Terms that identify inner surfaces (toward the tongue) of maxillary versus mandibular teeth
    C. Terms that differentiate biting surfaces of anterior versus posterior teeth
    D. Terms that differentiate approximating surfaces of teeth
    E. Divisions (thirds) of the crown or root (for purposes of description)
    F. Terms to denote tooth surface junctions or dimensions
    G. Root-to-crown ratio
IV. Terminology used to describe the morphology of a tooth
    A. Morphology of an anatomic crown
    B. External morphology of the anatomic root
    C. Relative size
    D. Cervical line (CEJ) curvature
V. Terminology related to the ideal tooth alignment of teeth in dental arches
    A. Root axis line
    B. Height of contour (crest of curvature)
    C. Contact areas (or proximal heights of contour)
    D. Embrasure spaces
VI. Ideal occlusion: inter (between) arch relationship of teeth
VII. Tooth development from lobes

OBJECTIVES

This chapter is designed to prepare the learner to perform the following:

- Use the Universal Numbering System to identify permanent and primary teeth.
- Recognize the Palmer and International Tooth Numbering Systems and "translate" them to the Universal System.
- Identify and describe the four tissues of a tooth and their location, mineral content, and function.
- Differentiate an *anatomic* crown and root from a *clinical* crown and root.
- Name each tooth surface for anterior and posterior teeth.
- From all views, divide a tooth crown and root into thirds and label each third.
- Define terms used to denote a specific dimension of a tooth.
- Describe and identify (by name) common tooth bumps, ridges, depressions, and grooves for each type of tooth.
- Describe and recognize the parts of a root.

- Describe and identify the attributes of ideal tooth alignment and embrasure spaces relative to other teeth within the arch, including the cusp or incisal edge position relative to the tooth's midroot axis line, location of heights of contour and proximal contacts, and relative sizes of embrasure spaces.
- Describe and identify the ideal interarch relationship of teeth in class I occlusion, especially the relationship of first molars and canines.
- Identify the number of developmental lobes that form each tooth and recognize the anatomic landmarks of a tooth that may result from these lobe divisions.

When we enter into any new field of study, it is initially necessary to learn the particular language of that field. Without an adequate vocabulary, we can neither understand nor make ourselves understood. Definitions and explanations of terms used in descriptive tooth morphology are the basic foundation for understanding subject matter presented in subsequent chapters of this text. You must learn a few basics, similar to learning a foreign language. You will soon become nearly as familiar with these dental terms as you are with your name, and you will continue to use the majority of them throughout your professional dental career.

SECTION I	TOOTH IDENTIFICATION SYSTEMS: UNIVERSAL, PALMER, AND INTERNATIONAL NUMBERING SYSTEMS

The making and filing of accurate dental records is an important task in any dental practice. To do so expeditiously, it is necessary to adopt a type of code or numbering system for teeth. Otherwise, for each tooth being charted, one must write something like "maxillary right second molar mesio-occlusodistal amalgam restoration with a buccal extension" (11 words, or 81 letters). Simplified by using the Universal Numbering System (and other standard abbreviations to denote tooth restoration surfaces described later in Chapter 12), this same information would be "2MODBA" (only six symbols). There are also two other numbering systems, the Palmer and the International Systems. As can be seen in *Table 3-1*, the tooth in the previous example (Universal number 2), using the Palmer Notation System, would be number 7⌋, and when using the International System the tooth would be number 17.

The **Universal Numbering System,** first suggested by Parreidt in 1882, was officially adopted by the American Dental Association in 1975. It is accepted by third-party providers and is endorsed by the American Society of Forensic Odontology. Basically, the Universal Numbering System uses numbers 1 through 32 for the **permanent dentition,** starting with 1 for the maxillary right third molar, going around the arch to the maxillary left third molar as 16; dropping down on the same side, the left mandibular third molar becomes 17, and then the numbers increase clockwise around the lower arch to 32, which is the lower right third molar. This numbering system is used for each permanent tooth in the illustration in *Figure 3-1*.

For the 20 teeth in the **primary dentition,** letters of the alphabet are used from A through T. The letter A represents the maxillary right second molar, sequentially around the arch and through the alphabet to J for the maxillary left second molar, then dropping down on the same side to K for the mandibular left second molar, and then clockwise around the lower arch to T for the lower right second molar. This system is used to identify each primary tooth in the illustration in *Figure 3-2*.

The **Palmer Notation System** utilizes four brackets (to denote each quadrant), which surround a number (denoting the tooth in that quadrant). The specific brackets are designed to represent each of the four quadrants of the dentition, as if you are facing the patient:

⌋　　is upper right
L　　is upper left
⌐　　is lower right
Γ　　is lower left

The **permanent teeth** in each quadrant are numbered from 1 (nearest to the arch midline) to 8 (farthest from the midline). For example, 1 is a central incisor, 2 is a lateral incisor, 3 is a canine, etc. This number is placed within the bracket that indicates its quadrant. For example, the lower left central incisor, lower left second

Table 3-1   MAJOR TOOTH IDENTIFICATION SYSTEMS

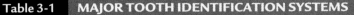

	TOOTH	UNIVERSAL		PALMER NOTATION		INTERNATIONAL (FDI)	
		Right	Left	Right	Left	Right	Left
DECIDUOUS DENTITION — MAXILLARY TEETH	Central incisor	E	F	A⌋	⌊A	51	61
	Lateral incisor	D	G	B⌋	⌊B	52	62
	Canine	C	H	C⌋	⌊C	53	63
	First molar	B	I	D⌋	⌊D	54	64
	Second molar	A	J	E⌋	⌊E	55	65
MANDIBULAR TEETH	Central incisor	P	O	A⌉	⌈A	81	71
	Lateral incisor	Q	N	B⌉	⌈B	82	72
	Canine	R	M	C⌉	⌈C	83	73
	First molar	S	L	D⌉	⌈D	84	74
	Second molar	T	K	E⌉	⌈E	85	75
PERMANENT DENTITION — MAXILLARY TEETH	Central incisor	8	9	1⌋	⌊1	11	21
	Lateral incisor	7	10	2⌋	⌊2	12	22
	Canine	6	11	3⌋	⌊3	13	23
	First premolar	5	12	4⌋	⌊4	14	24
	Second premolar	4	13	5⌋	⌊5	15	25
	First molar	3	14	6⌋	⌊6	16	26
	Second molar	2	15	7⌋	⌊7	17	27
	Third molar	1	16	8⌋	⌊8	18	28
MANDIBULAR TEETH	Central incisor	25	24	1⌉	⌈1	41	31
	Lateral incisor	26	23	2⌉	⌈2	42	32
	Canine	27	22	3⌉	⌈3	43	33
	First premolar	28	21	4⌉	⌈4	44	34
	Second premolar	29	20	5⌉	⌈5	45	35
	First molar	30	19	6⌉	⌈6	46	36
	Second molar	31	18	7⌉	⌈7	47	37
	Third molar	32	17	8⌉	⌈8	48	38

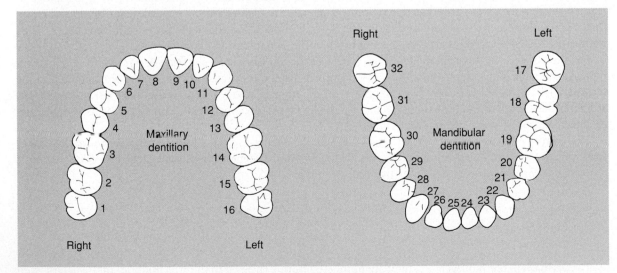

FIGURE 3-1. A drawing of the occlusal and incisal surfaces of the maxillary and mandibular adult dentition. The numerals 1 to 32 inside the arches give the **Universal numbering code** commonly used for record keeping.

DECIDUOUS TEETH

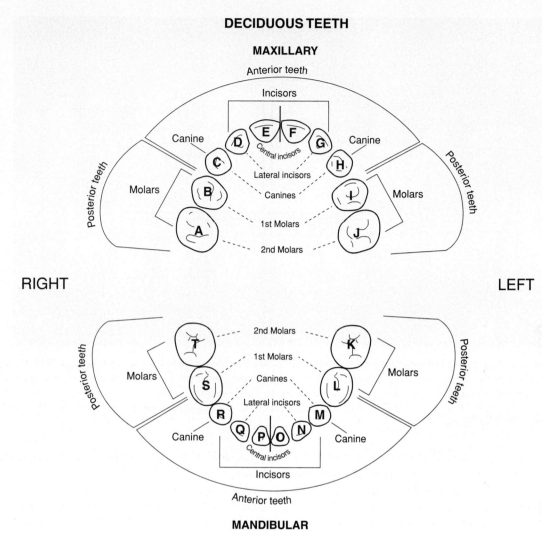

FIGURE 3-2. A drawing of the occlusal and incisal surfaces of the maxillary and mandibular deciduous or primary dentition. The letters A to T give the **Universal numbering code** commonly used for record keeping.

premolar, and upper right canine would be shown as ⎾1, ⎾5, and 3⏌, respectively. The quadrant symbols (brackets used to identify each quadrant as you are facing a patient) and the tooth numbers (1–8) within each quadrant are illustrated in *Figure 3-3*. For **primary teeth,** the same four brackets are used to denote the quadrants, but letters of the alphabet A through E represent the primary teeth (with A being a central incisor, B a lateral incisor, C a canine, etc.). If you are confused, refer to Table 3-1 for clarification.

The **International Tooth Numbering System** (Federation Dentaire Internationale [FDI]) uses two digits for each tooth, permanent or primary. The *first digit* denotes the quadrant (right or left) *and* arch (maxillary or mandibular) *and* dentition (permanent or primary) as follows:

1 = Permanent dentition, maxillary, right side
2 = Permanent dentition, maxillary, left side
3 = Permanent dentition, mandibular, left side
4 = Permanent dentition, mandibular, right side
5 = Primary dentition, maxillary, right side
6 = Primary dentition, maxillary, left side
7 = Primary dentition, mandibular, left side
8 = Primary dentition, mandibular, right side.

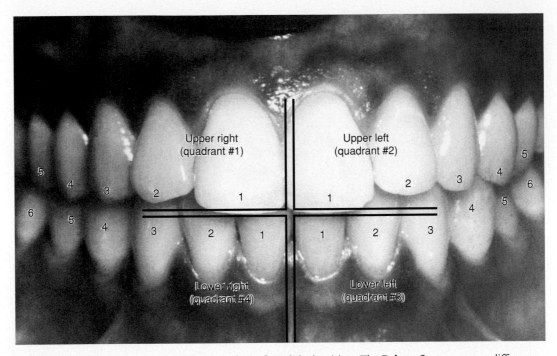

FIGURE 3-3. Two methods for denoting each quadrant for adult dentition. The **Palmer System** uses a different "bracket" shape for each quadrant, as indicated, whereas the **International System** uses the numbers 1 through 4 to denote each adult quadrant. The numbers on each tooth denote the method for identifying teeth within each quadrant beginning with #1 for the central incisors, #2 for lateral incisors, etc.

The adult quadrants labeled 1, 2, 3, and 4 and the tooth numbers (1–8) within each quadrant are illustrated in Figure 3-3, as they would be in the International Numbering System.

The *second digit* denotes the tooth position relative to the midline, from closest to farthest away (similar to the Palmer System). Therefore, the second digits 1 through 8 stand for the permanent central incisor through the third molar and 1 through 5 stand for the primary central incisor through the primary second molar. Combining the first and second digits using the International System, all numbers within the range 11 through 48 represent permanent teeth. For example, 48 is a permanent mandibular right third molar since the first digit, 4, indicates the mandibular right quadrant for a permanent tooth, and the second digit, 8, indicates the eighth tooth from the midline in that quadrant, namely, the third molar. Numbers within the range 51 through 85 represent primary teeth. For example, 51 is a primary maxillary right central incisor since the first digit, 5, indicates the maxillary right quadrant for a primary tooth, and the second digit, 1, indicates the first tooth from the midline in that quadrant, namely, the central incisor. All of the tooth numbers are shown in Table 3-1. You will find it easy to become familiar with any system by first learning (memorizing) the number or letters for key teeth, possibly the central incisors, canines, and first molars. **NOTE: Unless otherwise stated, the Universal System of tooth numbering is used throughout this text.**

SECTION II — TERMINOLOGY USED TO DESCRIBE THE PARTS OF A TOOTH

A. FOUR TISSUES OF A TOOTH

The tooth is made up of four tissues: enamel, dentin, cementum, and pulp. The first three of these are mostly inorganic or calcified (containing considerable mineral content) and surround the pulpal tissue where the nerves and blood supply are found. Only two tissues are normally visible in an intact extracted tooth: enamel and cementum. The other two tissues (dentin and pulp) are usually not visible unless the

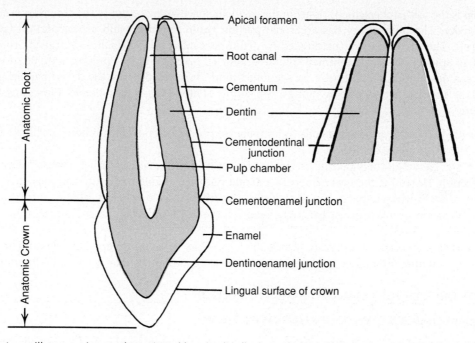

FIGURE 3-4. A maxillary anterior tooth sectioned longitudinally through the middle to show the distribution of the **tooth tissues** and the shape of the pulp cavity (made up of pulp chamber and root canal). On the right is a close-up of the apical portion depicting the usual expected constriction of the root canal near the apical foramen. The layer of cementum covering the root of an actual tooth is proportionately much *thinner* than seen in these drawings.

tooth is badly decayed, sectioned, or prepared with a bur, removing the outer layers. Refer to *Figure 3-4* while reading about each tissue.

Enamel [ee NAM el] is the white, protective external surface of the anatomic *crown*. It is highly calcified or mineralized and is the hardest substance in the body. The mineral content is 95% calcium hydroxyapatite (which is calcified and inorganic). The remaining substances include 4% water and 1% enamel matrix (organic matter). It develops from the enamel organ (ectoderm) and is a product of a specialized type of epithelial cell called **ameloblasts** [ah MEL o blasts].

Cementum [se MEN tum] is the dull yellow external layer of the anatomic tooth *root*. The cementum is very thin next to the cervical line, no thicker than a page in this text (only 50–100 μm thick). It is composed of 65% calcium hydroxyapatite (calcified and inorganic), 23% organic matter (collagen fibers), and 12% water and is about as hard as bone. [Another author, Melfi, states that the inorganic (mineral content) of cementum is about 50%.] It develops from the dental sac (mesoderm), and it is produced by cells called **cementoblasts** [se MEN toe blasts].

The **cementoenamel** [se MEN toe ehn AM el] **junction** (also called the **CEJ**) separates the enamel of the anatomic crown from the cementum of the anatomic root. This junction is also known as the **cervical** [SER vi kal] **line,** denoting that it surrounds the neck or **cervix** [SER viks] of the tooth.

Dentin [DEN tin] is the hard, yellowish tissue underlying the enamel and cementum making up the major bulk of the inner portion of each tooth crown and root. It extends internally from the pulp cavity in the center of the tooth outward to the inner surface of the enamel (on the crown) or cementum (on the root). Dentin is not normally visible except on a dental radiograph, on a sectioned tooth, or on a badly worn tooth. Mature dentin is composed of about 70% calcium hydroxyapatite (calcified and inorganic), 18% organic matter (collagen fibers), and 12% water, making it harder than cementum but softer than enamel. Dentin develops from the embryonic dental papilla (mesoderm). The cells that form dentin are called **odontoblasts** [o DON toe blasts] located at the junction between pulp and dentin.

The **dentinoenamel** [DEN tin o ehn AM el] **junction** is the inner surface of the enamel cap where enamel joins dentin (only visible on a cross section or when preparing a tooth for a restoration). The **cementodentinal** [se MEN toe DEN tin al] or **dentinocemental junction** is the inner surface of cementum lining the root (also only visible on teeth in cross section).

Pulp is the soft (not calcified) tissue in the cavity or space in the center of the crown and root called the **pulp cavity.** The pulp cavity has a coronal portion (**pulp chamber**) and a root portion (**pulp** or **root canal[s]**). The pulp cavity is surrounded by dentin, except at a hole (or holes) near the root tip (apex) called an **apical** [APE i kal] **foramen** (plural foramina). Like dentin, the pulp is normally not visible, except on a dental radiograph (x-ray) or sectioned tooth. It develops from the dental papilla (mesoderm). Pulp is soft connective tissue containing a rich supply of blood vessels and nerves. Functions of the dental pulp are:

- *Formative:* Dentin-producing cells (odontoblasts) produce dentin throughout the life of a tooth. This is called secondary dentin.
- *Sensory:* Nerve endings permit the sense of pain from heat, cold, drilling, sweet, decay, trauma, or infection. However, the nerve fibers in a dental pulp are unable to distinguish the cause of the pain.
- *Nutritive:* Pulp transports nutrients from the bloodstream to cells of the pulp that reach the osteoblasts in the dentin. Surprisingly, blood in the tooth pulp had passed through the heart only 6 seconds previously.
- *Defensive or protective:* Pulp responds to injury or decay by forming reparative dentin (by the odontoblasts). Undifferentiated mesenchymal cells serve to replace injured or destroyed odontoblasts.

B. ANATOMIC VERSUS CLINICAL CROWN AND ROOT

1. ANATOMIC CROWN AND ROOT DEFINITION

The **anatomic crown** is that part of the tooth (in the mouth or handheld) normally covered by an enamel surface (*Fig. 3-4*), and the **anatomic root** is the part of a tooth covered by a cementum surface. A cervical line (or cementoenamel junction) separates the anatomic crown from the anatomic root. This relationship does not change over a patient's lifetime.

2. CLINICAL CROWN AND ROOT (ONLY APPLIES WHEN THE TOOTH IS IN THE MOUTH AND AT LEAST PARTIALLY ERUPTED)

The **clinical crown** refers specifically to the amount of tooth visible in the oral cavity, and the **clinical root** refers to the amount of tooth that is *not* visible since it is beneath the gingiva. Clinically, the gingival margin in a 25-year-old patient with healthy gingiva approximately follows the curvature of the cervical line, and under these conditions, the clinical crown is essentially the same as the anatomic crown. However, the gingiva or gingival margin is not always at the level of the cervical line because of the eruption process early in life or due to recession of the gingiva later in life. For example, the gingiva on a partially erupted tooth of a 10 year old covers much of the enamel of the anatomic crown of the tooth, resulting in a clinical crown (exposed in the mouth) that is much shorter than the anatomic crown. The clinical root (not visible in the mouth) would be longer than the anatomic root (consisting of the anatomic root plus the part of the anatomic crown covered with gingiva).

In contrast, the gingival margin in a 60-year-old person may exhibit gingival recession, especially after having periodontal disease or periodontal therapy, exposing more of the anatomic root, and may result in a clinical crown that is longer than the anatomic crown (made up of all of the anatomic crown and part of the anatomic root that is exposed). In this situation, the clinical root is shorter than the anatomic root.

LEARNING EXERCISE

Examine the mouths of several persons of different ages to see if the cervical line is visible or hidden. As the individual grows older, the location of the margin of the gingiva may recede toward the root tip (apically) because of periodontal disease or injury (such as from the faulty use of oral hygiene aids). Of course, the location of the cervical line on the tooth remains the same. In other words, the distinction between the *anatomic* crown and root does not change over a lifetime.

SECTION III TERMINOLOGY USED TO DEFINE TOOTH SURFACES

A. TERMS THAT IDENTIFY OUTER SURFACES (TOWARD THE CHEEK OR LIPS) OF ANTERIOR VERSUS POSTERIOR TEETH

All teeth have surfaces that are named according to their usual alignment within the dental arch. Refer to Figure 3-3 when studying the terms to denote tooth surfaces. The **facial surface** of a tooth is the surface toward the face, that is, the outer surface of a tooth in the mouth resting against or next to the cheeks or lips. Facial may be used to designate this portion of any tooth, anterior or posterior. Another name for the facial surface of *posterior* teeth is **buccal** [BUCK k'l], located next to the cheek (labeled on tooth #3 in *Fig. 3-5*). It is incorrect to use this term when speaking about the incisors or canines because they do not approximate the cheeks. The facial surface of *anterior* teeth are properly called **labial** [LAY bee al] **surfaces,** located next to the lip (labeled on tooth #6 in *Fig. 3-5*). This term should not be used when referring to the premolars or the molars.

B. TERMS THAT IDENTIFY INNER SURFACES (TOWARD THE TONGUE) OF MAXILLARY VERSUS MANDIBULAR TEETH

The **lingual** [LIN gwal] **surface** is the surface of a maxillary or mandibular tooth nearest the tongue. In the maxillary arch, this surface can also be called the **palatal surface** due to its proximity with the palate (labeled on tooth #5 in *Fig. 3-5*). (Notice that the palatal surface of tooth #8 in *Fig. 3-5* has a structure labeled **cingulum** [SING gyoo lum], which is a bump located on the lingual surface near the cervical part of the crown of all anterior teeth.)

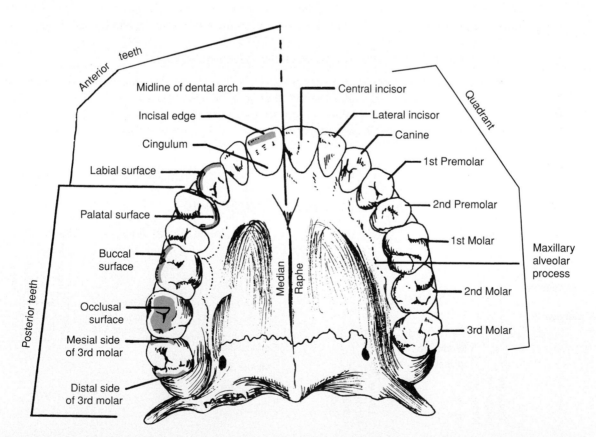

FIGURE 3-5. Maxillary dental arch of teeth with the **tooth surfaces** labeled. Remember that the labial surface of an anterior tooth and the buccal surface of a posterior tooth are both referred to as facial surfaces. Also, the mesial and distal sides or surfaces are correctly called proximal surfaces.

C. TERMS THAT DIFFERENTIATE BITING SURFACES OF ANTERIOR VERSUS POSTERIOR TEETH

The **occlusal** [ahk KLOO zal] **surface** is the chewing surface of a posterior tooth (labeled on tooth #2 in *Fig. 3-5*). Anterior teeth (incisors and canines) do not have an occlusal surface but do have an **incisal edge,** which is the cutting edge, ridge, or surface (labeled on tooth #8 in *Fig. 3-5*).

D. TERMS THAT DIFFERENTIATE APPROXIMATING SURFACES OF TEETH

The **proximal** [PROCK se mal] **surfaces** are the sides of a tooth generally next to an adjacent tooth. Depending on whether the tooth surface faces toward the arch midline between the central incisors or away from the midline, it is either a **mesial** [MEE zi al] **surface** (closer to the midline) or a **distal** [DIS tal] **surface** (farther from the midline). (Do not confuse the mesial surface of a tooth with medial aspect of the skull defined earlier in this text.) Mesial and distal surfaces are labeled on tooth #1 in Figure 3-5. Note that the mesial surface of all teeth touch, or are closest to, the distal surface of the adjacent tooth except between the central incisors where the mesial surface of one central incisor faces another mesial surface. Also, the distal surface of the last molar in each arch does not approximate another tooth. Proximal surfaces are generally not considered to be self-cleansing (by the action of the cheeks and lips and tongue) when compared to the facial, lingual, and occlusal surfaces, which are more self-cleansing.

E. DIVISIONS (THIRDS) OF THE CROWN OR ROOT (FOR PURPOSES OF DESCRIPTION)

A tooth can be divided into thirds in order to define more precisely the location of its specific landmarks. When viewing a tooth from the facial, lingual, mesial, or distal surface, *horizontal* lines can divide the tooth *crown* into thirds: cervical, middle, and occlusal (or incisal). Similarly, *horizontal* lines can divide the *root* into thirds: cervical, middle, and apical (toward the root tip or apex) (*Fig. 3-6*).

When viewing the tooth from the *facial (or lingual)* surface, *vertical* lines can be used to divide the crown or root into mesial, middle, and distal thirds. When viewing the tooth from the *proximal* (mesial or distal) surface, *vertical* lines can be used to divide the crown or root into facial, middle, and lingual thirds.

F. TERMS TO DENOTE TOOTH SURFACE JUNCTIONS OR DIMENSIONS

To describe the junction (line) where two surfaces meet (called an external **line angle**), the names for the two surfaces are combined by changing the "al" ending in the first surface to an "o." Examples of external line angles of a molar crown include mesio-occlusal, mesiolingual, mesiofacial, disto-occlusal, distolingual, distofacial, bucco-occlusal, and linguo-occlusal. Examples of these external line angles of the tooth are seen in Figure 3-7. **Point angles** are the junctions of three tooth surfaces at a point, such as a mesiobucco-occlusal point angle.

Arbitrary Division of teeth in thirds

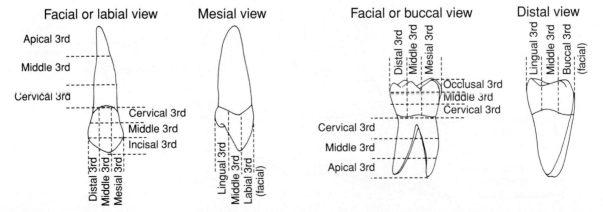

FIGURE 3-6. Diagram of a maxillary canine and a mandibular first molar to show the manner in which the crown or root may be divided into **thirds** from each view for purposes of describing the location of anatomic landmarks, contact areas, and so forth.

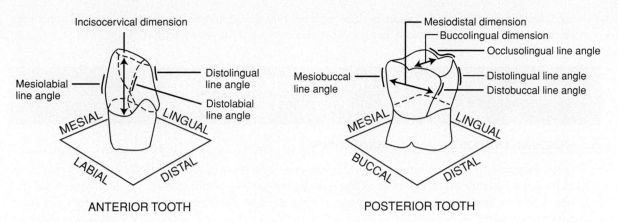

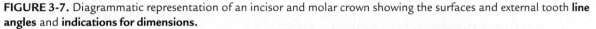

ANTERIOR TOOTH   POSTERIOR TOOTH

FIGURE 3-7. Diagrammatic representation of an incisor and molar crown showing the surfaces and external tooth **line angles** and **indications for dimensions.**

To describe a dimension of a tooth, combined terms can be used to denote the direction over which the dimension was taken. For example, the length of an incisor crown from the incisal edge to the cervical line could be called the incisocervical dimension or the dimension incisocervically (*Fig. 3-7*). Other similar terms used to describe a crown dimension include faciolingual or buccolingual, mesiodistal, and cervico-occlusal. Root dimensions could also be described as cervicoapical.

G. ROOT-TO-CROWN RATIO

If we know the length of a tooth root (from the cervical line to the tip of the root [or tip of the mesial or mesiobuccal root of teeth with multiple roots]) and the length of the crown (from the cervical line to the tip of the longest cusp or highest part of the incisal edge), we can calculate a **root-to-crown ratio** (or root length divided by crown length). Since the roots of teeth are normally longer than their crowns, the root-to-crown ratios for teeth are normally greater than 1.0. For example, the average root length of a maxillary central incisor is only 13.0 mm and the crown length is 11.2 mm; these lengths are really close to the same size length. The root-to-crown ratio is 13 divided by 11.2, which equals 1.16. This ratio of *close to 1* indicates that the root is not much longer than the crown. Contrast this with a maxillary canine, where the average root is much longer, at 16.5 mm, but the crown is only 10.6 mm, for a much larger root-to-crown ratio of 1.56. A larger ratio like this indicates that the root is over one and a half times longer than the crown. The obvious difference between the root-to-crown ratio on these two teeth is apparent in *Figure 3-8*. The ratio becomes clinically significant, since a tooth with a *small* root-to-crown ratio (closer to 1) is not a good

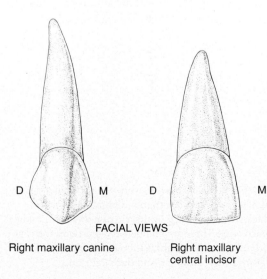

D   M   D   M

FACIAL VIEWS

Right maxillary canine   Right maxillary
                                central incisor

FIGURE 3-8. A comparison of the root-to-crown ratio of the maxillary central incisor (where the root is not much longer than the crown and the ratio is only 13 divided by 11.2, or 1.16) and the maxillary canine (where the root is considerably longer than the crown, and the ratio is much larger: 16.5 divided by 10.6, or 1.56).

candidate for attaching and supporting false teeth because the additional attached teeth would apply even more force on a tooth that already has a short root compared to its crown length.

SECTION IV   TERMINOLOGY USED TO DESCRIBE THE MORPHOLOGY OF A TOOTH

A. MORPHOLOGY OF AN ANATOMIC CROWN

Teeth are made up of many bumps, ridges, depressions, and grooves. Specific tooth structures that occur with some frequency on teeth within a class have been assigned specific names. To identify the following anatomic structures, reference will be made to representative drawings of various teeth seen in *Figures 3-9* through *3-15*.

1. BULGES (ROUNDED) AND RIDGES (LINEAR)

A **cusp** (with a **cusp tip**) is a pointed part, or peak, located on the occlusal surfaces of molar and premolar teeth and on the incisal edges of canines. Each cusp tip has four **cusp ridges** (linear prominences) of enamel converging toward it. These four ridges form the shape of a four-sided, somewhat rounded pyramid. If you were to draw a line along the greatest linear bulge of each of these four ridges, the lines would intersect at the cusp tip, forming a + shape seen by the dotted lines on the buccal cusp of the premolar in *Figure 3-9*. On this cusp, three of the ridges are named after the circumferential tooth surface they extend toward: the subtle *facial* (buccal or labial) ridge actually extends onto the facial surface, the *mesial* cusp ridge extends from the cusp tip toward the mesial surface, and the *distal* cusp ridge extends from the cusp tip toward the distal surface. The fourth ridge from the cusp tip to the faciolingual center of the tooth is called a *triangular* ridge.

Each cusp is named according to its location on the tooth. For example, on a two-cusped premolar, the two cusps are named after the adjacent surface for each cusp: buccal and lingual. On a four-cusped molar, the four cusps are named after the adjacent (corner) line angles: mesiobuccal, distobuccal, mesiolingual, and distolingual. Refer to *Figure 3-10* for examples of cusp names on teeth with two, three, and four cusps.

The **mesial and distal cusp ridges** are also known as **cusp slopes** or cusp arms. They are the inclined surfaces or slopes that converge at the cusp tip to form an angle when viewed from the facial or lingual aspect (seen on the facial view of a canine in *Fig. 3-11A*, on the facial surface of a premolar and molar in *Fig. 3-12*, and on the lingual cusp of a premolar from the occlusal view in *Fig. 3-14A*). Seen from the facial or lingual views, this cusp angle (how sharp or how blunt) is an important trait for certain classes or types of teeth.

On incisor and canine teeth, **marginal ridges** are located on the mesial and distal border of the lingual surface and converge toward the cingulum (seen on the proximal view of a canine in *Fig. 3-11B*

All cusps are basically a gothic pyramid

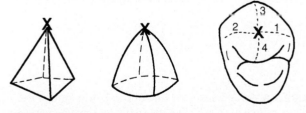

The cuspal gothic pyramid produces 4 ridges:
1. Mesial cusp ridge
2. Distal cusp ridge
3. Buccal cusp ridge (labial ridge on canines)
4. Triangular ridge on posterior teeth (lingual ridge on canines)

FIGURE 3-9. Buccal **cusp** showing the pyramidal design (actually, the pyramid with rounded sides is called a gothic pyramid) formed by the *four cusp ridges* that make up each cusp. These are numbered 1–4 around the cusp tip (*X*) on a maxillary right first premolar. (Courtesy of Drs. Richard W. Huffman and Ruth Paulson.)

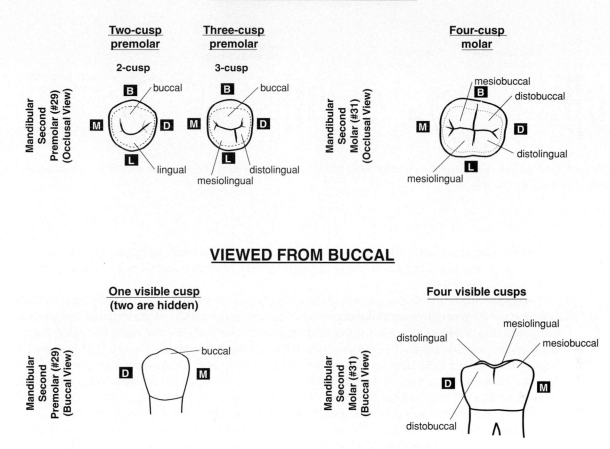

VIEWED FROM OCCLUSAL

Two-cusp premolar

2-cusp

Mandibular Second Premolar (#29) (Occlusal View)

B — buccal

M — D

L — lingual

Three-cusp premolar

3-cusp

B — buccal

M — D

L

mesiolingual — distolingual

Four-cusp molar

Mandibular Second Molar (#31) (Occlusal View)

mesiobuccal
B — distobuccal

M — D

distolingual

L

mesiolingual

VIEWED FROM BUCCAL

One visible cusp (two are hidden)

Mandibular Second Premolar (#29) (Buccal View)

D — buccal — M

Four visible cusps

Mandibular Second Molar (#31) (Buccal View)

distolingual — mesiolingual — mesiobuccal

D — M

distobuccal

FIGURE 3-10. Cusp names on a sampling of teeth (with two, three, and four cusps) viewed from the occlusal and buccal views. Notice that the cusps are named after the adjacent surface or line angle.

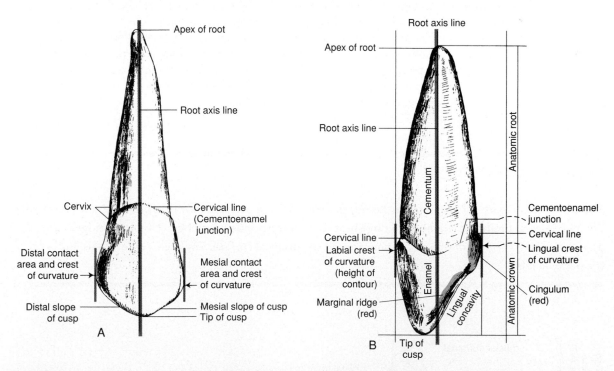

A

Apex of root

Root axis line

Cervix — Cervical line (Cementoenamel junction)

Distal contact area and crest of curvature — Mesial contact area and crest of curvature

Distal slope of cusp — Mesial slope of cusp — Tip of cusp

B

Root axis line

Apex of root

Root axis line

Cementum — Anatomic root

Cementoenamel junction

Cervical line

Cervical line — Lingual crest of curvature

Labial crest of curvature (height of contour)

Enamel — Cingulum (red)

Marginal ridge (red) — Lingual concavity — Anatomic crown

Tip of cusp

FIGURE 3-11. A. Labial surface of the maxillary right canine showing the **root axis** line determined by bisecting the root at the cervix. **B.** Mesial side of the same maxillary right canine. The root axis line bisects the root in the cervical area. Customarily, parts of the tooth are located or described relative to this line. For instance, the cusp tip of this canine is labial to the root axis line.

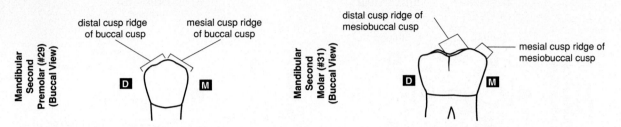

FIGURE 3-12. A sample of **cusp ridges** (cusp slopes) labeled on the facial cusp of a premolar and on the mesiobuccal cusp of a four-cusped molar.

and on the lingual surface of an incisor in *Fig. 3-13*). On posterior teeth, marginal ridges are located on the mesial and distal borders of the occlusal surface. The mesial marginal ridge on a premolar is shaded red in *Fig. 3-14A*.

Triangular ridges are located on each major cusp of *posterior* teeth. Each triangular ridge extends from a cusp tip generally toward the depression (sulcus) in the middle of the occlusal surface faciolingually (Fig. 3-14A and B). Each major cusp on all posterior teeth has one triangular ridge, except the mesiolingual cusp on maxillary molars, which has two triangular ridges *(Fig. 3-15)*. When one triangular ridge from a facial cusp tip joins with a triangular ridge from a lingual cusp tip, the two ridges together form a longer ridge called either a transverse or oblique ridge. A **transverse ridge** crosses the occlusal surface of posterior teeth in a more or less buccolingual direction (e.g., running between the buccal and lingual cusp on a premolar [Fig. 3-14A and B] or connecting the buccal and lingual cusps lined up across from one another on a molar [seen on the two-cusped premolar and mandibular first molar in Fig. 3-15]). An **oblique ridge** is a ridge found only on maxillary molars. It crosses the occlusal surface obliquely (diagonally) and is made up of one triangular ridge of the mesiolingual and the triangular ridge of the distobuccal cusp (seen on the maxillary first molar in Fig. 3-15). According to Ash,[1] the more distal triangular ridge of the mesiobuccal cusp (that forms the lingual half of the oblique ridge) may also be called the distal ridge of the mesiolingual cusp.

Perhaps the most indistinct ridge coming off of the cusp tip is the facial (labial or buccal) ridge. The **buccal** (cusp) **ridge** is a subtle ridge running cervico-occlusally in approximately the center of the buccal surface of premolars, more pronounced on the first premolars than on the second premolars (Figs. 3-9 and 3-14A). Similar in appearance to a buccal ridge on posterior teeth, a canine has a **labial ridge** that runs cervicoincisally and is most prominent on maxillary canines.

LEARNING EXERCISE

The diagram in *Figure 3-16* represents the ridges seen from the occlusal view that bound the occlusal table of a two-cusped premolar. Name each ridge next to its corresponding number. (Note that ridges labeled 1, 3, 4, 5, 6, and 7 form a continuous outline around the occlusal surface. The area inside of this line is called the **occlusal table**.)

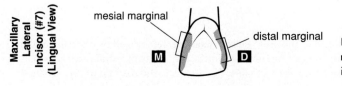

FIGURE 3-13. The mesial and distal **marginal ridges** shaded red on the lingual surface of an incisor [right maxillary lateral].

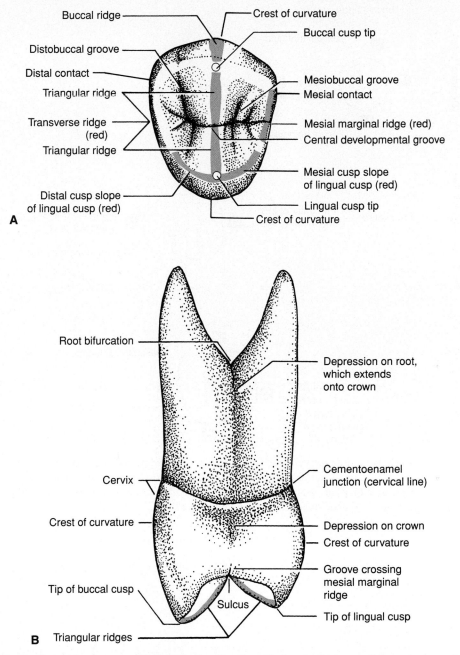

FIGURE 3-14. Maxillary right first premolar. **A.** Occlusal surface. Notice the **four cusp ridges:** the buccal and triangular ridges shaded red on the buccal cusp and the mesial and distal cusp ridges (slopes) [and triangular ridge] shaded red on the lingual cusp. One marginal ridge (the mesial) is also shaded red. The two connecting triangular ridges form one transverse ridge. **B.** Mesial surface. The two triangular ridges join at the occlusal sulcus to form one transverse ridge.

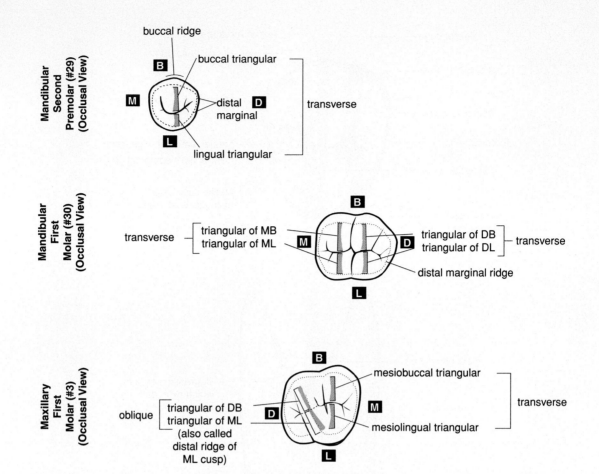

FIGURE 3-15. Three teeth showing **triangular ridges. Top:** Two triangular ridges on a two-cusped premolar form one transverse ridge. **Center:** Two pairs of triangular ridges on a mandibular molar form two **transverse ridges. Bottom:** One pair of triangular ridges on a maxillary molar is aligned buccolingually and forms one **transverse ridge,** and another pair of triangular ridges is aligned obliquely to form an **oblique ridge.**

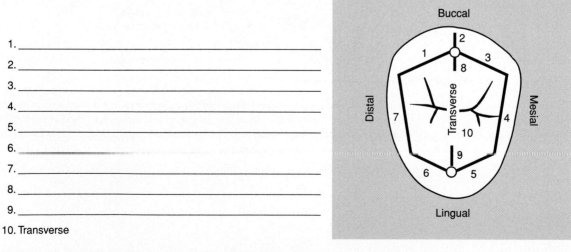

1. _____

2. _____

3. _____

4. _____

5. _____

6. _____

7. _____

8. _____

9. _____

10. Transverse

FIGURE 3-16. Identify the ridges numbered on this maxillary premolar.

ANSWERS: 1.–distal cusp ridge of buccal cusp; 2.–buccal (cusp) ridge; 3.–mesial cusp ridge of buccal cusp; 4.–mesial marginal ridge; 5.–mesial cusp ridge of lingual cusp; 6.–distal cusp ridge of lingual cusp; 7.–distal marginal ridge; 8.–triangular ridge of buccal cusp; 9.–triangular ridge of lingual cusp.

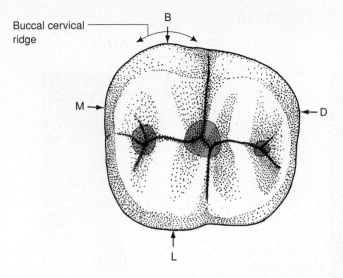

Buccal cervical ridge

B

M

D

L

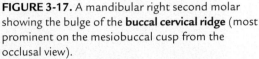

FIGURE 3-17. A mandibular right second molar showing the bulge of the **buccal cervical ridge** (most prominent on the mesiobuccal cusp from the occlusal view).

Other bulges or ridges can be seen on the cervical third of a tooth facially and lingually. On the lingual of all anterior teeth, the **cingulum** [SING gyoo lum] is the enlargement or bulge on the cervical third of the lingual surface of the crown on anterior teeth (incisors and canines) (*Fig. 3-11B*). Finally, found on the facial surface of permanent molars and all primary teeth, the **cervical ridge** is a subtle ridge running *mesiodistally* in the cervical one-third of the buccal surface of the crown (*Fig. 3-17*).

Mamelons are three small tubercles or scallops, each formed from one of the three facial developmental lobes on the incisal edges of newly erupted incisors (*Fig. 3-18*). (Lobes will be described in more detail in Section VII of this chapter.) Usually mamelons are not evident on adult dentition since they are worn off after the tooth comes into functional contact with its opposing tooth. If you have the opportunity, observe a 7-year-old smile to see these mamelons on newly erupted incisors. When mamelons remain on an adult, it is because these teeth do not contact opposing teeth in function, as may occur when maxillary and mandibular anterior teeth do not touch together during function (have an anterior open-bite relationship). When a patient desires, the dentist can reduce the mamelons to make the incisal edge more uniformly curved.

Finally, **perikymata** [pear i KY mah tah] are the numerous, minute horizontal ridges on the enamel of newly erupted permanent teeth (*Figs. 3-19 and 3-20*). They form from the overlapping of layers of enamel laid down

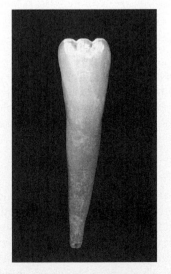

FIGURE 3-18. Example of three distinct unworn **mamelons** present on the incisal edge of a mandibular right central incisor, labial view.

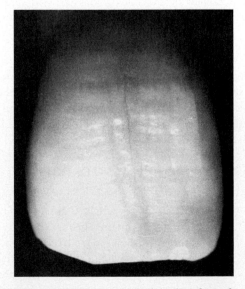

FIGURE 3-19. Perikymata on the labial surface of a maxillary right central incisor.

Perikymata

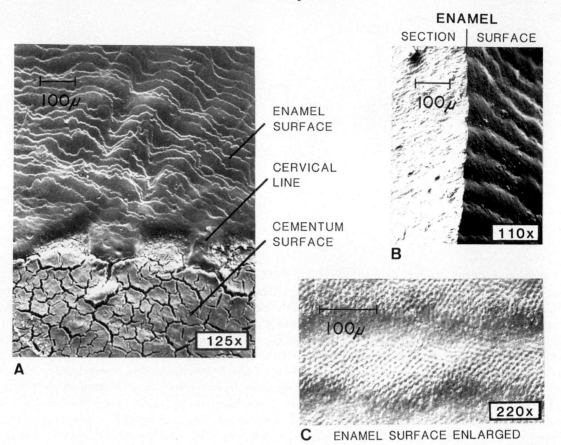

FIGURE 3-20. A. Magnified view of **perikymata** (imbrication lines) near the cementoenamel junction, where they are closest together. Notice their wave-like pattern. The cervical line is quite irregular at this magnification, and the cementum is thin, not necessarily extending to the enamel at every point. **B.** Cross section of enamel showing perikymata waves on the right and the long enamel rods packed tightly and extending inward from the surface on the left. **C.** Higher magnification (×220) of enamel surface shows enamel rod ends on the perikymata waves. Enamel rods are about 4 μm in diameter. (These scanning electron micrographs were kindly provided by Dr. Ruth B. Paulson, Associate Professor Emeritus, Division of Oral Biology, Ohio State University.)

during tooth formation. These lines are closer together in the cervical part of the crown than they are nearer the incisal edge. They are most easily seen on the labial surfaces of the anterior teeth because of their accessible location. Perikymata are more prominent on the teeth of young people than on the teeth of older persons because perikymata, like mamelons, wear away from ongoing abrasion due to eating and even tooth brushing with abrasive toothpastes.

2. DEPRESSIONS AND GROOVES

The tooth **sulcus** [SUL kuss] is the broad depression or valley on the occlusal surfaces of posterior teeth, the inclines of which are formed by triangular ridges that often converge at the depth of the sulcus in a developmental **groove** (see *Fig. 3-14B*). Grooves and their sulci are important escapeways for food morsels when the teeth of the mandible chew from side to side (lateral movements) and protrude forward (protrusive movements). Partially chewed food squirts out toward the tongue and cheeks.

Developmental grooves are sharply defined narrow linear depressions, short or long, formed during tooth development and usually separating the lobes or major portions of a tooth (described in Section VII of this chapter). Like cusps, the major grooves are named according to their location. For example, on the premolar in *Figure 3-21*, the *central* groove is located in the buccolingual center of the

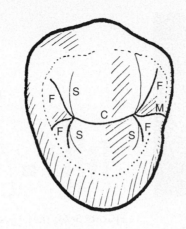

Central developmental groove (**C**)

Fossa developmental grooves (**F**)

Supplemental grooves (**S**)

Marginal ridge groove (**M**)

FIGURE 3-21. An occlusal surface of a maxillary right first premolar depicting developmental (major) and supplemental (extra) occlusal grooves. Some texts consider the fossa grooves as supplemental grooves. (Courtesy of Drs. Richard W. Huffman and Ruth Paulson.)

tooth sulcus and runs mesiodistally. At each end of the central groove both mesially and distally, *fossa developmental grooves* (*or triangular fossa grooves*) may be found splitting off toward the corners of the tooth. These grooves can be named for the corner of the tooth toward which they aim, for example, the mesiobuccal fossa developmental groove (sometimes just called mesiobuccal groove). On many molars and three-cusped premolars, major developmental grooves separate adjacent cusps. For example, on mandibular molars, a *buccal* groove runs from the central groove onto the buccal surface separating the mesiobuccal from distobuccal cusps, and on maxillary molars, a *lingual* groove extends from the central sulcus onto the lingual surface separating the mesiolingual from the distolingual cusps (*Fig. 3-22*).

Additional grooves that are not developmental grooves are called **supplemental grooves.** These small irregularly placed (extra) grooves on the occlusal surface do *not* occur at the junction of the lobes or major portions of the tooth (*Fig. 3-21*).

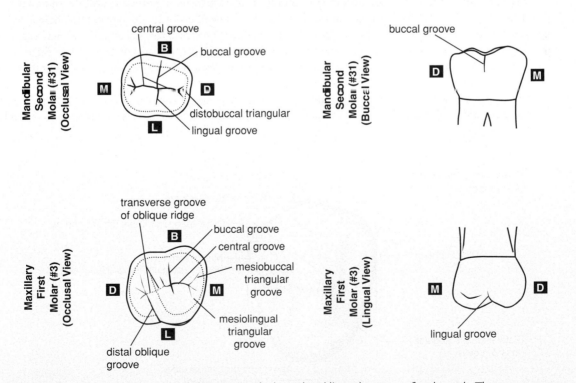

FIGURE 3-22. Grooves labeled on two molars. Notice the buccal and lingual grooves of each tooth. These grooves separate cusps. The buccal (developmental) groove extends onto the buccal surface on the mandibular molar, and the lingual (developmental) groove extends onto the lingual surface of the maxillary molar.

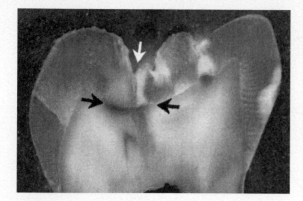

FIGURE 3-23. Cross section of a mandibular molar showing an occlusal groove (*white arrow*), which actually has a **fissure** (crack-like fault) extending through the outer enamel and into the dentin. The black arrows show the spread of dental decay in the dentin where the decay in the fissure joined the softer dentin.

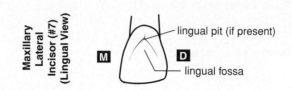

FIGURE 3-24. The lingual surface of an incisor [right maxillary lateral] showing the shallow **lingual fossa** and adjacent lingual pit.

A **fissure** is a very narrow cleft or crevice at the depth of any groove, caused by the incomplete fusion of enamel during tooth development (the white arrow in *Fig. 3-23*). Decay (dental **caries** [CARE eez]) often begins in the deepest part of a fissure (seen in dentin as the dark area between the two black arrows in *Fig. 3-23* and described in more detail in Chapter 13).

A **fossa** [FAH sah] (plural, fossae [FAH see]) is a small hollow or depression found between the marginal ridges on the lingual surfaces of anterior teeth (particularly maxillary incisors, *Fig. 3-24*) and on occlusal surfaces of posterior teeth (denoted by the circles in *Fig. 3-25*). **Pits** often occur at the depth of a fossa where two or more grooves join. For example, within the distal fossa on a premolar, there is a distal pit at the junction of the central groove with the distobuccal and distolingual fossa grooves (*Fig. 3-25*). Like fissures that are found at the depth of grooves, pits are enamel defects where dental decay may begin. Most two-cusped premolars have two fossae (mesial and distal), whereas most molars and three-cusped premolars have three fossae (mesial, central, and distal) seen in *Figure 3-26*.

Hint: In summary, if you compare tooth morphology to a mountain range, the mountain peak would be the cusp tip. Ridges emanating from the mountain peak are like the cusp ridges and triangular ridges. The depression between the height of the mountains (or cusps) is a valley, like the tooth occlusal sulcus. The dried riverbed at the bottom of the valley (sulcus) is like a groove (and if cracked

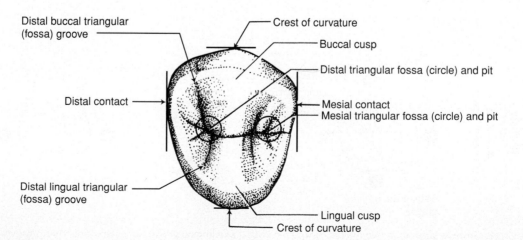

FIGURE 3-25. Maxillary right first premolar, occlusal surface. Notice the mesial and distal triangular fossae circled in red.

FOSSAE AND PITS

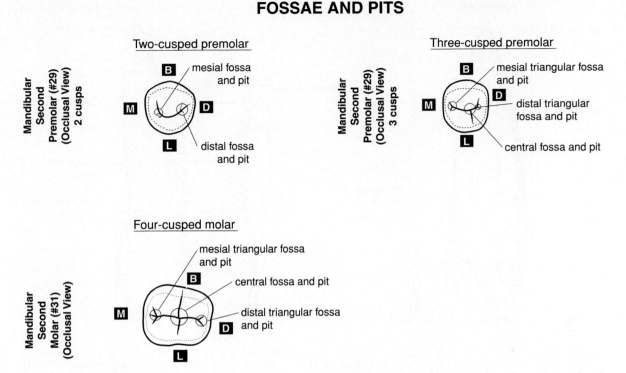

FIGURE 3-26. Fossae labeled on teeth with two, three, and four cusps. Two-cusped teeth have two fossae (mesial and distal), while three- or four-cusped teeth are more likely to have three fossae (mesial, central, and distal). (Maxillary molars have four fossae and will be discussed later.)

open, it is like a fissure). Where riverbeds converge, the whirlpools and eddies may have formed a depression, like a fossa, possibly with a pit at its depth. Needless to say, it is hard to define exactly where a mountain stops and a valley starts, just as it would be hard to point to exactly where a tooth cusp stops and a sulcus begins. Just realize that these terms are not precise but that they are helpful when learning how to reproduce tooth form during construction of crowns and placement of fillings or when learning to finish and polish an existing filling.

B. EXTERNAL MORPHOLOGY OF THE ANATOMIC ROOT

Refer to *Figure 3-27* while studying the external morphology of tooth roots. Recall that the anatomic root is the part of a tooth that has a cementum surface. The **apex** of the root is the tip or peak at the end of the root, often with visible openings called **apical foramina,** where the nerves and blood vessels enter into the tooth pulp. The **cervix** [SUR viks] or neck of the tooth is the slightly constricted region of union of the crown and the root.

Some new terms apply to multirooted teeth *(Fig. 3-27B)*. The **root trunk** or trunk base is the part of the root of a multirooted molar or two-rooted premolar next to the cementoenamel junction that has not yet split (like a stubby tree trunk before it gives off branches). The **furcation** [fur CAY shun] is the place on multirooted teeth where the root trunk divides into separate roots (called a **bifurcation** on two-rooted teeth and a **trifurcation** on three-rooted teeth). The **furcal region** or interradicular space is the region or *space* between two or more roots, apical to the place where the roots divide from the root trunk.

C. RELATIVE SIZE

Using a sample size of 4572 extracted teeth, the average dimensions of each type of tooth have been determined and serve as the basis for many statements made within this textbook. These data are presented in *Table 3-2* and are useful for determining the tooth with the longest crown, the longest overall length, the shortest root, and so forth. For example, note that, on average, the maxillary central incisor has the longest

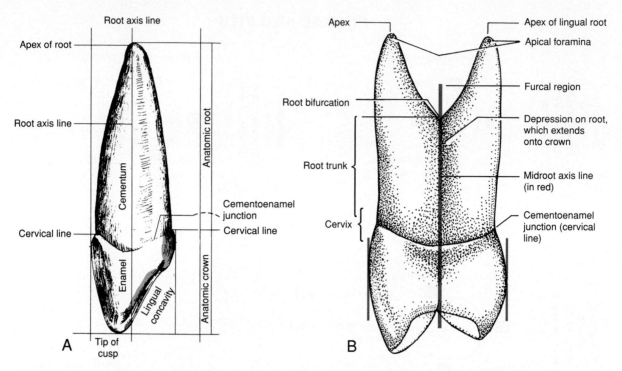

FIGURE 3-27. Root anatomy on a single-rooted canine **(A)** and bifurcated (split) root of a maxillary first premolar **(B)**.

crown, the maxillary canine is the longest tooth (overall length), the mandibular first molar has the widest crown, and the mandibular central incisor has the narrowest crown.

D.   CERVICAL LINE (CEJ) CURVATURE

When viewed from the mesial or distal aspect, the cervical line of a tooth curves (is convex) toward the incisal or occlusal surface *(Fig. 3-27)*. In general, the amount of curvature is greater on the mesial surface than on the distal surface of the same tooth, and the amount of curvature is greatest for central incisors and diminishes in size for each tooth when moving distally around each quadrant *(Table 3-3)*.

SECTION V	TERMINOLOGY RELATED TO THE IDEAL ALIGNMENT OF TEETH IN DENTAL ARCHES

When viewed from the occlusal aspect, each dental arch is somewhat U-shaped or parabolic like the famous arch in St. Louis (recall Fig. 3-1). The incisal edges and the buccal cusp tips follow a curved line around the outer edge of the dental arch; the lingual cusp tips of the posterior teeth follow a curved line nearly parallel to the buccal cusp tips. Between the buccal and lingual cusps is the **sulcular groove**, which runs anteroposteriorly the length of the posterior teeth in each quadrant.

When the arches are viewed *from the buccal aspect,* an **anteroposterior curve** (curve of Spee) is evident where the cusp tips of posterior teeth follow a gradual curve anteroposteriorly (see *Fig. 3-28*). The curve in the maxillary arch of teeth is convex, while that in the mandibular arch of teeth that fit together against the maxillary teeth is concave. A **mediolateral curve** (curve of Wilson) is a side-to-side curve (represented by the wax in *Fig. 3-29*). When viewed from the anterior aspect with the mouth slightly open (or seen posteriorly on models in *Fig. 3-29*), lingual cusps of the maxillary posterior teeth are longer than the buccal cusps, and the lingual cusps of mandibular posterior teeth appear to be shorter than the buccal cusps due to their alignment (lingual tip) within the mandible. When the buccal and lingual cusps of the molars or premolars on either side of the arch are connected forming one line from the left side to the right side, this curve is evident. The mediolateral curve of the maxillary arch is convex, whereas that of the mandibular arch is concave.

Table 3-2 — AVERAGE MEASUREMENTS ON 4572 EXTRACTED TEETH FROM OHIO FROM A STUDY BY DR. WOELFEL AND HIS FIRST-YEAR DENTAL HYGIENE STUDENTS OF THE OHIO STATE UNIVERSITY COLLEGE OF DENTISTRY, 1974–1979. SIZE RANGES ARE SHOWN IN TABLES IN EACH CHAPTER

		CROWN LENGTH (mm)	ROOT LENGTH (mm)	ROOT-TO-CROWN RATIO	OVERALL LENGTH (mm)	CROWN WIDTH MD (mm)	CERVIX WIDTH MD (mm)	CROWN WIDTH FL (mm)	CERVIX WIDTH FL (mm)	MESIAL CERVICAL CURVE (mm)	DISTAL CERVICAL CURVE (mm)
MAXILLARY TEETH											
Central incisor (398)		11.2*	13.0	1.16	23.6	8.6	6.4	7.1	6.3	2.8	2.3
Lateral incisor (295)		9.8	13.4	1.37	22.5	6.6	4.7	6.2	5.8	2.5	1.9
Canine (321)		10.6	16.5	1.56	26.3**	7.6	5.6	8.1	7.6	2.1	1.4
First premolar (234)		8.6	13.4	1.56	21.5	7.1	4.8	9.2	8.2	1.1	0.7
Second premolar (224)		7.7	14.0	1.82	21.2	6.6	4.7	9.0	8.1	0.9	0.6
First molar (308)	MB	7.5	12.9	1.72	20.1	10.4	7.9	11.5	10.7	0.7	0.3
	DB		12.2								
	L		13.7								
Second molar (309)	MB	7.6	12.9	1.70	20.0	9.8	7.6	11.4	10.7	0.6	0.2
	DB		12.1								
	L		13.5								
Third molar (305)	MB	7.2	10.8	1.49	17.5	9.2	7.2	11.1	10.4	0.5	0.2
	DB		10.1								
	L		11.2								
Avg. 2392 Upper teeth		8.77	13.36	1.55	21.59	8.23	6.11	9.20	8.48	1.40	0.97
MANDIBULAR TEETH											
Central incisor (226)		8.8	12.6	1.43	20.8	5.3***	3.5	5.7	5.4	2.0	1.6
Lateral incisor (234)		9.4	13.5	1.43	22.1	5.7	3.8	6.1	5.8	2.1	1.5
Canine (316)		11.0	15.9	1.45	25.9	6.8	5.2	7.7	7.5	2.4	1.6
First premolar (238)		8.8	14.4	1.64	22.4	7.0	4.8	7.7	7.0	0.9	0.6
Second premolar (227)		8.2	14.7	1.80	22.1	7.1	5.0	8.2	7.3	0.8	0.5
First molar (281)	M	7.7	14.0	1.83	20.9	11.4****	9.2	10.2	9.0	0.5	0.2
	D		13.0								
Second molar (296)	M	7.7	13.9	1.82	20.6	10.8	9.1	9.9	8.8	0.5	0.2
	D		13.0								
Third molar (262)	M	7.5	11.8	1.57	18.2	11.3	9.2	10.1	8.9	0.4	0.2
	D		10.8								
Avg. 2180 Lower teeth		8.62	13.85	1.62	21.61	8.17	6.24	8.22	7.44	1.20	0.80

* = longest crown; ** = longest tooth overall length; *** = narrowest crown mesiodistally; **** = widest crown mesiodistally. D, distal; DB, distobuccal; FL, faciolingually; L, lingual; M, mesial; MB, mesiobuccal; MD, mesiodistal.

Table 3-3	SUMMARY OF CURVATURES OF THE CEMENTOENAMEL JUNCTION	
CERVICAL LINE (CEMENTOENAMEL JUNCTION) CURVATURES	Proximal surfaces: mesial curvature versus distal curvature	Generally, teeth have a greater proximal cervical line curvature on the mesial than the distal.
	Proximal surfaces: anterior teeth versus posterior teeth	Proximal cervical line curvatures are greatest on the mesial surfaces of central incisors and tend to get smaller when moving toward the last molar, where there may be no curvature at all.
	Posterior teeth: facial versus lingual surface	On many posterior teeth, the cervical line is in a more occlusal position on the lingual than on the facial.

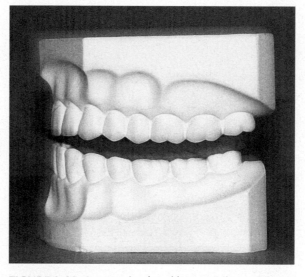

FIGURE 3-28. A wax strip placed between the maxillary and mandibular teeth of stone models demonstrates the **anteroposterior curve (curve of Spee),** which is concave in the mandibular arch and convex in the maxillary arch.

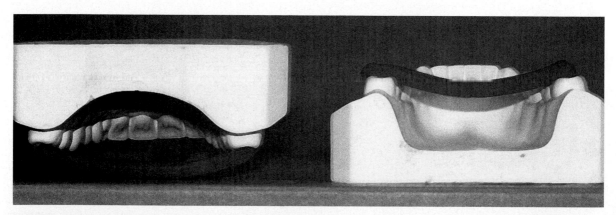

FIGURE 3-29. Dental stone casts from the distal surface with strips of wax placed to demonstrate the **mediolateral curve (of Wilson).** It is convex in the maxillary arch but concave in the mandibular arch.

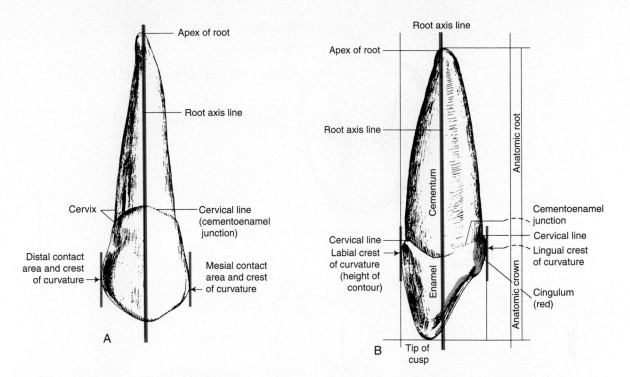

FIGURE 3-30. Maxillary right canine. **A.** Labial surface showing the **mesial and distal contact areas** (heights of contour) or contact areas. **B.** Mesial side of the same maxillary right canine. The **facial and lingual crests of curvature** (touching the lines parallel to the axis line) are in the cervical third on both the facial and lingual (on the cingulum) surfaces. This is typical of anterior teeth.

A. ROOT AXIS LINE

The **root axis line** is an imaginary line through the center of the tooth root. It can be visualized on the facial or lingual surface as a line that divides the tooth at the cervix into mesial and distal halves (*Fig. 3-30A*). When viewing the mesial or distal surface, it divides the tooth at the cervix into facial and lingual halves (*Figs. 3-30B* and *3-31B*). It is an important reference line for describing the location of tooth landmarks. For example, you will learn that the incisal edge of many mandibular anterior teeth is more likely to be lingual to the root axis line, whereas for many maxillary anterior teeth, the incisal edge is more likely to be labial to the root axis line (as seen on a maxillary canine in *Figure 3-30B*).

B. HEIGHT OF CONTOUR (CREST OF CURVATURE)

The shape and height of the greatest curvature or convex bulge on tooth surfaces helps determine the direction of food particles as they are pushed cervically over the tooth surfaces during mastication. When we are chewing food, these natural tooth convexities divert food away from the collar of tissue (gingiva) surrounding the neck of the tooth and toward the buccal vestibule and toward the palate or tongue, thus preventing trauma to the gingiva. If teeth were flat in their middle and cervical thirds, a great deal of food would lodge and remain near the gingival margin and sulcus until removed by a toothpick or toothbrush or by dental floss. Needless to say, it would behoove the dentist, dental hygienist, and/or dental technician to reproduce and maintain these natural convexities when restoring a tooth, when finishing and polishing fillings near the gum line, or when replacing a tooth with a bridge or dental implant. Thus, the restored or replaced tooth will be more self-cleansing and protect the adjacent gingiva.

Refer to Figures 3-30B and 3-31B while reading the following. The **height of contour (crest of curvature)** is the greatest amount of a curve, or greatest convexity or bulge, farthest from the root axis line. The height of contour on the facial or lingual surfaces of the crown is where this greatest bulge would be touched by

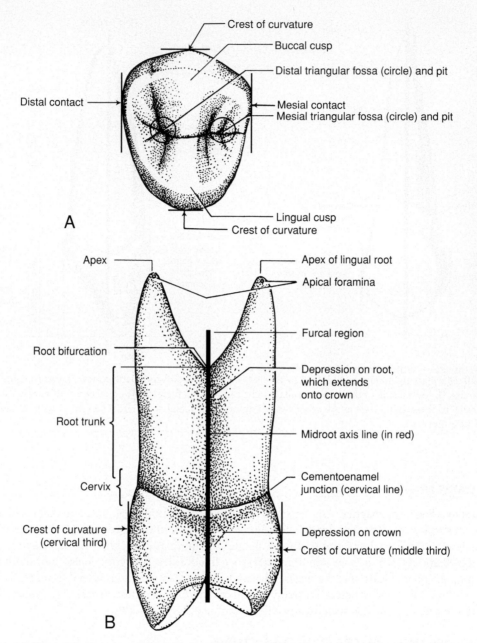

FIGURE 3-31. Maxillary right first premolar. **A.** Occlusal surface. Notice the mesial and distal contact area located buccal from the center of the tooth buccolingually. **B.** Mesial surface. Notice the **buccal height of contour** (crest of curvature) located near the cervical third, while the **lingual height of contour** (crest of curvature) is located more occlusally, in the middle third. This is typical of posterior teeth.

a tangent line drawn parallel to the root axis line. The location of the height of contour on the facial and lingual surfaces of the crowns of teeth can be best seen from the mesial or distal views and is usually located in either the cervical third or the middle third (never the occlusal or incisal third).

The location of the height of contour on the *facial* surface of *all* crowns is located in or near the cervical third. The location of the lingual height of contour differs, depending on whether the tooth is anterior or posterior. The *lingual* height of contour on *anterior* teeth is on the cingulum *(Fig. 3-30B)*, which is in the cervical third. The *lingual* height of contour on *posterior* teeth is more likely to be located in the middle third *(Fig. 3-31B)*. Refer to *Table 3-4* for a summary of the location of the facial and lingual heights of contour for anterior teeth compared to posterior teeth.

Table 3-4	SUMMARY OF THE LOCATION OF FACIAL AND LINGUAL HEIGHTS OF CONTOUR (GREATEST BULGE) OF CROWN (BEST SEEN FROM PROXIMAL VIEW)	
	FACIAL (HEIGHT OF CONTOUR)	**LINGUAL** (HEIGHT OF CONTOUR)
Anterior teeth (incisors and canines)	Cervical third	Cervical third (on cingulum)
Posterior teeth (premolars and molars)	Cervical third	At or near middle third

General Learning Guidelines:
1. **Facial** crest of curvature for all teeth is in **cervical** third (closer to cementoenamel junction for maxillary and mandibular incisors, mandibular first premolars, and mandibular second molars).
2. **Lingual** crest of curvature for all **anterior** teeth is in the **cervical** third (on the cingulum).
3. **Lingual** crest of curvature for **posterior** teeth is in the **middle** third (slightly more occlusal in mandibular teeth due to lingual tilt).

C. CONTACT AREAS (OR PROXIMAL HEIGHTS OF CONTOUR)

When the teeth are in normal, ideal alignment within an arch, the location of the mesial and distal heights of contour (when viewed directly from the facial or lingual sides) is essentially the same location as contact areas (seen from the facial view in *Fig. 3-30A* and from the occlusal view in *Fig. 3-31A*). **Contact areas** are the greatest heights of contour or location of the greatest bulges on the proximal surfaces of tooth crowns, where one tooth touches an adjacent tooth. Floss must pass through contact areas to clean the proximal surfaces, which are otherwise inaccessible to the toothbrush.

In a young person, contact areas on teeth start off between recently erupted teeth as contact *points*. Then, as the teeth rub together in function, these points become somewhat flattened and truly become contact *areas*. It has been shown by careful measurements that, by age 40 in a healthy mouth with a complete dentition, 10 mm of enamel has been worn off the contact areas of the teeth in an entire arch. This averages 0.38 mm per contact area on each tooth and certainly emphasizes the amount of proximal wear (attrition) that occurs. Therefore, we would expect contact areas on teeth of older people to be large and somewhat flattened.

When viewing teeth from the facial view, contact areas are characteristically located in the incisal or occlusal third, in the middle third, or at the junction of the incisal and middle (or occlusal and middle) thirds. Contact points are not normally cervical to the middle of the tooth crown and are therefore never located in the cervical third. When viewing posterior teeth from the occlusal view, contact points are often located slightly to the facial of the tooth midline buccolingually *(Fig. 3-31A)*. The contact of each tooth with the adjacent teeth has important functions:

- The combined anchorage of all teeth within each arch making positive contact with each other *stabilizes* the position of teeth within the dental arches.
- Contact helps *prevent food impaction,* which can contribute to decay and gum and bone disease (periodontal disease).
- Contact *protects the interdental papillae* of the gingiva by shunting food toward the buccal and lingual areas.

Refer to *Table 3-5* for a summary of the relative position of proximal contacts when moving from anterior teeth to posterior teeth. A **diastema** [di ah STEE mah] is a space between two adjacent teeth that do not contact each other (seen between teeth #23, 24, and 25 in *Fig. 3-33*).

D. EMBRASURE SPACES

When adjacent teeth contact, the continuous *space* that surrounds each contact area can be divided into four separate triangular **embrasure spaces** *(Fig. 3-32)*. These spaces are narrowest closest to the contact area where the teeth are in tight contact, and widen facially to form a **buccal or labial embrasure,** widen lingually to form a **lingual embrasure,** and widen occlusally (or incisally) to form an **occlusal or incisal embrasure.** The fourth space, cervical to the contact area and between two adjacent teeth, is properly called the interproximal space.

Table 3-5	SUMMARY OF CURVATURES OF PROXIMAL HEIGHTS OF CONTOUR (PROXIMAL CONTACTS)	
PROXIMAL CONTACTS (PROXIMAL HEIGHT OF CONTOUR) VIEWED FROM THE FACIAL ASPECT	All teeth: relative height of distal versus mesial contacts	Distal contacts are more cervical than mesial contacts (EXCEPT mandibular first premolars where the mesial is more cervical and mandibular central incisors where mesial and distal contacts are at the same level).
	Anterior teeth: relative height moving distally from the midline	Mesial contact areas of the central incisors are most incisally positioned. The distal of the maxillary canine is most cervically positioned of the anterior teeth.
	Anterior teeth: location of proximal contacts	Anterior contacts are in the incisal third (EXCEPT the distal surface of the maxillary lateral incisor and maxillary canine, which may be located in the middle third).
	Anterior teeth: contact location viewed from the incisal	Tooth contacts are nearly centered faciolingually.
	Posterior teeth: relative height moving from more anterior to posterior teeth	Mesial and distal contact areas become more cervical toward the distal of the arch (accentuated by shorter and slightly titled crowns), but mesial and distal contacts are more nearly at the same level than for anterior teeth.
	Posterior teeth: location of proximal contacts	Contacts are in the middle third or near the junction of the middle and occlusal thirds (EXCEPT the mesial of the mandibular first premolar, which may be in the occlusal third).
	Posterior teeth: contact location viewed from the occlusal	Contact areas are larger than anterior contact areas and tend to be slightly buccal to the middle of the tooth buccolingually.

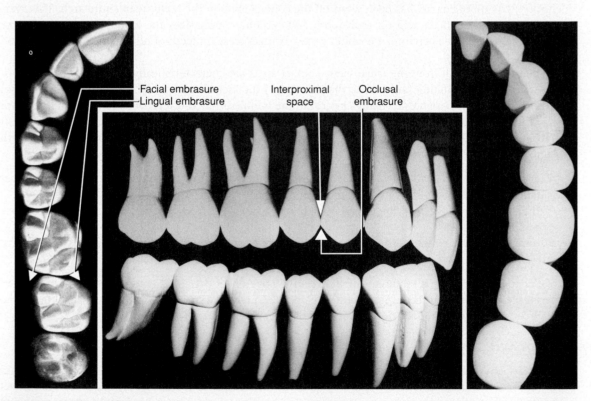

FIGURE 3-32. These photographs are of large plastic tooth models and give an indication of the location of **contact points** between adjacent teeth. The quadrant of teeth on the left contains the occlusal and incisal surfaces of the permanent maxillary dentition; on the right is the mandibular dentition. White triangles fill the facial and lingual **embrasure spaces** (seen from the occlusal or incisal view) and occlusal (incisal) embrasure spaces and interproximal spaces (seen from the facial view).

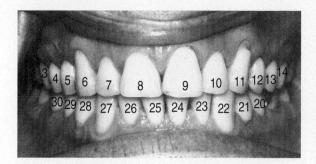

FIGURE 3-33. Maxillary and mandibular teeth of the permanent dentition are in the maximum intercuspal position. Observe the **interproximal spaces** filled with the **interdental papillae** between each pair of teeth. Notice how each tooth is in contact with adjacent teeth, except between tooth numbers 24 and 25 and between tooth numbers 23 and 24. When adjacent teeth do not contact, the resultant space is called a **diastema.** Note how the incisal edges and cusp tips of maxillary teeth overlap and hide the incisal edges and cusp tips of the mandibular teeth, and how the greater width of the maxillary central incisors causes each of them to overlap not only the mandibular central incisor, but also half of the mandibular lateral incisor. The numbers depict the Universal Tooth Identification System.

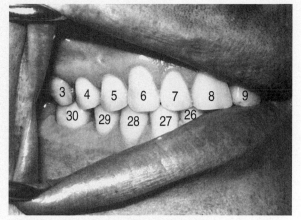

FIGURE 3-34. The subject is the same as in Figure 3-33, but here the right cheek is drawn back. Notice how each maxillary tooth overlaps two mandibular teeth, and the mesiobuccal cusp of the maxillary first molar (just visible on tooth #3) appears to be in occlusion with the mesiobuccal area (groove) on the opposing mandibular first molar, tooth #30.

The **interproximal space,** when viewed from the facial or lingual, is a triangular embrasure space between adjacent teeth located cervical to their contact area. The sides of the triangle are formed by the proximal surfaces of adjacent teeth, with the apex of the triangle at the contact between two teeth. This space is occupied in periodontally healthy persons by the interdental papilla (see *Figs. 3-33* and *3-34*). Sometimes this interproximal space is referred to as the **cervical or gingival embrasure.**

The **lingual embrasure** is ordinarily *larger* than the **facial embrasure** because most teeth are narrower on the lingual side than on the facial side and because their contact points are located facial to the faciolingual midline of the crown. The triangles in Figure 3-32 illustrate these embrasure spaces.

The **occlusal or incisal embrasure** is usually shallow from the occlusal surface or incisal edge to the contact areas and is narrow faciolingually on anterior teeth but broad on posterior teeth. The occlusal embrasure is the area between the marginal ridges on two adjacent teeth and occlusal to their contact area. This is where we place the dental floss before passing it through the contact area to clean tooth surfaces in the interproximal space.

Embrasures surrounding good proximal contact areas serve as spillways to direct food away from the gingiva. When the occlusal embrasure is incorrectly shaped in a dental restoration (amalgam, composite, or gold), fibrous food will readily lodge in the interproximal spaces and can be removed only with dental floss. This food impaction is not only an annoyance, but it can contribute to the formation of dental decay and periodontal disease (bone loss).

SECTION VI IDEAL OCCLUSION: INTER (BETWEEN) ARCH RELATIONSHIP OF TEETH

It is important to learn the relationships of teeth in ideal occlusion in order to identify malocclusions that could contribute to dental problems. **Occlusion** [ah KLOO zhun] is contacting of occlusal and incisal surfaces of opposing maxillary and mandibular teeth. To occlude literally means to close, as in shutting your mouth and closing your teeth together. The importance of proper occlusion cannot be overestimated. It is essential to both general and dental health and to a patient's comfort and ability to speak, chew, and enjoy food. Understanding occlusion requires not only a knowledge of the relation of the mandible to the maxillae, but also of the tem-

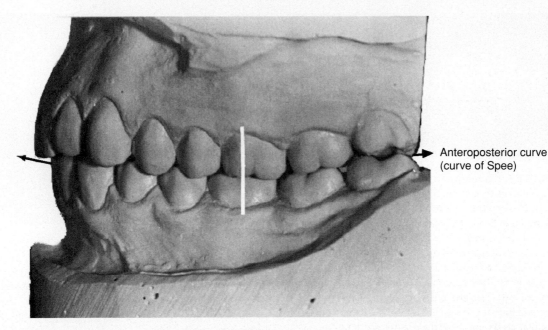

Anteroposterior curve
(curve of Spee)

FIGURE 3-35. Dental stone casts with adult teeth fitting together in the maximum intercuspal position (tightest fit). Notice that, from this view, each tooth has the potential for contacting two opposing teeth except the maxillary third molar. The vertical white line marks the **relationship of first molars in class I occlusion**; the mesiobuccal cusp of the maxillary first molar occludes in the mesialbuccal groove of the mandibular first molar.

poromandibular joints, their complexities, and the muscles, nerves, ligaments, and soft tissues that affect the position of the mandible. These topics were briefly covered in Chapters 1 and 2. The arrangement of teeth within the dental arches (alignment, proximal contacts, and embrasure spaces) was discussed in the last section, and the *ideal* relationship of the mandibular dental arch of teeth to the maxillary dental arch of teeth will be presented in this section.

Ideal tooth relationships were described and classified in the early 1900s by Edward H. Angle. He classified ideal occlusion as class I and defined it based on the relationship between the maxillary and mandibular dental arches. When closed together, the teeth are in their **maximal intercuspal position,** or *best fitting together* of the teeth, as shown in Figures 3-33, 3-34, and 3-35. This relationship can be achieved on handheld models when the maxillary teeth fit as tightly as possible against the mandibular teeth (i.e., are most stable). The following specific tooth relationships define class I ideal occlusion:

- **Horizontal overlap of anterior teeth:** The incisal edges of maxillary anterior teeth overlap the mandibular teeth such that the incisal edges of maxillary teeth are labial to the incisal edges of mandibular teeth (best seen in *Fig. 3-35*).
- **Vertical overlap of anterior teeth:** The incisal edges of the maxillary anterior teeth extend below (overlap) the incisal edges of the mandibular teeth so that, when viewed from the facial, the incisal edges of mandibular incisors are hidden from view by the overlapping maxillary incisors (*Fig. 3-33*).
- **Relationship of posterior teeth:** The maxillary *posterior* teeth are slightly buccal to the mandibular posterior teeth (*Figs. 3-33* and *3-34*) so that:
  - The buccal cusps and buccal surfaces of the maxillary teeth are buccal to those in the mandibular arch.
  - The lingual cusps of maxillary teeth rest in occlusal fossae of the mandibular teeth.
  - The buccal cusps of the mandibular teeth rest in the occlusal fossae of the maxillary teeth.
  - The lingual cusps and lingual surfaces of the mandibular teeth are lingual to those in the maxillary arch.
- **Relative alignment:** The vertical (long) axis midline of each maxillary tooth is slightly distal to the vertical axis of its corresponding mandibular tooth type (*Figs. 3-33* and *3-34*) so that:
  - The tip of the mesiobuccal cusp of the maxillary first molar is aligned directly over the mesiobuccal groove on the mandibular first molar (*Fig. 3-35*). This relationship of first molars (the first permanent teeth to erupt) is a *key factor* in the definition of class I occlusion. Further, the maxillary canine fits into the facial embrasure between the mandibular canine and first premolar.

- Each tooth in a dental arch has the potential for occluding with two teeth in the opposing arch, except the mandibular central incisor (which is narrower than the maxillary central incisor) and the maxillary last molar. For example, the distal surface of the maxillary first molar in Figure 3-35 is posterior to the distal surface of the mandibular first molar, and therefore occludes with both the mandibular first and second molars.

To summarize, *ideal occlusion* involves a class I relationship between the maxillary and mandibular first molars in maximum intercuspal position. Further, only the canines touch when the mandible moves to either side, without molar and premolar contacts. Finally, ideally there should be *no* large facets and/or bruxing habits, bone loss, crooked teeth, loose teeth, or joint pain.[1] Other classes of occlusion (malocclusion) will be discussed in detail in Chapter 11.

SECTION VII　TOOTH DEVELOPMENT FROM LOBES

In terms of the evolution of the dentition, tooth crowns are said to have developed from **lobes** or primary growth centers (*Fig. 3-36*). All *normal* teeth show evidence of having developed from three or more lobes. As a general rule, the facial portion of incisors and canines and premolars forms from three lobes, and the cin-

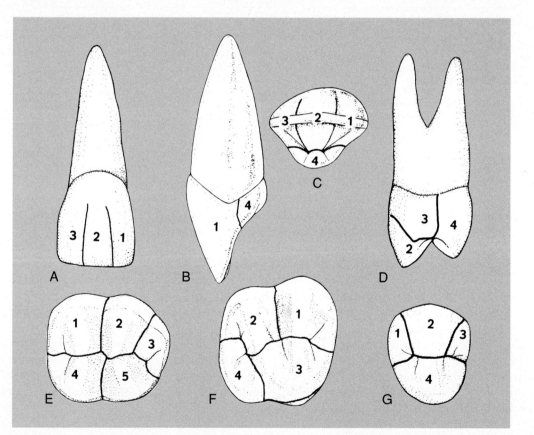

FIGURE 3-36. Lobes or primary anatomic divisions on teeth. Drawings **A, B,** and **C** are the facial, mesial, and incisal views, respectively, of a maxillary central incisor that, like all anterior teeth, has *four* lobes. The lingual cingulum develops from one lobe (labeled 4) seen in view B and C. Mamelons may appear on the incisal edge of newly erupted incisors, an indication of the three labial lobes. Drawings **D** and **G** are the mesial and occlusal views, respectively, of a maxillary first premolar that also forms from *four* lobes. Here the lingual lobe forms the lingual cusp. The divisions between the facial and lingual lobes are evidenced by the marginal ridge developmental grooves. Drawing **E** is a mandibular first molar with five lobes, three buccal and two lingual, which is one lobe per cusp. Drawing **F** is a maxillary first molar with three larger lobes and one smaller lobe, or one per cusp. The Carabelli cusp, when present, may form from a part of the large mesiolingual lobe or may form from a separate lobe.

Table 3-6	GUIDELINES FOR DETERMINING THE NUMBER OF LOBES FORMING EACH TOOTH	

TOOTH NAME (ANTERIOR OR PREMOLAR)	# LINGUAL CUSPS Or CINGULUM	# LOBES
Maxillary central incisor	Cingulum	3 + 1 = **4**
Maxillary lateral incisor	Cingulum	3 + 1 = **4**
Maxillary canine	Cingulum	3 + 1 = **4**
Maxillary 1 premolar	1 lingual	3 + 1 = **4**
Maxillary 2 premolar	1 lingual	3 + 1 = **4**
Mandibular central incisor	Cingulum	3 + 1 = **4**
Mandibular lateral incisor	Cingulum	3 + 1 = **4**
Mandibular canine	Cingulum	3 + 1 = **4**
Mandibular 1 premolar	1 lingual	3 + 1 = **4**
Mandibular 2 premolar	1 or 2 lingual	3 + 1 = **4** or 3 + 2 = **5**

Guideline for determining the number of lobes for anterior teeth and premolars:
Number of lobes = 3 facial lobes + 1 lobe per lingual cusp or cingulum

MOLAR NAME	# TOTAL CUSPS	# LOBES
Maxillary 1 molar	4 (or **5** if Carabelli)	4 (maybe **5** if Carabelli)
Maxillary 2 molar	4	4
Mandibular 1 molar	5	5
Mandibular 2 molar	4	4

Guideline for determining the number of molar lobes:
Number of molar lobes = 1 per cusp (including Carabelli)

gulum area and lingual cusp(s) each form from one lobe. Therefore, incisors develop from four lobes: *three facial* lobes forming three incisally located mamelons and *one lingual* lobe forming the cingulum area. Canines and most premolars also develop from four lobes: *three facial* lobes forming the facial portion and *one lingual* lobe forming the cingulum area on the canine and the one lingual cusp. An EXCEPTION is the *three-cusp* type (mandibular second) premolar, which has one buccal and two lingual cusps, and therefore forms from five lobes: three forming the facial cusp and two (one each) forming the two lingual cusps. The three lobes of the facial surface of anterior teeth and premolars are usually evidenced by the three very subtle vertical ridges separated by two depressions.

As a general rule, each molar cusp forms from one lobe. For example, the mandibular first molar has five cusps (three buccal and two lingual) and develops from five lobes. Only some maxillary third molars have as few as three lobes forming three cusps. Two types of tooth anomalies, peg-shaped maxillary lateral incisors and some extra teeth (also called supernumerary teeth), form from less than three lobes. Guidelines for determining the number of lobes that form each tooth is presented in Table 3-6.

LEARNING EXERCISE

Sketch a tooth and adjacent gingiva in cross section (as in Fig. 3-4) and label the following structures: enamel, dentin, cementum, pulp cavity, pulp chamber, apical foramen location, dentinoenamel junction, cementoenamel junction, dentinocemental junction, periodontal ligament space, alveolar bone, gingiva, gingival sulcus, anatomic crown, and anatomic root.

LEARNING QUESTIONS

These questions were designed to help you confirm that you understand the terms and concepts presented in this chapter. Answer each question by circling the letter (or letters) of the correct answer (or answers). More than one answer may be correct.

1. If you read an article in a British dental journal that refers to tooth #48, you would suspect that the authors were using the International Numbering System. What universal number (or letter) would they be talking about?
   a. 25
   b. J
   c. 30
   d. T
   e. 32

2. Using the Universal Numbering System, what numbers are used to identify maxillary canines?
   a. 6
   b. 8
   c. 10
   d. 11
   e. 27

3. Which tooth junctions are NOT normally visible on a handheld intact tooth?
   a. cementoenamel junction
   b. dentinoenamel junction
   c. dentinocemental junction
   d. dentinopulpal junction

4. Which statement(s) is (are) likely to be true on a person with a barely erupted tooth #9?
   a. The clinical crown is larger than the anatomic crown
   b. The clinical crown is smaller than the anatomic crown
   c. The clinical root is larger than the anatomic root
   d. The clinical root is smaller than the anatomic root

5. Which tooth surface(s) face(s) the lips or cheeks?
   a. facial
   b. distal
   c. buccal
   d. occlusal
   e. labial

6. Which pairs of teeth have a mesial surface touching a mesial surface?
   a. 25 and 26
   b. 16 and 17
   c. 7 and 8
   d. 1 and 32
   e. 8 and 9

7. When viewing tooth #8 from the distal view, it can be divided into thirds from the incisal to the cervical and from the facial to the lingual. Which third is NOT possible to see from the distal view?
   a. facial
   b. cervical
   c. middle
   d. mesial
   e. incisal

8. If you were observing the *faciolingual* length of a tooth, what surface(s) could you be viewing?
   a. mesial
   b. occlusal
   c. proximal
   d. labial
   e. distal

9. If the root-to-crown ratio of a maxillary molar (#14) is 1.72 and that of another molar, #16, is 1.49, which tooth has the longest *root* relative to its shorter *crown*?
   a. #14
   b. #16
   c. More information is required in order to answer this question

10. Which of the following bumps or ridges is NOT likely to be found on a maxillary premolar?
    a. oblique ridge
    b. cingulum
    c. mesial marginal ridge
    d. transverse ridge
    e. triangular ridge

11. Which ridges may help *surround* the perimeter of the occlusal surface of a premolar?
    a. mesial marginal ridge
    b. distal marginal ridge
    c. mesial cusp ridge of the buccal cusp
    d. distal cusp ridge of the lingual cusp
    e. transverse ridge

12. What is the correct order of anatomic landmarks of a tooth with two roots from the cementoenamel junction to the root tip?
    a. cervix, trunk, furcation, apex
    b. trunk, cervix, furcation, apex
    c. trunk, furcation, cervix, apex
    d. cervix, trunk, apex, furcation
    e. furcation, trunk, cervix, apex

13. When viewed from the proximal views, what is the location of the greatest bulge (crest of curvature or height of contour) on the *facial* surface of *all* teeth?
    a. occlusal third
    b. lingual third
    c. buccal third
    d. middle third
    e. cervical third

14. Which space(s) contain(s) the part of the gingiva known as the interdental papilla?
    a. the buccal embrasure
    b. occlusal embrasure
    c. lingual embrasure
    d. cervical embrasure
    e. interproximal space

15. Ideal class I occlusion involves an important first permanent molar relationship where the mesiobuccal cusp of the maxillary first molar is located within the:
    a. mesiobuccal groove of the mandibular first molar
    b. distobuccal groove of the mandibular first molar
    c. buccal groove of the mandibular second molar
    d. mesiobuccal groove of the mandibular second molar
    e. distobuccal groove of the mandibular second molar

16. Where do *lingual* cusps of *maxillary* teeth occlude in ideal class I occlusion?
    a. in the buccal embrasure space between mandibular teeth
    b. in the lingual embrasure space between mandibular teeth
    c. in the occlusal embrasure space between mandibular teeth
    d. in occlusal fossae of mandibular teeth

17. How many developmental lobes form a premolar with two cusps (one buccal cusp and one lingual cusp)?
    a. 1
    b. 2
    c. 3
    d. 4
    e. 5

ANSWERS: 1-e; 2-a, d; 3-b, c, d; 4-b, c; 5-a, c; 6-e; 7-d; 8-a, b, c, e; 9-a; 10-a, b; 11-a, b, c, d; 12-a; 13-e; 14-d, e; 15-a; 16-d; 17-d.

REFERENCES

1. Ash MM. Wheeler's dental anatomy, physiology, and occlusion. 7th ed. Philadelphia: W.B. Saunders, 1993.

GENERAL REFERENCES

Jordan R, Abrams L, Kraus B. Kraus' dental anatomy and occlusion. St. Louis: Mosby Year Book, 1992.

Melfi RC. Oral embryology and microscopic anatomy, a textbook for students in dental hygiene. 8th ed. Philadelphia: Lea and Febiger, 1988.

Renner RP. An introduction to dental anatomy and esthetics. Chicago: Quintessence Publishing, 1985.

4

Morphology of the Permanent Incisors

Topics covered within the three sections of this chapter include the following:

I. General description of incisors
   - A. Functions of incisors
   - B. Morphology of incisors
   - C. Class traits for all incisors
   - D. Arch traits that distinguish maxillary from mandibular incisors
II. Maxillary incisor type traits: similarities and differences useful to distinguish maxillary central incisors from maxillary lateral incisors (from all views)
   - A. Maxillary incisors from the *labial view*
   - B. Maxillary incisors from the *lingual view*
   - C. Maxillary incisors from the *proximal views*
   - D. Maxillary incisors from the *incisal view*
   - E. Variations in maxillary incisors
III. Mandibular incisor type traits: similarities and differences useful to distinguish mandibular central incisors from mandibular lateral incisors (from all views)
   - A. Mandibular incisors from the *labial view*
   - B. Mandibular incisors from the *lingual view*
   - C. Mandibular incisors from the *proximal views*
   - D. Mandibular incisors from the *incisal view*
   - E. Variations in mandibular incisors

Using the maxillary right lateral incisor as a representative example for all incisors, refer to page 1 of the Appendix while reading Section I of this chapter. Within this text, the word "Appendix" followed by a number and letter (e.g., Appendix 1a) is used to denote the appendix page (number 1) and item (letter a) being referenced. The appendix pages are designed to be torn out to facilitate study and minimize page turns as you read the main text. Other appendix pages will be referred to throughout this and several chapters that follow. Notice that the trait being demonstrated by each letter on the appendix pages is described on the back of each appendix page.

SECTION I GENERAL DESCRIPTION OF INCISORS

OBJECTIVES

This section is designed to prepare the learner to perform the following:

- Describe the functions of incisors.
- List class traits common to all incisors.
- List arch traits that can be used to distinguish maxillary from mandibular incisors.
- From a selection of all teeth, select and separate out the incisors.
- Divide a selection of all incisors into maxillary and mandibular (using arch traits).

Refer to *Figure 4-1* or, better yet, to a model of the complete set of permanent teeth while becoming familiar with the location and universal number of each incisor. There are four maxillary incisors: two central incisors (first maxillary incisors: universal numbers 8 and 9) and two lateral incisors (second maxillary incisors: numbers 7 and 10). There are four mandibular incisors: two central incisors (first mandibular incisors: numbers 24 and 25) and two lateral incisors (second mandibular incisors: numbers 23 and 26).

Central incisors are located on either side in their respective arch (maxillary or mandibular) with their mesial surfaces next to one another at the midline, usually in contact. (If there is a space between these or other teeth, it is called a **diastema** [die a STEE mah].) Their distal surfaces contact the mesial surfaces of the lateral

144

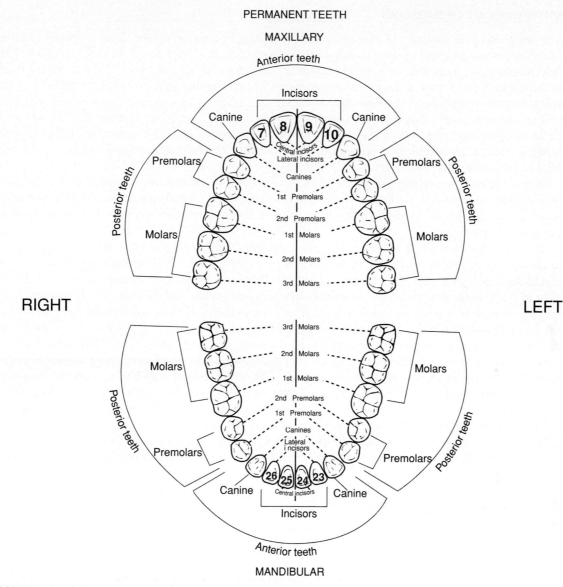

PERMANENT TEETH

MAXILLARY

FIGURE 4-1. Adult dentition with Universal numbers on the incisors highlighted in red.

incisors. Lateral incisors are therefore just distal to central incisors, while their mesial surfaces are in contact with the distal surfaces of the adjacent central incisors. Their distal surfaces contact the canines. (Did you know that the tusks on an elephant are maxillary central incisors? [Recall Table 1-1.] Elephants have the largest diastema in the world, large enough for the massive trunk between their central incisors.)

A. FUNCTIONS OF INCISORS

The mandibular incisors function with the maxillary incisors to (a) cut food (mandibular incisors are moving blades against the stationary maxillary incisors), (b) enable articulate speech (consider the enunciation of a toothless person), and (c) help to support the lip and maintain an esthetic appearance. By current standards, a person lacking one or more incisors has an undesirable appearance. (Did you ever hear the song "All I want for Christmas are my two front teeth"?) Their fourth function, by fitting the incisal edges of the mandibular incisors against the lingual surfaces of the maxillary incisors, is to (d) help guide the mandible posteriorly during the final phase of closing just before the posterior teeth contact.

B. MORPHOLOGY OF INCISORS

The morphology, or anatomy, of a tooth can best be studied by considering the shape (outline) and contours (ridges and grooves) visible on each tooth surface. All tooth crowns have five surfaces, that is, four side surfaces plus a chewing or cutting surface or edge, depending on whether it is a posterior tooth (chewing in the back part of the mouth) or an anterior tooth (cutting in the front of the mouth). In the study of tooth morphology, the description and location of the ridges, grooves, convexities, and concavities on each tooth surface should be well fixed in your mind in order to describe and identify teeth by arch, class, type, and side of the mouth; to reproduce tooth contours when constructing crowns, bridges, and fillings; to remove deposits (tartar and calculus) skillfully from crowns and roots; or to finish and polish existing restorations.

When discussing traits, the external morphology of an incisor is customarily described from each of five views: (a) **facial** (or labial), (b) **lingual** (tongue side), (c) **mesial,** (d) **distal,** and (e) **incisal.** Due to similarities between the mesial and distal, these surfaces will be discussed together in this text under the heading of **proximal** surfaces.

In the study of any single type of human tooth, such as the maxillary central incisor, it is necessary to realize that this tooth varies in form in different people as much as facial features vary from one person to another. One study of a collection of 100 maxillary central incisors showed considerable difference in such characteristics as size, relative proportions, and color.[1] Information in this text on crown length, crown width, and root length is taken from measurements of extracted teeth by Dr. Woelfel and his dental hygiene students at Ohio State University between 1974 and 1979. Teeth were collected from dentists in Ohio. The ranges indicate how greatly the same tooth can vary in size. Study *Table 4-1A* and *B* to compare average measurements. Notice that the crown of the maxillary central incisor is longer than all other incisor crowns, and the mesiodistal width of the roots of mandibular incisors are considerable narrower (ribbon-like) compared to maxillary incisors. Also, notice the range of difference between measurements for the same tooth type. For example, among the 398 maxillary central incisors measured, one central incisor was 16 mm longer than the shortest one. There was a lesser, but still considerable, range in crown length (6 mm) and in crown width (3 mm) from the smallest to the largest tooth found in this sample. *Specific data collected from Dr. Woelfel's studies are presented throughout the text in brackets [like this].*

C. CLASS TRAITS FOR ALL INCISORS

First, consider the class traits of incisors, that is, traits that apply to *all* incisors.

Developmental lobes: Recall from Chapter 3 that the *facial* surface of all anterior teeth forms from three labial portions called the mesial, middle, and distal lobes. Incisors usually have two shallow vertical developmental depressions separating the parts of the facial surface formed by these three lobes. These depressions are denoted by the subtle shading on the drawings in Figure 4-4. The three lobes also contribute to three rounded "bumps" on the incisal edge called **mamelons,** located on the incisal edges of newly erupted incisor teeth (*Fig. 4-2*). Finally, remember that a fourth (*lingual*) lobe forms the

Table 4-1A	SIZE OF MAXILLARY INCISORS (MILLIMETERS)				
	398 CENTRALS			**295 LATERALS**	
DIMENSION MEASURED	Average	Range	Average	Range	
Crown length	11.2	8.6–14.7	9.8	7.4–11.9	
Root length	13.0	6.3–20.3	13.4	9.6–19.4	
Overall length	23.6	16.5–32.6	22.5	17.7–28.9	
Crown width (mesiodistal)	8.6	7.1–10.5	6.6	5.0–9.0	
Root width (cervix)	6.4	5.0–8.0	4.7	3.4–6.4	
Faciolingual crown size	7.1	6.0–8.5	6.2	5.3–7.3	
Faciolingual root (cervix)	6.4	5.1–7.8	5.8	4.5–7.0	
Mesial cervical curve	2.8	1.4–4.8	2.5	1.3–4.0	
Distal cervical curve	2.3	0.7–4.0	1.9	0.8–3.7	

Table 4-1B   SIZE OF MANDIBULAR INCISORS (MILLIMETERS)

DIMENSION MEASURED	226 CENTRALS		234 LATERALS	
	Average	Range	Average	Range
Crown length	8.8	6.3–11.6	9.4	7.3–12.6
Root length	12.6	7.7–17.9	13.5	9.4–18.1
Overall length	20.8	16.9–26.7	22.1	18.5–26.6
Crown width (mesiodistal)	5.3	4.4–6.7	5.7	4.6–8.2
Root width (cervix)	3.5	2.7–4.6	3.8	3.0–4.9
Faciolingual crown size	5.7	4.8–6.8	6.1	5.2–7.4
Faciolingual root (cervix)	5.4	4.3–6.5	5.8	4.3–6.8
Mesial cervical curve	2.0	1.0–3.3	2.1	1.0–3.6
Distal cervical curve	1.6	0.6–2.8	1.5	0.8–2.4

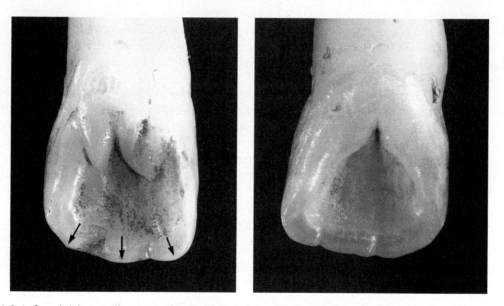

FIGURE 4-2. Left and right maxillary central incisors, *lingual views.* Both teeth are "*shovel shaped*" due to their deep lingual fossae along with pronounced lingual marginal ridges and cingula. Both teeth have three rounded protuberances on their incisal edge called *mamelons* (*arrows*). The right tooth has a stained *pit* on the incisal border of the cingulum where caries can penetrate without being easily noticed.

Table 4-2   GUIDELINE FOR DETERMINING THE NUMBER OF LOBES FOR INCISORS*

TOOTH NAME (ANTERIOR OR PREMOLAR)	CINGULUM?	# LOBES
Maxillary central incisor	Yes	3 + 1 = 4
Maxillary lateral incisor	Yes	3 + 1 = 4
Mandibular central incisor	Yes	3 + 1 = 4
Mandibular lateral incisor	Yes	3 + 1 = 4

* Number of lobes = 3 facial lobes + 1 lobe per cingulum

lingual bulge called a cingulum. See *Table 4-2* for a summary of the number of lobes forming each type of incisor.

1. CHARACTERISTICS OF ALL INCISORS FROM THE FACIAL VIEW

Refer to page 1 of the Appendix while studying the similarities of *all* incisors. (Note that there may be exceptions to the general incisor traits presented here, and these are noted in capital letters.)

All incisor *crowns,* when viewed from the *facial,* have a relatively straight or slightly curved incisal edge (versus all other teeth that have one or more pointed cusp tips). Their crowns are relatively rectangular, longer incisogingivally than wide mesiodistally (Appendix 1a). They taper (narrower) from the widest mesiodistal areas of proximal contact toward the cervical line and are therefore narrowest in the cervical third and broader toward the incisal third (Appendix 1b). Incisor crown outlines are more convex on the distal than on the mesial sides EXCEPT the mandibular central, which is symmetrical (Appendix 1c). Incisor mesioincisal angles are more acute (sharper) than distoincisal angles EXCEPT on the symmetrical mandibular central incisors, where the angles are not noticeably different (Appendix 1d). Incisor crown contact areas (greatest height of contour proximally) on mesial surfaces are located in the incisal third. On the distal surfaces, the contact areas are more cervical than the mesial EXCEPT on the distal of the mandibular central, which is at the same level as the mesial due to its symmetry (Appendix 1e). Before wear, the incisal edge of all incisors EXCEPT the symmetrical mandibular central slopes cervically (appears shorter) toward the distal. Finally, the cervical line curves toward the apex in the middle of the facial (and lingual) sides (Appendix 1l).

Incisor *roots,* when viewed from the *facial,* taper (become more narrow) from the cervical line to the apex (Appendix 1f). They are wider faciolingually than mesiodistally EXCEPT that maxillary central incisors, where the mesiodistal width is approximately the same as the faciolingual thickness (compare the widths of facial and mesial root surface by viewing the facial and mesial root views in Appendix 1g). Incisor roots may bend in the apical one-third EXCEPT maxillary central incisor roots, which are not as likely to bend; this bend is more often toward the distal (Appendix 1h). Incisor roots are longer than the crowns (Appendix 1i).

2. CHARACTERISTICS OF ALL INCISORS FROM THE LINGUAL VIEW

Incisor *crowns,* when viewed from the *lingual,* have a narrower lingual surface because the mesial and distal sides converge lingually (best appreciated from the incisal view, Appendix 1j). The mesial and distal marginal ridges converge toward the lingual cingulum (Appendix 1k).

3. CHARACTERISTICS OF ALL INCISORS FROM THE PROXIMAL VIEWS

Incisor *crowns,* when viewed from the *proximal,* are wedge shaped or triangular (Appendix 1m). They have a *facial* height of contour (greatest bulge) that is in the cervical third just incisal to the cervical line and are therefore more convex cervically than incisally on their labial surfaces (Appendix 1n). The *lingual* height of contour is also in the cervical third on the cingulum, but the contour of the incisal two-thirds of the lingual surface is concave from cingulum area to the incisal edge. Therefore, the lingual outline is S-shaped, being convex over the cingulum and concave from the cingulum nearly to the incisal edge (Appendix 1p). The lingual concavity on the maxillary anterior teeth is a most important guiding factor in the closing movements of the lower jaw because the mandibular incisors fit into this concavity and against marginal ridges of the maxillary incisors as maximum closure or occlusion is approached. The cervical line proximally curves toward the incisal edge. The resultant curve is greater on the mesial surface than on the distal (compare the mesial and distal views in Appendix 1o).

The incisor *roots,* when viewed from the *proximal,* are widest at the cervical and gradually taper to a rounded apex (Appendix 1f). All may have a longitudinal depression in the middle third of the *mesial* root surface, but the mesial root depression is most evident on mandibular incisors, and is minimal or not present on the mesial root surface of a maxillary incisor. (Only mandibular central and lateral incisors also have a prominent longitudinal depression on the *distal* root surface.)

4. CHARACTERISTICS OF ALL INCISORS FROM THE INCISAL VIEW

The *crowns*, when viewed from the *incisal*, have a lingual fossa that is concave just incisal to the cingulum. They have an incisal ridge that terminates mesiodistally at the widest portion of the crown (Appendix 1q). The labial outline is broader and less curved than the convex lingual outline (Appendix 1r). Marginal ridges converge toward the cingulum (Appendix 1k), and the crown outline tapers from proximal contact area toward the cingulum (Appendix 1j), resulting in a narrower lingual than labial side.

D. ARCH TRAITS THAT DISTINGUISH MAXILLARY FROM MANDIBULAR INCISORS

Refer to page 2 of the Appendix while reading about these arch traits that can be used to distinguish mandibular incisors from maxillary incisors.

The **mandibular incisors** (relative to the maxillary incisors) are generally smaller than maxillary incisors. Mandibular central and lateral incisors look more alike and are more nearly the same size in the same mouth, compared to greater differences between maxillary central and lateral incisors. *Mandibular* incisor crowns are flatter than maxillary incisor crowns on the mesial and distal sides (Appendix 2q) and have contact areas located nearer the incisal ridge than maxillary incisors (Appendix 2r and 2i). *Mandibular* incisor crowns are relatively wider faciolingually than mesiodistally compared to maxillary central incisors, which are wider mesiodistally (Appendix 2h). *Mandibular* incisor crowns also have smoother lingual surfaces with less prominent anatomy than maxillary crowns, which have deeper fossae and more pronounced marginal ridges (Appendix 2m). Finally, *mandibular* incisor roots are longer in proportion to their crowns than are maxillary incisors.

Incisal edges of *mandibular incisors* are usually positioned lingual to the root axis line, whereas the incisal edges of *maxillary incisors* are more often on or labial to the root axis line (best seen from the proximal views on Appendix 2o). Attrition on the incisal edges of incisors that occurs when shearing or incising food results in tooth wear that is in a different location on maxillary incisors compared to mandibular incisors (*Fig. 4-3*). This wear occurs when the labial part of the incisal edges of mandibu-

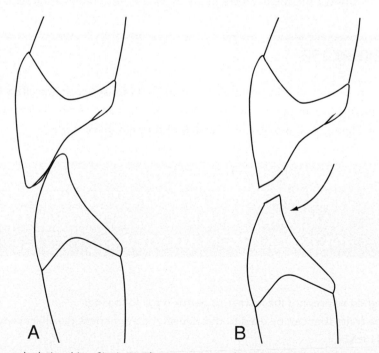

FIGURE 4-3. A. The normal relationship of incisors when posterior teeth are biting tightly together. **B.** The arrow indicates the direction of movement of the mandibular incisor moving forward with the mandible (protruding), so the incisors work edge to edge during incision. The resultant *wear pattern* or facets on the incisal edges of *maxillary* incisors occurs more onto the lingual surface (wear facets slope cervically toward the lingual), whereas wear occurs primarily on the facial surface of *mandibular* incisors (wear facets slope cervically toward the labial).

Table 4-3	MAJOR ARCH TRAITS THAT DISTINGUISH MAXILLARY FROM MANDIBULAR INCISORS	

	MAXILLARY INCISORS	MANDIBULAR INCISORS
LABIAL VIEW	Wider crowns mesiodistally Less symmetrical crown More rounded mesial (M) and distal (D) incisal angles Contact areas more cervical	Narrower crowns mesiodistally More symmetrical crowns More square M and D incisal angles Contact areas very incisal

LINGUAL VIEW	Lingual anatomy more distinct:
	    Pronounced marginal ridges
	    Deeper lingual fossa
	    Sometimes lingual pits
	    Larger cingulum
		Lingual surface smoother:
		    Almost no marginal ridges
		    Shallower lingual fossa
		    No pits
		    Smaller cingulum

PROXIMAL VIEWS	Incisal edge on or labial to root axis line Facets on lingual slope of incisal edge Mesial root surfaces are more convex	Incisal edge on or lingual to root axis line Facets on labial slope of incisal edge Mesial root surfaces have depressions
INCISAL VIEW	Crowns wider mesiodistally (MD) than faciolingually (FL) Plus the five traits seen from lingual view can also be seen from the incisal view	Crowns wider FL than MD

lar incisors slides forward and downward while contacting the lingual surface and part of the incisal edge of opposing maxillary incisors. The wear results in a shiny, flat, polished surface of enamel on the incisal edge called a **facet** [FAS it]. Assuming a normal tooth relationship, facets that commonly form on mandibular incisors are more on the labial slope of the incisal edge, sloping cervically toward the labial. In contrast, facets on *maxillary incisors* occur more on the lingual slope of the incisal edge, sloping cervically toward the lingual fossa and may occur on the lingual marginal ridges.

LEARNING EXERCISE

Refer to *Table 4-3* for a summary of the noticeable arch traits that distinguish maxillary from mandibular incisors and see how many of them can be used to differentiate the rows of maxillary and mandibular incisors from various views in Figures 4-4, 4-5, 4-7, 4-9, and 4-13 through 4-16.

SECTION II	MAXILLARY INCISOR TYPE TRAITS: SIMILARITIES AND DIFFERENCES USEFUL TO DISTINGUISH MAXILLARY CENTRAL INCISORS FROM LATERAL INCISORS (FROM ALL VIEWS)

OBJECTIVES

This section is designed to prepare the learner to perform the following:
- Describe the type traits that can be used to distinguish the permanent maxillary central incisor from the maxillary lateral incisor.
- Describe and identify the labial, lingual, mesial, distal, and incisal surfaces for all maxillary incisors.
- Assign a universal number to maxillary incisors present in a mouth (or on a model) with complete dentition. If possible, repeat this on a model with one or more maxillary incisors missing.
- Select and separate maxillary incisors from a selection of all teeth on a bench top.

- Holding a maxillary incisor, determine whether it is a central or a lateral and right or left. Then assign a universal number to it.

Within this section, the maxillary central and lateral incisors will be compared for similarities and differences. These differences are presented for each view of the tooth: facial, lingual, proximal (mesial and distal), and incisal.

A. MAXILLARY INCISORS FROM THE LABIAL VIEW

LEARNING EXERCISE

Examine several extracted maxillary central and lateral incisors and/or tooth models as you read. Hold these teeth root up and crown down, as they are positioned in the mouth. Also, tear out and refer to Appendix page 2 and refer to *Figure 4-4* as you study about the labial traits of incisors.

1. CROWN SHAPE OF MAXILLARY INCISORS FROM THE LABIAL VIEW

The *crown* of the **maxillary central incisor** is the longest [average: 11.2 mm] of all human tooth crowns (although maxillary canines are the longest teeth overall) and is also the widest of all incisors. (One text states that the mandibular canine crown is the longest crown overall.[9]) The crown is usually longer (incisogingivally) than wide (mesiodistally) [averaging 2.6 mm longer] (Appendix 2a). The crown is narrowest in the cervical third and becomes broader toward the incisal third.

There is great morphologic variation in the **maxillary lateral incisor.** It may be missing altogether; it may resemble a small slender version of a maxillary central incisor; it may be quite asymmetrical; or it may be peg shaped (as seen later in Chapter 12). Normally, the labial surface of the maxillary lateral incisor is much like that of the central incisor, but it is more convex or less flat mesiodistally and overall it appears narrower mesiodistally. Mamelons, and particularly labial depressions, are less prominent and less common than on the central incisor.

The crown of the average *maxillary lateral incisor* is narrower [about 2 mm] than the crown of the central incisor, and the root is longer [about 0.5 mm], giving this entire tooth a long, slender look (Appendix 2a and 2d). The crown outline is less symmetrical than the central incisor.

2. MAXILLARY INCISOR INCISAL-PROXIMAL CROWN ANGLE FROM THE LABIAL VIEW

On **maxillary central incisors,** the corner or angle formed by the mesial and incisal surfaces (called the mesioincisal angle) forms nearly a right angle. The distoincisal corner is more rounded, and the angle is slightly obtuse or greater than a right angle (Appendix 2b).

On **maxillary lateral incisors,** both the mesioincisal and distoincisal angles are more rounded than on the central incisor (Appendix 2b). The mesioincisal angle is more acute than the distoincisal angle, accentuated by the incisal edge sloping cervically toward the distal (more so than on the maxillary central incisor) (Appendix 2c).

3. PROXIMAL CONTACT AREAS OF MAXILLARY INCISORS FROM THE LABIAL VIEW

For all human teeth, contact areas are located in one of three places: in the incisal (occlusal) third, at the junction of the incisal and middle thirds, or in the middle third of the crown. Tooth contact areas are not normally located in the cervical third of teeth. The *mesial* contacts of *both* a maxillary central and lateral incisor are in the incisal third, very near the incisal edge for the central and slightly more cervical for the lateral. The *distal* contacts of *both* incisors are more cervical than the mesial: for a **maxillary central incisor**, it is near the junction of the incisal and the middle thirds; for the **maxillary lateral incisor** it is even more cervical, sometimes in the middle third (making this contact the most cervical for any incisor).

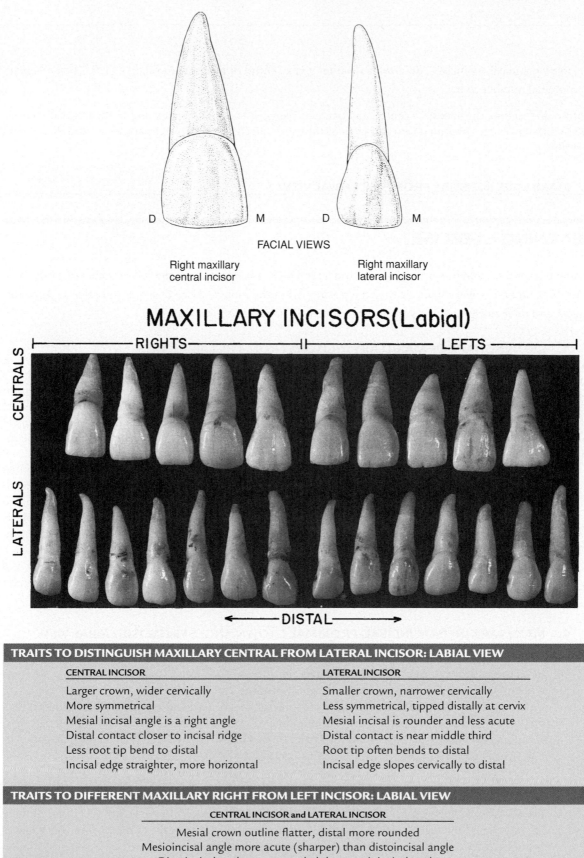

FACIAL VIEWS

Right maxillary
central incisor

Right maxillary
lateral incisor

MAXILLARY INCISORS (Labial)

RIGHTS — LEFTS

CENTRALS

LATERALS

DISTAL

TRAITS TO DISTINGUISH MAXILLARY CENTRAL FROM LATERAL INCISOR: LABIAL VIEW	
CENTRAL INCISOR	**LATERAL INCISOR**
Larger crown, wider cervically	Smaller crown, narrower cervically
More symmetrical	Less symmetrical, tipped distally at cervix
Mesial incisal angle is a right angle	Mesial incisal is rounder and less acute
Distal contact closer to incisal ridge	Distal contact is near middle third
Less root tip bend to distal	Root tip often bends to distal
Incisal edge straighter, more horizontal	Incisal edge slopes cervically to distal

TRAITS TO DIFFERENT MAXILLARY RIGHT FROM LEFT INCISOR: LABIAL VIEW
CENTRAL INCISOR and LATERAL INCISOR
Mesial crown outline flatter, distal more rounded
Mesioincisal angle more acute (sharper) than distoincisal angle
Distoincisal angle more rounded than mesioincisal angle
Distal contact more cervical than mesial contact

FIGURE 4-4. Maxillary central and lateral incisors, **labial views,** with type traits that distinguish maxillary central from lateral incisors and traits that distinguish right and left sides.

4. ROOT-TO-CROWN PROPORTIONS OF MAXILLARY INCISORS FROM THE LABIAL VIEW

On a **maxillary central incisor,** the root is only slightly longer than the crown [root-to-crown ratio is 1.16:1] (Appendix 2d). The **maxillary lateral incisor** root is longer than on the central [by 0.4 mm with a root-to-crown ratio of 1.37, comparing measurements of 398 maxillary central incisors and 295 lateral incisors]. This results in a root that appears longer in proportion to the crown than on the maxillary central incisor.

5. ROOT SHAPE OF MAXILLARY INCISORS FROM THE LABIAL VIEW (COMPARED WITH THE PROXIMAL VIEW)

The root of the **maxillary central incisor** is thick in the cervical third and narrows through the middle to a blunt apex. Its outline and shape is much like an ice cream cone. An apical bend is *not* common in the maxillary central incisor. The central incisor root is the only maxillary tooth that is as thick at the cervix mesiodistally as faciolingually [6.4 mm]. Compare the root width seen on the proximal view to the root width seen on the labial view in Appendix 2n. The seven other types of maxillary teeth have roots that are thicker faciolingually than mesiodistally [ranging from 1.1 to 3.4 mm thicker for the lateral incisors and premolars, respectively]. Because of its shortness and conical shape, the maxillary central incisor root may be a poor risk to support a replacement tooth as part of a dental bridge (that is, a replacement tooth crown attached to, and supported by, two adjacent teeth).

The root of a **maxillary lateral incisor** tapers evenly toward the rounded apex, and the apical end is commonly bent distally [12 of the 14 maxillary lateral incisors in *Fig. 4-4,* lower row).

B. MAXILLARY INCISORS FROM THE LINGUAL VIEW

Refer to *Figure 4-5* while studying about the lingual traits of maxillary incisors.

1. LINGUAL FOSSAE OF MAXILLARY INCISORS FROM THE LINGUAL VIEW

The large lingual fossa is located immediately incisal to the cingulum and bounded by two marginal ridges. The fossae of both maxillary incisors may be either shallow or deep, but either way they are usually deeper than fossae in *mandibular* incisors. Maxillary incisors with a deep lingual fossa and prominent mesial and distal marginal ridges are called "shovel-shaped incisors" (as seen in Fig. 4-2).[2–6] [Dr. Woelfel examined the maxillary incisors on casts of 715 dental hygiene students and found that 32% of the central incisors and 27% of the lateral incisors have some degree of shoveling. The rest had smooth concave lingual surfaces without prominent marginal ridges or deep fossae.] The lingual fossa of the *maxillary lateral incisor,* although smaller in area, is often even more pronounced than on the central incisor. Note the deeper lingual fossae on many maxillary lateral incisors compared to central incisors in Figure 4-5.

2. CINGULUM OF MAXILLARY INCISORS FROM THE LINGUAL VIEW

The cingulum on the **maxillary central incisor** is usually well developed and is located off-center, distal to the root axis line that bisects the root longitudinally. (This can also be seen from the incisal view.) The cingulum of the **maxillary lateral incisor** is narrower than on the central, and it is almost centered on the root axis line (Appendix 2e).

3. MARGINAL RIDGES OF MAXILLARY INCISORS FROM THE LINGUAL VIEW

The mesial and distal marginal ridges vary in prominence on *all maxillary incisors* from one person to another. They may be prominent or inconspicuous. They may also have been worn smooth (forming facets) from attrition or chewing by the mandibular incisors. Due to the distal placement of the cingulum and incisal edge slope cervically toward the distal, the mesial marginal ridge of the **maxillary central incisor** (from proximal contact area to cingulum) is longer than its distal marginal ridge. On the **maxillary lateral incisor,** the distal marginal ridge is also shorter than the mesial, because the incisal edge slopes cervically from mesial to distal, even more so than on the central (Appendix 2f). The longer mesial marginal ridge of the maxillary lateral incisor outline is nearly

Maxillary Incisors (Lingual)

Lefts　　　　　　　　　　　　　　　　**Rights**

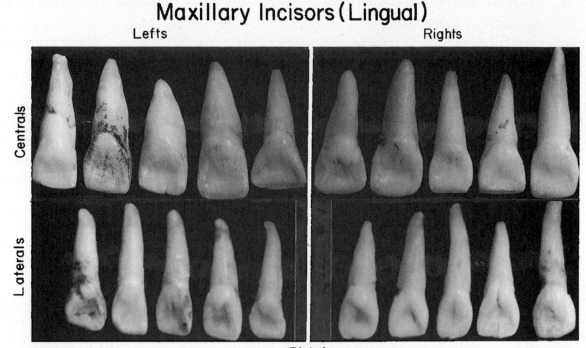

Centrals

Laterals

← Distal →

TRAITS TO DISTINGUISH MAXILLARY CENTRAL FROM LATERAL INCISOR: LINGUAL VIEW	
CENTRAL INCISOR	**LATERAL INCISOR**
Larger shallow lingual fossa	Deep but small fossa
Cingulum distally positioned	Cingulum centered
Less frequent lingual pits	More common lingual pits
Plus six outline characteristics seen from facial apply to lingual outline	

TRAITS TO DIFFERENTIATE MAXILLARY RIGHT FROM LEFT INCISOR: LINGUAL VIEW	
CENTRAL INCISOR	**LATERAL INCISOR**
Cingulum toward distal	Longer and straighter mesial (M) marginal ridge
	Distal marginal ridge more curved than M
Longer mesiolingual marginal ridge	
Plus four outline characteristics from facial also apply to lingual outline	

FIGURE 4-5. Maxillary central and lateral incisors, **lingual views,** with type traits that distinguish maxillary central from lateral incisors and traits that distinguish right and left sides.

straight, while the shorter distal marginal ridge outline is curved cervicoincisally, as on the central incisor. Note the shorter, more rounded distal marginal ridges compared to mesial marginal ridges in most lateral incisors in Figure 4-5.

4. MAXILLARY INCISOR PITS AND ACCESSORY RIDGES FROM THE LINGUAL VIEW

The lingual anatomy of the **maxillary central incisor** is variable. Its fossa may be deep but smooth, that is, with no lingual ridges bordering the fossa. Accessory lingual ridges, if present, are small or narrow, and extend vertically from the cingulum toward the center of the fossa. Accessory ridges may be one, two, three, or four in number (on *Fig. 4-6* tooth #9 shows these accessory ridges most clearly). Tiny grooves separate these ridges. [Inspection of 506 maxillary central incisors by Dr. Woelfel revealed 36% with none of these ridges, 27% with one small ridge, 28% with two accessory ridges, 9% with three ridges, and only three teeth with four small ridges.]

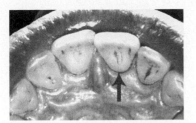

FIGURE 4-6. The lingual surfaces of these maxillary incisors reveal accessory ridges, especially on tooth #9 (at the *arrow*).

The **maxillary lateral incisor** may also have small vertical accessory lingual ridges on and incisal to the cingulum, only they are fewer in number and less common. [Inspection of 488 maxillary lateral incisors by Dr. Woelfel revealed 64% with none of these small ridges, 32% with one small accessory ridge, and only 4% with two ridges.]

On *both* maxillary incisors, but more frequently in lateral incisors, a lingual pit may be detectable at the incisal border of the cingulum where the mesial and distal marginal ridges converge. This pit may need to be restored or filled by the dentist to arrest decay, especially on maxillary lateral incisors. (Notice the deep lingual pits in several maxillary lateral incisors in *Fig. 4-5*.)

5. ROOT SHAPE OF MAXILLARY INCISORS FROM THE LINGUAL VIEW

The root contour of *all maxillary incisors,* like all anterior teeth, is convex and tapers, becoming narrower toward the lingual side *(Fig. 4-5)*.

C. MAXILLARY INCISORS FROM THE PROXIMAL VIEWS

Refer to *Figure 4-7* while studying about the proximal traits of maxillary incisors.

1. INCISAL EDGE OF MAXILLARY INCISORS FROM THE PROXIMAL VIEWS

On *both* maxillary incisors, the incisal edge is commonly just *labial* to the root axis line or may be on the root axis line (Appendix 2o). When viewed from the distal, the distoincisal edge (corner) of the **maxillary central incisor** is on or just *lingual* to the axis line because of a slight distolingual twist of the incisal edge (seen incisally in Appendix 2g).

2. CERVICAL LINE OF MAXILLARY INCISORS FROM THE PROXIMAL VIEWS

As on all anterior teeth, the cervical line of all maxillary incisors curves incisally on the mesial and distal tooth surfaces, and this curvature is greater on the mesial surface than on the distal surface (as seen in *Fig. 4-8* where a drawing of a mandibular canine is used to demonstrate this concept for all anterior teeth). This difference is most pronounced on the anterior teeth. The *mesial* curvature of the cervical line of the **maxillary central incisor** is larger than for any other tooth [average: 2.8 mm] extending incisally one-fourth of the crown length, whereas the *distal* cervical line curves less [on average 2.3 mm]. The curvature of the *mesial* cervical line of the **maxillary lateral incisor** is also considerable but slightly less than on the central [averaging 2.5 mm or one-fourth of the crown length].

3. HEIGHT (CREST) OF CONTOUR OF MAXILLARY INCISORS FROM THE PROXIMAL VIEWS

On the labial outline, the height of contour on *all* maxillary incisors is in the cervical third, just incisal to the cervical line. The outline becomes nearly flat in the middle and incisal thirds. On the lingual, the height of contour is also in the cervical third, on the cingulum.

4. MAXILLARY INCISOR ROOT AND ROOT DEPRESSIONS FROM THE PROXIMAL VIEWS

The root of the **maxillary central incisor** is wide faciolingually at the cervix and tapers to a rounded apex. The lingual outline is nearly straight in the cervical third, then curves labially toward the tip in the middle and apical thirds. The labial outline is less convex (more nearly straight). In contrast, the

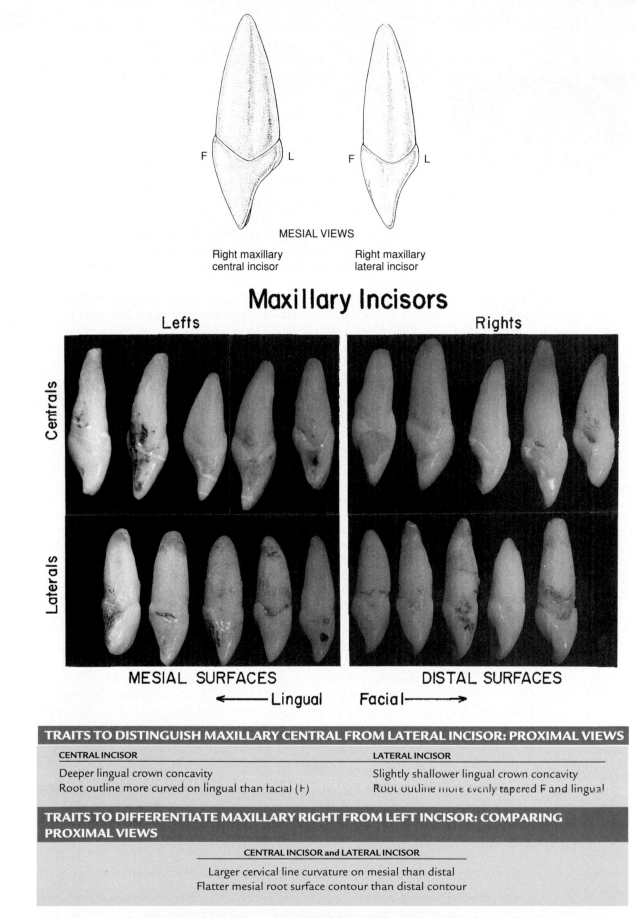

MESIAL VIEWS

Right maxillary
central incisor

Right maxillary
lateral incisor

Maxillary Incisors

Lefts

Rights

Centrals

Laterals

MESIAL SURFACES

DISTAL SURFACES

⟵ Lingual

Facial ⟶

TRAITS TO DISTINGUISH MAXILLARY CENTRAL FROM LATERAL INCISOR: PROXIMAL VIEWS	
CENTRAL INCISOR	**LATERAL INCISOR**
Deeper lingual crown concavity	Slightly shallower lingual crown concavity
Root outline more curved on lingual than facial (F)	Root outline more evenly tapered F and lingual

TRAITS TO DIFFERENTIATE MAXILLARY RIGHT FROM LEFT INCISOR: COMPARING PROXIMAL VIEWS
CENTRAL INCISOR and LATERAL INCISOR
Larger cervical line curvature on mesial than distal
Flatter mesial root surface contour than distal contour

FIGURE 4-7. Maxillary central and lateral incisors, **proximal views,** with type traits that distinguish maxillary central from lateral incisors and traits that distinguish right and left sides.

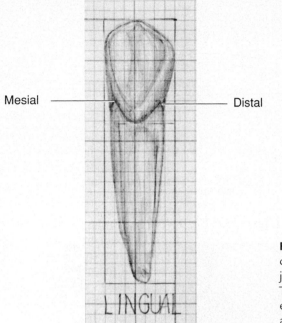

Mesial —————— ———— Distal

LINGUAL

FIGURE 4-8. Lingual view of a mandibular canine shows the difference in the amount of curvature of the cementoenamel junction (CEJ) on the mesial versus distal surface of the tooth. The CEJ on the mesial surface curves more toward the incisal edge than it does on the distal surface. This trait is evident on all incisors and canines (and most posterior teeth as well).

root of the **maxillary lateral incisor** tapers more evenly throughout the root toward the blunt apex. From the proximal view, this flatter facial root outline and more convex lingual root outline is evident in many incisors (especially the central incisors) in Figure 4-7.

The *mesial* root surface of *all* maxillary incisors is likely to have a slight depression or be nearly flat, but the *distal* root surface is likely to be convex, without a longitudinal depression. The mesial longitudinal depression, when present, is in the middle third cervicoapically and slightly lingual to the center faciolingually. This mesial root depression is discernible in the shaded line drawings in Figure 4-7.

D. MAXILLARY INCISORS FROM THE INCISAL VIEW

Refer to *Figure 4-9* when studying the incisal view. To follow this description, a maxillary incisor should be held in such a position that the incisal edge is toward you, the labial surface is at the top, and you are looking *exactly along the root axis line*. You should see slightly more lingual surface than labial surface if the incisal ridge is located somewhat labial to the root axis line (as in many teeth, especially the lateral incisors, in *Fig. 4-9*).

1. MAXILLARY INCISOR CROWN PROPORTION FACIOLINGUALLY VERSUS MESIODISTALLY FROM THE INCISAL VIEW

The crown outline of the **maxillary central incisor** is noticeably wider mesiodistally than faciolingually [by an average of 1.5 mm] (Appendix 2h). The mesiodistal measurement of the **lateral incisor** crown is also greater than the labiolingual measurement but less so than on the central incisor [averaging only 0.4 mm greater]. On some lateral incisors, the two dimensions of the crown are almost the same size faciolingually as mesiodistally (Appendix 2h). Notice this difference in the proportion of maxillary central incisors (relatively wider mesiodistally) compared to lateral incisors in Figure 4-9.

2. OUTLINE SHAPE OF MAXILLARY INCISOR CROWNS FROM THE INCISAL VIEW

The crown shape of the **maxillary central incisor** is roughly triangular, with a broadly curved labial outline forming the base that converges toward the cingulum. As was seen from the lingual view, the cingulum of the *maxillary central incisor* is slightly off-center to the distal, resulting in the mesial marginal ridge measuring longer than the distal marginal ridge (seen best from the lingual view in Appendix 2f).

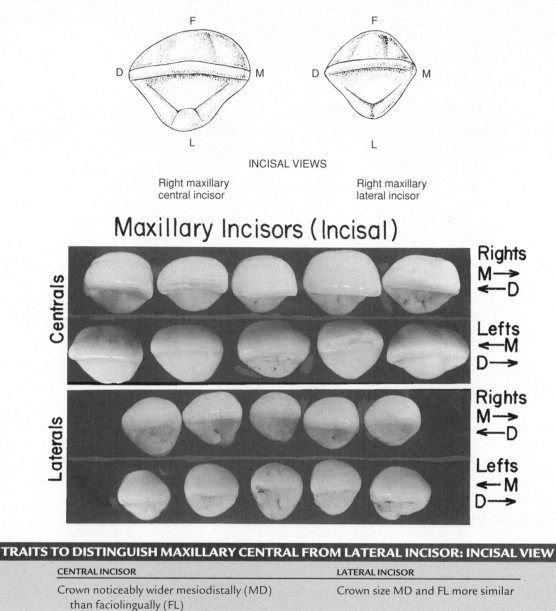

INCISAL VIEWS

Right maxillary
central incisor

Right maxillary
lateral incisor

Maxillary Incisors (Incisal)

TRAITS TO DISTINGUISH MAXILLARY CENTRAL FROM LATERAL INCISOR: INCISAL VIEW	
CENTRAL INCISOR	**LATERAL INCISOR**
Crown noticeably wider mesiodistally (MD) than faciolingually (FL)	Crown size MD and FL more similar
Crown outline roughly triangular	Crown outline more round or oval
Cingulum off center to distal	Cingulum centered
Incisal edge curves mesiodistally	Incisal edge straighter mesiodistally

TRAITS TO DIFFERENTIATE MAXILLARY RIGHT FROM LEFT INCISOR: INCISAL VIEW	
CENTRAL INCISOR	**LATERAL INCISOR**
Cingulum more distal	Distal crown outline more rounded

FIGURE 4-9. Maxillary central and lateral incisors, **incisal views,** with type traits that distinguish maxillary central from lateral incisors and traits that distinguish right and left sides.

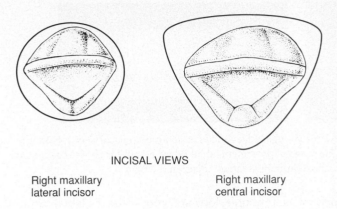

INCISAL VIEWS

Right maxillary
lateral incisor

Right maxillary
central incisor

FIGURE 4-10. The geometric outline of the incisal views of a maxillary lateral incisor on the left and a maxillary central incisor on the right. Notice that the outline of the maxillary lateral incisor is almost *round* or slightly *oval* (slightly wider mesiodistally than faciolingually), whereas the outline of the maxillary central incisor is more *triangular* in shape.

The crown of the **lateral incisor** resembles the central incisor from this aspect, but its outline is more round or oval than triangular. The cingulum of the *lateral incisor* is nearly centered mesiodistally. Compare the triangular shape of the maxillary central incisor to the more round or slightly oval shape of the maxillary lateral incisor in *Figure 4-10*. These differences in outline shape are evident when comparing many central incisors (triangular) with lateral incisors (oval or round) in Figure 4-9.

3. INCISAL RIDGE CONTOUR OF MAXILLARY INCISORS FROM THE INCISAL VIEW

The incisal ridge or edge of the **maxillary central incisor** is 1.5–2 mm thick faciolingually and is slightly curved from mesial to distal, the convexity being on the labial side. It terminates mesially and distally at the widest portion of the crown (Appendix 1q). The position of the distoincisal angle is slightly more lingual than the position of the mesioincisal angle, which then gives the incisal edge its slight distolingual twist as though someone took the distal half of the incisal edge and twisted it to the lingual (Appendix 2g). The incisal ridge of the **lateral incisor** is straighter mesiodistally than on the central incisors.

Be aware that for maxillary central incisors, the two traits just discussed (the cingulum displaced to the distal and the distolingual twist of the incisal edge) are dependent on how the tooth is held. When viewed from the incisal, the distolingual twist of the incisal edge is more obvious when the cingulum is aligned vertically (Appendix 2g), whereas the displacement of the cingulum to the distal is more obvious when the incisal edge is aligned horizontally (Appendix 2e). This is why these two traits are shown on page 2 of the Appendix, showing two views of the same tooth, each having a slightly different alignment to accentuate the trait being discussed.

4. LABIAL CONTOUR OF MAXILLARY INCISORS FROM THE INCISAL VIEW

The labial outline of the **maxillary central incisor** crown usually appears broadly convex, but on some teeth, the center portion may be nearly flat. The labial outline of the **lateral incisor** is noticeably more convex than that of the central incisor. This characteristic difference is clearly seen in many teeth in Figure 4-9.

LEARNING EXERCISE

In determining a right from a left central incisor when it is not in the mouth (as on the bracket table with other incisors after multiple extractions), you need to distinguish the mesial from the distal surface. If you look at the facial surface of a tooth with its root aligned correctly for the correct arch and are able to identify the mesial or distal surface, you can place the tooth in its correct quadrant (right or left) and assign its Universal number. Evaluate the photographs of maxillary incisors in the figures in this chapter and, using the chart in each figure, see how many "mesial versus distal" traits can be used to differentiate the mesial from

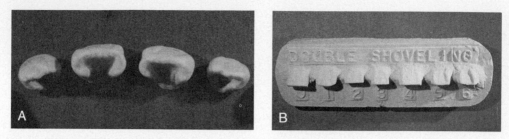

FIGURE 4-11. A. Shovel-shaped permanent incisors from a young Native American dentition (incisal views). Note the prominent marginal ridges on the lingual surface. **B.** The range of prominent labial ridges on double shovel-shaped incisors varies from barely discernible labial ridges on the left to prominent labial ridges on the right.

the distal surfaces and therefore right from left incisors. For example, look at Figure 4-4 at the labial surfaces for the shape of the incisal angles (more rounded on distal) and the position of the contact areas (more cervical on distal), or look at Figure 4-7 for the amount of cervical line curvature on the mesial and distal sides (more curved on mesial), as well as the flatter or concave mesial versus convex distal root surfaces. From the lingual view, look at Figure 4-5 for the length of the marginal ridges (mesial is longer, especially noticeable on maxillary lateral incisors), and from the incisal view on the maxillary central (*Fig. 4-9*), look for the distal location of the cingulum on most maxillary central incisors.

E. VARIATIONS IN MAXILLARY INCISORS

Racial differences in the maxillary incisor teeth have been reported in dental literature. For example, a high incidence of shovel-shaped incisors has been observed in Mongoloid people, including many groups of American Indians.[2,4,5,7] (Mongoloid pertains to a major racial division marked by a fold from the eyelid over the inner canthus, prominent cheekbones, straight black hair, small nose, broad face, and yellowish complexion. Included are Mongols, Manchus, Chinese, Koreans, Eskimos, Japanese, Siamese, Burmese, Tibetans, and American Indians.) White and black people are reported to have less frequent occurrences of this characteristic. Shovel-shape is the term commonly used to designate incisor teeth that have prominent marginal ridges and a deep fossa on their lingual surfaces (*Fig. 4-11A*).

A study of the skulls of American Indians who lived in Arizona about 1100 AD has disclosed the occurrence of incisor teeth that have a mesial marginal ridge on the *labial* surface and a depression, or concavity, on the mesial part of the *labial* surface just distal to this ridge.[8] In these teeth, the distal part of the labial surface is rounded in an unusual manner. Such teeth have been referred to as "three-quarter double shovel-shaped," a descriptive, if ponderous, term. Labial "shoveling" has also been reported in some Eskimo people (see Figure 4-11B).

Other anomalies will be presented in Chapter 12, such as palatal gingival grooves and peg-shaped lateral incisors.

SECTION III	MANDIBULAR INCISOR TYPE TRAITS: SIMILARITIES AND DIFFERENCES USEFUL TO DISTINGUISH MANDIBULAR CENTRAL INCISORS FROM LATERAL INCISORS (FROM ALL VIEWS)

OBJECTIVES

This section is designed to prepare the learner to perform the following:
- Describe the type traits that can be used to distinguish the permanent mandibular central incisor from the mandibular lateral incisor.
- Describe and identify the labial, lingual, mesial, distal, and incisal surfaces for mandibular lateral incisors, and the labial, lingual, and incisal surfaces for the symmetrical mandibular central incisor (where the mesial may be difficult to distinguish from the distal).

- Assign a Universal number to mandibular incisors present in a mouth (or on a model) with complete dentition. If possible, repeat this on a model with one or more mandibular incisors missing.
- Select and separate mandibular incisors from a selection of all teeth on a bench top.
- Holding a mandibular incisor, determine whether it is a central or a lateral and right or left. Then assign a Universal number to it.

A. MANDIBULAR INCISORS FROM THE LABIAL VIEW

Examine several extracted teeth and/or models as you read. Also, refer to page 2 of the Appendix and Figure 4-13 while you study the labial surface of mandibular incisors. Hold mandibular teeth with the root down and crown up, the position of the teeth in the mouth.

1. CROWN SHAPE OF MANDIBULAR INCISORS FROM THE LABIAL VIEW

Mamelons are usually present on newly emerged mandibular incisors and reflect the formation of the facial surface by three labial lobes (*Fig. 4-12*). Ordinarily, they are soon worn off by functional contacts against the maxillary incisors (attrition).

All mandibular incisor crowns are quite narrow relative to their crown length, but the **mandibular central incisor** crown is the narrowest crown in the mouth and is considerably narrower than the *maxillary* central incisor [on average only five-eighths, or 62%, as wide] (Appendix 2p). Unlike *maxillary* incisor crowns in the same mouth where the central is larger than the lateral, the *mandibular lateral incisor* crown is a little larger in all dimensions than the mandibular central incisor in the same mouth, as seen when comparing many central and lateral incisors in *Figure 4-13*. Further, the mandibular central incisor is so *symmetrical* that it is difficult to tell lefts from rights unless on full arch models or in the mouth. About the only difference to be found is the greater mesial than distal curvature of the cervical line (normally visible only on extracted teeth). This trait would *not* be helpful in identifying one remaining central incisor after an orthodontist has realigned the teeth and closed the spaces on either side. The fairly straight mesial and distal crown outlines taper, becoming narrower toward the convex cervical line.

The crown of the **mandibular lateral incisor** resembles that of the mandibular central incisor, but it is slightly wider and is not as bilaterally symmetrical. Its crown tilts distally on the root, giving the impression that the tooth has been bent at the cervix (Appendix 2l). This makes the curved distal outline of the crown (from proximal contact area to cervical line) shorter than the flatter mesial crown outline. Look at the incisors in Figure 4-13 and notice the lack of symmetry of most mandibular lateral incisors relative to the symmetry of the central incisors.

The labial surface of the *all mandibular incisors* is nearly smooth, but about half may have two shallow developmental depressions in the incisal third if you examine the surface closely. [Dr. Woelfel found these depressions on 48% of 793 centrals and on 51% of 787 lateral incisors.] The labial con-

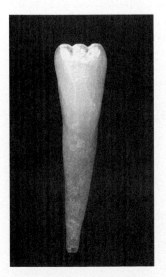

FIGURE 4-12. Example of a mandibular central incisor with three distinct **mamelons** that reflect the formation of the labial surface of incisors from three labial lobes (plus one lingual lobe forming the cingulum).

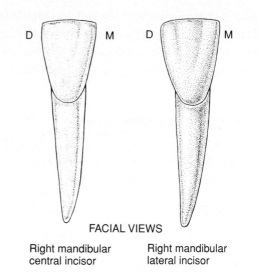

FACIAL VIEWS

| Right mandibular central incisor | Right mandibular lateral incisor |

Facial

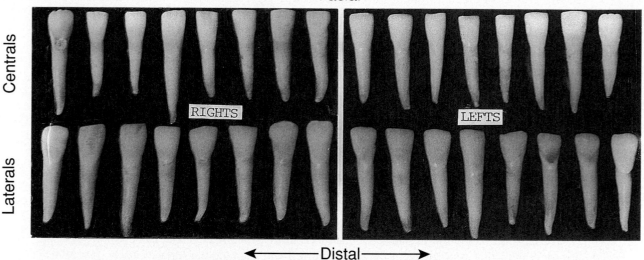

Centrals

Laterals

RIGHTS

LEFTS

←——— Distal ———→

TRAITS TO DIFFERENTIATE MANDIBULAR CENTRAL FROM LATERAL INCISOR: LABIAL VIEW

CENTRAL INCISOR	LATERAL INCISOR
More symmetrical crown	Less symmetrical crown, tips to distal
No distal side bulge on crown	Distal side bulge on crown
Proximal contacts at same level mesial and distal	Mesial proximal contact more incisal
Smaller than lateral in same mouth	Larger than central in same mouth

TRAITS TO DIFFERENTIATE MANDIBULAR RIGHT FROM LEFT INCISOR: LABIAL VIEW

CENTRAL INCISOR	LATERAL INCISOR
Very symmetrical: cannot tell right from left	Crown tips to distal
	Distal crown outline bulges more than mesial
	Distal proximal contact more cervical

FIGURE 4-13. Mandibular central and lateral incisors, **labial views,** with type traits that distinguish mandibular central from lateral incisors and traits that distinguish right and left sides.

tour of all mandibular incisor crowns is convex mesiodistally in the cervical third (best viewed from the incisal) but nearly flat in the incisal third (feel it).

LEARNING EXERCISE

Look at your mouth in the mirror while you place your anterior maxillary and mandibular teeth edge to edge, and align the arch midlines (the proximal contacts between central incisors) over one another. Notice that the distal outline of each maxillary central incisor extends distal to its opposing mandibular central incisor because the maxillary central is wider by about 3.3 mm. Also, notice that the maxillary central incisors are wider and larger than the maxillary lateral incisors and both of the mandibular incisors but that the mandibular central incisors appear smaller than the adjacent mandibular lateral incisors.

2. INCISAL PROXIMAL ANGLES OF MANDIBULAR INCISORS FROM THE LABIAL VIEW

The crown of the **mandibular central incisor** is nearly bilaterally symmetrical, so the mesioincisal and distoincisal angles are very similar: very slightly rounded, forming nearly right angles (Appendix 2j). The distoincisal angle may barely be more rounded than the mesioincisal angle. The distoincisal angle of the **mandibular lateral incisor,** however, is noticeably more rounded than the mesioincisal angle (Appendix 2j). This helps to distinguish rights from lefts prior to attrition (wear).

3. PROXIMAL CONTACT AREAS OF MANDIBULAR INCISORS FROM THE LABIAL VIEW

The mesial and distal contact areas of the **mandibular central incisor** are at the same level: in the incisal third (Appendix 2i) almost level with the incisal edge. The mesial and distal contact areas of the **lateral incisor** are *not* at the same level (Appendix 2i). Although both the mesial and distal contacts are in the incisal third fairly near the incisal edge, the distal contact is noticeably cervical to the level of the mesial contact on lateral incisors. Refer to *Table 4-4* for a summary of the location of proximal contacts for all incisors.

4. ROOT-TO-CROWN PROPORTIONS OF MANDIBULAR INCISORS FROM THE LABIAL VIEW

Long incisocervically but thin mesiodistally, mandibular incisor roots appear proportionally longer compared to their crown length than the maxillary incisors. Therefore, the root-to-crown ratio is

Table 4-4	LOCATION OF PROXIMAL CONTACTS (PROXIMAL HEIGHT OF CONTOUR) ON INCISORS*	
	MESIAL SURFACE (WHICH THIRD OR JUNCTION?)	**DISTAL SURFACE (WHICH THIRD OR JUNCTION?)**
MAXILLARY CROWNS Central incisor	Incisal third (near incisal edge)	Incisal/middle junction
Lateral incisor	Incisal third	Middle third (most cervical of incisor contacts)
MANDIBULAR CROWNS Central incisor	Incisal third (near incisal edge)	Incisal third (near incisal edge; same as mesial)
Lateral incisor	Incisal third (near incisal edge)	Incisal third (but more cervical)

* Seen best from facial view.
General Learning Guidelines:
1. Distal proximal contacts are more cervical than mesial contacts EXCEPT for mandibular central incisors, where the mesial and distal contacts are at the same height, and mandibular first premolars, where the mesial contact is more cervical than the distal.
2. For **anterior teeth,** most contacts are in the incisal third EXCEPT the *distal* of maxillary lateral incisors and canines that are more in the middle third.

larger for both mandibular incisors [both ratios are 1.43] compared to maxillary central and lateral incisors [1.16 and 1.37, respectively].

5. ROOT SHAPE OF MANDIBULAR INCISORS FROM THE LABIAL VIEW

The roots of *all* mandibular incisors appear very narrow mesiodistally but wide faciolingually (ribbonlike) (compare proximal to labial surfaces in Appendix 2n) and taper uniformly on both sides from the cervical line to the apex. The apical end may curve slightly to the distal (seen in some incisors in *Fig. 4-13*).

B. MANDIBULAR INCISORS FROM THE LINGUAL VIEW

Refer to *Figure 4-14* while studying the lingual surface of mandibular incisors.

1. LINGUAL ANATOMY (MARGINAL RIDGES, FOSSAE, AND CINGULUM) OF MANDIBULAR INCISORS FROM THE LINGUAL VIEW

The lingual fossae of *all* mandibular incisors are barely visible, smooth (without grooves, accessory ridges, or pits), and shallow, just slightly concave in the middle and incisal thirds (Appendix 2m). The adjacent marginal ridges, if distinguishable, are scarcely discernible, unlike with the maxillary incisors, where they are more likely to be quite prominent.

Mandibular Incisors (Lingual)

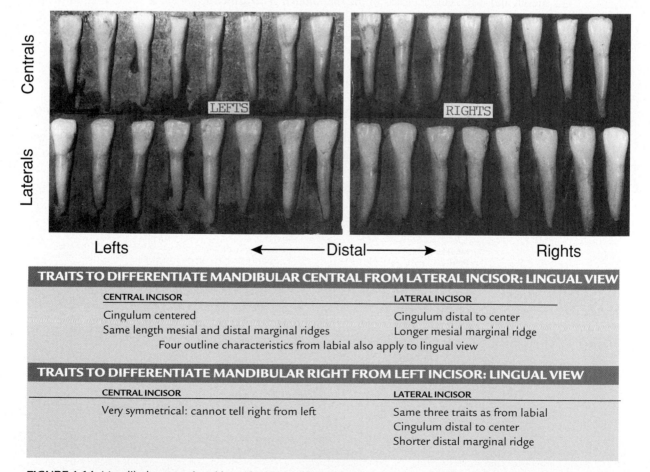

Centrals

Laterals

Lefts ←————— Distal —————→ Rights

TRAITS TO DIFFERENTIATE MANDIBULAR CENTRAL FROM LATERAL INCISOR: LINGUAL VIEW	
CENTRAL INCISOR	**LATERAL INCISOR**
Cingulum centered	Cingulum distal to center
Same length mesial and distal marginal ridges	Longer mesial marginal ridge
Four outline characteristics from labial also apply to lingual view	

TRAITS TO DIFFERENTIATE MANDIBULAR RIGHT FROM LEFT INCISOR: LINGUAL VIEW	
CENTRAL INCISOR	**LATERAL INCISOR**
Very symmetrical: cannot tell right from left	Same three traits as from labial
	Cingulum distal to center
	Shorter distal marginal ridge

FIGURE 4-14. Mandibular central and lateral incisors, **lingual views,** with type traits that distinguish mandibular central from lateral incisors and traits that distinguish right and left sides.

2. CINGULUM OF MANDIBULAR INCISORS FROM THE LINGUAL VIEW

As seen from the lingual view (or from the incisal view in Appendix 2k), the cingulum of the **mandibular central incisor** is convex, small, and centered on the axis line of the root. The cingulum of the **lateral incisor** lies slightly distal to the axis line of the root (similar to the *maxillary* central incisor), making the mesial marginal ridge slightly longer than the distal marginal ridge.

3. ROOT SHAPE OF MANDIBULAR INCISORS FROM THE LINGUAL VIEW

As with other incisor roots, the roots of *all* mandibular incisors are in general convex and slightly narrower on the lingual side than on the labial side. There are longitudinal depressions on *both* the mesial and distal sides of mandibular incisor roots (unlike the *maxillary* incisors, which normally only have mesial root depressions).

C. MANDIBULAR INCISORS FROM THE PROXIMAL VIEWS

Refer to *Figure 4-15* while studying the proximal surfaces of the mandibular incisors.

1. INCISAL EDGE ON MANDIBULAR INCISORS FROM THE PROXIMAL VIEWS

The incisal edges of *both types* of mandibular incisors are normally located on or lingual to the midroot axis (Appendix 2o). From the mesial side, the distolingual twist of the incisal ridge of the **mandibular lateral incisor** places the distal portion at the ridge even somewhat more lingual than on the mesial, unlike the mandibular central, which has no twist. Recall that the maxillary central incisor also exhibits a slight distolingual twist of the incisal edge.

2. CERVICAL LINE ON MANDIBULAR INCISORS FROM THE PROXIMAL VIEWS

The cervical line on the mesial of *all* mandibular incisors normally has a relatively large curvature of about 2 mm, extending incisally over one-fourth of the short crown length. As on other anterior teeth, the curvature on the distal is less [an average of 0.4 mm less on mandibular central incisors and 0.6 mm less on the mandibular lateral incisors for 234 teeth measured].

3. HEIGHT (CREST) OF CONTOUR OF MANDIBULAR INCISORS FROM THE PROXIMAL VIEWS

Like the other anterior teeth, the heights of contour or greatest bulge on the *labial* surface of *all* mandibular incisors are in the cervical third, just incisal to the cervical line. The labial contour of the crown from the height of contour to the incisal edge is so slightly curved that it often appears nearly flat, especially in the incisal half.

The *lingual* contours or outlines of *all* mandibular incisors are convex over the cingulum but concave in the middle third and straightening out in the incisal third (a shallow S outline), similar to all anterior teeth. The height of contour of the lingual surface is in the cervical third on the cingulum.

4. ROOTS AND ROOT DEPRESSIONS OF MANDIBULAR INCISORS FROM THE PROXIMAL VIEWS

The relatively large faciolingual dimension of the root at the cervix is very apparent from the proximal view. The cervical portion of the roots on the mandibular incisors is 2 mm wider faciolingually than mesiodistally. The facial and lingual outlines of the roots of *all* mandibular incisors are nearly straight from the cervical line to the middle third; then the root tapers with its apex on the axis line (seen in most roots in *Fig. 4-15*).

The root contours of *all* mandibular incisors are noticeably less convex on their mesial and distal sides than the maxillary incisors (arch trait). In fact, there is usually a slight longitudinal depression on the middle third of the mesial *and* distal root surfaces, with the distal depression somewhat more distinct. See *Table 4-5* for a summary of incisor root depressions.

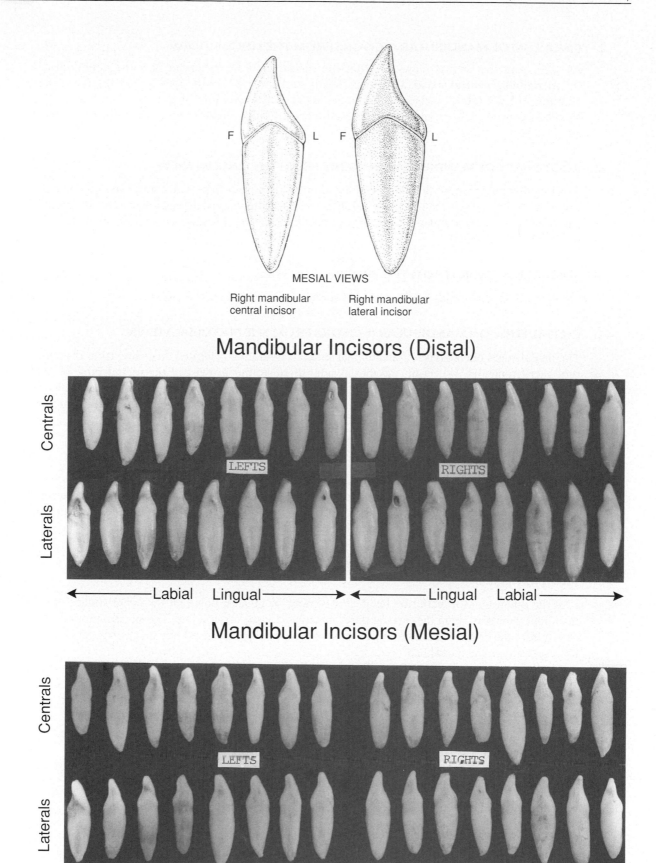

MESIAL VIEWS

Right mandibular
central incisor

Right mandibular
lateral incisor

Mandibular Incisors (Distal)

Centrals

Laterals

LEFTS   RIGHTS

◄——Labial   Lingual——►   ◄——Lingual   Labial——►

Mandibular Incisors (Mesial)

Centrals

Laterals

LEFTS   RIGHTS

◄——Lingual   Labial——►   ◄——Labial   Lingual——►

FIGURE 4-15. Mandibular central and lateral incisors, **proximal views,** with type traits that distinguish mandibular central from lateral incisors and traits that distinguish right and left sides.

TRAITS TO DIFFERENTIATE MANDIBULAR CENTRAL FROM LATERAL INCISOR: PROXIMAL VIEWS

CENTRAL INCISOR and LATERAL INCISOR
This view is not good to differentiate central from lateral incisor

TRAITS TO DIFFERENTIATE MANDIBULAR RIGHT FROM LEFT INCISOR: COMPARING PROXIMAL VIEWS

CENTRAL INCISOR	LATERAL INCISOR
Distal incisal ridge even with mesial incisal ridge	Distal incisal ridge may be more lingual
Mesial cervical line curve greater than distal on both central and lateral incisors	

D. MANDIBULAR INCISORS FROM THE INCISAL VIEW

To follow this description, the tooth should be held in such a position that the incisal edge is toward the observer, the labial surface is at the top, and the observer is looking *exactly along the root axis line* as in *Figure 4-16*. You will see slightly more of the labial than the lingual surface if the incisal ridge is just lingual to the root axis line.

1. CROWN PROPORTIONS OF MANDIBULAR INCISORS FROM THE INCISAL VIEW

The labiolingual measurements of *all* mandibular incisor crowns are greater than the mesiodistal measurement [by about 0.4 mm]. This is different from the measurements of the maxillary incisors, especially maxillary central incisors, which are considerably wider mesiodistally than faciolingually.

2. CROWN OUTLINE OF MANDIBULAR INCISORS FROM THE INCISAL VIEW

The **mandibular central incisor** is practically bilaterally symmetrical with little to differentiate the mesial half from the distal half. The greatest height of contour labially and lingually is centrally located. The **mandibular lateral incisor** is not bilaterally symmetrical (the cingulum is located distal to the mesiodistal midline, Appendix 2k), and this asymmetry makes it easy to select rights from lefts and to distinguish mandibular centrals from laterals, especially from this view (Fig. 4-16).

Table 4-5	PRESENCE AND RELATIVE DEPTH OF LONGITUDINAL ROOT DEPRESSIONS ("ROOT GROOVES") ON INCISORS		
	TOOTH	MESIAL ROOT DEPRESSION?	DISTAL ROOT DEPRESSION?
MAXILLARY TEETH	Maxillary central incisor	No (or slight or flat)	No (convex)
	Maxillary lateral incisor	Yes (sometimes no)	No (convex)
MANDIBULAR TEETH	Mandibular central incisor	Yes	Yes (deeper)
	Mandibular lateral incisor	Yes	Yes (deeper)

General Learning Guidelines:
1. **Maxillary incisors** are not likely to have root depressions.
2. **Mandibular incisors** have deeper distal root depressions.

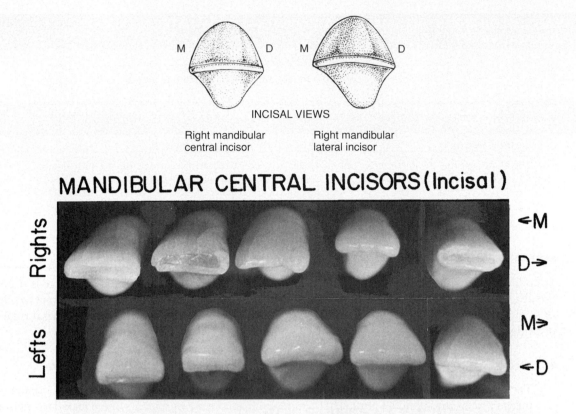

MANDIBULAR CENTRAL INCISORS (Incisal)

Mandibular Lateral Incisors (Incisal)

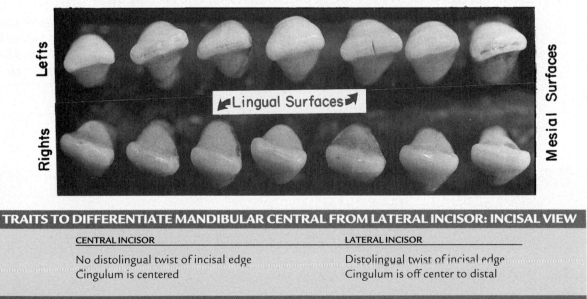

TRAITS TO DIFFERENTIATE MANDIBULAR CENTRAL FROM LATERAL INCISOR: INCISAL VIEW

CENTRAL INCISOR	LATERAL INCISOR
No distolingual twist of incisal edge	Distolingual twist of incisal edge
Cingulum is centered	Cingulum is off center to distal

TRAITS TO DIFFERENTIATE MANDIBULAR RIGHT FROM LEFT INCISOR: INCISAL VIEW

CENTRAL INCISOR	LATERAL INCISOR
Very symmetrical: cannot tell right from left	Distolingual twist of incisal edge
	Cingulum is off center to distal

FIGURE 4-16. Mandibular central and lateral incisors, **incisal views,** with type traits that distinguish mandibular central from lateral incisors and traits that distinguish right and left sides.

3. **INCISAL RIDGE CONTOUR (ALIGNMENT) OF MANDIBULAR INCISORS FROM THE INCISAL VIEW**

The incisal ridge or edge of the **mandibular central incisor** is at right angles to the labiolingual root axis plane. It is nearly 2 mm thick and runs in a straight line mesiodistally toward the contact areas. The ridge is lingual to the midroot axis. If you hold an extracted mandibular incisor with the root facing directly away from your sight line, slightly more of the labial than lingual surface is visible because of the lingually positioned incisal ridge.

If you were to align a **mandibular lateral incisor** with its lingual *cingulum directly exactly downward* or vertically (represented roughly by the dotted vertical line with the arrow in Appendix 2k), the distal half of the incisal edge would be perceived as twisted lingually (called a distolingual twist). The twist of the incisal edge corresponds to the curvature of the mandibular dental arch; a tooth on the right side of the arch is twisted clockwise; one on the left is twisted counterclockwise. This twist is evident in most mandibular lateral incisors in Figure 4-16 and is an excellent way to distinguish mandibular central from lateral incisors, and to distinguish the right from left mandibular lateral incisor.

4. **CINGULUM OF MANDIBULAR INCISORS FROM THE INCISAL VIEW**

If, instead of aligning the tooth with the labiolingual root axis exactly vertical you were to align the incisal edge of a lateral incisor exactly horizontal, the cingulum of the **mandibular lateral incisor** would be slightly off center to the distal (Appendix 2k). Recall that this was also seen on the maxillary central incisor. In comparison, the cingulum on the **mandibular central incisor** is centered, smooth, and makes a narrow convex outline.

5. **LABIAL CONTOUR OF MANDIBULAR INCISORS FROM THE INCISAL VIEW**

The labial surfaces of *all* mandibular incisors are only slightly convex in the incisal third labial to the incisal edge, but the outline in the cervical third is decidedly convex.

E. **VARIATIONS IN MANDIBULAR INCISORS**

There is more uniformity of shape in the mandibular incisor teeth than in other teeth. In some Mongoloid people, the cingulum of mandibular incisors is characteristically marked by a short deep groove running cervicoincisally. This groove is often a site of dental caries. In Chapter 12 on anomalies, you will see fused mandibular incisors, missing central incisors, and even a lateral incisor emerged distally to the canine.

LEARNING EXERCISE

Assign a Universal number to a handheld incisor:

Suppose a patient just had all of his or her permanent teeth extracted. Imagine being asked to find tooth #8 from among a pile of 32 extracted teeth on the oral surgeon's tray because you wanted to evaluate a lesion seen on the radiograph on the root of that incisor. How might you go about it? Try the following steps:

- From a selection of all permanent teeth (extracted teeth or tooth models), select only the incisors (based on class traits).
- Determine whether each incisor is maxillary or mandibular. Review Table 4-3 if needed. *You should never rely on only one characteristic difference* between teeth to name them; rather, make a list of many traits that suggest that the tooth is a maxillary incisor, as opposed to only one trait that makes you think it belongs in the maxilla. This way you can play detective and become an expert at recognition at the same time.

- If you determine that the tooth is maxillary, position the root up; if it is mandibular, position the root down.
- Next, using type traits, determine the type of incisor you are holding (central or lateral). Refer to the tables and teeth in the figures throughout this chapter as needed.
- Use characteristic traits for each surface to identify the facial surface. This will permit you to view the tooth as though you were looking into a patient's mouth.
- Finally, determine which surface is the mesial. Refer to figures throughout this chapter as needed. While viewing the incisor from the facial and picturing it within the appropriate arch (upper or lower), the mesial surface can be positioned toward the midline in only one quadrant, the right or left.
- Once you have determined the quadrant, assign the appropriate Universal number for the incisor in that quadrant. For example, the central incisor in the upper right quadrant is tooth #8.

LEARNING QUESTIONS

For each of the traits listed below, select the letter(s) of the permanent incisor(s) that normally exhibit(s) that trait. More than one answer may apply.

- a. Maxillary central incisor
- b. Maxillary lateral incisor
- c. Mandibular central incisor
- d. Mandibular lateral incisor

1. Mesiodistal dimension is larger than the labiolingual dimension.   a   b   c   d

2. Incisal ridge exhibits a distolingual twist.   a   b   c   d

3. Root is very narrow mesiodistally with mesial and distal root depressions.   a   b   c   d

4. Incisal edge is positioned more to the lingual of the root axis line.   a   b   c   d

5. The distal proximal height of contour is more cervical than the mesial height of contour.   a   b   c   d

6. It has the widest (mesiodistally) incisor crown.   a   b   c   d

7. It has the shortest *root* relative to its crown.   a   b   c   d

8. It is the most symmetrical incisor.   a   b   c   d

9. It has the largest curvature of the mesial cervical line.   a   b   c   d

10. It has the narrowest incisor crown (mesiodistally).   a   b   c   d

ANSWERS: 1-a, b; 2-a, d; 3-c, d; 4-c, d; 5-a, b, d; 6-a; 7-a; 8-c; 9-a; 10-c

REFERENCES

1. Hanihara K. Racial characteristics in the dentition. J Dent Res 1967;46:923–926.
2. Carbonelli VM. Variations in the frequency of shovel-shaped incisors in different populations. In: Brothel DR, ed. Dental anthropology. London: Pergamon Press, 1963:211–234.
3. Brabant H. Comparison of the characteristics and anomalies of the deciduous and the permanent dentitions. J Dent Res 1967;48:897–902.
4. De Voto FCH. Shovel-shaped incisors in pre-Columbian Tastilian Indians. J Dent Res 1971;50:168.
5. De Voto FCH, Arias NH, Ringuelet S, et al. Shovel-shaped incisors in a northwestern Argentine population. J Dent Res 1968;47:820.
6. Taylor RMS. Variations in form of human teeth: I. An anthropologic and forensic study of maxillary incisors. J Dent Res 1969;48:5–16.

7. Dahlberg AA. The dentition of the American Indian. In: Laughlin WS, ed. The physical anthropology of the American Indian. New York: The Viking Fund, 1949.

8. Snyder RG. Mesial marginal ridging of incisor labial surfaces. J Dent Res 1960;39:361.

9. Ash MM, Nelson SJ. Wheeler's dental anatomy, physiology and occlusion. Philadelphia: Saunders 2003.

GENERAL REFERENCE

Goose DH. Variability of form of maxillary permanent incisors. J Dent Res 1956;35:902.

Web site: http://animaldiversity.ummz.umich.edu/site/topics/mammal_anatomy/gallery_of_incisors.html—University of Michigan Museum of Zoology Animal Diversity Web Gallery of Incisors

5 Morphology of the Permanent Canines

Topics covered within the three sections of this chapter include the following:

I. General description of canines
   A. Functions
   B. General characteristics or class traits (similarities) of canines (both maxillary and mandibular)

II. Arch traits for canines: how to distinguish maxillary from mandibular canines (from each view)
   A. Canines from the labial view
   B. Canines from the lingual view
   C. Canines from the proximal views
   D. Canines from the incisal view

III. Variations in canine teeth

As in Chapter 4, "Appendix" followed by a number and letter (for example, "Appendix 3a") is used to denote reference to the page (number 3) and item (letter a) being referred to on that Appendix page. The appendix pages are designed to be torn out to facilitate study and minimize page turns as you read the main text. This chapter will focus on Appendix pages 3 and 4.

SECTION I   GENERAL DESCRIPTION OF CANINES

OBJECTIVES

This section is designed to prepare the learner to perform the following:
- Describe the functions of canines.
- List the class traits that apply to all canines. Include the incisor class traits that also apply to the canines.
- From a selection of all permanent teeth (or from drawings or photographs of all teeth from various views), select and separate out the canines.

Use a cast of all permanent teeth and/or *Figure 5-1* while studying about the position of the canines within the arch. There are four canines: one on either side in the maxillary arch (Universal numbers 6 and 11) and one on either side of the mandibular arch (numbers 22 and 27). They are the longest of the permanent teeth [26.3 mm and 25.9 mm, respectively]. The canines are distal to the lateral incisors and are the third teeth from the midline. The mesial surface of the canine is in contact with the distal surface of the lateral incisor. The distal surface of each canine contacts the mesial surface of the first premolar.

The four canines are justifiably considered cornerstones of the arches, as they are located at the corners of the mouth or dental arches. They are often referred to as cuspids, eyeteeth, and fangs (nicknames and slang terminology). The use of such slang terminology should be discouraged. Frequently, the canines are the last teeth to be lost from dental disease (decay and/or periodontal problems). Have you known or seen an elderly person who is edentulous (toothless), except for one or more of the canines?

The name canine is of Greek origin and is found in the writings of Hippocrates and Aristotle of 2350 years ago. Aristotle first described canine anatomy, stressing the intermediate nature of it between incisors and molars: it is sharp like an incisor but broader at the base like a molar. Celsus was the first writer to mention the roots of teeth, saying the canine was monoradicular (that is, normally having one root).[1,2]

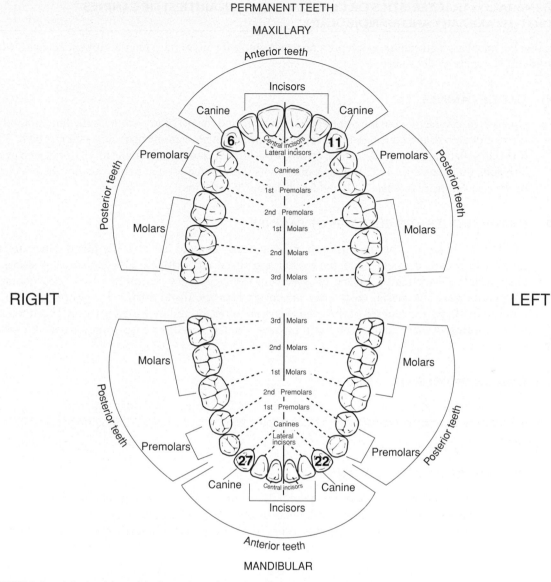

FIGURE 5-1. Adult dentition with the Universal numbers for canines highlighted in red.

A. FUNCTIONS

In dogs, cats, and other animals with long, prominent canine teeth, the functions of these teeth are catching and tearing food and defense. As a matter of fact, *caninus* in Latin means "dog." Canines are essential to their survival. In human beings, these teeth usually function with the incisors (a) to support the lips and the facial muscles and (b) to cut, pierce, or shear food morsels. A steep overlap of the maxillary and mandibular canines, when present, serves as (c) a protective mechanism since the longer, opposing canines ride up over each other when the mandible moves to either side, causing all of the posterior teeth to separate (disocclude). This canine guidance (also known as canine-protected occlusion) relieves the premolars and molars from potentially damaging horizontal forces while chewing.

Canines, because of their large, long roots, are good anchor teeth (abutments) for a fixed dental bridge or removable partial denture attachments (clasps) when other teeth have been lost. As such, they often continue to function as a prime support for the replacement teeth for many years.

B. GENERAL CHARACTERISTICS OR CLASS TRAITS (SIMILARITIES) OF CANINES (BOTH MAXILLARY AND MANDIBULAR)

Using the maxillary right canine as a representative example for all canines, refer to Appendix page 3 while studying the traits of all canines.

1. SIZE OF CANINES

On average, canines are the longest *teeth* in each arch, and the maxillary canine is the longest tooth in the mouth even though the mandibular canine crown is longer than the maxillary canine crown. (One text states that the mandibular canine crown is the longest crown in the mouth.[3]) They have particularly long roots [average: 16.2 mm] and thick roots (faciolingually) that help to anchor them securely in the alveolar process. *Table 5-1* provides all canine dimensions.

2. INCISAL RIDGES AND CUSP TIPS OF CANINES

The incisal ridges of a canine, rather than being nearly straight horizontally like the incisors, are divided into two inclines called the mesial and distal cusp ridges (also called cusp slopes or cusp arms). Subsequently, canine crowns from the facial view resemble a five-sided pentagon (Appendix 3a). The mesial cusp ridge is shorter than the distal cusp ridge (Appendix 3b). In older individuals, the lengths of the cusp ridges are often altered by wear (attrition). Canine teeth do not ordinarily have mamelons but may have a notch on either cusp ridge, as seen clearly in *Figure 5-2*.

3. LABIAL CONTOUR OF CANINES

The labial surface of a canine is prominently convex with a vertical labial ridge (Appendix 3c). Canines are the only teeth with a *labial* ridge, although premolars have a similar-looking ridge called a *buccal* ridge.

4. CROWN PROPORTIONS OF CANINES

The measurement of a maxillary or mandibular canine crown is greater labiolingually than it is mesiodistally [on maxillary canines by 0.5 mm and on mandibular canines by 0.9 mm; averages from 637 teeth] (Appendix 3d). Recall that this proportion (greater labiolingually than mesiodistally) also applied to both types of mandibular incisors. The root cervix measurements are even more oblong fa-

Table 5-1	SIZE OF CANINES (MEASURED BY DR. WOELFEL AND HIS DENTAL HYGIENE STUDENTS, 1974–1979)			
	321 MAXILLARY CANINES		**316 MANDIBULAR CANINES**	
DIMENSION MEASURED	AVERAGE (MM)	RANGE (MM)	AVERAGE (MM)	RANGE (MM)
Crown length	10.6	8.2–13.6	11.0	6.8–16.4
Root length	16.5	10.8–28.5	15.9	9.5–22.2
Overall length	26.4	20.0–38.4	25.9	16.1–34.5
Crown width (mesiodistal)	7.6	6.3–9.5	6.8	5.7–8.6
Root width (cervix)	5.6	3.6–7.3	5.2	4.1–6.4
Faciolingual crown size	8.1	6.7–10.7	7.7	6.4–9.5
Faciolingual root (cervix)	7.6	6.1–10.4	7.5	5.8–9.4
Mesial cervical curve	2.1	0.3–4.0	2.4	0.2–4.8
Distal cervical curve	1.4	0.2–3.5	1.6	0.2–3.5

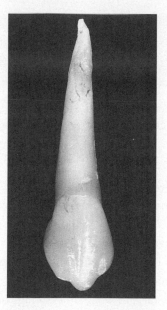

FIGURE 5-2. *Labial view* of a maxillary right canine with a prominent labial ridge and notches on mesial and distal cusp ridges.

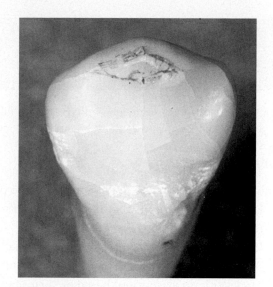

FIGURE 5-3. Maxillary canine (incisal view) showing a characteristic pattern of incisal wear that is diamond shaped.

ciolingually [greater faciolingually by 2.0 mm on maxillary canines and 2.3 mm on mandibular canines]. (Compare the facial and mesial views in Appendix 3i.)

5. CANINE TRAITS THAT ARE SIMILAR TO INCISOR TRAITS

Similar to most incisors (EXCEPT the mandibular central, where contacts are at the same level), the distal contact area is more cervical in position than the mesial contact area (Appendix 3g), and the crown outline is more convex on the distal than on the mesial surface (Appendix 3f). From the *proximal views,* canine crowns are wedge, or triangular, shaped (Appendix 3o). The height of contour on the facial surface is in the cervical third, and on the lingual surface is on the cingulum, which makes up the cervical third of the crown length (Appendix 3p). The remaining outline of the lingual surface (lingual ridge) is slightly concave in the middle third and is straight or slightly convex in the incisal third. Combined, the lingual outline is S-shaped, as on all other anterior teeth (Appendix 3q). Further similarities with incisors include the following: crowns taper, narrowing from the contact areas toward the cervix (Appendix 3e); cervical lines curve more on the mesial than on the distal surface (compare mesial and distal views in Appendix 3n); and marginal ridges (as well as crowns) taper lingually from the contact areas toward the cingulum (Appendix 3l), so the crown is narrower on the lingual half than on the facial half. From the incisal view, facial outlines are less convex than lingual outlines (Appendix 3s), and the incisal edges extend from mesial to distal contact areas (Appendix 3r). Further, roots taper, narrower on the lingual half than on the facial half, and taper narrower from the cervix toward the apex (Appendix 3h), with the root tip or apex often bending to the distal (Appendix 3j). Roots are also longer than crowns (Appendix 3k) [with the root-to-crown ratio of 1.56 for maxillary canines and 1.45 for mandibular canines].

The location of incisal edge tooth wear on canines is similar to wear on incisors. Facets on the mandibular canine cusp tip and cusp ridge normally form more on the labial border, not the lingual border of the cusp ridge as occurs on the maxillary canine. If you find wear facets on the lingual surface of a mandibular canine or on the labial surface of a maxillary canine, it is probably because the teeth were not aligned with the normal overlapping of anterior teeth described in Chapter 3. Refer back to Figure 4-3 for an illustration of this concept on incisors. (Further, maxillary canines viewed incisally often have a characteristic diamond-shape wear pattern that does not occur on other anterior teeth as seen in *Fig. 5-3.*)

| SECTION II | ARCH TRAITS FOR CANINES: HOW TO DISTINGUISH MAXILLARY FROM MANDIBULAR CANINES (FROM EACH VIEW) |

Unlike incisors where there are two types, a central and a lateral, there is only one type of canine. Therefore, type traits do not apply to canines, but arch traits are useful to distinguish maxillary from mandibular canines.

OBJECTIVES

This section is designed to prepare the learner to perform the following:
- Describe the arch traits that can be used to distinguish the permanent maxillary canines from mandibular canines.
- Describe and identify the labial, lingual, mesial, distal, and incisal surfaces for all canines.
- Assign a Universal number to canines present in a mouth with a complete permanent dentition (or on a model or in an illustration) based on their shape and position in the quadrant.
- Holding a canine, determine whether it is a maxillary or mandibular and whether it belongs on the right or left side. Then picture it within the appropriate quadrant and assign a Universal number to it.

A. CANINES FROM THE LABIAL VIEW

Examine several extracted canines and/or models as you study this section. As you examine them, hold maxillary canines with crowns down and mandibular canines with crowns up. This is the way they are oriented in the mouth. Also, while reading this section, tear out and refer to the Appendix study page 4 on canines.

1. CANINE MORPHOLOGY FROM THE LABIAL VIEW

Along with the tooth models and the Appendix pages 3 and 4 available, refer to *Figure 5-4* for viewing similarities and the range of differences of canines from the labial view.

The facial side of any canine crown is formed from three labial lobes like the incisors. (The cingulum on the lingual side of the crown is from the fourth lobe.) The middle lobe on the facial forms the *labial ridge* (Appendix 3c), which can be quite prominent on the maxillary canine. The labial ridge runs cervicoincisally near the center of the crown in the middle and incisal thirds. Shallow depressions lie mesial and distal to the labial ridge. See *Table 5-2* for a summary of the number of lobes that form canines.

The labial surface of mandibular canines is more smooth and convex. A labial ridge is often present but not as pronounced as on the maxillary canines. In the incisal third, the labial crown surface is convex but slightly flattened mesial to the labial ridge and even a little more flattened distal to the ridge. (Feel it.)

2. CANINE SHAPE AND SIZE FROM THE LABIAL VIEW

The outline of the *mesial* half of the maxillary canine crown is broadly convex in the middle third, becoming nearly flat in the cervical third (Appendix 4b). The outline of the *distal* portion of this crown forms a shallow S shape, being convex in the middle third (over the height of contour or proximal contact area) and slightly concave in the cervical third.

The mandibular canine crown appears longer and narrower than the crown of the maxillary canine (Appendix 4a). [The mandibular canine crown is actually 0.4 mm longer and 0.8 mm narrower; averages from 637 teeth.] The *mesial* outline of the mandibular crown is almost flat to slightly convex, *nearly in line* with the mesial side of the root, and not projecting beyond it (Appendix 4b). This conspicuous feature is quite evident in most mandibular canines in Figure 5-4 but is not seen on maxillary canines. In other words, the mesial side of the mandibular canine crown does not bulge or project beyond the adjacent root outline. The *distal* side of the crown may be slightly concave in the cervical third; it is con-

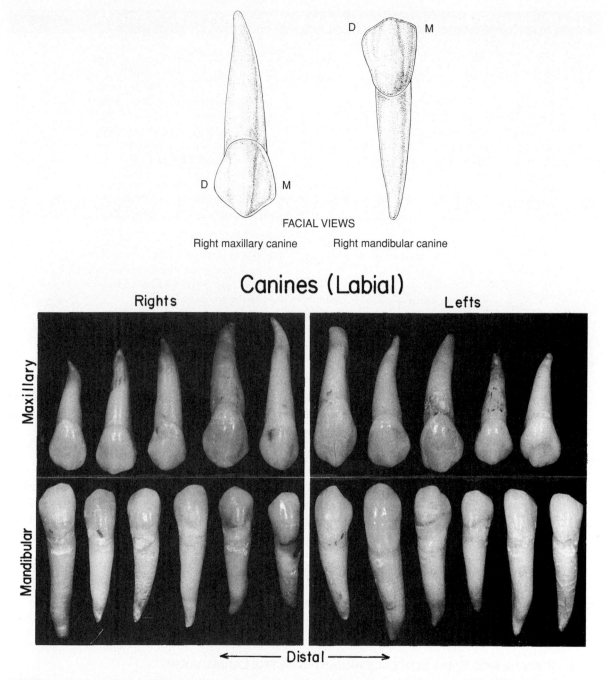

FACIAL VIEWS

Right maxillary canine   Right mandibular canine

FIGURE 5-4. Labial views of canines with traits to distinguish maxillary from mandibular canines and traits to distinguish rights from lefts.

TRAITS TO DISTINGUISH MAXILLARY FROM MANDIBULAR CANINE: LABIAL VIEW

MAXILLARY CANINE	MANDIBULAR CANINE
Cusp angle sharper, more acute (105°)	Cusp angle more blunt (120°)
	Mesial cusp ridge almost horizontal
Mesial (M), distal (D) contacts more cervical	M, D proximal contacts more incisal
Crown wider mesiodistally (MD)	Crown narrower MD
Mesial cusp ridge shorter than distal	Mesial cusp ridge *much* shorter than distal
Mesial of crown bulges beyond root outline	Mesial crown-to-root outline continuous
More pronounced labial ridge	Less pronounced labial ridge
More pointed root tip	Blunter root tip

TRAITS TO DIFFERENTIATE RIGHT FROM LEFT CANINES: LABIAL VIEW

MAXILLARY CANINE	MANDIBULAR CANINE
Mesial crown outline less curved than distal	Mesial crown outline flatter than distal
Mesial crown outline bulges beyond root	Mesial crown outline is in line with root
	Mesial cusp ridge more horizontal

Distal crown outline curves more than mesial crown outline
Distal contact more cervical than mesial contact
Mesial cusp ridge shorter than distal

FIGURE 5-4. (continued).

vex in the incisal two-thirds. There is noticeably more of the crown distal to the root axis line than mesial to it. This often makes the lower canine crown appear to be tilted or bent distally when the root is held in a vertical position (similar to the mandibular lateral incisor just mesial to it).

3. CANINE CUSP TIP AND INCISAL RIDGES FROM THE LABIAL VIEW

Recall that the mesial ridges are normally shorter than the distal ridges for *all* canines. The cusp ridges and the cusp of the maxillary canine make up nearly one-third of the cervicoincisal length of the crown, because the angle formed by the cusp ridges is relatively sharp, slightly more than a right angle (105°) (Appendix 4c). Compare this to the cusp tip of the mandibular canine, where cusp ridges form a less sharp, more obtuse (blunt) angle (120°) (Appendix 4c). The *mesial* cusp ridge of the mandibular canine is also almost horizontal compared to its longer distal cusp ridge, which slopes more steeply in an apical direction. Shorter, more horizontal mesial cusp ridges are seen clearly on most mandibular canines in Figure 5-4. Wear on the incisal edge may alter the length of the cusp slopes, sometimes even completely obliterating the cusp, resulting in an appearance from the facial that is similar to an incisor.

4. CANINE PROXIMAL CONTACT AREAS FROM THE LABIAL VIEW

The *mesial* contact area of the maxillary canine is located at the junction of the incisal and middle thirds. The *distal* contact area of the maxillary canine, like all anterior teeth, is in a more cervical

Table 5-2	GUIDELINE FOR DETERMINING THE NUMBER OF LOBES FOR CANINES*	
TOOTH NAME	**CINGULUM?**	**# LOBES**
Maxillary canine	Yes	3 + 1 = 4
Mandibular canine	Yes	3 + 1 = 4

* Number of lobes = 3 facial lobes + 1 lobe per cingulum

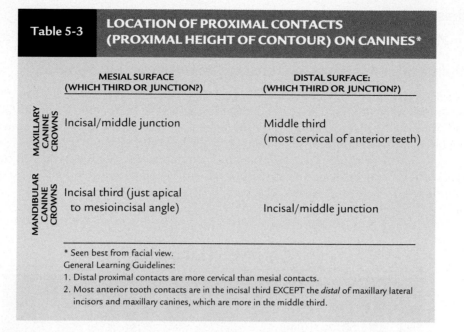

Table 5-3	LOCATION OF PROXIMAL CONTACTS (PROXIMAL HEIGHT OF CONTOUR) ON CANINES*	
	MESIAL SURFACE (WHICH THIRD OR JUNCTION?)	**DISTAL SURFACE:** (WHICH THIRD OR JUNCTION?)
MAXILLARY CANINE CROWNS	Incisal/middle junction	Middle third (most cervical of anterior teeth)
MANDIBULAR CANINE CROWNS	Incisal third (just apical to mesioincisal angle)	Incisal/middle junction

* Seen best from facial view.
General Learning Guidelines:
1. Distal proximal contacts are more cervical than mesial contacts.
2. Most anterior tooth contacts are in the incisal third EXCEPT the *distal* of maxillary lateral incisors and maxillary canines, which are more in the middle third.

location on the distal side than on the mesial side. It is located in the middle third, just cervical to the junction of the incisal and middle thirds (recall Appendix 3g). This is the only canine proximal contact area (mesial or distal) located in the middle third.

The *mesial* contact area of the mandibular canine is in a more incisal position than on the maxillary canine due to its nearly horizontal mesial cusp ridge. It is in the incisal third just cervical to the mesioincisal angle. The *distal* contact area is, as expected, more cervical than the mesial, at the junction of the middle and incisal thirds. See *Table 5-3* for a summary of the location of contact areas on canines.

5. CANINE TOOTH PROPORTIONS FROM THE LABIAL VIEW

The maxillary canine crown is nearly as long as the maxillary central incisor crown, but the root of the canine is much longer [3.5 mm longer than the average on 719 teeth] making the maxillary canine, on average, the *longest tooth* in the mouth (Appendix 3k). The mandibular canine is considerably larger than either of the mandibular incisors, particularly in length [by 4.1 mm] and mesiodistal width [1.3 mm]. It is, on average, the longest mandibular tooth.

6. CANINE ROOT CONTOUR FROM THE LABIAL VIEW

The labial surface of a canine root is normally convex. The root of the maxillary canine is long, slender, and conical. The apical third is narrow mesiodistally, and the apex may be pointed or sharp. The apical third of the root often bends distally (Appendix 3j). [On 100 maxillary canines examined by Dr. Woelfel, 58 bent distally, 24 were straight, and 18 had the apical end of their roots bending slightly toward the mesial.] Only three maxillary canine roots can be seen bending mesially in Figure 5-4.

The mandibular canine root tapers apically to a somewhat more blunt apex. The apical end of the root is more often straight rather than curving toward the mesial or distal sides. [On 100 mandibular canines inspected by Dr. Woelfel, 45 had absolutely straight roots, 29 had the apical third bending mesially, and 26 bent slightly toward the distal.] Therefore, on mandibular canines, the root curvature should not be used to differentiate rights and lefts. Mandibular canine roots are shorter than the roots of maxillary canines [0.6 mm shorter on 637 teeth].

B. CANINES FROM THE LINGUAL VIEW

Refer to *Figure 5-5* while studying similarities and differences of canines from the lingual view.

1. CANINE LINGUAL RIDGES AND FOSSAE FROM THE LINGUAL VIEW

The maxillary canine has a prominent lingual ridge running cervicoincisally from the cusp to the cingulum (Appendix 4d). Mesial and distal lingual fossae lie on either side of the lingual ridge and are usually shallow. Sometimes the lingual surface of the maxillary canine is naturally smooth or worn smooth from attrition so that the lingual ridge and the two fossae on either side of it are not easily discernible. By examining a number of specimens, you will find some with considerable wear or attrition on the lingual surface, sometimes entirely obliterating the lingual ridge.

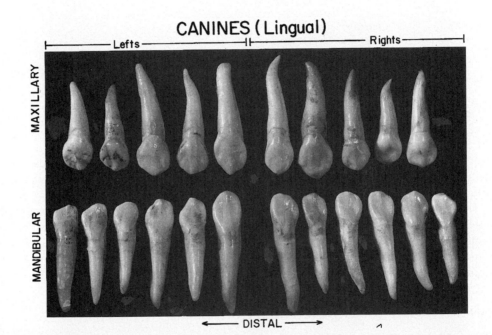

TRAITS TO DISTINGUISH MAXILLARY FROM MANDIBULAR CANINE: LINGUAL VIEW	
316 MAXILLARY CANINES	**316 MANDIBULAR CANINES**
More prominent anatomy on lingual:	Smoother lingual surface:
Lingual marginal ridges pronounced	Lingual marginal ridges less pronounced
Prominent lingual ridge and fossae	Less prominent ridge and fossae
Most prominent lingual ridge (46%)	Most prominent distal ridge (63%)
Cingulum centered	Cingulum centered or to distal
Also, six outline traits from facial view also apply to lingual view	

TRAITS TO DIFFERENTIATE RIGHT FROM LEFT CANINES: LINGUAL VIEW	
MAXILLARY CANINE	**MANDIBULAR CANINE**
Cingulum distal to center	
Outline traits that are seen from facial view also are seen from lingual view	
Mesial marginal ridge longer than distal marginal ridge	

FIGURE 5-5. Lingual views of canines with traits to distinguish maxillary from mandibular canines and traits to distinguish rights from lefts.

With normal occlusion, the lingual surface of the mandibular canine is not subject to lingual wear as on the maxillary canine, but even without wear, the lingual ridge and fossae are normally less prominent.

2. CANINE CINGULUM FROM THE LINGUAL VIEW

The maxillary canine cingulum is large. Its incisal border is sometimes pointed in the center, resembling a small cusp or tubercle (seen in the far right maxillary canine in *Fig. 5-4*). The cingulum and the tip of the cusp are usually centered mesiodistally (seen best from the incisal view in Appendix 4e). The cingulum of the mandibular canine is low, less bulky, and less prominent than on maxillary canines. Unlike maxillary canines, the cingulum lies just distal to the root axis line. This is most apparent from the incisal view in Appendix 4e. (Recall that the distal-to-midline location of the cingulum is also apparent on maxillary central incisors and mandibular lateral incisors.)

3. CANINE MARGINAL RIDGES FROM THE LINGUAL VIEW

The elevated mesial and distal marginal ridges of the maxillary canines are usually of moderate size, and the *lingual ridge* is often most prominent. The distal marginal ridge is slightly more elevated than the mesial marginal ridge (prior to attrition). [Dr. Woelfel's dental hygiene students inspected 455 maxillary canines on dental stone casts. The lingual ridge was found to be the most elevated of the three lingual ridges 46% of the time, the distal ridge was most elevated 36% of the time, and the mesial marginal ridge was most elevated only 18% of the time.] The mesial marginal ridge (extending from the proximal contact area to the cingulum) is longer than the distal marginal ridge because of the shorter mesial cusp slope and the more incisally located mesial contact area.

The marginal ridges of mandibular canines are not prominent, and much of the lingual surface appears smooth when compared to that of the maxillary canines (an arch trait). The somewhat inconspicuous mesial marginal ridge may be longer and straighter than the shorter, more elevated, and curved distal marginal ridge. The *distal marginal ridge* is usually slightly more prominent or elevated than either the lingual ridge or the mesial marginal ridge. [Of 244 mandibular canines on dental stone casts inspected by dental hygiene students, the distal marginal ridge was the most prominent of the three lingual ridges on 63% of the teeth and the mesial marginal ridge was the most prominent on only 18%. The lingual ridge was most prominent only on 19% of these unworn lingual surfaces.]

4. CANINE ROOTS FROM THE LINGUAL VIEW

Maxillary and mandibular canine roots are usually convex on the lingual surface and are narrower mesiodistally on the lingual half than on the labial half. Therefore, it is often possible to see both mesial and distal sides of the root and one or both of the proximal longitudinal root depressions from this view.

C. CANINES FROM THE PROXIMAL VIEWS

Refer to *Figure 5-6* while studying the similarities and differences of canines from the mesial or distal views.

1. CANINE OUTLINE FROM THE PROXIMAL VIEWS

The wedge- or triangular-shaped maxillary canine crown from this view has a bulky (thick) cusp because of the prominent labial and lingual ridges. The mandibular canine crown is also wedge shaped but thinner in the incisal portion than the crown of the maxillary canine because of a less bulky lingual ridge. Observe this difference in cusp thickness in the canines in Figure 5-6.

2. INCISAL RIDGE AND CUSP TIP OF CANINES FROM THE PROXIMAL VIEWS

The incisal ridge and cusp tip of a maxillary canine are usually located *labial* to the midroot axis line. The incisal ridge and cusp tip of the mandibular canine are most often located slightly *lingual* to the root axis line, but it may be centered over it (Appendix 4h). This is a good distinguishing trait between

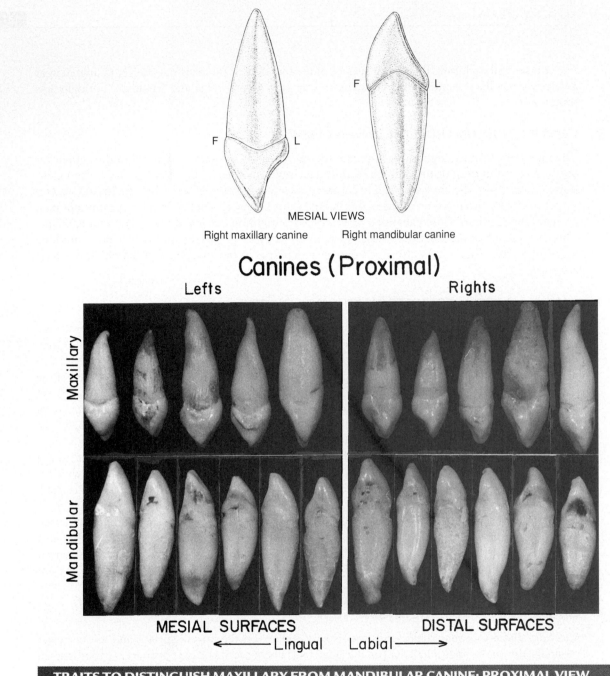

MESIAL VIEWS

Right maxillary canine   Right mandibular canine

Canines (Proximal)

Lefts   Rights

Maxillary

Mandibular

MESIAL SURFACES   DISTAL SURFACES

← Lingual   Labial →

TRAITS TO DISTINGUISH MAXILLARY FROM MANDIBULAR CANINE: PROXIMAL VIEW

MAXILLARY CANINE	MANDIBULAR CANINE
Cingulum more prominent	Cingulum less prominent
Cusp tip labial to root axis line	Cusp tip lingual to root axis line
Labial height of contour less cervical	Labial height of contour closer to cervical line
Labial height of contour more pronounced	Labial height of contour less pronounced
Incisal wear is more lingual, even in fossa	Incisal wear more labial
Cusp tip appears thicker faciolingually (FL)	Cusp tip appears less thick FL

TRAITS TO DIFFERENTIATE RIGHT FROM LEFT CANINES: COMPARING PROXIMAL VIEWS

MAXILLARY CANINE	MANDIBULAR CANINE
Cervical line curves more on the mesial than distal surface	
Distal root depression is more distinct than mesial	

FIGURE 5-6. Proximal views of canines with traits to distinguish maxillary from mandibular canines and traits to distinguish rights from lefts.

mandibular and maxillary canines. Observe this difference in cusp tip location (more labial on the maxillary canine and more lingual on mandibular canines) in a majority of canines in Figure 5-6. Further, the distoincisal angle of the mandibular canine is slightly more lingual in position than the cusp tip because of the distolingual twist of the crown so that much of the lingual surface is visible from the mesial aspect, similar to the adjacent mandibular lateral incisors (best appreciated from the incisal view on Appendix 4f).

3. CANINE HEIGHT OF CONTOUR FROM THE PROXIMAL VIEWS

As with all teeth, the *facial* height of contour of the maxillary canine is in the cervical third of the crown, but it may not be as close to the cervical line as the corresponding curvature on the incisor teeth or on the mandibular canine. The labial surface is much more convex than on the incisors. (Feel it and compare the curvatures of the incisors and the canines.)

The height of contour of the *labial* surface of the mandibular canine crown is closer to the cervical line than on a maxillary canine. There is an almost continuous crown–root outline on mandibular canines with minimal facial or lingual (cingulum) crown bulge when viewed from the proximal aspects. This lack of discernible cervical crown bulge beyond the root facially and lingually is clearly evident in many mandibular canines in Figure 5-6. This feature can be helpful when distinguishing mandibular from maxillary canines.

As with all anterior teeth, the *lingual* heights of contour of *all canines* are usually in the cervical third, on the cingulum.

4. CANINE CERVICAL LINE FROM THE PROXIMAL VIEWS

The cervical lines of *all canines* from the proximal views usually curve incisally quite a bit (over 2 mm on maxillary canines). As on incisors, the curvature is greater on the mesial surface than on the distal surface, but the difference is less on the canines than on the incisors. [Of the 321 maxillary canines measured by Dr. Woelfel's dental hygiene students, the *mesial* cervical curvature averaged 2.1 mm, with a range from 0.3 to 4.0 mm; the *distal* curvature averaged 1.4 mm, with a range of 0.2 to 3.5 mm. Such wide variability is not unusual.]

The mandibular canine cervical line appears to curve more incisally than on maxillary canines. The fact that the mandibular canine crown is narrower faciolingually than the maxillary canine [by 0.4 mm] and has a greater mesial cervical line curve [by 0.3 mm] accentuates the apparent greater depth of the curve [averages from 637 canines]. However, the amount of curvature of the cervical lines of the mandibular canines varied considerably [from 4.8 mm to 0.2 mm, one that was almost flat]. So, once again, a tremendous variation is evident between the same type of teeth. As with most other teeth, the cervical line curves less on the distal surface than on the mesial surface [by 0.8 mm; of the 316 mandibular canines measured, the *mesial* curvature averaged 2.4 mm; the *distal* curvature averaged 1.6 mm].

5. CANINE ROOT SHAPE AND DEPRESSIONS FROM THE PROXIMAL VIEWS

The labial outlines of the roots of *maxillary and mandibular canines* are often *slightly* convex with the lingual outline more convex, although this varies. *Both maxillary and mandibular canine* roots usually have vertical longitudinal (cervicoapical) depressions on the mesial *and* distal surfaces, and the distal depression is usually more distinct (deeper), especially on the lowers. [Mesial: on 100 *maxillary* canines examined by Dr. Woelfel, 70 had a longitudinal depression on the *mesial* root surface (six fairly deep), 23 were flat, and only 8 had convex mesial middle third root surfaces with no depression. On 100 *mandibular* canines examined by Dr. Woelfel, 88 had a longitudinal *mesial* root depression (28 were fairly deep), 8 were flat, and 4 were considered to be convex. Distal: on 100 *maxillary* canines examined by Dr. Woelfel, 90 had a longitudinal depression on the *distal* surface (20 were rather deep), and only 10 had no distal root depression. Of 100 *mandibular* canines examined by Dr. Woelfel, 97 had a longitudinal depression on the *distal* surface (40 were fairly deep), and only 3 had flat distal root surfaces. None of the distal root surfaces was judged to be convex on the middle third of the root.] A summary of the location and relative depth of root depressions on canines is presented in *Table 5-4*.

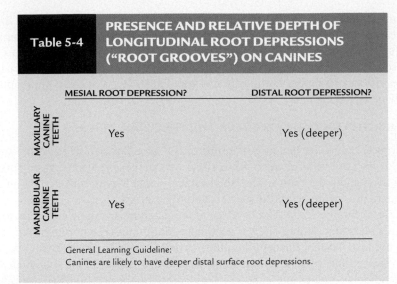

Table 5-4	PRESENCE AND RELATIVE DEPTH OF LONGITUDINAL ROOT DEPRESSIONS ("ROOT GROOVES") ON CANINES	
	MESIAL ROOT DEPRESSION?	DISTAL ROOT DEPRESSION?
MAXILLARY CANINE TEETH	Yes	Yes (deeper)
MANDIBULAR CANINE TEETH	Yes	Yes (deeper)

General Learning Guideline:
Canines are likely to have deeper distal surface root depressions.

D. CANINES FROM THE INCISAL VIEW

Refer to *Figure 5-7* for a comparison of similarities and differences of canines from the incisal view. To follow this description, the tooth should be held so that the incisal edge (cusp tip) is toward the observer, the labial surface is at the top, and the observer is looking *exactly down the midroot axis line*. You should see more of the lingual surface of the maxillary canine since the cusp tip and the cusp ridges are usually labial to the midroot axis line, and you should see more of the labial surface of mandibular canines when the cusp ridges are lingual to the midroot axis line, as seen on most canines in Figure 5-7.

1. CANINE CROWN PROPORTIONS FROM THE INCISAL VIEW

The maxillary canine crown outline is not symmetrical. The faciolingual dimension of the maxillary canine crown is slightly greater than the mesiodistal dimension [by 0.5 mm] (recall Appendix 3d). This is similar to the *mandibular* anterior teeth but uncharacteristic of the *maxillary incisors,* which are usually wider mesiodistally than faciolingually. The labiolingual dimension of the mandibular canine crown is noticeably greater than the mesiodistal measurement [by an average of 0.9 mm on 316 teeth]. This characteristic oblong faciolingual outline is seen on many mandibular canines in Figure 5-7.

2. CANINE INCISAL EDGE (CUSP TIP) CONTOUR FROM THE INCISAL VIEW

The incisal edge (made up of the cusp tip and thick mesial and distal cusp ridges) of the maxillary canine is located slightly labial to the labiolingual center of the root, and this edge is aligned almost horizontally (Appendix 4f).

The cusp tip of the mandibular canine is near the center labiolingually, or it may be lingual to the center. When the tooth is held with the faciolingual axis of the cervix of the root exactly vertical, the distal cusp ridge is directed slightly lingually from the cusp tip, placing the distoincisal angle in a position somewhat lingual to the position of the cusp tip (Appendix 4f). This lingual placement of the distoincisal angle gives the incisal part of the crown a slight distolingual twist (similar to the adjacent mandibular lateral incisor). From this view, the *distolingual twist* of the crown appears to "bend" to follow the curvature of the dental arch.

3. CANINE CINGULUM AND MARGINAL RIDGES FROM THE INCISAL VIEW

The maxillary canine cingulum is large and is located in the center mesiodistally (Appendix 4e). On the lingual outline of the mandibular canine, the height (crest) of contour of the cingulum is centered or slightly distal to the centerline (Appendix 4e). The mesial marginal ridge (extending from the con-

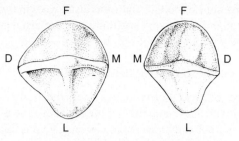

INCISAL VIEWS

Right maxillary canine   Right mandibular canine

CANINES (Incisal)
Facial Surfaces

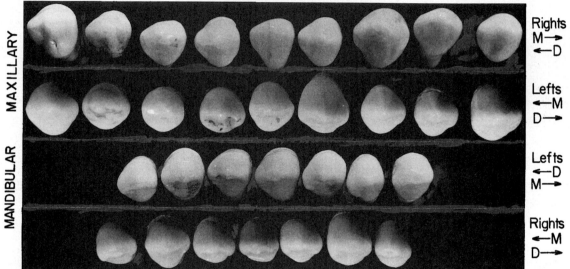

Lingual Surfaces

TRAITS TO DISTINGUISH MAXILLARY FROM MANDIBULAR CANINE: INCISAL VIEW

MAXILLARY CANINE	MANDIBULAR CANINE
More asymmetrical crown outline	More symmetrical crown outline
Slightly greater faciolingually (FL) than mesiodistally (MD)	Much greater FL compared to MD
Distal half of crown pinched in FL	Distal crown pinch FL not as evident
Cingulum centered	Cingulum to distal (or centered)
Incisal edge more horizontal mesiodistally	Incisal edge with distolingual twist
Facets on lingual-incisal or lingual surface	Facets on labial-incisal of cusp ridge
Contour traits noted from lingual view are also seen from incisal view	

TRAITS TO DIFFERENTIATE RIGHT FROM LEFT CANINES: INCISAL VIEW

MAXILLARY CANINE	MANDIBULAR CANINE
More faciolingual bulk in mesial half	Cingulum often to distal
	Incisal ridge more lingual on distal half
Distal half of crown pinched faciolingually	Distal half of crown may be pinched faciolingually
Contour traits seen from lingual are also viewed from incisal	

FIGURE 5-7. Incisal views of canines with traits to distinguish maxillary from mandibular canines and traits to distinguish rights from lefts.

tact area to the cingulum) appears longer than the distal marginal ridge because of the slight distal placement of the cingulum and the lingual positioning of the distal cusp ridge, placing it closer to the cingulum. This may be better appreciated from the lingual view.

4. CANINE LABIAL CONTOUR FROM THE INCISAL VIEW

The labial outline of the maxillary canine is convex, more than either maxillary incisor, since the labial ridge is often quite prominent. The *mesial* half of the labial outline is quite convex, whereas the *distal* half of the labial outline is frequently somewhat concave, giving this distal portion of the crown the appearance that it has been "pinched in" on the facial (Appendix 4g). This observation is most helpful and is a reliable guide in determining right from left maxillary canines and is seen on many upper canines in the top row in Figure 5-7.

The outline of the mandibular canine crown is more symmetrical than a maxillary canine. However, the labial crown outline mesial to the centerline is noticeably more convex, whereas the labial outline distal to the center is more flat, or even slightly concave.

5. CANINE LINGUAL CONTOUR FROM THE INCISAL VIEW

The lingual ridge of the maxillary canine divides the lingual surface in half with a shallow fossa on each side. This ridge and fossae are less evident on the mandibular canine.

LEARNING EXERCISES

Assign a Universal number to a handheld tooth:

A patient just had all of his permanent teeth extracted. Imagine being asked to find tooth #6 from among a pile of 32 extracted teeth on the oral surgeon's tray because you want to evaluate a lesion on the root of that canine. How might you go about it? Try the following steps:

- From a number of extracted teeth or tooth models, select the canines based on class traits.
- Determine whether the canine is maxillary or mandibular. You should never rely on only one characteristic difference between teeth to name them; rather, make a list of many traits that suggest the tooth is a maxillary canine as opposed to only one trait that makes you think it belongs in the mandible. Refer to the arch traits in Figures 5-4 through 5-7 as needed.
- If you determine that the tooth is maxillary, position the root up; if it is mandibular, position the root down.
- With the tooth aligned correctly, use characteristic traits for each surface to identify the facial surface. This will permit you to view the tooth as though you were looking into a patient's mouth.
- Finally, determine which surface is the mesial. (Refer to the right/left traits in *Figs. 5-4* through *5-7* as needed.) While viewing the tooth from the facial and picturing it within the appropriate arch (upper or lower), the mesial surface can be positioned toward the midline in only one quadrant, the right or left.
- Once you have determined the quadrant, assign the appropriate Universal number for the canine in that quadrant. For example, the canine in the upper right quadrant is tooth #6.

SECTION III VARIATIONS IN CANINE TEETH

Probably the most conspicuous variation in canine teeth is found in the mandibular canine. For example, although it is rare to find a maxillary canine tooth with the root divided, this division is known to occur. The division results in labial and lingual roots and may be split only in the apical third, or it may extend into the cervical third of the root (*Fig. 5-8*).

Observe the enormous variation in size and shape among several maxillary and mandibular canines in *Figure 5-9*. Referring to the measurements of 637 canines in Table 5-1 under the range column, maxillary canine crowns from shortest to longest varied by 5.4 mm, root length differed by 17.7 mm, and overall length differed

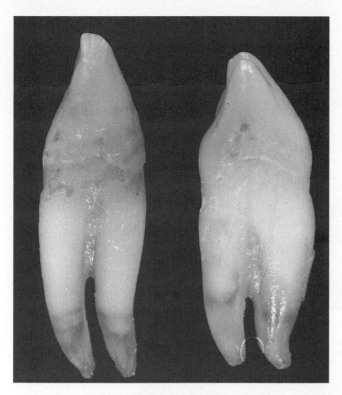

FIGURE 5-8. Two mandibular canines, each with a split (bifurcated) root that has a facial and lingual root tip.

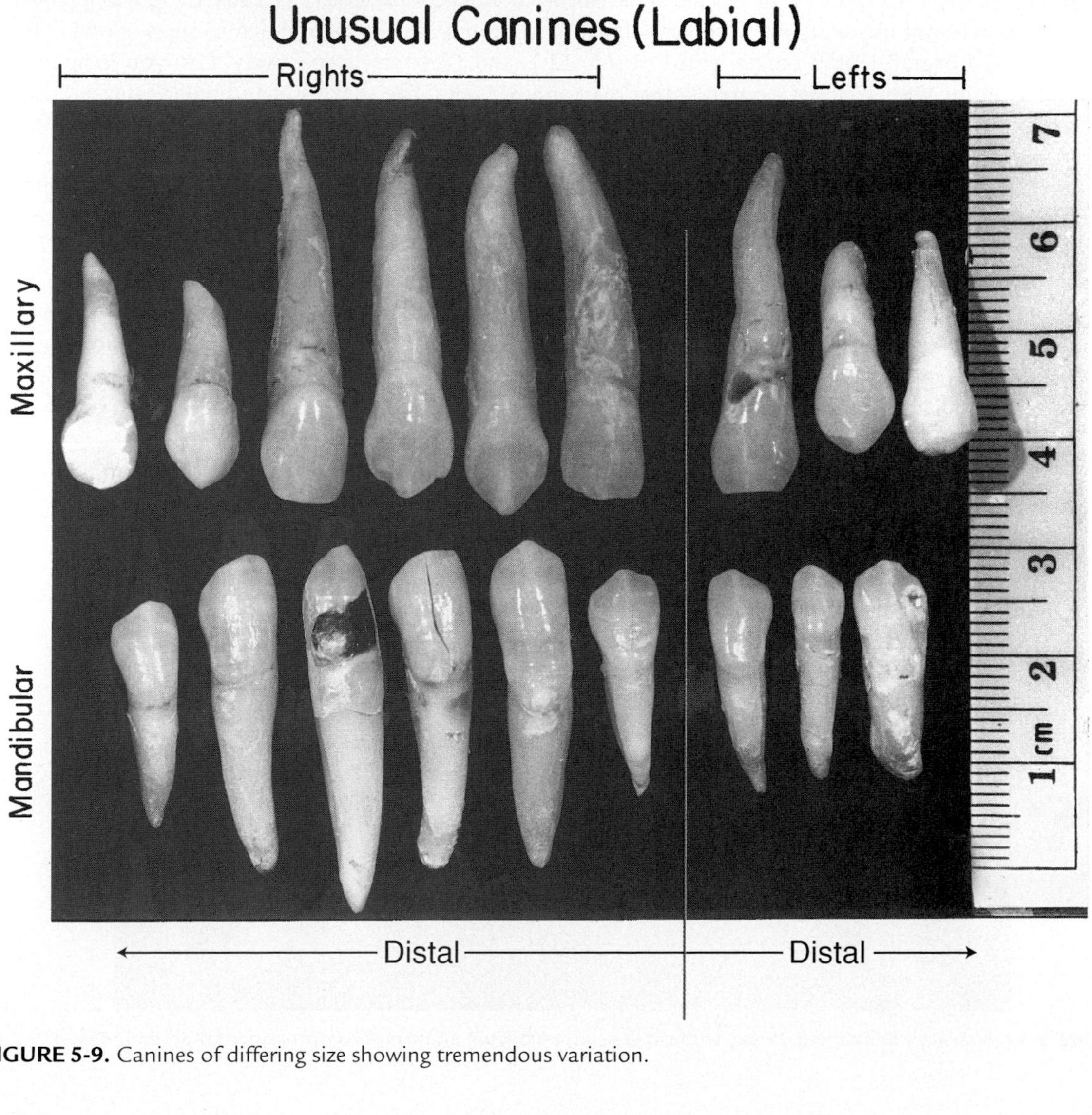

Unusual Canines (Labial)
Rights
Lefts
Maxillary
Mandibular
Distal
Distal
1cm
2
3
4
5
6
7

FIGURE 5-9. Canines of differing size showing tremendous variation.

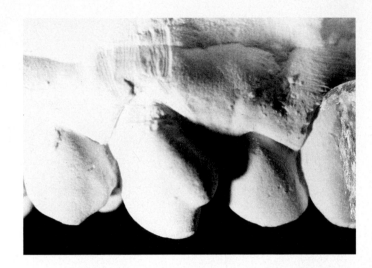

FIGURE 5-10. Maxillary right canine with a deep notch in the mesial cusp ridge.

by 18.4 mm. In the 1962 issue of the *Journal of the North Carolina Dental Society* (46:10), there was a report of an extraction, without incident, of a maxillary left canine 47 mm long. On mandibular canines, crown length, root length, and overall length ranges varied by 9.6, 12.7, and 18.4 mm, respectively. Can you imagine one mandibular canine with a crown 9.6 mm longer than another one? The shortest mandibular canine (cusp tip to root apex) was only 16.1 mm long. Two of the mandibular canine crowns in Figure 5-9 are that long. See if you can spot these teeth.

A maxillary canine with an unusual notch on its mesial cusp slope is seen in *Figure 5-10*. An unusual canine with a shovel-shaped lingual surface is evident in *Figure 5-11*. Other anomalies will be described in Chapter 12. Perhaps the most unique canines of all occur on the male Babirusa (type of wild boar) seen in *Figure 5-12*. Its two enormous maxillary canines curve backward, piercing the upper lip and bony snout on each side. Then they curve in a large arc upward, backward, and finally down toward the forehead. These unusual maxillary canines serve only to protect the boar's eyes and upper face. The Babirusa's mandibular canines are also very large and tusk-like, and curve up and back, possibly serving to protect the side of his face and for fighting or piercing food when his jaw is opened wide.

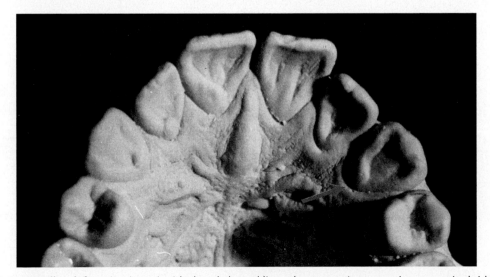

FIGURE 5-11. Maxillary left canine (*arrow*) with shovel-shaped lingual anatomy (very prominent marginal ridges).

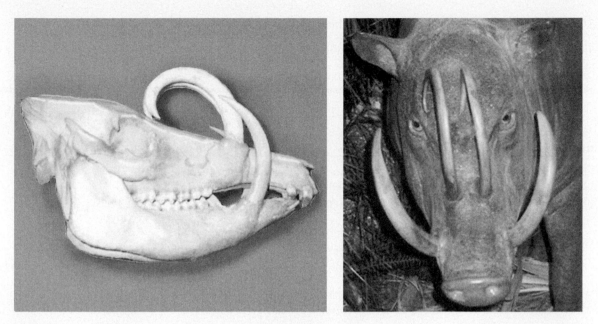

FIGURE 5-12. A male Babirusa (type of wild boar) with extremely unique canines that actually pierce the upper lip and bony snout on each side.

LEARNING QUESTIONS

For each trait described below, indicate the letter of the best response from the five selections provided. Each trait has only one best answer.

    a. Maxillary central incisor
    b. Maxillary canine
    c. Mandibular canine
    d. All of the above
    e. None of the above

1. This tooth exhibits less cervical line curvature on the distal aspect than on the mesial aspect. a b c d e

2. The cingulum is centered mesiodistally. a b c d e

3. There is an almost continuous crown-root outline on the mesial surface of this tooth. a b c d e

4. The mesial contact area is located more incisally than the distal contact area on the same tooth. a b c d e

5. The cusp tip is positioned lingual to the midroot axis line from the proximal view. a b c d e

6. Mamelons could be observed on this tooth. a b c d e

7. On which tooth is the cusp angle most acute? a b c d e

8. The mesiodistal width of this tooth is greater than its labiolingual width. a b c d e

9. The mesial and distal marginal ridges are aligned more vertically than horizontally on the lingual surface. a b c d e

10. The tooth (teeth) develop(s) from four lobes.   a   b   c   d   e

11. The tooth (teeth) develop(s) from three lobes.   a   b   c   d   e

ANSWERS: 1–d; 2–b; 3–c; 4–d; 5–c; 6–a; 7–b; 8–a; 9–d; 10–d; 11–e

REFERENCES

1. Cootjans G. The cuspid in Greaco-Latin literature. Rev Belge Med Dent 1971;26(3):387–392.
2. Year Book of Dentistry. Chicago: Year Book Medical Publishers, 1973:354.
3. Ash MM, Nelson SJ. Wheeler's dental anatomy, physiology and occlusion. Philadelphia: Saunders 2003.

GENERAL REFERENCES

Taylor RMS. Variations in form of human teeth: II. An anthropologic and forensic study of maxillary canines. J Dent Res 1969;48:173–182.

Web site: http://animaldiversity.ummz.umich.edu/site/topics/mammal_anatomy/gallery_of_canines.html—University of Michigan Museum of Zoology Animal Diversity Web Gallery of Canines

Morphology of Premolars

Topics covered within the three sections of this chapter include the following:

I. Overview of premolars
   A. General description of premolars
   B. Functions of premolars
   C. Class traits of premolars (including traits similar to anterior teeth)
   D. Arch traits that differentiate maxillary from mandibular premolars
II. Type traits that differentiate maxillary first from maxillary second premolars
   A. Type traits of maxillary premolars from the buccal view
   B. Type traits of maxillary premolars from the lingual view
   C. Type traits of maxillary premolars from the proximal views
   D. Type traits of maxillary premolars from the occlusal view
III. Type traits that differentiate mandibular first from second premolars
   A. Type traits of mandibular premolars from the buccal view
   B. Type traits of mandibular premolars from the lingual view
   C. Type traits of mandibular premolars from the proximal views
   D. Type traits of mandibular premolars from the occlusal view

SECTION I   OVERVIEW OF PREMOLARS

OBJECTIVES

This section is designed to prepare the learner to perform the following:

- Describe the functions of premolars.
- List class traits common to all premolars.
- List arch traits that can be used to distinguish maxillary from mandibular premolars.
- From a selection of all teeth, select and separate out the premolars.
- Divide a selection of all premolars into maxillary and mandibular.

Using the maxillary right second premolar as a representative example for all premolars, refer to the Appendix, page 5, while reading Section I of this chapter. Throughout this chapter, "Appendix" followed by a number and letter (e.g., Appendix 5a) is used to denote reference to the page (number 5) and item (letter a) being referred to on that appendix page. The appendix pages are designed to be torn out to facilitate study and minimize page turns.

A. GENERAL DESCRIPTION OF PREMOLARS

The term premolar is used to designate any tooth in the permanent (secondary) dentition of mammals that replaces a primary molar. There are eight premolars: four in the maxillary arch and four in the mandibular arch (*Fig. 6-1*). They are the fourth and fifth teeth from the midline in each quadrant. The maxillary premolars can be identified by the Universal Numbering System as teeth numbers 5 and 12 (maxillary right and left *first* premolars, respectively) and numbers 4 and 13 (maxillary right and

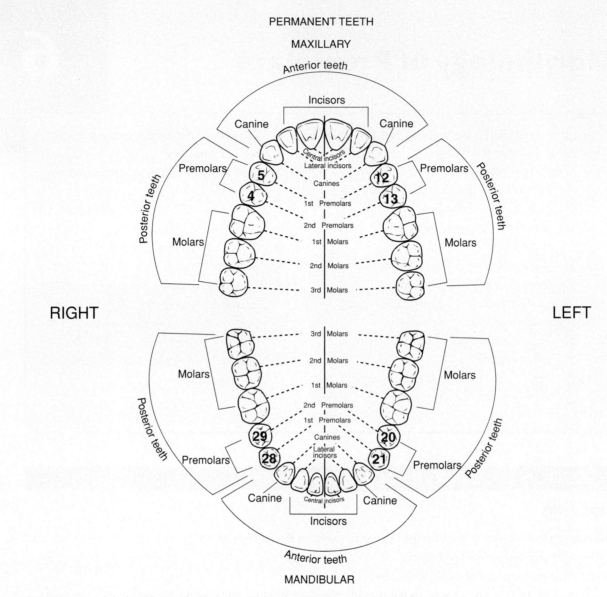

FIGURE 6-1. Adult dentition with the Universal numbers for premolars highlighted in red.

left *second* premolars, respectively). The mandibular right and left *first* premolars are numbers 28 and 21, respectively, with the mandibular right and left *second* premolars numbered 29 and 20, respectively.

The mesial surfaces of first premolars contact the distal surfaces of adjacent canines, whereas distal surfaces contact the mesial surfaces of adjacent second premolars. The distal sides of second premolars are in contact with the mesial sides of adjacent first molars.

B. FUNCTIONS OF PREMOLARS

The premolars (upper and lower) function with the molars (a) in the mastication of food and (b) in maintaining the vertical dimension of the face. The first premolars (c) assist the canines in shearing or cutting food morsels, and all premolars (d) support the corners of the mouth and cheeks to keep them from sagging. This is more discernible in older people. Patients who unfortunately have lost all of their molars can still masticate or chew quite well if they still have four to eight occluding

Table 6-1	GUIDELINE FOR DETERMINING THE NUMBER OF LOBES FOR PREMOLARS*	
TOOTH NAME	**# CUSPS**	**# LOBES**
Maxillary 1 premolar	2 (1 lingual)	3 + 1 = 4
Maxillary 2 premolar	2 (1 lingual)	3 + 1 = 4
Mandibular 1 premolar	2 (1 lingual)	3 + 1 = 4
Mandibular 2 premolar	2 or 3 (1 or 2 lingual)	3 + 1 = 4 or 3 + 2 = 5

* Number of lobes = 3 facial lobes + 1 lobe per lingual cusp

premolars. However, it is very noticeable when a person smiles and is missing one or more maxillary premolars.

C. CLASS TRAITS OF PREMOLARS

1. CLASS TRAITS SIMILAR TO ANTERIOR TEETH

Consider first the similarities between premolars and anterior teeth by examining models of the entire maxillary and mandibular arches as you read the following:

Number of Developmental Lobes: Like anterior teeth, the facial (or buccal) surfaces of all premolars develop from three *facial* lobes, usually evidenced by two shallow, vertical depressions separating a center buccal ridge on the facial surface of the crown from mesial and distal portions (Appendix 5a). This centered buccal ridge is more conspicuous on first than second premolars, and is more pronounced on maxillary than mandibular premolars. (The prominent buccal ridge on the maxillary first premolar is similar to the pronounced labial ridge on the maxillary canine.) Also, the lingual surfaces of most premolars (like anterior teeth) develop from one *lingual* lobe. In premolars, this lobe forms one lingual cusp; in anterior teeth, it forms the cingulum (recall *Fig. 3-36*). An EXCEPTION occurs in a common variation of the mandibular second premolar, the three-cusped type, which develops from three facial and *two* (not one) *lingual* lobes, forming two lingual cusps. Due to this variation of the mandibular second premolar with three cusps, the term bicuspid (referring to *two* cusps) is hardly appropriate for this group of teeth. See *Table 6-1* for a summary of the number of lobes forming each type of premolar.

Crowns Taper Toward the Cervical: From the facial, crowns are narrower in the cervical third than occlusally (Appendix 5m). This is because the widest *proximal* heights (crests) of contour (or contact areas) are located in the occlusal to middle thirds on posterior teeth (similar to the location on anterior teeth in the incisal to middle thirds).

Cervical Lines: Similar to all anterior teeth, cervical lines, when viewed from the proximal, curve toward the biting surfaces (occlusal or incisal) (Appendix 5o), and the amount of curvature is slightly greater on the mesial than on the distal surface. When viewed from the facial or lingual, cervical lines are curved toward the apex (Appendix 5n).

Root Shape: Like anterior teeth, facial and lingual root surfaces are convex, and roots taper apically (Appendix 5q). Also, the root tapers toward the lingual, resulting in a narrower lingual side of the root mesiodistally. The apical third is usually bent distally (Appendix 5p). Notice the similarity in root and crown taper and cervical line curvature on incisors, canines, and premolars when much of the incisal/occlusal third has been removed in *Figure 6-2*.

2. CLASS TRAITS THAT DIFFER FROM ANTERIOR TEETH

Tooth Surface Terminology: Compared to the anterior teeth, the facial surfaces of the posterior teeth are called *buccal* (resting against the cheeks) instead of *labial,* and posterior teeth have

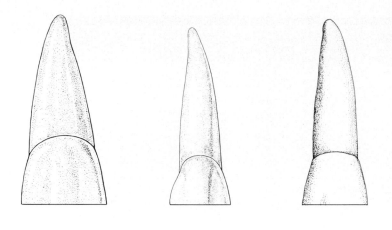

Right maxillary
central incisor

Right maxillary canine

Right maxillary
second premolar

FIGURE 6-2. Facial views of an incisor, canine, and premolar with the incisal/occlusal thirds of the crowns removed. Notice the similarities in crown taper toward the cervical line, root taper toward the apex, and cervical line contour on these three classes of teeth.

occlusal surfaces instead of *incisal* edges. Occlusal surfaces have cusps, ridges, and grooves on the occlusal surface that are basically oriented in a horizontal plane.

Occlusal Cusps Versus Incisal Edges: Unlike anterior teeth with incisal edges or ridges and a cingulum, premolars have one buccal (or facial) cusp, and most have one lingual cusp (Appendix 5b). The EXCEPTION is the mandibular second premolar, which often has two lingual cusps [54% of the time].

Marginal Ridges: The marginal ridges of premolars are oriented in a horizontal plane versus a more lingually sloping plane in the anterior teeth (Appendix 5c). However, the mesial marginal ridge of the mandibular first premolar is an EXCEPTION since it is aligned almost halfway between horizontal and vertical (Appendix 6s).

Crown and Root Length: Premolar crowns are shorter than *anterior* tooth crowns [maxillary premolar crowns are 0.8–3.5 mm shorter and mandibular premolars are 0.3–2.5 mm shorter]. Maxillary premolar roots are about the same length as maxillary incisor roots [within 1 mm], but are shorter than the roots of maxillary canines [by 2.5–3.1 mm for 1472 teeth]. Mandibular premolar roots are longer than mandibular incisor roots [by 1–1.9 mm] but are shorter than the mandibular canine root [by 1.3 mm]. First premolar crowns in both arches are slightly longer than second premolars (just think of the gradation in size as a transition from the long canine

Table 6-2A	SIZE OF MAXILLARY PREMOLARS (MILLIMETERS) (MEASURED BY DR. WOELFEL AND HIS DENTAL HYGIENE STUDENTS, 1974–1979)			
	234 FIRST PREMOLARS		**224 SECOND PREMOLARS**	
DIMENSION MEASURED	Average	Range	Average	Range
Crown length	8.6	7.1–11.1	7.7	5.2–10.5
Root length	13.4	8.3–19.0	14.0	8.0–20.6
Overall length	21.5	15.5–28.9	21.2	15.2–28.4
Crown width (mesiodistal)	7.1	5.5–9.4	6.6	5.5–8.9
Root width (cervix)	4.8	3.6–8.5	4.7	4.0–5.8
Faciolingual crown size	9.2	6.6–11.2	9.0	6.9–11.6
Faciolingual root (cervix)	8.2	5.0–9.4	8.1	5.8–10.5
Mesial cervical curve	1.1	0.0–1.7	0.9	0.4–1.9
Distal cervical curve	0.7	0.0–1.7	0.6	0.0–1.4

Table 6-2B	SIZE OF MANDIBULAR PREMOLARS (MILLIMETERS) (MEASURED BY DR. WOELFEL AND HIS DENTAL HYGIENE STUDENTS, 1974–1979)			
	238 FIRST PREMOLARS		**227 SECOND PREMOLARS**	
DIMENSION MEASURED	Average	Range	Average	Range
Crown length	8.8	5.9–10.9	8.2	6.7–10.2
Root length	14.4	9.7–20.2	14.7	9.2–21.2
Overall length	22.4	17.0–28.5	22.1	16.8–28.1
Crown width (mesiodistal)	7.0	5.9–8.8	7.1	5.2–9.5
Root width (cervix)	4.8	3.9–7.3	5.0	4.0–6.8
Faciolingual crown size	7.7	6.2–10.5	8.2	7.0–10.5
Faciolingual root (cervix)	7.0	5.5–8.5	7.3	6.1–8.4
Mesial cervical curve	0.9	0.0–2.0	0.8	0.0–2.0
Distal cervical curve	0.6	0.0–1.6	0.5	0.0–1.3

crowns to the shorter molar crowns). However, roots of second premolars are slightly longer than first premolars. This is reflected in a root-to-crown ratio that is greater on second premolars than on firsts. Complete data can be found in Table 6-2A and B.

Height (Crest) of Contour: From both mesial and distal aspects, the *facial* heights of contour of premolar crowns are in the cervical third, like on anterior teeth. However, the heights of contour are more occlusal in position than the corresponding heights of contour on the anterior teeth (Appendix 5d). In other words, the greatest facial bulge is farther from the cervix on premolars. An EXCEPTION is the buccal height of contour of the mandibular first premolar, which may be located as far cervically as on anterior teeth. The location of the *lingual* height of contour for premolars is also farther from the cervix relative to anterior teeth. Lingually, it is located in the *middle third* occlusocervically compared to the cervical third as on anterior teeth.

Contact Areas: The proximal contact areas are more cervically located and broader than on anterior teeth.

3. OTHER CLASS TRAITS CHARACTERISTIC OF MOST PREMOLARS

Evaluate the similarities of all premolars while comparing models or extracted specimens of all four types of premolars from the views indicated. Also, use the study pages from the Appendix to identify the class traits. It is important to note that although general characteristics are described in this book, there is considerable variation from these descriptions in nature.[1–3] Please remember when studying the *maxillary* premolars to hold them with their crowns down and roots upward. With *mandibular* premolars, have the crowns upward and the roots below. In this manner, the teeth will be oriented as they were in the mouth.

a. Class Traits of Most Premolars From the Buccal View

Crown Outline Shape: The crown from the buccal view is broadest at the level of the contact areas and more narrow at the cervix: shaped roughly like a five-sided pentagon, similar to the canine crown shape (Appendix 5g). The mesial and distal outlines of the crown are nearly straight or slightly convex from contact areas to the cervical line.

Contact Areas: Both mesial and distal sides of the crown are convex around the contact areas, similar to canines. *Mesial* proximal contacts are near the junction of the occlusal and middle thirds, and the *distal* contacts are normally slightly more cervical, in the middle third (Appendix 5e), EXCEPT on mandibular first premolars, where mesial contacts are usually more cervical than the distal contacts.

Cusp Ridge Size: As with canines, when viewed from the facial, the tip of the facial cusp is often slightly mesial to the vertical root axis line of the tooth (Appendix 5h), with the *mesial* cusp ridge of the buccal cusp shorter than the *distal* ridge (Appendix 5i). The EXCEPTION to this general rule is the maxillary first premolar, where the buccal cusp tip is located slightly to the distal of the root axis line and the mesial cusp ridge is *longer* (Appendix 6e).

b. Class Traits of Most Premolars From the Lingual View

Crown Shape (Outline): The crown is narrower on the lingual side than on the buccal side, EXCEPT some three-cusped mandibular second premolars that may be wider on the lingual half. The lingual surface is convex.

c. Class Traits of Most Premolars From the Proximal Views

Marginal Ridges: The relative height of the mesial and distal marginal ridge is similar to the relative height of the proximal contact areas. The *mesial* marginal ridge is more occlusally positioned than the *distal* marginal ridge, so if you first look at the mesial side and then the distal side of this tooth, you should be able to see a little less of the triangular ridges from the mesial view (compare mesial and distal surfaces in Appendix 5j). An EXCEPTION is the mandibular first premolar, where the *distal* marginal ridge is in a more occlusal position than the *mesial* marginal ridge.

d. Class Traits of Most Premolars From the Occlusal View

Tooth Proportions: Like the majority of anterior teeth (except maxillary central and lateral incisors), all types of premolars, on average, are wider faciolingually than mesiodistally (Appendix 5k). [Measuring 923 premolars, their crowns were wider faciolingually by 1.2 mm and their roots by 2.8 mm.]

Cusp Ridges and Marginal Ridges Bound the Occlusal Table: Like canine cusps, both the buccal and lingual premolar cusps have mesial and distal cusp ridges. On premolars, these merge

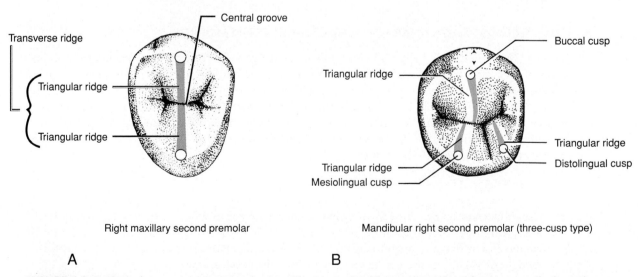

Right maxillary second premolar

Mandibular right second premolar (three-cusp type)

A

B

FIGURE 6-3. A. Typical two-cusp type premolar (maxillary second) with two **triangular ridges** (one on the buccal cusp and one on the lingual cusp) joining to form one longer **transverse ridge. B.** The mandibular second premolar, three-cusp type, is the EXCEPTION since it is the only premolar that has three triangular ridges (one per cusp) that do NOT join to form a transverse ridge.

laterally with the marginal ridges to surround the portion of the tooth known as the **occlusal table** (inside of the dotted lines on Appendix 5-l).

Triangular Ridges Form Transverse Ridges: The triangular ridges of the buccal and lingual cusps slope toward the occlusal sulcus and converge at the central groove (see *Fig. 6-3A*). On premolars with only two cusps, the two triangular ridges (one buccal and one lingual) join together to form a transverse ridge, which can be best observed from the occlusal aspect. An EXCEPTION: The three triangular ridges on the three-cusped mandibular second premolar do *not* meet so do *not* form a transverse ridge (*Fig. 6-3B*).

Grooves and Fossae: A groove (or grooves) runs mesiodistally across the occlusal surface on most premolars. (EXCEPTION: the mandibular first premolar has a pronounced transverse ridge, often without a groove running mesiodistally across it.) This groove (or grooves), when present, ends mesially in the mesial fossa and distally in the distal fossa. These fossae are bounded on one side by the buccal and lingual triangular ridges and on the other side by a marginal ridge. A central groove is labeled in Figure 6-3A.

Proximal Contacts Viewed from the *Occlusal View:* Proximal contacts from the occlusal view are either on or most often slightly buccal to the faciolingual midline of the crown (Appendix 5f).

D. ARCH TRAITS THAT DIFFERENTIATE MAXILLARY FROM MANDIBULAR PREMOLARS

Refer to Appendix page 6 while reading about differences between maxillary and mandibular premolars.

Relative Shape and Size: The maxillary first and second premolars appear more alike than the mandibular premolars (yet the *maxillary first* premolar crown is larger than the second in all dimensions).

Lingual Crown Tilt in Mandibular Premolars: From either proximal aspect, the **mandibular** premolar crowns appear to be *tilted* lingually relative to their roots (the first premolar noticeably more than the second). This lingual tilting of the crown is characteristic for all mandibular posterior teeth and enables their buccal cusps to fit and function both beneath and lingual to the **maxillary** buccal cusps, which are aligned more directly over their roots. This difference is easy to recognize when comparing the proximal views of maxillary and mandibular premolars in Appendix 6j, maxillary, and 6a, mandibular.

Cusp Size and Location: The buccal cusp is larger, and longer, than the lingual cusp (or cusps) on all premolars, but the difference is minimal on maxillary second premolars and is much more evident on **mandibular** premolars (compare Appendix 6c, maxillary, and 6p, mandibular). *Lingual cusp* tips are positioned off center *to the mesial* most often on maxillary premolars and may be centered or positioned to the mesial on mandibular first and second (two-cusp) premolars (seen from lingual views in Appendix 6i and 6q).

Distal Crown Tilt on Mandibular Premolars: From the buccal and lingual aspects, many mandibular premolar crowns, especially mandibular first premolars, appear to be tilted somewhat distally at the cervix. This distal tilting is characteristic of all *mandibular posterior* teeth (including the three molars) and the mandibular canines.

Buccal Ridge Prominence: The buccal ridge is more prominent on the maxillary first premolar than on the mandibular first premolar.

Crown Proportions: From the occlusal view, **maxillary** premolars are more *oblong* or rectangular (considerably wider faciolingually than mesiodistally), whereas **mandibular** premolars are more *square* (closer to equal dimension faciolingually as mesiodistally) (*Fig. 6-4*). This difference may be even more apparent when comparing the shape of the occlusal table (the area bounded by a perimeter of ridges: mesial and distal cusp ridges of each cusp, and mesial and distal marginal ridges). This difference is also apparent when comparing the dimensions of the occlusal views of maxillary and mandibular premolars in Appendix 6d.

Now is a good time to review major differences between maxillary and mandibular premolars highlighted in *Table 6-3*.

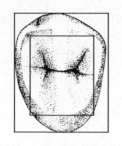
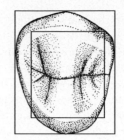

Right maxillary second premolar   Right maxillary first premolar

MAXILLARY PREMOLARS (OCCLUSAL)

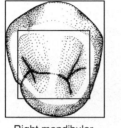
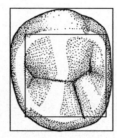
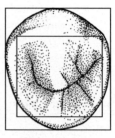

Right mandibular   Three-cusp type   Two-cusp type
first premolar

Right mandibular second premolar

MANDIBULAR PREMOLARS (OCCLUSAL)

FIGURE 6-4. ARCH DIFFERENCES BETWEEN PREMOLARS: all types of premolars with an outer box highlighting the proportion of the entire occlusal outline of each tooth and an inner box highlighting the proportion of its occlusal table. Notice that, even though all premolar types are longer faciolingually than mesiodistally, the shapes of the maxillary premolars are much more rectangular (more obviously longer faciolingually) compared to the shape of mandibular premolars, which are closer to square.

Table 6-3	MAJOR ARCH TRAITS THAT DISTINGUISH MAXILLARY FROM MANDIBULAR PREMOLARS	
	MAXILLARY PREMOLARS	**MANDIBULAR PREMOLARS**
BUCCAL VIEW	Buccal ridge is more prominent	Buccal ridge is less prominent
	No distal crown tilt relative to root	Crown exhibits slight distal tilt on root
LINGUAL VIEW	Lingual cusps relatively longer than mandibular lingual cusps	Lingual cusps relatively shorter than maxillary lingual cusps
	Tip of lingual cusp toward mesial	Lingual cusp tip centered or two lingual cusps
PROXIMAL VIEWS	Crown tips aligned over root	Crown tilts to lingual relative to root
	Lingual cusp is just slightly shorter than buccal	Lingual cusp is much shorter than buccal
OCCLUSAL VIEW	Crown shape oval or rectangular	Crown shape closer to square
	Crown considerably wider faciolingually (FL) than mesiodistally	Crown less oblong FL

SECTION II	TYPE TRAITS THAT DIFFERENTIATE MAXILLARY FIRST FROM MAXILLARY SECOND PREMOLARS

OBJECTIVES

This section prepares the reader to perform the following:

- Describe the type traits that can be used to distinguish the permanent maxillary first premolar from the maxillary second premolar.
- Describe and identify the labial, lingual, mesial, distal, and occlusal surfaces for all maxillary premolars.
- Assign a Universal number to maxillary premolars present in a mouth (or on a model of the teeth) with complete dentition. If possible, repeat this on a model with one or more maxillary premolars missing.
- Holding a maxillary premolar, determine whether it is a first or a second and right or left. Then assign a Universal number to it.

A. TYPE TRAITS OF MAXILLARY PREMOLARS FROM THE BUCCAL VIEW

From the buccal view, compare the maxillary first and second premolars in *Figure 6-5*. Compare tooth models and/or extracted maxillary premolars as you read the following characteristics, holding the crowns down and roots up, just as they are oriented in the mouth.

1. RELATIVE SIZE OF MAXILLARY PREMOLAR CROWNS FROM THE BUCCAL VIEW

The *crown* of the *maxillary first premolar* is larger than the maxillary second premolar [wider by 0.5 mm and longer by 0.9 mm], but the root is shorter overall [by 0.6 mm; measurements on 458 teeth]. The **shoulders** (junction of cusp slopes and proximal surfaces) seem more broad, bulging, and angular (especially on the mesial) on the first premolar than on the more gently convex second premolar.

The mesial and distal sides of the crown, from the contact areas to the cervical line, converge more noticeably on the maxillary first premolar than second premolar. This makes the cervical portion of the crown of the second premolar appear relatively wider. Observe the more prominent mesial shoulders and increased crown taper on many maxillary first premolars in Figure 6-5.

2. LOCATION OF PROXIMAL CONTACTS FOR MAXILLARY PREMOLARS FROM THE BUCCAL VIEW

For *both* types of maxillary premolars, mesial contacts are usually in the middle third, near the junction of the occlusal and middle thirds. As on anterior teeth, distal contacts are slightly more cervical. Distal contacts of premolars are in the middle third (recall Appendix 5e).

3. LOCATION OF THE BUCCAL CUSP TIP OF MAXILLARY PREMOLARS FROM THE BUCCAL VIEW

The *maxillary first premolar* has its buccal cusp tip placed slightly to the *distal* of the vertical midroot axis line with a longer mesial cusp ridge, as compared to the distal cusp ridge (Appendix 6e and most maxillary first premolars in *Fig. 6-5*). This is an EXCEPTION to all other premolars (including maxillary second premolars) and canines, which have their buccal cusp tip placed more to the mesial, or centered, with their mesial cusp ridge shorter than their distal.

4. SHAPE OF THE BUCCAL CUSP OF MAXILLARY PREMOLARS FROM THE BUCCAL VIEW

The buccal cusp of the **maxillary first premolar** is relatively long and pointed or sharp (Appendix 6f), resembling a maxillary canine, with the mesial and distal slopes meeting at almost a right angle

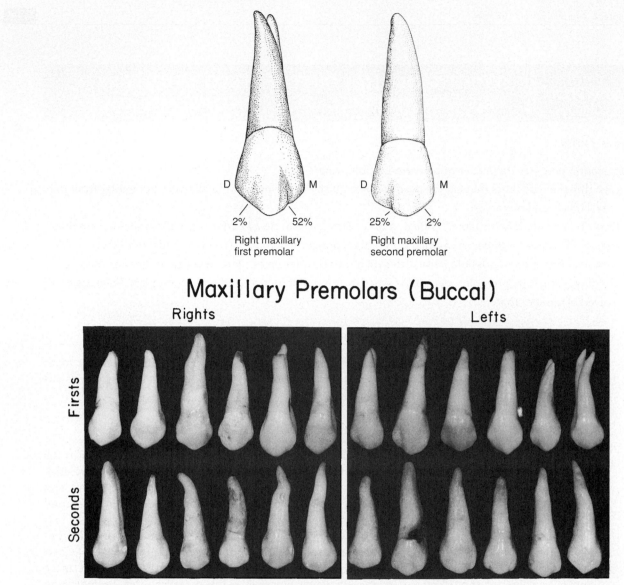

Maxillary Premolars (Buccal)

Right maxillary first premolar
2%   52%
D   M

Right maxillary second premolar
25%   2%
D   M

Rights   Lefts

Firsts

Seconds

← Distal →

TRAITS TO DISTINGUISH MAXILLARY FIRST FROM SECOND PREMOLAR: BUCCAL VIEWS

MAXILLARY FIRST PREMOLAR	MAXILLARY SECOND PREMOLAR
Mesial buccal ridge depression [52%]	Distal buccal ridge depression [25%]
Sharper buccal cusp angle (105°)	More blunt buccal cusp angle (125°)
Bulging shoulders and angular outline	Narrow, more rounded shoulders
Tapers more from contacts cervically	Less taper from contacts cervically
Mesial cusp arm longest	Distal cusp arm longest
Prominent buccal ridge	Less prominent buccal ridge

TRAITS TO DIFFERENTIATE MAXILLARY RIGHT FROM LEFT PREMOLARS: BUCCAL VIEWS

MAXILLARY FIRST PREMOLAR	MAXILLARY SECOND PREMOLAR
Longer mesial cusp ridge	Shorter mesial cusp ridge
Depression mesial to buccal ridge [52%]	Depression distal to buccal ridge [25%]

Root often, but not always, curves to distal for both

FIGURE 6-5. Buccal views of maxillary premolars with type traits to distinguish maxillary first from second premolars and traits to distinguish rights from lefts. Percentages give the frequency of deeper depressions on the occlusal third of the buccal crown surface.

(100–110°), compared to the **second premolar,** which is less pointed and more obtuse (125–130°), as seen on most second premolars in Figure 6-5.

5. BUCCAL RIDGE AND DEPRESSIONS OF MAXILLARY PREMOLARS FROM THE BUCCAL VIEW

The buccal ridge is prominent on the **maxillary first premolar** (Appendix 6g). A shallow vertical depression mesial to the buccal ridge in the occlusal third of the crown was found about half of the time in the first premolars [52% of 452], but rarely on the distal [2%]. The buccal ridge is less prominent on the *maxillary* **second premolar,** and depressions were found only 27% of the time on second premolars, more often in the distal [506 teeth]. The most common location of these depressions is depicted in the drawings in Figure 6-5.

6. ROOTS OF MAXILLARY PREMOLARS FROM THE BUCCAL VIEW

Most of the time, the **maxillary first premolar** has a divided root with buccal and lingual portions or roots coming off a common trunk in the apical third (seen best from the proximal view in Appendix 6h, but both root tips may also be seen from the buccal view). [On 200 teeth, 61% had two roots, 38% had one root, and 1% had three roots.] The buccal and lingual roots are usually relatively straight except for a frequent distal curve of the buccal root near the apex. Sometimes you can see the tip of the lingual root when it is straighter or bends in a different direction than the buccal root. This is evident in several maxillary first premolars in Figure 6-5.

The single root of the **second premolar** is longer on the average than on the first premolar [by 0.6 mm] and is nearly twice as long as the crown. The root-to-crown ratio is 1.8:1, which is the highest for any maxillary tooth. This means that the root is 1.8 times the length of the crown.

The apical end of the root of *all* premolars frequently bends distally [58% of 343 second premolars and 66% of 426 first premolars], but these roots may also be straight or bend mesially.

B. TYPE TRAITS OF MAXILLARY PREMOLARS FROM THE LINGUAL VIEW

Compare the lingual view of maxillary first and second premolars in *Figure 6-6.*

1. RELATIVE CUSP SIZE OF MAXILLARY PREMOLARS FROM THE LINGUAL VIEW

The lingual cusp is shorter than the buccal cusp, considerably more so on the maxillary first premolar. The cusps of the maxillary second premolar are nearly the same length. This trait is seen in almost all first premolars in Figure 6-6 and is evident on the lingual views of maxillary premolars on Appendix page 6. [Maxillary *first* premolar lingual cusps were 1.3 mm shorter on the average, ranging from 0.3 to 3.3 mm shorter on 317 teeth; *second* premolar lingual cusps averaged only 0.4 mm shorter on 300 teeth.] The crown is a little narrower on the lingual side than on the buccal side, more obviously so on the first premolar than on the second premolar.

2. CUSP RIDGES OF MAXILLARY PREMOLARS FROM THE LINGUAL VIEW

The mesial and distal ridges of the *lingual* cusp of the **maxillary first premolars** meet at the cusp tip at a somewhat rounded angle, but the angle is still sharp or steep compared to the molar cusps. The tip of the lingual cusp of the **second premolar** is relatively sharper.

3. LINGUAL CUSP POSITION FOR MAXILLARY PREMOLARS FROM THE LINGUAL VIEW

The tips of the unworn lingual cusps of *both* maxillary premolars are consistently positioned to the *mesial* of the midroot axis line (Appendix 6i). This trait is an excellent way to tell rights from lefts, especially for the maxillary second premolar, which is, in most other ways, nearly symmetrical.

4. MARGINAL RIDGES OF MAXILLARY PREMOLARS FROM THE LINGUAL VIEW

From the lingual view, differences in marginal ridge heights are apparent on handheld teeth when rotating the tooth just enough one way to see the mesial ridge height, then just enough in the opposite

MAXILLARY PREMOLARS (Lingual)

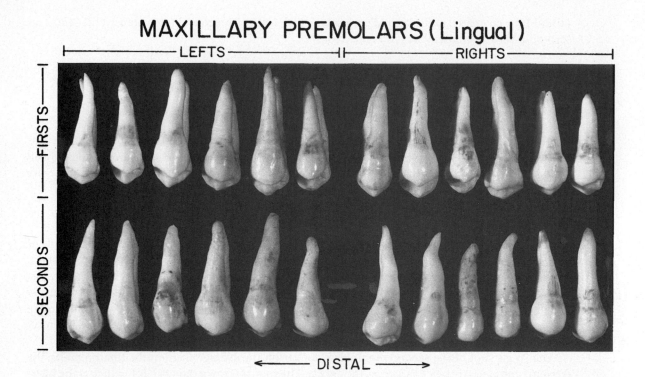

FIGURE 6-6. Lingual views of maxillary premolars with type traits to distinguish maxillary first from second premolars and traits to distinguish rights from lefts.

TRAITS TO DISTINGUISH MAXILLARY FIRST FROM SECOND PREMOLAR: LINGUAL VIEWS	
MAXILLARY FIRST PREMOLAR	**MAXILLARY SECOND PREMOLAR**
Lingual cusp shorter: see both cusps	Buccal and lingual cusps same length and width
Crown narrower on lingual	Less taper toward lingual
Outline traits visible from buccal view are also visible from lingual view	

TRAITS TO DIFFERENTIATE MAXILLARY RIGHT FROM LEFT PREMOLARS: LINGUAL VIEWS	
MAXILLARY FIRST PREMOLAR	**MAXILLARY SECOND PREMOLAR**
Lingual cusp tip is bent toward the mesial for both	
Length of buccal cusp ridges: mesial longest on first and distal longest on second	

direction to compare the distal ridge height. The *distal* marginal ridges of *both* types of maxillary premolars are more cervical in position than the mesial marginal ridge (recall Appendix 5j). (This relative positioning is true of all posterior teeth, with the EXCEPTION of the *mandibular* first premolar, where the distal marginal ridge is the more occlusal one.)

5. ROOTS OF MAXILLARY PREMOLARS FROM THE LINGUAL VIEW

The lingual root of a two-rooted maxillary *first premolar* is usually shorter than the buccal root [0.8 mm for 93 teeth]. The apical end of the lingual root of the teeth may bend toward either the mesial or the distal. *Both* first and second premolar roots taper narrower to the lingual.

C. TYPE TRAITS OF MAXILLARY PREMOLARS FROM THE PROXIMAL VIEWS

Compare the proximal views of maxillary first and second premolars in *Figure 6-7*.

1. CROWN SHAPE AND MORPHOLOGY OF MAXILLARY PREMOLARS FROM THE PROXIMAL VIEWS

All maxillary premolars are shaped like a trapezoid from the proximal view (Appendix 6b). A trapezoid is a four-sided figure with two parallel sides and two nonparallel sides. **Maxillary first premolars** have a prominent mesial concavity cervical to the contact area; **second premolars** do not (Appendix 6j). This unique *mesial crown concavity* is perhaps the most consistent and obvious trait of the maxillary first premolar crown that can be used to distinguish it from a maxillary second premolar and can be used to confirm the mesial surface on the maxillary first premolar. It is important to remember the location of this unique crown concavity when restoring the contours of this surface, or when detecting and removing calcified deposits on this root.

2. RELATIVE CUSP HEIGHT OF MAXILLARY PREMOLARS FROM THE PROXIMAL VIEWS

From this view, as from the lingual, the buccal cusp is noticeably longer than the lingual cusp on **maxillary first premolars,** compared to the **second premolar,** which has two cusps of nearly equal length (Appendix 6c). This difference is obvious when comparing first and second premolars in Figure 6-7. From this view, it is a challenge telling buccal from lingual on the mandibular second premolar based solely on the cusp heights, since the cusp heights are so similar. Differences in the heights of contour, however (described next) will be useful for distinguishing buccal from lingual surfaces on these teeth.

3. HEIGHT (CREST) OF CONTOUR OF MAXILLARY PREMOLARS FROM THE PROXIMAL VIEWS

Like all teeth, the *facial* height of contour of maxillary premolars is located in the cervical third. Specifically, it is near the junction of the middle and cervical third. Lingually (like other posterior teeth) it is more occlusal, in the middle third (near the center of the crown). This trait helps distinguish the buccal from lingual surfaces on the majority of maxillary premolars from the proximal views in Figure 6-7.

4. DISTANCE BETWEEN CUSPS ON MAXILLARY PREMOLARS FROM THE PROXIMAL VIEWS

The average distance between the buccal and lingual cusp tips of maxillary first and second premolars is about the same [5.9 mm and 5.7 mm, respectively, or 65–67% of the faciolingual dimension for 243 teeth]. However, both cusp tips are located over the root and *well within the boundary of the root contour,* an important relationship imparting good functional support for a large chewing area.

5. MARGINAL RIDGE GROOVES OF MAXILLARY PREMOLARS FROM THE PROXIMAL VIEWS

The *mesial* marginal ridge of **maxillary first premolars** is almost always crossed by a developmental groove called a marginal ridge groove [on 97% of 600 maxillary first premolars]. This marginal ridge groove serves as a spillway for food during mastication (best seen from the occlusal view in Appendix 6k). The *distal* marginal ridge groove occurs less frequently [39% of 600 teeth]. Short mesial *and* distal marginal ridge grooves were even less likely to be found crossing the ridges of **second premolars** [only present on 37% of 641 mesial marginal ridges and 30% of distal marginal ridges of maxillary second premolars].

6. CERVICAL LINES OF MAXILLARY PREMOLARS WHEN COMPARING PROXIMAL VIEWS

The cervical line on the *mesial* of the **maxillary first premolar** curves occlusally in a broad but shallow arc [averaging only 1.1 mm high on 234 teeth]. As on anterior teeth, the mesial curvature is slightly greater than on the distal side [by 0.4 mm on maxillary premolars]. The cervical line on

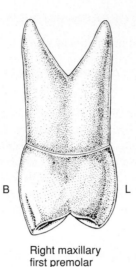

B   L

Right maxillary
first premolar

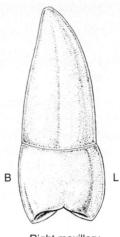

B   L

Right maxillary
second premolar

MESIAL VIEWS

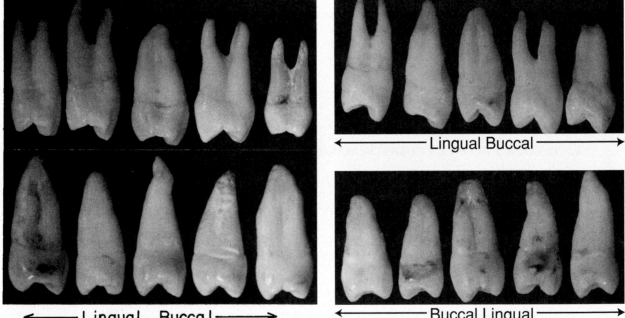

Maxillary Left Premolars
Mesial Surfaces

← Lingual   Buccal →

Maxillary Right Premolars
Distal Surfaces

← Lingual Buccal →

← Buccal Lingual →

FIGURE 6-7 Proximal views of maxillary premolars with type traits to distinguish maxillary first from second premolars and traits to distinguish rights from lefts.

TRAITS TO DISTINGUISH MAXILLARY FIRST FROM SECOND PREMOLAR: COMPARE PROXIMAL VIEWS

MAXILLARY FIRST PREMOLAR	MAXILLARY SECOND PREMOLAR
Buccal cusp longer than lingual [1.3 mm]	Buccal and lingual cusps same length
Cusp tips closer together	Cusp tips farther apart
Mesial crown and root depression	Mesial root but not crown depression
Mesial root depression deeper than distal	Distal root depression deeper than mesial
Divided or two roots [62%]	Single root
Mesial marginal ridge groove [97%]	Less likely mesial marginal ridge [37%]

TRAITS TO DIFFERENTIATE MAXILLARY RIGHT FROM LEFT PREMOLARS: PROXIMAL VIEWS

MAXILLARY FIRST PREMOLAR	MAXILLARY SECOND PREMOLAR
Mesial crown depression	No mesial crown depression
Mesial root depression at cervix	Flat/convex mesial root surface at cervix
Deeper mesial than distal root depression	Deeper distal than mesial root depression
Mesial marginal ridge groove [97%]	Mesial marginal ridge groove [only 37%]
Greater mesial than distal cervical line curvature for both	
Distal marginal ridge is more cervical than mesial for both	

FIGURE 6-7. (continued).

the *lingual* surface is in a more occlusal position than on the buccal surface. This accentuates the appearance that the lingual cusp is definitely shorter than the buccal cusp. The cervical line curvature on the mesial of the **second premolar** is also greater than on the distal [by 0.3 mm].

7. ROOTS AND ROOT DEPRESSIONS OF MAXILLARY PREMOLARS FROM THE PROXIMAL VIEWS

The roots of the maxillary premolars, when viewed from the mesial or distal aspect, often have root depressions of varying depths. Knowledge of the frequency with which these depressions occur, as well as the relative location and depth of these depressions, can be helpful clinically when using special instruments under the gingiva to detect and remove calcified deposits that contribute to periodontal disease, and when identifying areas of decay on the roots.

The **maxillary first premolar,** as stated previously, is the only premolar with an obvious concavity or depression on the mesial surface of the *crown,* and this depression continues onto the *root* [100% of teeth studied]. This important type trait is seen clearly on the mesial views of all maxillary first premolars in Figure 6-7. Recall that this tooth usually has two roots [61% of 100 teeth] with the lingual root slightly shorter [by 0.8 mm] than the buccal root. A bifurcation (split into two roots) occurs in the apical third of the root. Even when there is only one root, there is a prominent *mesial* root and adjacent crown depression. There is also a *distal* root depression found on both double- and single-rooted teeth [100% of 100 teeth]. This depression is located on the middle third of the undivided portion of the root. Near the cervix, however, the distal side of the root is usually convex or flat with little or *no* depression. The root of the maxillary first premolar is UNIQUE in that it is the only premolar type where the *mesial*-side longitudinal root depression is deeper than on the distal side.

The **maxillary second premolar** usually has one root, but like the maxillary first premolar, it also has root depressions on both sides. However, the longitudinal depression on the *mesial* root surface [78% of 100 teeth] does *not* extend onto the crown. The longitudinal depression on the *distal* root surface is located in the middle third of the root, and is usually *deeper than on the mesial root surface*. This feature is the opposite from the maxillary first premolar, which usually has the deeper midroot depression on the mesial.

D. TYPE TRAITS OF MAXILLARY PREMOLARS FROM THE OCCLUSAL VIEW

Compare occlusal views of maxillary first and second premolars in *Figure 6-8*. To follow this description, the teeth or tooth models you are using should be held as those displayed in Figure 6-8, so that the buccal surface is at the top and you are sighting down along the vertical midroot axis.

1. RELATIVE SIZE OF MAXILLARY PREMOLARS FROM THE OCCLUSAL VIEWS

In the same mouth, the *maxillary first premolar* was judged to be larger than the second premolar in 55% of the specimens examined and smaller than the second premolar in only 18% [1392 comparisons were done on dental stone casts].

2. GROOVES AND FOSSAE OF MAXILLARY PREMOLARS FROM THE OCCLUSAL VIEW

Characteristically, central developmental grooves run mesiodistally across the center of *both* maxillary premolars with a pit at both ends. The length of the central groove of the **maxillary first premolar** is more than one-third the mesiodistal width of the occlusal surface [average length was 2.7 mm of 408 teeth]. The groove of the **second premolar** averaged only 2.1 mm, shorter than on first premolars [by 0.6 mm based on 818 teeth] (Appendix 6l). This longer central groove is one of the distinguishing characteristics of the maxillary first premolar, compared to the central groove length of the second premolar, and is quite obvious when comparing the maxillary premolars in Figure 6-8.

Because the central groove is longer on the *maxillary first premolar,* the mesial and distal pits are relatively closer to the marginal ridges than on maxillary second premolars. In other words, the pits are farther apart on maxillary first premolars.

There are fewer supplemental grooves on **maxillary first premolars** than on maxillary second premolars. On **second premolars,** there are usually supplementary grooves radiating buccally and lingually from the pit at the depth of each triangular fossa.

As was seen from the mesial view of the **maxillary first premolar,** a mesial marginal ridge groove almost always crosses the mesial marginal ridge and connects with the central groove in the mesial triangular fossa (seen on the drawing in *Fig. 6-8*). The mesial marginal groove is one of the distinguishing characteristics of the maxillary first premolar, where it occurs with much greater frequency [97% of 600 first premolars] than on **second premolars** [only 37%]. Distal marginal grooves were also less common [30–39% of second and first premolars, respectively].

On about half of all maxillary premolars, the distal triangular fossae are larger than the mesial fossae. [The distal triangular fossa was larger on 55% of the 184 maxillary *first* premolars and 53% of 209 maxillary *second* premolars. The mesial triangular fossa was considered to be larger on 27% of first premolars and 17% of second premolars.]

3. RELATIVE PROPORTIONS OF MAXILLARY PREMOLARS FROM THE OCCLUSAL VIEW

The oblong (rectangular) outline of the maxillary premolar crown is greater buccolingually than mesiodistally [by 2.1 mm on 234 maxillary first premolars, and by 2.4 mm on second premolars]. This is obvious in all maxillary premolars in Figure 6-8.

4. OUTLINE OF MAXILLARY PREMOLARS FROM THE OCCLUSAL VIEW

On *both* types of maxillary premolars, the lingual half of the tooth is narrower mesiodistally than the buccal half, more so on first premolars.

From the occlusal aspect, the outline of the buccal surface of the **maxillary first premolar** is a rounded and inverted V-shape because of the prominent buccal ridge, but is less prominent on the second premolar as seen in Figure 6-8. This is the only part of the occlusal outline that looks symmetrical. The lingual three-fourths of the tooth seems to be bent slightly mesially. This is due in part to the buccal cusp tip location distal to the midline (UNIQUE to the maxillary first premolar with its mesial cusp ridge longer than its distal cusp ridge) and the lingual cusp tip mesial to the midline (*Fig. 6-9*). This *asymmetrical occlusal outline* is a distinguishing feature of maxil-

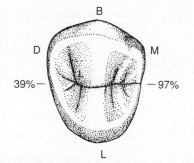

Right maxillary first premolar

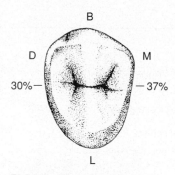

Right maxillary second premolar

Maxillary Premolars (Occlusal)

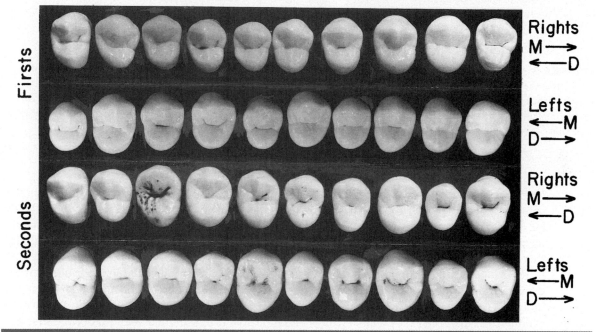

TRAITS TO DISTINGUISH MAXILLARY FIRST FROM SECOND PREMOLAR: OCCLUSAL VIEWS

MAXILLARY FIRST PREMOLAR	MAXILLARY SECOND PREMOLAR
Crown asymmetrical, more hexagonal	Crown symmetrical and more oval
Mesial side concave or flat	Mesial side more convex
Proximal surfaces converge lingually	Little tapering toward lingual
Longer central groove	Shorter central groove
Triangular fossae closer to marginal ridge	Triangular fossae closer to tooth center
Mesial marginal ridge groove [97%]	Less common mesial marginal ridge [37%]
More prominent buccal ridge	Less prominent buccal ridge
Fewer supplemental grooves	More supplemental grooves

TRAITS TO DIFFERENTIATE MAXILLARY RIGHT FROM LEFT PREMOLARS: OCCLUSAL VIEWS

MAXILLARY FIRST PREMOLAR	MAXILLARY SECOND PREMOLAR
Distal contact is more buccal	Mesial contact is more buccal
Mesial marginal ridge groove [97%]	Mesial marginal ridge groove less [37%]
Mesial crown outline is concave or flat	Mesial crown outline is convex
Mesiobuccal (MB) corner is a right angle	MB corner is obtuse angle
Lingual cusp tipped toward mesial for both	
Distal marginal ridge longer than mesial for both	

FIGURE 6-8. Occlusal views of maxillary premolars with type traits to distinguish maxillary first from second premolars and traits to distinguish rights from lefts. Percentages on the top drawings give the frequency of marginal ridge grooves crossing each marginal ridge.

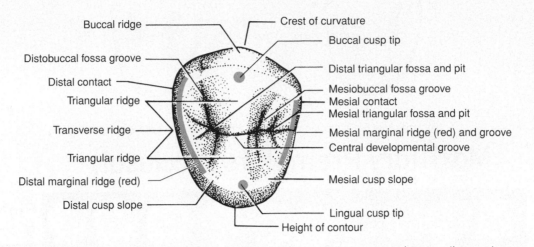

FIGURE 6-9. Maxillary right first premolar, occlusal surface, with anatomic structures that contribute to its asymmetry. Notice the proximal contact locations (the distal contact of this tooth is more buccal than the mesial), the relative length of the marginal ridges (mesial is shorter), and the location of the cusp tips where the buccal tip is distal to the middle, making the mesial cusp ridge of the buccal cusp longer than the distal cusp ridge (UNIQUE to maxillary first premolars) and the lingual cusp tip is mesial to the middle.

lary first premolars and is not found on most second premolars (compare outline shapes in Appendix 6m). The mesiobuccal cusp ridge joins the mesial marginal ridge at an almost right angle (not so on second premolars). The *mesial* outline of the *maxillary first premolar* and the *mesial marginal ridge* form a nearly straight or concave (bent inward) outline buccolingually. Recall that this mesial surface also has the mesial marginal ridge groove, and a mesial crown concavity next to the root. This mesial marginal ridge is shorter buccolingually than the longer, more convex distal marginal ridge (note this characteristic on the occlusal surfaces of most maxillary first premolars) (Fig. 6-8). Seen from the occlusal aspect, the **second premolar** is typically much more symmetrical than the first premolar. Its occlusal outline is less angular than that of the first premolar, and it has an oblong or oval shape. This smoother, more symmetrical outline is obvious on the maxillary second premolars in Figure 6-9.

5. CONTACT AREAS AND HEIGHTS OF CONTOUR OF MAXILLARY PREMOLARS FROM THE OCCLUSAL VIEW

Mesial contacts for *both* types of maxillary premolars are near or at the junction of the buccal and middle thirds (slightly more buccal on first premolars) *(Fig. 6-9)*. Recall that one-third of the tooth from this aspect means one-third of the total buccolingual measurements of the crown, rather than one-third of the occlusal surface measurement. *Distal* contacts are in the middle third on **maxillary second premolars,** located more lingually than mesial contacts. Just the opposite is true on **first premolars** with their asymmetry, where the distal contact is more buccal than the mesial contact *(Fig. 6-9)*. Picture this asymmetry when viewing the hexagon outline presented in Appendix 6m for the maxillary first premolar.

The *lingual* height of contour is usually *mesial* to the center line of the tooth for *both* first and second premolars, with the tip of the *lingual cusp always mesial to the center* of the tooth.

LEARNING EXERCISE

Review the summary tables of type traits that differentiate the maxillary first from second premolars and maxillary right from left premolars in Figures 6-5 through 6-8.

| SECTION III | TYPE TRAITS THAT DIFFERENTIATE MANDIBULAR FIRST FROM MANDIBULAR SECOND PREMOLARS |

OBJECTIVES

The section prepares the reader to perform the following:

• Describe the type traits that can be used to distinguish the permanent mandibular first premolar from the mandibular second premolar.

• Describe and identify the labial, lingual, mesial, distal, and occlusal surfaces for all mandibular premolars on a photograph, model, or extracted tooth.

• Assign a Universal number to mandibular premolars present in a mouth (or on a model of the teeth) with complete dentition. If possible, repeat this on a model with one or more mandibular premolars missing.

• Holding a mandibular premolar, determine whether it is a first or a second and right or left. Then assign a Universal number to it.

For this section, compare mandibular first and second premolars on Appendix page 6. To appreciate differences in mandibular first and second premolars, it is first important to know that there are two common types of mandibular second premolars[3]: a two-cusp type with one buccal and one lingual cusp and a three-cusp type with one buccal and two lingual cusps (seen from the occlusal sketches in *Fig. 6-15*). The frequency of these two types on 808 dental hygiene students from Ohio is given in *Table 6-4*.

LEARNING EXERCISE

Look in your own mouth and determine which of these categories matches your mandibular second premolars. The three-cusp type occurs with only slightly greater frequency than the two-cusp type [54.2% of 532 teeth for the three-cusp type versus 43% for the two-cusp type].

The morphologic details of mandibular premolars are a challenge to describe because of the great amount of variation. To list all of the frequent variations would lead to confusion rather than to clarification. Bear in mind while studying these teeth that one description will not exactly fit every tooth.[1–3] Most descriptions in

| Table 6-4 | OCCURRENCE OF LINGUAL CUSPS ON MANDIBULAR SECOND PREMOLARS (808 FEMALES, 1532 TEETH) |

NUMBER AND FREQUENCY	PERCENTAGE	COMMENT
Two lingual cusps on both sides	44.2%	Almost half
One lingual cusp on both sides	34.2%	One-third
Two lingual cusps on one side	18.2%	One-fifth
Three lingual cusps on both sides	1.7% ⎫	
Three lingual cusps on one side	1.7% ⎭	1 in 29
Overall frequency	⎧ 3-cusp type 54.2% ⎫ ⎨ 2-cusp type 43.0% ⎬ ⎩ 4-cusp type 2.8% ⎭	1532 teeth
Same type on both sides	80.1% ⎫	
Different type on each side	19.9% ⎭	702 comparisons

this book are for unworn teeth. Most extracted tooth specimens will have signs of attrition, and some will show evidence of tooth decay (caries) or wear from bruxing or grinding teeth.

Examine several extracted mandibular premolars or models as you read, and have Appendix pages 5 and 6 available. Hold them with the crowns up and the roots down.

A. TYPE TRAITS OF MANDIBULAR PREMOLARS FROM THE BUCCAL VIEW

Refer to views from the buccal of mandibular first and second premolars in *Figure 6-10*.

1. RELATIVE CROWN SHAPE AND SIZE OF MANDIBULAR PREMOLARS FROM THE BUCCAL VIEW

As with all premolars and canines, the premolar crown shape from the facial view is roughly a five-sided pentagon (Appendix 5g). From this view, *both* types of mandibular premolars appear nearly symmetrical except for the shorter mesial than distal cusp ridge and the greater distal bulge of the crown. The greater distal bulge gives the appearance of a slight distal tilt of the crown relative to the midroot axis.

The crown of the **mandibular first premolar** bears some resemblance from this aspect to the second premolar, but there are differences that make first premolars distinguishable. The buccal cusp of the mandibular first premolar crown appears longer, is centered over the root, and resembles a maxillary canine from this aspect. In general, the first premolar is slightly longer overall than the second with a longer crown [by 0.6 mm] and a shorter root [by 0.3 mm average for 465 teeth]. Just like maxillary premolars, the mandibular *first* premolar has a sharper buccal cusp [110°] than the *second*. The crown of the **mandibular second premolar** also has a pentagon shape but appears closer to square than the first premolar because it is shorter overall, it is wider in the cervical third, and its buccal cusp is less pointed than on the mandibular first premolar, with cusp slopes meeting at an angle of about 130° (Appendix 6n). The shape of the buccal surface of the second premolar is similar on both *two-cusp* and *three-cusp* types.

Cusp ridge notches: Shallow *notches* are commonplace on both cusp ridges on unworn premolars. These notches serve as spillways for food during mastication (sometimes called Thomas notches, named after Peter K. Thomas, who recommended carving them in all occlusal restorations and crowns because spillways for food are so important). The most common occurrence and frequency of such notches and of depressions in the occlusal third of the buccal surface on the cusp ridges is evident in *Figure 6-11*. On the **mandibular first premolar,** the shorter *mesial* cusp ridge of the buccal cusp is more likely to have a notch [65% of 1348 teeth] than the longer distal cusp ridge [46% of 1348 teeth]. On the **second premolar,** the frequency of notches is reversed. Its crown is more likely to have a notch on the *distal* cusp ridge [66% of 1522 teeth] than on the mesial cusp ridge [43% of 1522 teeth].

2. MORPHOLOGY OF MANDIBULAR PREMOLARS FROM THE BUCCAL VIEW

The buccal ridge and adjacent depressions of *both* types of mandibular premolars are less discernible than on the maxillary premolars. However, when vertical depressions on either side of the indistinct buccal ridge are present on the mandibular *first* premolar, the *mesial* crown depression is more likely to be deeper, whereas on the mandibular *second* premolar, the *distal* crown depression is more likely to be deeper (*Fig. 6-11*). [Of 285 mandibular *first* premolars, 80% had a smooth buccal surface in the occlusal third without depressions, 17% had a deeper depression on the *mesial* side of the buccal ridge, and only 3% had a deeper *distal* depression. Of mandibular *second* premolars, 74% had no discernible depressions, 25% had a deeper *distal* than mesial depression, and only 1% had a deeper mesial depression.] The location of these deeper depressions (mesial or distal) is consistent with the location of cusp ridge notches.

3. CERVICAL LINES OF MANDIBULAR PREMOLARS FROM THE BUCCAL VIEW

The cervical line on the buccal surface of the first premolar curves more mesiodistally than on second premolars.

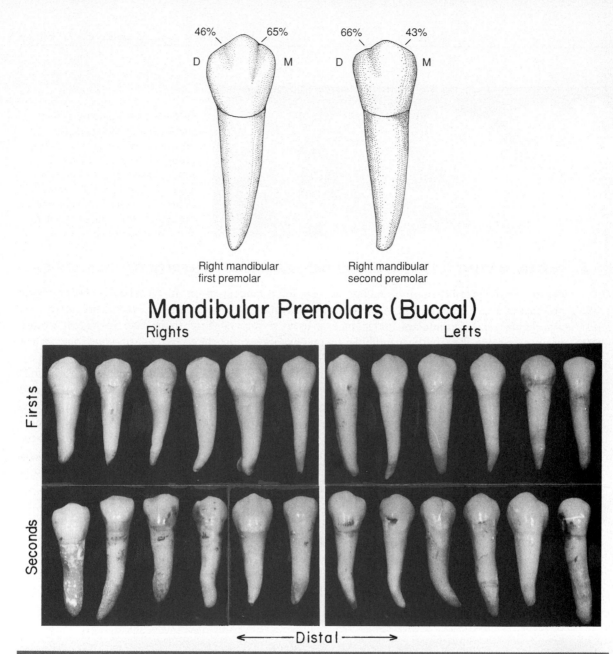

46% 65%
D   M

66% 43%
D   M

Right mandibular
first premolar

Right mandibular
second premolar

Mandibular Premolars (Buccal)
Rights   Lefts

Firsts

Seconds

←——— Distal ———→

TYPE TRAITS TO DISTINGUISH MANDIBULAR FIRST FROM SECOND PREMOLARS: BUCCAL VIEWS

MANDIBULAR FIRST PREMOLAR	MANDIBULAR SECOND PREMOLAR
Longer crown	Shorter wider crown
More crown taper from contact to cervix	Crown relatively wider at cervix
More pointed cusp (110°)	Less pointed cusp (130°)
More prominent buccal ridge	Less prominent buccal ridge
Shorter root with pointed apex	Longer root with blunt apex

TRAITS TO DIFFERENTIATE MANDIBULAR RIGHT FROM LEFT PREMOLARS: BUCCAL VIEWS

MANDIBULAR FIRST PREMOLAR	MANDIBULAR SECOND PREMOLAR
Mesial cusp ridge notch more common [65%]	Distal cusp ridge notch more common [66%]
Lower mesial than distal contact	Lower distal than mesial contact
Mesial cusp ridge is shorter than distal on both mandibular premolars	

FIGURE 6-10. Buccal views of mandibular premolars with type traits to distinguish mandibular first from second premolars and traits to distinguish rights from lefts. Percentages give the frequency of notches on each cusp ridge.

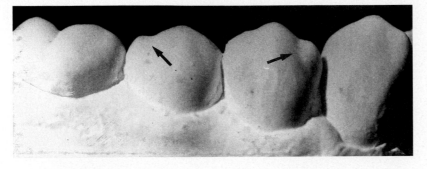

FIGURE 6-11. Mandibular first and second premolars depicting the most common type of notch location on the buccal cusp ridges with a shallow depression beneath it on the buccal surface (see arrows). Depressions were found in these locations on 17% of first premolars and 25% of second premolars.

4. PROXIMAL CONTACT AREAS OF MANDIBULAR PREMOLARS FROM THE BUCCAL VIEW

Because of the greater length of the buccal cusp, the contact areas on the **mandibular first premolar** are located more cervically from the cusp tip than they are on mandibular second premolars. On **mandibular second premolars,** both contact areas are positioned closer to the cusp tip or are in a more occlusal position than on the mandibular first premolars because the second's cusp ridges join at a less steep angle.

Mesial contacts of *both* types of mandibular premolars are near the junction of the occlusal and middle thirds (slightly more occlusal on second premolars). The *distal* contact of the **mandibular second premolar** follows the general rule: distal contact is slightly *cervical* to the mesial contact area (Appendix 6o). The distal contact area of the **mandibular first premolar** is an EXCEPTION to most other teeth; here the distal contact is slightly more *occlusal* in position than the mesial contact area (Appendix 6o). (The mandibular first premolar is one of only two teeth that have a more occlusally [incisally] located distal than mesial contact; the other tooth is the primary maxillary canine). A summary of the location of contact areas in all types of premolars is presented in *Table 6-5*.

5. ROOTS OF MANDIBULAR PREMOLARS FROM THE BUCCAL VIEW

The roots of mandibular premolars taper gradually to the apex. The roots are noticeably more blunt on mandibular second premolars than on first premolars. As with most roots, there is a tendency for the apical third of the root to bend distally [on 58% of 424 teeth mandibular first premolars and 62% of 343 teeth mandibular second premolars; the tendency for a mesial bend was 23% and 17% on first and second premolars, respectively].

Table 6-5	PREMOLARS: LOCATION OF PROXIMAL CONTACTS (PROXIMAL HEIGHT OF CONTOUR) IN PREMOLARS*	
	MESIAL SURFACE (WHICH THIRD OR JUNCTION?)	**DISTAL SURFACE** (WHICH THIRD OR JUNCTION?)
MAXILLARY CROWNS 1st Premolar	Middle third or occlusal/ middle junction	Middle (but more cervical than on mesial)
2nd Premolar	Middle third (near occlusal/ middle junction)	Middle (but more cervical than on mesial)
MANDIBULAR CROWNS 1st Premolar	Occlusal/middle junction or middle third	Occlusal third (more occlusal than on mesial = exception to the rule)
2nd Premolar	Occlusal/middle junction	Middle third (which is more cervical than on the mesial)

* Seen best from facial view.
General Learning Guidelines:
1. For premolars, the mesial and distal contacts are closer to the middle of the tooth and are more nearly at the same level.
2. Distal proximal contacts of premolars are more cervical than mesial contacts EXCEPT for mandibular first premolars where the mesial contact is more cervical than the distal.

The root of the *mandibular second premolar* appears only slightly thicker [0.2 mm wider mesiodistally] and is slightly longer [0.3 mm] than the root of the first premolar. The root of the mandibular second premolar is nearly twice as long as the crown, with a root-to-crown ratio of 1.80:1.

B.   TYPE TRAITS OF MANDIBULAR PREMOLARS FROM THE LINGUAL VIEW

For the lingual aspect, refer to lingual views of mandibular first and second premolars in *Figure 6-12*.

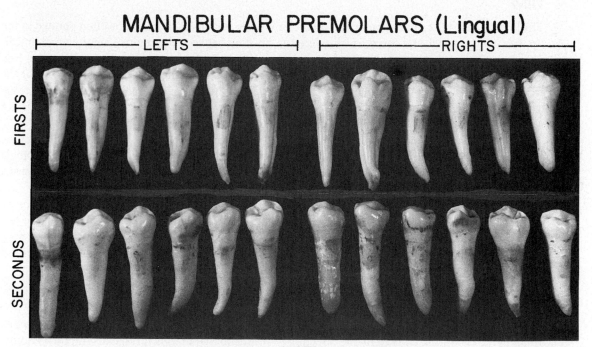

TYPE TRAITS TO DISTINGUISH MANDIBULAR FIRST FROM SECOND PREMOLARS: LINGUAL VIEWS

MANDIBULAR FIRST PREMOLAR	MANDIBULAR SECOND PREMOLAR
Crown much narrower on lingual	Crown quite wide on lingual
Lingual cusp very short, narrow	If one lingual cusp, not as short as first
One nonfunctional lingual cusp	Many have two functional lingual (L) cusps
Mesial marginal ridge with mesiolingual groove	Lingual groove between two L cusps
Mesial marginal ridge lower than distal	Distal marginal ridge lower than mesial
Buccal outline traits also apply since lingual cusps are short	

TRAITS TO DIFFERENTIATE MANDIBULAR RIGHT FROM LEFT PREMOLARS: LINGUAL VIEWS

MANDIBULAR FIRST PREMOLAR	MANDIBULAR SECOND PREMOLAR
Mesial marginal ridge lower than distal	Distal marginal ridge lower than mesial
Mesiolingual groove present [67%]	If three-cusp type, mesiolingual cusp larger
More occlusal visible on mesial	More occlusal visible on distal
Buccal outline traits also apply from this view	

FIGURE 6-12. **Lingual views** of mandibular premolars with type traits to distinguish mandibular first from second premolars and traits to distinguish rights from lefts.

1. **CROWN SHAPE OF MANDIBULAR PREMOLARS FROM THE LINGUAL VIEW**

On **mandibular first premolars,** as on most teeth, the crown is much narrower mesiodistally on the lingual half than on the buccal half. This can also be seen on second **premolars** with *one* lingual cusp. However, the width of the lingual half of a second premolar with *two* lingual cusps is usually as wide or wider mesiodistally than the buccal half. ONLY this three-cusp mandibular second premolar and some maxillary first molars have their crowns wider on the lingual half than on the buccal half.

2. **LINGUAL CUSPS AND GROOVES OF MANDIBULAR PREMOLARS FROM THE LINGUAL VIEW**

The lingual cusp of the **mandibular first premolar** is quite small and short, and is often pointed at the tip. It is *nonfunctional,* and could be considered a transition between the canine cingulum and prominent lingual cusp or cusps of the second premolar (best appreciated from the proximal views in Fig. 6-14). Much of the occlusal surface of this tooth can be seen from the lingual aspect because of the most obvious shortness of the lingual cusp. [Of 321 first premolars measured, the lingual cusp averaged 3.6 mm shorter than the buccal cusp (range from 1.7 to 5.5 mm shorter).] This tooth may have almost no lingual cusp or as many as four lingual cusplets.

On **mandibular second premolars** with *one lingual cusp,* the single lingual cusp is smaller than the buccal cusp, but it is larger (longer and wider) than the lingual cusp of the first premolar. This single lingual cusp is either just mesial to (often) or on the center line of the root (Appendix 6q). The mesial and distal cusp ridges of the lingual cusp merge into the mesial and distal marginal ridges.

In the *two lingual cusp* variation, there is one large buccal and two smaller lingual cusps. The mesiolingual cusp is almost always larger and longer than the distolingual cusp [90% of 818 teeth; the two lingual cusps were rarely equal in size, only on 3%, and the distolingual cusp was rarely larger, only 7%]. The longer mesiolingual cusp tip is mesial to the center line of the root, similar to the one cusp tip of the two-cusp type.

3. **MARGINAL RIDGES OF MANDIBULAR PREMOLARS FROM THE LINGUAL VIEW**

From the lingual view, differences in marginal ridge heights are apparent on handheld teeth when rotating the tooth first enough in one direction to see the mesial marginal ridge height, then enough in the opposite direction to compare the distal ridge height. As with most other posterior teeth, the *distal* marginal ridges of the **mandibular second premolars** are slightly more cervically located than the mesial marginal ridges (evident on all mandibular second premolars in *Fig. 6-12*). An EXCEPTION to all other adult teeth is the **mandibular first premolar,** the only adult tooth where the *mesial* marginal ridge is more cervically located than the distal marginal ridge (evident in *Fig. 6-12* for many mandibular first premolars). This is similar to the UNIQUE relative location of the mesial proximal contact of the mandibular first premolar (more cervical) and the distal proximal contact (more occlusal).

4. **GROOVES ON MANDIBULAR PREMOLARS FROM THE LINGUAL VIEW**

On **mandibular second premolars** with *two lingual cusps* [present 54% of the time], a *lingual groove* passes between the mesiolingual and distolingual cusps and extends slightly onto the lingual surface of the crown (seen occlusally in *Fig. 6-13*). On **mandibular first premolars,** there is frequently a *mesiolingual groove* separating the mesial marginal ridge from the mesial slope of the small lingual cusp (Appendix 6r) [present in 67% of 609 first premolars]. Rarely, a similar groove might be present between the distal marginal ridge and the distal slope of the lingual cusp [8% of these 609 first premolars]. This difference in grooves extending onto the lingual surfaces of first and second mandibular premolars is presented in *Fig. 6-13*.

5. **ROOTS OF MANDIBULAR PREMOLARS FROM THE LINGUAL VIEW**

The roots of second mandibular premolars are tapered and only slightly longer than the roots of first premolars [0.3 mm longer on average for 465 teeth].

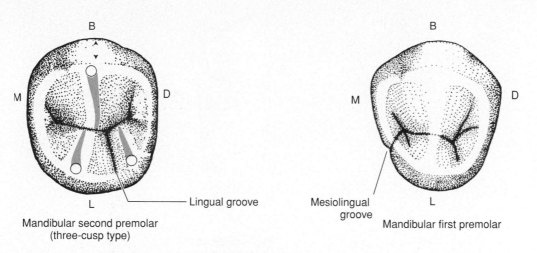

FIGURE 6-13. Variations in grooves extending onto the lingual surfaces of mandibular first and second (three-cusp type) premolars. The **mandibular second premolar with two lingual cusps** has a **lingual groove** that separates the two lingual cusps, and the **mandibular first premolar** often [67%] has a **mesiolingual groove** that separates the mesial marginal ridge from the lingual cusp and is located on the "pushed in" mesiolingual surface.

C. TYPE TRAITS OF MANDIBULAR PREMOLARS FROM THE PROXIMAL VIEWS

When studying the proximal views of mandibular first and second premolars, refer to *Figure 6-14*.

1. CROWN SHAPE OF MANDIBULAR PREMOLARS FROM THE PROXIMAL VIEWS

Mandibular premolars are shaped like a rhomboid from the proximal view (Appendix 6b). A rhomboid is a four-sided figure with opposite sides parallel to one another, like a parallelogram. As on all mandibular posterior teeth, the crown of the **mandibular first premolar** tilts noticeably toward the lingual surface at the cervix (much more than any other premolar). This tilt places the tip of the buccal cusp almost over the midroot axis line (obvious on all mandibular first premolars in *Fig. 6-14*). As was also seen from the lingual aspect, the lingual cusp of the mandibular first premolar is considerably shorter than the buccal cusp by more than one-third of the total crown length [3.6 mm average for 321 teeth]. By virtue of being so short and narrow mesiodistally, it is a *nonfunctioning* cusp (Appendix 6p). The tip of the short lingual cusp results in the cusp tip location usually being in line vertically with the lingual outline of the cervical portion of the root. The short lingual cusp also results in an occlusal plane than approaches 45° relative to the long axis of the root.

The **mandibular second premolar** crown (both types) also tips lingually, but not as much as the mandibular first premolar. The tip of the buccal cusp of the *mandibular second premolar* is usually located on a line that would divide the crown vertically between the buccal and middle thirds. As with the first premolar, the tip of the lingual cusp (or of the mesiolingual cusp) of this second premolar is usually about on a line with the lingual surface of the root at the cementoenamel junction (CEJ).

The lingual cusps (or mesiolingual cusps for three-cusp types) of *second premolars* are closer in length to the buccal cusp than on first premolars [average of only 1.8 mm shorter than the buccal cusp; range of 0.1 to 3.8 mm for 317 teeth]. From the mesial view, the mesiolingual cusp conceals the shorter distolingual cusp, while looking from the distal, both lingual cusp tips are usually visible (as seen on several mandibular second premolars viewed from the distal in *Fig. 6-14*).

2. MARGINAL RIDGES OF MANDIBULAR PREMOLARS FROM THE PROXIMAL VIEWS

The *mesial* marginal ridge of the **mandibular first premolar** slopes cervically from the buccal toward the center of the occlusal surface at nearly a 45° angle and is nearly parallel to the triangular ridge of the buccal cusp (Appendix 6s, and mesial views of the mandibular first premolars in *Fig. 6-14*). The

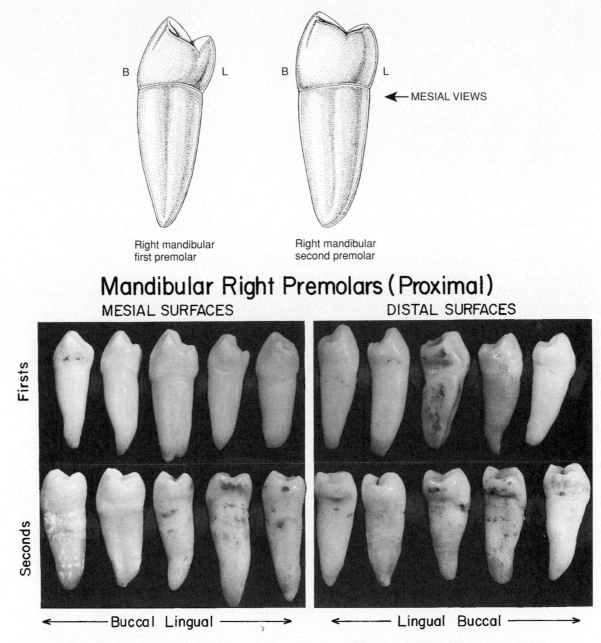

B   L   B   L   ← MESIAL VIEWS

Right mandibular   Right mandibular
first premolar   second premolar

Mandibular Right Premolars (Proximal)
MESIAL SURFACES   DISTAL SURFACES

Firsts

Seconds

←—— Buccal Lingual ——→   ←—— Lingual Buccal ——→

FIGURE 6-14. **Proximal views** of mandibular premolars with type traits to distinguish mandibular first from second premolars and traits to distinguish rights from lefts.

TYPE TRAITS TO DISTINGUISH MANDIBULAR FIRST FROM SECOND PREMOLARS: PROXIMAL VIEWS

MANDIBULAR FIRST PREMOLAR	MANDIBULAR SECOND PREMOLAR
Severe lingual crown tip	Less lingual crown tip
Lingual (L) cusp much shorter than buccal (B) cusp	L cusp slightly shorter than B cusp
Mesial (M) marginal ridge parallel to B cusp ridge	M marginal ridge higher and horizontal
Can see much of occlusal from mesial	Cannot see much of occlusal from mesial
Mesiolingual groove on most [67%]	Lingual groove on three-cusp type
No lingual groove	No mesiolingual groove
Root may be divided in apical third	Root not divided
Mesial root depression [45%]	Mesial root flat or convex [81%]

TRAITS TO DIFFERENTIATE MANDIBULAR RIGHT FROM LEFT PREMOLARS: PROXIMAL VIEWS

MANDIBULAR FIRST PREMOLAR	MANDIBULAR SECOND PREMOLAR
Mesial marginal ridge is lower than distal	Distal marginal ridge is lower than mesial
Deeper distal root depression [69%]	No mesial root depression [81%] but distal
More occlusal is visible from mesial	More occlusal is visible from distal
Mesial marginal ridge parallel to buccal triangle ridge	Mesiolingual cusp larger [90%] on three-cusp type

FIGURE 6-14. (continued).

distal marginal ridge of the *mandibular first premolar* is in a more horizontal position compared to the *mesial marginal* ridge, and is longer from buccal to lingual than the mesial marginal ridge. The difference in marginal ridge angle is most helpful in differentiating rights from lefts (by identifying the more downward sloping mesial marginal ridge). Also, the *triangular* ridge of the *lingual* cusp is short and is in a nearly horizontal plane.

The more horizontal *mesial* marginal ridge of the **second premolar** is occlusally located, hiding much of the occlusal surface when viewed from the mesial. The *distal* marginal ridge is more concave, somewhat longer buccolingually, and definitely in a more cervical position than the mesial marginal ridge (compare mesial and distal views in Fig. 6-14).

3. MARGINAL RIDGE GROOVES AND MESIOLINGUAL GROOVES ON MANDIBULAR PREMOLARS FROM THE PROXIMAL VIEWS

When present [67% of the teeth studied], the *mesiolingual grooves* on **mandibular first premolars** lie between the mesial marginal ridge and the mesial slope of the lingual cusp in the lingual third of the tooth (Appendix 6r). There is seldom a groove between the *distal* marginal ridge and the distal slope of the lingual cusp [8% of 609 mandibular first premolars]. Mesiolingual grooves are *not* present on mandibular second premolars, and the *mesial* marginal ridges of these teeth are *not* frequently crossed by a marginal ridge groove [only 21 of 100 teeth]. Only rarely is the *distal* marginal ridge crossed by a marginal ridge groove [4 of 100 teeth]. The **three-cusp type of mandibular second premolars** have a *lingual* groove separating the two lingual cusps. (Recall the occlusal views in Fig. 6-13.)

4. HEIGHT (CREST) OF CONTOUR OF MANDIBULAR PREMOLARS FROM THE PROXIMAL VIEWS

As on all teeth, the height of contour of *both* types of mandibular premolar crowns on the *facial* surface is in the cervical third. On the **mandibular first premolar,** the *buccal* height of contour of the crown is just occlusal to the cervical line, like the mandibular canine next to it (Fig. 6-14). The buccal height of contour on **second premolars** is near the junction of the cervical and middle thirds. The *buccal* crown outline of the second premolar is flatter or less convex than on the first mandibular premolar from the height of contour to the cusp tip.

For *all* mandibular premolars, the height of contour of the *lingual* surface of the crown is in the middle third, about in the center of the total crown length. On the mandibular first premolar, this is not far from the cusp tip of the lingual cusp (clearly seen on mandibular first premolars in *Fig. 6-14*). Because of the extreme lingual tilting of the crown, the lingual surfaces of *all* mandibular premolar crowns extend lingually beyond the lingual surface of the root.

5.   CERVICAL LINES OF MANDIBULAR PREMOLARS FROM THE PROXIMAL VIEWS

Similar to other teeth, the occlusal curve of the cervical line on the proximal surfaces of premolars is greater on the mesial surface than on the distal. [The *mesial* cervical line of the mandibular *first* premolar curves an average of 0.9 mm for 238 teeth versus 0.6 mm on the *distal;* the *mesial* of *second* mandibular premolar curves occlusally an average of 0.8 mm for 227 teeth versus 0.5 mm (almost flat) on the *distal.*] The cervical line is also located more occlusally on the lingual than on the buccal [by as much as 2 mm on first premolars]. This makes the crowns appear to be quite short on the lingual side.

6.   ROOTS OF MANDIBULAR PREMOLARS FROM THE PROXIMAL VIEWS

Both types of mandibular premolar roots taper apically, with the least taper in the cervical third. Rarely, an anomaly occurs where a mandibular premolar has a furcated root (i.e., the apical part of the root is divided into a buccal and lingual portion [discussed later in Chapter 12 on anomalies]).

7.   ROOT DEPRESSIONS OF MANDIBULAR PREMOLARS FROM THE PROXIMAL VIEWS

Mandibular first premolars have a shallow longitudinal depression in the apical and middle thirds of the *mesial* root surface about half of the time [45 of 100 teeth], but are even more likely to have a longitudinal depression on the *distal* surface [86 of 100 teeth], which is deeper than on the mesial [69% of the time]. The relative depths of the depressions on mesial and distal root surfaces of this tooth are not a reliable basis on which to determine rights from lefts.

Most **mandibular second premolars** [81%] have *no* depression on the mesial root surface, but are likely to have a longitudinal depression in the middle third of the *distal* root surface [73% of 100 teeth].

To summarize, all types of premolars, on average, are likely to have a deeper root depression on the distal root surface than on the mesial EXCEPT the maxillary first premolar. See *Table 6-6* for a summary of the location and relative depth of root depressions on all types of premolars.

Table 6-6	PRESENCE AND RELATIVE DEPTH OF LONGITUDINAL ROOT DEPRESSIONS ("ROOT GROOVES") IN PREMOLARS	
TOOTH	**MESIAL ROOT DEPRESSION?**	**DISTAL ROOT DEPRESSION?**
MAXILLARY PREMOLARS — Maxillary 1st premolar	Yes (deeper, extends onto mesial of crown) = UNIQUE	Yes
Maxillary 2nd premolar	Yes	Yes (deeper)
MANDIBULAR PREMOLARS — Mandibular 1st premolar	Yes (or no: about 50%)	Yes (deeper)
Mandibular 2nd premolar	No (unlikely)	Yes (deeper)

General Learning Guideline:
Premolars (EXCEPT maxillary first premolars) are likely to have deeper distal surface root depressions.

D. TYPE TRAITS OF MANDIBULAR PREMOLARS FROM THE OCCLUSAL VIEW

For the occlusal view of mandibular first and second premolars, refer to *Figure 6-15*. To follow this description, the teeth or tooth models should be held with the occlusal surface toward the observer and the buccal surface up, and the observer looking exactly along the vertical midroot axis.

1. OUTLINE SHAPE OF MANDIBULAR PREMOLARS FROM THE OCCLUSAL VIEW

There is much variation in the occlusal morphology of the **mandibular first premolar.**[2] The outline of the crown is *not* symmetrical (more bulk in the distal half) as seen in practically all mandibular first premolars in Figure 6-15. It often looks as though the mesiolingual corner of the crown has been *pushed inward on the mesiolingual corner* (Appendix 6u). This results in a somewhat diamond-shaped outline (also Appendix 6u). This "pushed in" mesiolingual surface is a reliable trait to identify the mesial surface of a mandibular first premolar.

The distal marginal ridge is often nearly at right angles to the distal cusp ridge of the buccal cusp, whereas the mesial marginal ridge meets the mesiobuccal cusp ridge at a more acute angle on the first premolars. The cusp ridges of the buccal cusp are in a nearly straight line mesiodistally. The contact areas, as seen from the occlusal view, are at the point of broadest mesiodistal dimension just lingual to the line of the buccal cusp ridges and cusp tip.

Sometimes the mesial and distal marginal ridges may converge symmetrically to the lingual in such a way that the occlusal table (surface) is nearly an equilateral triangle with the base made up of the buccal cusp ridges, and the apex is the lingual cusp tip. On this symmetrical type of mandibular first premolar, it is more difficult to determine right from left by only looking at the occlusal design.

On **mandibular first premolars,** the buccal ridge is not prominent, and the buccal crest of contour is slightly mesial to center. The crest of contour of the lingual surface is often distal to the center line of the tooth. Much of the buccal surface is visible from this view since the tip of the buccal cusp is slightly buccal to tooth center from this view (clearly seen in almost all mandibular first premolars in *Fig. 6-15*).

On the **two-cusp mandibular second premolars,** the crown is round or oval shaped, but with a relatively square occlusal table. The crown outline tapers to the lingual, so the crown outline is more broadly curved on the buccal side than on the lingual side. The lingual cusp tip of often off center toward the mesial half of the crown.

On the **three-cusp second premolars,** the occlusal surface is more nearly square than is the occlusal surface of the two-cusp type because the crown is wider with two cusps on the lingual side. When the lingual cusps are large, the occlusal surface is broader mesiodistally on the lingual half than on the buccal half (seen on a number of three-cusp premolars in *Fig. 6-15* and in the mouth in *Fig. 6-16*). This is quite different than the two-cusp mandibular premolars. Three-cusp premolar teeth often have greater faciolingual bulk in the distal than mesial half of the crown (tapering from distal to mesial), which is an EXCEPTION to the normal taper to the distal. [This was true on 56% of 229 specimens examined, but more than one-third (38%) tapered the more conventional way (mesial to distal), like two-thirds of the two-cusp type.] Examples of differences in crown taper are seen on mandibular second premolars in Figure 6-15. The mesiolingual cusp is most often larger than the distolingual cusp [90% of 818 teeth]. This difference in size may be little or great. Distinguishing differences between the occlusal outlines of mandibular premolars are highlighted in *Figure 6-17*.

2. OCCLUSAL MORPHOLOGY OF MANDIBULAR PREMOLARS FROM THE OCCLUSAL VIEW

a. Ridges, Fossae, and Grooves of the Mandibular First Premolars From the Occlusal View

Due to the much larger buccal than lingual cusp on the *mandibular first premolars,* the triangular ridge of the buccal cusp is long and slopes lingually from the cusp tip to where it joins the very short triangular ridge of the lingual cusp. Most often the two triangular ridges unite smoothly near the center of the occlusal surface and form an uninterrupted pronounced *transverse ridge* that completely separates the mesial and distal circular fossae.

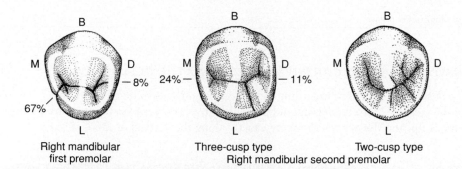

Right mandibular
first premolar

Three-cusp type
Right mandibular second premolar

Two-cusp type

Mandibular Premolars (Occlusal)

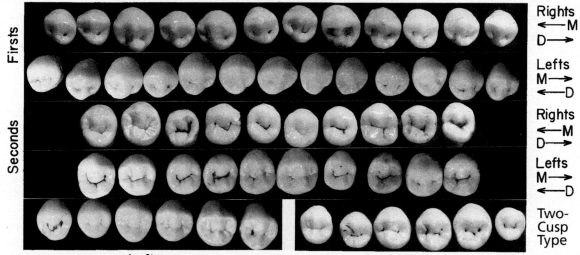

Firsts — Rights ←M D→

Lefts M→ ←D

Seconds — Rights ←M D→

Lefts M→ ←D

Two-Cusp Type

Lefts   Rights

TYPE TRAITS TO DISTINGUISH MANDIBULAR FIRST FROM SECOND PREMOLARS: OCCLUSAL VIEWS

MANDIBULAR FIRST PREMOLAR	MANDIBULAR SECOND PREMOLAR
Nonsymmetric crown outline	Outline nearly square
Small, nonfunctional occlusal table	Larger, functional occlusal table
Converges toward lingual, especially on mesial	Crown may be wider on lingual
Mesiolingual groove common [67%]	Lingual groove on three-cusp type
Two circular fossae (mesial and distal)	Two circular fossae (mesial and distal) on two-cusp type
Definite transverse ridge	Three-cusp type has no transverse ridge
Mesial and distal grooves run buccolingually	"Y" groove pattern on three-cusp type

TRAITS TO DIFFERENTIATE MANDIBULAR RIGHT FROM LEFT PREMOLARS: OCCLUSAL VIEWS

MANDIBULAR FIRST PREMOLAR	MANDIBULAR SECOND PREMOLAR
Asymmetric crown outline: convex on distal; mesiolingual (ML) "corner" flat (chopped off)	Wider faciolingual on distal than mesial
ML groove common [67%]	Lingual groove on three-cusp type with ML cusp
	Lingual cusp mesial or centered (three-cusp)
Distal fossa larger than mesial fossa [82%]	Distal fossa larger (two-cusp type)
	Distal fossa smallest, central fossa largest (three-cusp type)
Shorter mesiobuccal cusp ridge on both	

FIGURE 6-15. Occlusal views of mandibular premolars with type traits to distinguish mandibular first from second premolars and traits to distinguish rights from lefts. Percentages on the top drawings give the frequency of marginal ridge grooves crossing each marginal ridge.

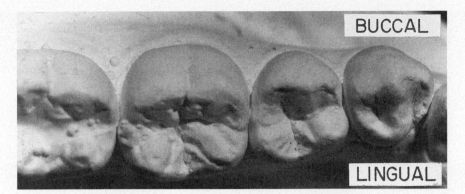

FIGURE 6-16. Mandibular second premolar (three-cusp type) and first molar (four-cusp type), which are both wider lingually than buccally. Note that the distolingual cusp on the second premolar is almost wider than the mesiolingual cusp (found on only 7%) and that the second premolar is larger than the first premolar (a common occurrence unlike the maxillary premolars). Also observe the pronounced mesiolingual groove on the first premolar.

On the *mandibular first premolar,* there is a mesial fossa and a distal fossa; both are called *circular,* not triangular; the mesial fossa is more linear buccolingually. Each fossa has a pit. Both of these deep pits are susceptible to decay (caries) and are therefore often restored with two separate restorations *(Fig. 6-18).* The distal fossa is usually larger or deeper [largest of 82 of 100 teeth examined, with the mesial fossa largest on only 8 teeth].

Only rarely is the pronounced transverse ridge of the *mandibular first premolar* crossed by a fissured central groove, which may extend from the mesial pit across the transverse ridge to the distal pit. More commonly, there are *mesial* and *distal* developmental grooves running in a nearly buccolingual direction, flaring buccally from the mesial and distal fossae *(Fig. 6-19).* The mesial groove is continuous with the mesiolingual groove (when present). The grooves on the first premolars are fewer in number but may be deeper than those on the second premolars.

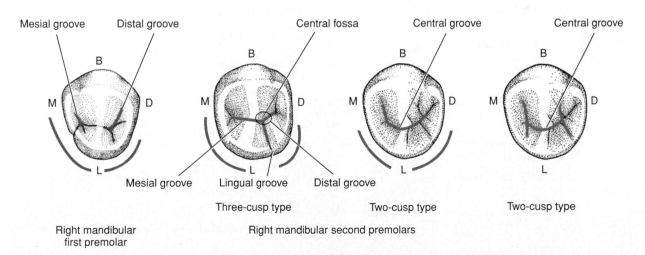

MANDIBULAR PREMOLARS (OCCLUSAL)

FIGURE 6-17. Occlusal views of three types of mandibular premolars. Red lines accentuate the unique **occlusal outlines and groove patterns** of each type. The **mandibular first premolar** has a lack of symmetry on the lingual half because the mesiolingual surface is "pushed in" or flattened, and is often crossed by a mesiolingual groove. It often has two separate pits that are not joined by a central groove due to the prominence of the transverse ridge. The **three-cusp type mandibular second premolar** can be as wide in the lingual half (or even wider) as on the buccal half due to having two lingual cusps. The groove pattern is Y-shaped with a central fossa and pit where the lines of the "Y" intersect. The **two-cusp type mandibular second premolar** is the most symmetrical of the three types, and has a groove pattern that is U- or H-shaped.

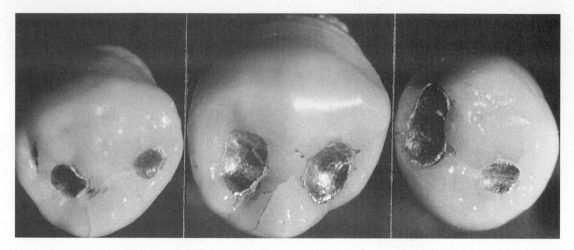

FIGURE 6-18. Two left and one smaller right mandibular first premolars that have amalgam restorations in the mesial and distal fossae. These restorations are sometimes nicknamed "snake eyes."

b. **Ridges, Fossae, and Grooves of the Two-cusp Mandibular Second Premolars From the Occlusal View**

Mandibular second premolars (two-cusp type), as on maxillary second premolars, have more numerous supplemental grooves on their occlusal surfaces than do first premolars.[4] On the *two-cusp* type mandibular second premolar, the lingual cusp is smaller than the buccal cusp. There is a large triangular ridge on the buccal cusp and a correspondingly smaller one on the lingual cusp that join to form a transverse ridge (unlike the three-cusp type). There is a curved *central developmental groove* but no lingual groove on the two-cusp type of second mandibular premolar. The central groove extends mesiodistally across the occlusal surface. Sometimes this groove is short

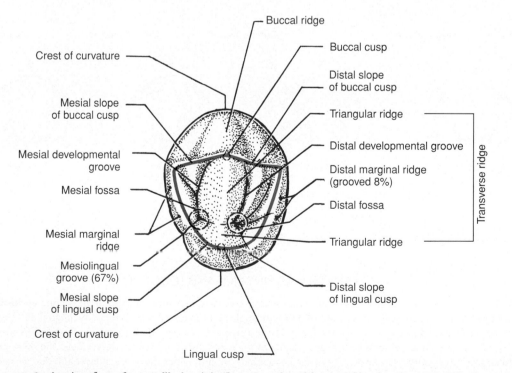

FIGURE 6-19. Occlusal surface of **a mandibular right first premolar with normal** landmarks. Notice the flatter (almost concave) mesiolingual outline compared to the distal lingual outline. Also notice the somewhat triangular shape of the occlusal table (outlined in red).

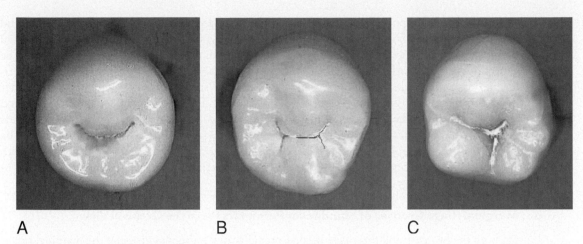

A   B   C

FIGURE 6-20. Variations in mandibular second premolars (occlusal views). A. Mandibular left second premolar (two-cusp type): buccal above and mesial at right. The single lingual cusp is slightly mesial to the center line. The central groove is U-shaped. **B.** Mandibular left second premolar (two-cusp type): with H-shaped groove pattern. **C.** Mandibular left second premolar (three-cusp type) with Y-shaped groove pattern.

and nearly straight with mesial and distal fossa grooves that together form an "H" shape; sometimes the grooves form a "U" shape or are like a crescent, with the open end directed buccally, or even form an "H" shape (*Figs. 6-17* and *6-20*). It may be interrupted near its center by a union of the buccal and lingual triangular ridges as they form the transverse ridge. The central groove ends in the *circular* mesial and circular distal fossae, where it often joins a mesiobuccal and distobuccal groove. The distal fossa is generally larger than the mesial fossa.

c. Ridges, Fossae, and Grooves of the Three-cusp Mandibular Second Premolar

On the *three-cusp* type of *mandibular second premolar*, there are three triangular ridges: one on each of the two lingual cusps and one on the buccal cusp. These three ridges converge toward the central fossa (*Fig. 6-21*) but do not connect to form a transverse ridge. This tooth has mesial and distal fossae like all other premolars, but it is the ONLY PREMOLAR to also have a *central fossa*. The large central fossa is located quite distal to the center of the occlusal surface and in the middle buccolingually. Comparing size and depth of the mesial triangular fossa and central fossa, the central fossa was usually largest [on 65% of 200 teeth; the mesial fossa was largest on only 25% of the teeth].

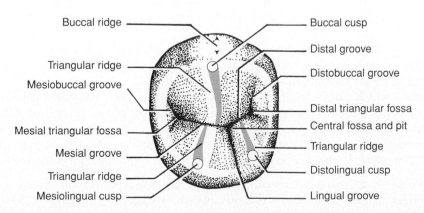

Buccal ridge — — Buccal cusp

— Distal groove

Triangular ridge — — Distobuccal groove

Mesiobuccal groove —

— Distal triangular fossa

— Central fossa and pit

Mesial triangular fossa — — Triangular ridge

Mesial groove — — Distolingual cusp

Triangular ridge —

Mesiolingual cusp — — Lingual groove

FIGURE 6-21. Mandibular right second premolar (three-cusp type). Occlusal surface with normal landmarks. Note that triangular ridges do **not** join to form a transverse ridge. Also, the groove that runs between the mesial and distal pits join at a central pit, so the longer groove mesial to the central pit is called mesial groove and the shorter groove distal to the central pit is called the distal groove.

The *three-cusp* type of *mandibular second premolar* does *not,* by definition, have a central groove. Rather, what appears similar to a central groove is more precisely the joining of a mesial and distal groove. The longer *mesial* groove extends from a small mesial *triangular* fossa to the central fossa. The shorter *distal* groove continues from the central fossa to the minute distal *triangular* fossa (*Fig. 6-21*). The distal triangular fossa is so small that it appears to be in the outer edge of the central fossa. A *lingual groove* (also UNIQUE to this three-cusp mandibular second premolar) begins in the central fossa at the junction of the mesial and distal grooves, and extends lingually between the mesiolingual and distolingual cusps and onto the lingual surface. The junction of three grooves forms a Y-shaped occlusal groove pattern found only on this tooth (*Fig. 6-21*). Differences of occlusal groove patterns on mandibular premolars are highlighted in Figure 6-17.

d. Marginal Ridge Grooves of Mandibular Premolars From the Occlusal View

On both the *two-cusp* and *three-cusp* second premolar types, grooves crossing the marginal ridges (that is, marginal ridge grooves) are not commonplace. [On the mesial marginal ridge, only 24% of 200 teeth had grooves crossing them, compared to distal marginal ridge grooves on only 11%.] The first premolar is much more likely to have a mesiolingual groove.

LEARNING EXERCISE

1. First, review all arch traits that differentiate the maxillary from the mandibular premolars in Table 6-3. Then review the summary tables of type traits that differentiate the first from second premolars and the right from left premolars.
2. Assign a Universal number to a handheld premolar:

Suppose a patient just had all of his or her permanent teeth extracted and you were asked to find tooth #4 from among a pile of 32 extracted teeth on the oral surgeon's tray because you wanted to evaluate a lesion on the root of that premolar that had been seen on the radiograph. How might you go about it? Try the following steps:

- From a selection of all permanent teeth (extracted teeth or tooth models), select only the premolars (based on class traits).
- Determine whether each premolar is maxillary or mandibular. *You should never rely on only one characteristic difference* between teeth to name them; rather, make a list of many traits that suggest the tooth is a maxillary premolar, as opposed to only one trait that makes you think it belongs in the mandible. This way you can play detective and become an expert at recognition at the same time.
- If you determine that the tooth is maxillary, position the root up; if it is mandibular, position the root down.
- Next, using type traits, determine the type of premolar you are holding (first or second).
- Use characteristic traits for each surface to identify the buccal surface. This will permit you to view the tooth as though you were looking into a patient's mouth.
- Finally, determine which surface is the mesial. While viewing the premolar from the facial and picturing it within the appropriate arch (upper or lower), the mesial surface can be positioned toward the midline in only one quadrant, the right or left.
- Once you have determined the quadrant, assign the appropriate Universal number for the premolar in that quadrant. For example, the second premolar in the upper right quadrant is tooth #4.

3. A. Name the ridges on this mandibular second premolar, two-cusp type, in *Figure 6-22A.*
   B. Name the ridges on this mandibular second premolar, three-cusp type, in Figure 6-22B.
4. What problem do you see in *Figure 6-23?*

A summary of the geometric outline shapes of premolars is presented in *Figure 6-24.*

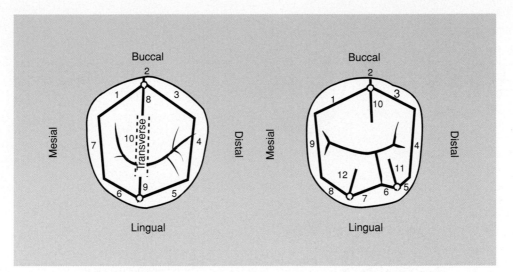

A. Name the ridges

B. Name the ridges

Ridges	Name
1. _____
2. _____
3. _____
4. _____
5. _____
6. _____
7. _____
8. _____
9. _____
10. _____

Ridges	Name
1. _____
2. _____
3. _____
4. _____
5. _____
6. _____
7. _____
8. _____
9. _____
10. _____
11. _____
12. _____

FIGURE 6-22. A. Mandibular second premolar, two-cusp type. **B.** Mandibular second premolar, three-cusp type. Write the name of each ridge denoted on these teeth.

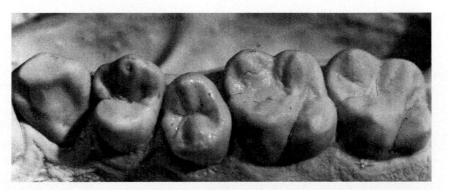

FIGURE 6-23. What is wrong with the teeth in this photograph? ANSWER: The maxillary second premolar is rotated, so its lingual surface is facing in a buccal direction. You can tell this by the taper of the tooth (which should be from buccal to lingual).

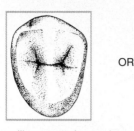   OR 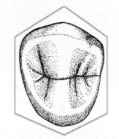

Right maxillary second premolar   Right maxillary first premolar

Rectangular or hexagon outline:
Occlusal views of maxillary premolars

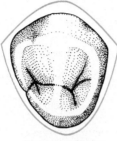

Right mandibular
first premolar

Diamond outline:
Occlusal views of mandibular first premolars

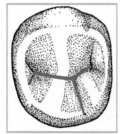   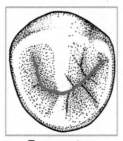

Three-cusp type   Two-cusp type

Right mandibular second premolar

Close to square outline:
Occlusal views (or especially occlusal table) of mandibular premolars
Y-shaped groove pattern:
On three-cusp type mandibular second premolar
U-shaped groove pattern:
On two-cusp type mandibular second premolar

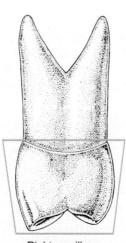

Right mandibular
second premolar   Right maxillary
first premolar

Rhomboid (parallelogram)-shaped outline:
Proximal view of mandibular premolars
Trapezoid-shaped outline:
Proximal view of maxillary premolars

FIGURE 6-24. Examples of **geometric outlines** of premolars from the occlusal and proximal views.

12.–triangular ridge of mesiolingual cusp.

9.–mesial marginal ridge; 10.–triangular ridge of buccal cusp; 11.–triangular ridge of distolingual cusp;

tolingual cusp; 7.–distal cusp ridge of mesiolingual cusp; 8.–mesial cusp ridge of mesiolingual cusp.

buccal cusp; 4.–distal marginal ridge; 5.–distal cusp ridge of distolingual cusp; 6.–mesial cusp ridge of dis-

B.   Ridges for three-cusp type: 1.–mesial cusp ridge of buccal cusp; 2.–buccal ridge; 3.–distal cusp ridge of

10.–transverse ridge.

cusp; 7.–mesial marginal ridge, 8.–triangular ridge of buccal cusp; 9.–triangular ridge of lingual cusp;

buccal cusp; 4.–distal marginal ridge; 5.–distal cusp ridge of lingual cusp; 6.–mesial cusp ridge of lingual

A.   Ridges for two-cusp type: 1.–mesial cusp ridge of buccal cusp; 2.–buccal ridge; 3.–distal cusp ridge of

ANSWERS TO LEARNING EXERCISE QUESTION 3

LEARNING QUESTIONS

Maxillary and Mandibular First and Second Premolars

For each of the following traits or statements, circle the letter (or letters) of the premolars (if any) that apply. More than one answer may be correct.

- a. Maxillary first premolar
- b. Maxillary second premolar
- c. Mandibular first premolar
- d. Mandibular second premolar (two-cusp type)
- e. Mandibular second premolar (three-cusp type)

1. Mesial ridge of the buccal cusp is longer than the distal cusp ridge. a b c d e

2. Has a nonfunctioning lingual cusp. a b c d e

3. Two premolars that most frequently have a groove crossing the mesial marginal ridge or one groove just lingual to it. a b c d e

4. Has a depression in the cervical one-third of the mesial side of the crown and root. a b c d e

5. Maxillary premolar that has the longer sharper buccal cusp. a b c d e

6. Largest maxillary premolar. a b c d e

7. Mandibular premolar with the longest and sharpest buccal cusp. a b c d e

8. Maxillary premolar that is most symmetrical (occlusal view). a b c d e

9. Two premolars without a central groove. a b c d e

10. Crowns tipped lingually with respect to the root axis line (proximal view). a b c d e

11. From buccal view, crown is tipped distally from the root axis. a b c d e

12. Mesial marginal ridge is more cervically located than its distal marginal ridge. a b c d e

13. Has no transverse ridge. a b c d e

14. Has the longer central groove. a b c d e

15. Has two major cusps almost the same size and length. a b c d e

16. Has a central fossa.   a b c d e

17. Premolars with two circular fossae.   a b c d e

18. Premolars with only two triangular fossae.   a b c d e

19. Has a central fossa and two triangular fossae.   a b c d e

20. Has a lingual groove.   a b c d e

ANSWERS: 1-a; 2-c; 3-a, c; 4-a; 5-a; 6-a; 7-c; 8-b; 9-c, e; 10-c, d, e; 11-c, d, e; 12-c; 13 e; 14-a; 15-b; 16-e; 17-c, d; 18-a, b; 19-e; 20-e.

REFERENCES

1. Morris DH. Maxillary premolar variations among Papago Indians. J Dent Res 1967;46:736–738.
2. Kraus BS, Furr ML. Lower first premolars. Part I. A definition and classification of discrete morphologic traits. J Dent Res 1953;32:554.
3. Ludwig FJ. The mandibular second premolar: morphologic variations and inheritance. J Dent Res 1957;36:263–273.
4. Brand RW, Isselhard DE. Anatomy of orofacial structures. St. Louis: C.V. Mosby, 1998.
5. Takeda Y. A rare occurrence of a three-root mandibular premolar. Ann Dent 1988;44:43–44.
6. Osborn JR, ed. Dental anatomy and embryology. Oxford: Blackwell Scientific Publications, 1981:133.
7. Palmer RS. Elephants. In: World Book Encyclopedia, Vol. 6. 1979:178c.
8. Brant D. Beaver. In: World Book Encyclopedia, Vol. 2. 1979:147.
9. Zoo Books: Elephants. Wildlife Education Ltd. San Diego: Frye & Smith, 1980:14.

GENERAL REFERENCES

Grundler H. The study of tooth shapes: a systematic procedure. (Weber L, trans.) Berlin: Buch-und Zeitschriften-Verlag "Die Quintessenz," 1976.

Oregon State System of Higher Education. Dental anatomy: a self-instructional program. 9th ed. East Norwalk: Appleton-Century-Crofts, 1982.

Renner RP. An introduction to dental anatomy and esthetics. Chicago: Quintessence Publishing, 1985.

Morphology of Permanent Molars

7

Topics covered within the four sections of this chapter include the following:

I. Overview of molars
   A. General description of molars
   B. Functions of molars
   C. Class traits of all molars
   D. Arch traits that differentiate maxillary from mandibular molars

II. Type traits that differentiate mandibular second molars from mandibular first molars
   A. Type traits of mandibular molars from the buccal view
   B. Type traits of mandibular molars from the lingual view
   C. Type traits of mandibular molars from the proximal views
   D. Type traits of mandibular molars from the occlusal view

III. Type traits that differentiate maxillary second molars from maxillary first molars

A. Type traits of the maxillary first and second molars from the buccal view
B. Type traits of maxillary molars from the lingual view
C. Type traits of first and second maxillary molars from the proximal views
D. Type traits of maxillary molars from the occlusal view

IV. Maxillary and mandibular third molar type traits
   A. Type traits of all third molars (different from first and second molars)
   B. Size and shape of third molars
   C. Similarities and differences of third molar crowns compared with first and second molars in the same arch
   D. Similarities and differences of third molar roots compared with first and second molars in the same arch

Using the mandibular right second molar as a representative example for all molars, refer to the Appendix, page 7, while reading Section I of this chapter. Throughout this chapter, "Appendix" followed by a number and letter (e.g., Appendix 7a) is used within the text to denote reference to the page (number 7) and item (letter a) being referred to on that appendix page. The Appendix pages are designed to be torn out to facilitate study and minimize page turns. Other appendix pages will be referred to throughout this chapter.

SECTION I   OVERVIEW OF MOLARS

OBJECTIVES

This section is designed to prepare the learner to perform the following:
- Describe the functions of molars.
- List class traits common to all molars.
- List arch traits that can be used to distinguish maxillary from mandibular molars.
- From a selection of all teeth, select and separate out the molars.
- Divide a selection of all molars into maxillary and mandibular.

A. GENERAL DESCRIPTION OF MOLARS

Use a cast of all permanent teeth or *Figure 7-1* while learning the position of molars in the arch. There are 12 permanent molars—six maxillary and six mandibular. The six permanent molars in each arch are the first, second, and third molars on either side of the arch. They are the sixth, seventh, and eighth teeth from the midline. Using the Universal Numbering System, the maxillary molars are numbers 1, 2, and 3 for the right third, second, and first molars, and numbers 14, 15, and 16 for the left first, second, and third molars, respectively. The mandibular molars are numbers 17, 18, and 19 for the left third, second, and first molars, and numbers 30, 31, and 32 for the right first, second, and third molars, respectively.

In the adult dentition, first molars are distal to second premolars. The permanent first molars are located near the center of each arch, anteroposteriorly. This is one reason that their loss is so devastating to arch continuity (allowing movement and tipping of the teeth on either side). They are the largest and strongest teeth in each arch. The second molars are distal to the first molars, and the third molars are distal to the second molars. Said another way, in the complete adult dentition the mesial surface of the first molar contacts the distal surface of the second premolar, the mesial surface of the second molar contacts the distal of the first molar, and the mesial surface of the third molar contacts the distal of the second molar.

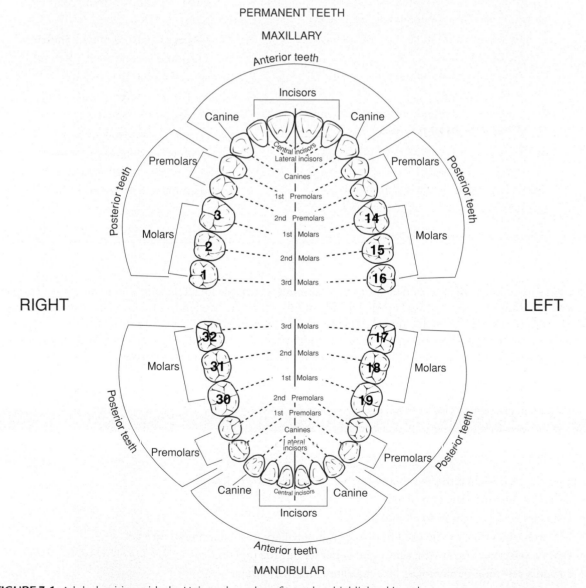

FIGURE 7-1. Adult dentition with the Universal numbers for molars highlighted in red.

The third molar is the last tooth in the arch, and its distal surface is not in contact with any other tooth. Unfortunately, this tooth's nickname is "wisdom tooth." It also has unfairly been given a bad reputation for having soft enamel, not serving any function, readily decaying, and causing crowding of the anterior teeth and other dental problems. The reason for this bad reputation is probably its posterior location that makes it difficult to keep clean. Frequently, one or more of the third molars are congenitally missing (never develop); this occurs in nearly 20% of the population.

The combined mesiodistal width of the three mandibular molars on one side makes up over half (51%) of the mesiodistal dimension of their quadrant. The maxillary molars constitute 44% of their quadrant's mesiodistal dimension, still a significant portion.

B. FUNCTIONS OF MOLARS

The permanent molars, like the premolars, (a) play a major role in the mastication of food (chewing and grinding to pulverize) and (b) are most important in maintaining the vertical dimension of the face (preventing a closing of the bite or vertical dimension, a protruding chin, and a prematurely aged appearance). They are also (c) important in maintaining continuity within the dental arches, thus keeping other teeth in proper alignment. You may have seen someone who has lost all 12 molars (six upper and six lower) and has sunken cheeks. The molars therefore have (d) at least a minor role in esthetics or keeping the cheeks normally full or supported, as well as keeping the chin a proper distance from the nose.

The loss of a first molar is really noticed and missed by most people when it has been extracted. More than 80 mm^2 of efficient chewing surface is gone; the tongue feels the huge space between the remaining teeth; and during mastication of coarse or brittle foods, the attached gingiva in the region of the missing molar often becomes abraded and uncomfortable. Loss of six or more molars would also predispose to problems in the temporomandibular joints.

C. CLASS TRAITS OF ALL MOLARS

Refer to Appendix page 7 while reading about the following class traits of all molars.

1. CROWN SIZE FOR ALL MOLARS

Molars have an occlusal (chewing) surface with three to five cusps, and their chewing surfaces are larger than the other teeth in their respective arches. (Refer to *Tables 7-1* and *7-2* for the average and

Table 7-1	SIZE OF MAXILLARY MOLARS (MILLIMETERS) (MEASURED BY DR. WOELFEL AND HIS DENTAL HYGIENE STUDENTS, 1974–1979)					
	308 FIRST MOLARS		309 SECOND MOLARS		303 THIRD MOLARS	
Dimension Measured	Average	Range	Average	Range	Average	Range
Crown length*	7.5	6.3–9.6	7.6	6.1–9.4	7.2	5.7–9.0
Root length						
Mesiobuccal*	12.9	8.5–18.8	12.9	9.0–18.2	10.8	7.1–5.5
Distobuccal	12.2	8.9–15.5	12.1	9.0–16.3	10.1	6.9–14.5
Lingual	13.7	10.6–17.5	13.5	9.8–18.8	11.2	7.4–15.8
Overall length*	20.1	17.0–27.4	20.0	16.0–26.2	17.5	14.0–22.5
Crown width (M–D)	10.4	8.8–13.3	9.8	8.5–11.7	9.2	7.0–11.1
Root width (cervix)	7.9	6.4–10.9	7.6	6.2–8.4	7.2	5.3–9.4
Faciolingual crown size	11.5	9.8–14.1	11.4	9.9–14.3	11.1	8.9–13.2
Faciolingual root (cervix)	10.7	7.4–14.0	10.7	8.9–12.7	10.4	7.5–12.5
Mesial cervical curvature	0.7	0.0–2.1	0.6	0.0–2.2	0.5	0.0–2.0
Distal cervical curvature	0.3	0.0–1.4	0.2	0.0–1.0	0.2	0.0–1.7

* Overall length from mesiobuccal root apex to tip of mesiobuccal cusp. Root length is from cervical line center to root apex. Crown length is from cervical line to tip of mesiobuccal cusp (slanted).

Table 7-2 — SIZE OF MANDIBULAR MOLARS (MILLIMETERS) (MEASURED BY DR. WOELFEL AND HIS DENTAL HYGIENE STUDENTS, 1974–1979)

Dimension Measured	281 FIRST MOLARS Average	Range	296 SECOND MOLARS Average	Range	262 THIRD MOLARS Average	Range
Crown length*	7.7	6.1–9.6	7.7	6.1–9.8	7.5	6.1–9.2
Root length						
Mesial*	14.0	10.6–20.0	13.9	9.3–18.3	11.8	7.3–14.6
Distal	13.0	8.1–17.7	13.0	8.5–18.3	10.8	5.2–14.0
Overall length*	20.9	17.0–27.7	20.6	15.0–25.5	18.2	14.8–22.0
Crown width (M–D)	11.4	9.8–14.5	10.8	9.6–13.0	11.3	8.5–14.2
Root width (cervix)	9.2	7.7–12.4	9.1	7.4–10.6	9.2	6.4–10.7
Faciolingual crown size	10.2	8.9–13.7	9.9	7.6–11.8	10.1	8.2–13.2
Faciolingual root (cervix)	9.0	7.3–11.6	8.8	7.1–10.9	8.9	7.0–11.5
Mesial cervical curvature	0.5	0.0–1.6	0.5	0.0–1.4	0.4	0.0–1.4
Distal cervical curvature	0.2	0.0–1.2	0.2	0.0–1.2	0.2	0.0–1.0

* Overall length from mesial root apex to tip of mesiobuccal cusp. Root length is from cervical line center to root apex. Crown length is from cervical line to tip of mesiobuccal cusp.

range in size of maxillary and mandibular molars in all dimensions.) They have broader occlusal surfaces than other posterior teeth (i.e., the premolars) both faciolingually and mesiodistally [averaging 2.2 mm and 3.0 mm, respectively, in maxillary molars and 2.1 mm and 3.2 mm, respectively, in mandibular molars]. However, molar crowns are shorter cervico-occlusally than all other crowns. The crowns of *both* the mandibular and maxillary molars are wider mesiodistally than long cervico-occlusally (Appendix 7a).

2. TAPER FROM BUCCAL TO LINGUAL FOR ALL MOLARS

From the occlusal view, molar crowns taper (get narrower) from the buccal to the lingual. That is, the mesiodistal width on the buccal half is wider than on the lingual half (Appendix 7b), EXCEPT on maxillary first molars with large distolingual cusps, where crowns actually taper narrower from lingual toward the buccal.

3. TAPER TO THE DISTAL FOR ALL MOLARS

For both arches, molar crowns from the occlusal view tend to taper distally, so that the distal side is narrower buccolingually than the mesial side (Appendix 7c). Also, from the buccal (or lingual) views, all molar occlusal surfaces slope toward the cervix (get shorter) from mesial to distal (Appendix 7d). This, along with the more cervical placement of the distal marginal ridge, makes more of the occlusal surface visible from the distal aspect than from the mesial aspect (compare mesial to distal views in Appendix page 7).

4. HEIGHT (CREST) OF CONTOUR FOR ALL MOLARS

As with premolars, the height of contour on the buccal of molars viewed from the proximal is in the cervical third; on the lingual, it is in the middle third (Appendix 7e).

5. CONTACT AREAS FOR ALL MOLARS

The contact areas of all molars viewed from the buccal (or lingual) views are at or near the junction of the occlusal and middle thirds mesially and are more cervical on the distal, near the middle of the tooth (Appendix 7f).

D. ARCH TRAITS THAT DIFFERENTIATE MAXILLARY FROM MANDIBULAR MOLARS

Compare extracted maxillary and mandibular molars and/or tooth models while reading about these differentiating arch traits. Also refer to page 8 in the Appendix.

1. CROWN OUTLINE TO DISTINGUISH MAXILLARY FROM MANDIBULAR MOLARS

From the occlusal view, the crowns of **mandibular molars** are oblong: they are characteristically much wider mesiodistally than faciolingually [by 1.2 mm on 839 teeth]. This is just the opposite of the **maxillary molars,** which have their greater dimension faciolingually [by 1.2 mm on 920 teeth]. From the occlusal view, *maxillary* molars have a more square or twisted parallelogram shape; *mandibular* molars have a somewhat rectangular shape (or even a pentagon shape on mandibular first molars). Compare the outline shapes in Appendix 8a (somewhat rectangular outline of mandibular molars) and 8k (a parallelogram outline for maxillary molars and a rectangular or pentagon outline for mandibular molars). Also, refer to a summary of geometric outlines of molars later in this chapter in Figure 7-27.

2. NUMBER AND RELATIVE SIZE OF CUSPS (AND NUMBER OF LOBES)

Mandibular molar crowns have four relatively large cusps: two buccal (mesiobuccal and distobuccal) and two lingual (mesiolingual and distobuccal). On most mandibular first molars and some third molars, there is often an additional fifth, smaller cusp called a distal cusp, located on the buccal surface just distal to the distobuccal cusp. The two mandibular lingual cusps are of nearly equal size (much different from the maxillary molars). The crowns of **maxillary molars** have three larger cusps (mesiobuccal, distobuccal, and mesiolingual) with a fourth cusp of lesser size (distolingual). The longest and largest mesiolingual cusp is connected by an *oblique ridge* to the distobuccal cusp (unique to maxillary molars) (Appendix 8d). A fifth, much smaller cusp (cusp of Carabelli) is often found on the lingual surface of the mesiolingual cusp of maxillary first molars (Appendix 8i). The number of lobes forming molars is one per cusp. See *Table 7-3* for a summary of the number of lobes forming first and second molars.

3. LINGUAL AND DISTAL TILT THAT DISTINGUISHES MAXILLARY FROM MANDIBULAR MOLARS

When examined from the mesial or distal views, **mandibular molar** crowns appear to be tilted lingually (true for all mandibular posterior teeth), whereas the crowns of **maxillary molars** are centered over their roots (Appendix 8b). *Mandibular* molar crowns also appear to tip distally relative to the long axis of the root due in part to the increased taper from the distal contact to the cervical line (see Appendix 8g where the distal crown bulge beyond the root can be seen).

4. ROOTS TO DISTINGUISH MAXILLARY FROM MANDIBULAR MOLARS

Perhaps the most obvious trait to differentiate *extracted* maxillary from mandibular molars is the number of roots. **Maxillary molars** have *three* relatively long roots: mesiobuccal, distobuccal, and lingual (palatal). [The average root-to-crown ratio is 1.72 and 1.70 for the maxillary first and second molars,

Table 7-3	MOLARS: GUIDELINES FOR DETERMINING NUMBER OF LOBES FOR MOLARS	
MOLAR NAME	**# CUSPS**	**# LOBES**
Maxillary 1 molar	4 (or **5** if Carabelli)	**4** (or **5** if Carabelli)
Maxillary 2 molar	4	**4**
Mandibular 1 molar	5	**5**
Mandibular 2 molar	4	**4**

Number of lobes = 1 per cusp (including Carabelli)

| Table 7-4 | ARCH TRAITS TO DISTINGUISH MANDIBULAR FROM MAXILLARY MOLARS |

	MAXILLARY MOLARS	MANDIBULAR MOLARS

BUCCAL VIEW	Two buccal cusps:
	  Mesiobuccal (MB) and distobuccal (DL)
	  Mesiolingual (ML) cusp tip visible from buccal
	One buccal groove
	Three roots (two buccal and one lingual)
	Root trunk longer
	Crown centered over root
		Two or three buccal cusps:
		  MB, DB, and distal
		  Both lingual cusp tips visible from buccal
		Two buccal grooves on first molars [81%]
		Two roots (one mesial and one distal)
		Root trunk shorter
		Crown tipped distally on root

LINGUAL VIEW	Lingual groove off center ML cusp much larger than distolingual (DL) cusp Cervix of crown tapers more to lingual Cusp of Carabelli or groove on 70% of first molars	Lingual groove centered ML and DL cusps size and height more equal Cervix of crown tapers less to lingual No Carabelli cusp
PROXIMAL VIEWS	Crown more centered over root DL cusp on second molars [62%] or no DL cusp [38%]	Crown tipped more lingually over root Distal cusp (third buccal cusp) seen from distal on first molars [81%]

OCCLUSAL VIEW	Crowns wider faciolingually than mesiodistal (MD)
	Oblique ridge present from ML to DB
	One transverse ridge MB to ML
	Parallelogram (or square) shape crown:
	  Three-cusp seconds are heart shaped
	Four fossae: including large central and cigar-shaped distal
	Central groove in mesial half does not cross oblique ridge
	First molars have four cusps plus Carabelli cusp/groove [70%]
	First molars wider on lingual than buccal
	Second molars have four cusps [62%] or three cusps (heart shaped) [38%]
	ML cusp much larger than DL
		Crowns wider mesiodistally than faciolingual (FL)
		No oblique ridge
		Two transverse ridges MB–ML and DB–DL
		Pentagon or rectangular shape crown:
		  Second molars are rectangular
		Three fossae: central fossa is large
		
		Central pit with Y or + groove pattern
		
		Five cusps on first [81%] (distal cusp is fifth cusp)
		
		First molars wider on buccal than lingual
		Second molars have four cusps:
		
		ML cusp slightly larger than DL

respectively.] The lingual root is usually the longest; the distobuccal root the shortest. The roots converge into a broad cervical root trunk. **Mandibular molars** have only *two* roots: a long mesial root and a slightly shorter distal root [mesial roots averaged 1 mm longer than the distal roots for 839 mandibular molars]. [The average root-to-crown ratio for mandibular molars is the greatest of all teeth: 1.83 and 1.82 for the first and second molars, respectively.] The root furcation on lower molars is usually close to the cervical line (especially on first molars), making the root trunk shorter than on the maxillary molars (see Appendix 8c).

Table 7-4 includes a summary of arch traits that can be used to differentiate maxillary from mandibular molars.

SECTION II   TYPE TRAITS THAT DIFFERENTIATE MANDIBULAR SECOND MOLARS FROM MANDIBULAR FIRST MOLARS

OBJECTIVES

This section prepares the reader to perform the following:

• Describe the type traits that can be used to distinguish the permanent mandibular first molar from the mandibular second molar.

- Describe and identify the buccal, lingual, mesial, distal, and occlusal surfaces for all mandibular molars.
- Assign a Universal number to mandibular molars present in a mouth (or on a model) with complete dentition. If possible, repeat this on a model with one or more mandibular molars missing.
- Holding a mandibular molar, determine whether it is a first or a second and right or left. Then assign a Universal number to it.

Mandibular first and second molars have specific traits that can be used to distinguish one from the other. The third molars vary considerably, often resembling a first or a second molar while still having their own unique traits that will be discussed later in Section IV. For this section, hold a mandibular first and second molar in front of you (with crowns up, roots down) and refer to Appendix page 8 while making the following comparisons.

A.   TYPE TRAITS OF MANDIBULAR MOLARS FROM THE BUCCAL VIEW

Refer to *Figure 7-2* for similarities and differences of mandibular first and second molars.

1.   CROWN PROPORTIONS FROM THE BUCCAL VIEW

For *both* types of mandibular molars, the crowns are wider mesiodistally than high cervico-occlusally, but more so on the larger first molars [3.7 mm larger on first molars versus 3.1 mm for second molars].

2.   RELATIVE NUMBER AND SIZE OF MANDIBULAR MOLAR CUSPS (AND GROOVES THAT SEPARATE THEM) FROM THE BUCCAL VIEW

The crown of the **mandibular first molar** is usually larger than the crown of the second molar in the same mouth. [In one study, second *mandibular* molars were larger than first molars in only 10% of Ohio Caucasians and in 19% of Pima Indians.[23] In contrast, Dr. Woelfel examined more than 600 sets of complete dentition casts of young dental hygienists' mouths and found only a few where *mandibular* second molars were slightly larger than the first molars. There were a few more in which the mandibular third molar crowns were as large as the first molars and larger than the mandibular second molars.]

The *mandibular first molar* has the largest mesiodistal dimension [11.4 mm] of any tooth [includes measurements of 2392 maxillary and 2180 mandibular teeth].

The mandibular first molar usually has *five* cusps: three buccal [81% of the time] and two lingual (*Fig. 7-3A* and *B*). They are, in order from longest to shortest, mesiolingual, distolingual, mesiobuccal, distobuccal, then the smallest distal cusp. The mesiobuccal cusp is the largest, widest, and highest cusp *on the buccal* side of the tooth. [The mesiobuccal cusp was widest in 61%, compared to only 17% for the distobuccal cusp, for 1367 *mandibular first molars*.] The *distobuccal* cusp is slightly smaller and shorter and may be sharper than the *mesiobuccal* cusp. [After examination of 430 teeth, it was considered to be sharper than the mesiobuccal cusp 55% of the time, compared to only 17% for the mesiobuccal cusp. The rest were equally sharp.] The smallest (minor) *distal* cusp, present about 81% of the time, is located on the distobuccal angle of the crown. It is the smallest of the five cusps. [In Mongoloid peoples, this cusp is often positioned lingually. It may also be split into two parts by a fissure.[1]]

The *mesiolingual* cusp of the *mandibular first molar*, which is the highest or longest of all the cusps of the mandibular first molar, is just visible behind the mesiobuccal cusp even from the buccal view. The *distolingual* cusp is visible behind the distobuccal cusp and is usually the second highest cusp when the tooth is oriented vertically. This is clearly seen in the first molars in Figure 7-2. Even though the lingual cusps are higher than buccal cusps when viewing extracted teeth with the root axis held vertically, the lingual cusp tips are at a lower level than the buccal cusps *in the mouth* due to the lingual tilt of the root axis in the mandible (creating the curve of Wilson shown earlier in *Fig. 3-29*).

When there are three buccal cusps on the *mandibular first molar*, there are two buccal grooves: the longer mesiobuccal and shorter distobuccal. The *mesiobuccal groove* on the buccal surface separates the mesiobuccal cusp from the distobuccal cusp. There may be a deep pit at the cervical end of the mesiobuccal groove. This pit is sometimes a site of caries. (This pit is common in the teeth of Mongoloid persons.) Six of the *mandibular first molars* in Figure 7-2 have pits at the end of the

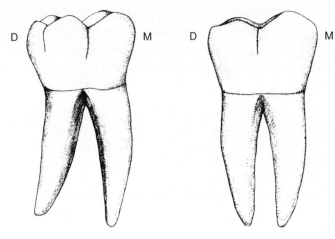

Right mandibular first molar   Right mandibular second molar

Mandibular Molars (Buccal)

Rights   Lefts

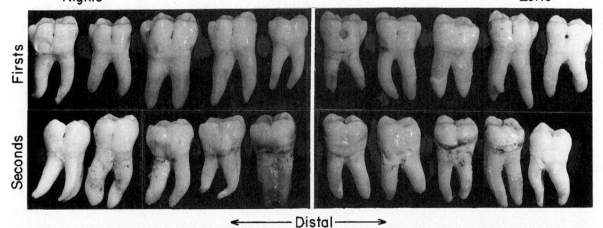

← Distal →

TRAITS TO DISTINGUISH MANDIBULAR FIRST MOLARS FROM SECOND MOLARS: BUCCAL VIEW

MANDIBULAR FIRST MOLAR	MANDIBULAR SECOND MOLAR

Three buccal cusps [81%]:
  Mesiobuccal (MB), distobuccal (DB), and distal
  Two buccal grooves
Crowns tipped less distally on root
Wider root spread, shorter trunk
Roots more curved
	Two buccal cusps:
	  MB and DB
	  One buccal groove
	Crowns tipped distally on root
	Less root spread, longer trunk
	Straighter, less curved roots

TRAITS TO DISTINGUISH MANDIBULAR RIGHT FROM LEFT MOLARS: BUCCAL VIEW

MANDIBULAR FIRST MOLAR	MANDIBULAR SECOND MOLAR
Distal cusp is smallest buccal cusp	Distobuccal cusp is smaller than mesiobuccal
Crown tapers and is shorter toward distal	
Distal contact more cervical than mesial contact	
Crown appears to tilt distally on its root	
Mesiobuccal root is longer than distobuccal root	

FIGURE 7-2. Buccal views of mandibular molars with type traits to distinguish mandibular first from second molars and traits to distinguish rights from lefts.

CUSPS

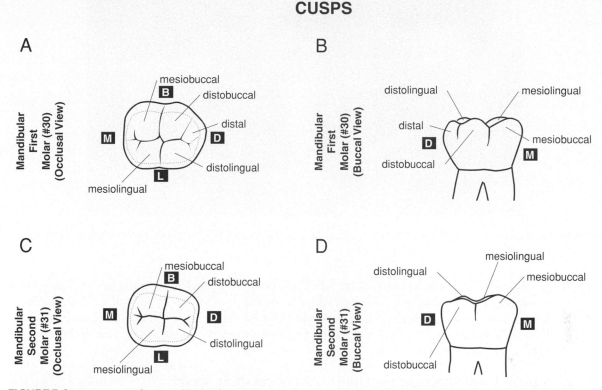

FIGURE 7-3. Cusp names for mandibular first and second molars showing relative location and size (occlusal and buccal views).

mesiobuccal groove, and a seventh has an amalgam restoration. The *distobuccal groove* separates the distobuccal cusp from the distal cusp. It is shorter than the mesiobuccal groove [70% of the time on 720 molars] and is *not* frequently pitted. One of the *mandibular first molars* in Figure 7-2 has this pit; can you find it?

The **mandibular second molar** has *four* cusps: two buccal and two lingual (*Fig. 7-3C and D*). These cusps, in order from longest to shortest, are the mesiolingual, distolingual, mesiobuccal, and distobuccal, the same order as for the four major cusps of the mandibular first molar. As on the first molar, the mesiobuccal cusp is usually wider mesiodistally than the distobuccal cusp. [The mesiobuccal cusp was considered widest on 66%, compared to only 19% with a wider distobuccal cusp, for 1514 mandibular second molars examined on dental stone casts.] As on the first molar, the lingual cusp tips are visible from the buccal side. The tips of the slightly longer mesiolingual and distolingual cusps are seen behind the mesiobuccal and distobuccal cusps (seen in most teeth in *Fig. 7-2*).

Mandibular second molars have only one *buccal* groove, separating the mesiobuccal and the distobuccal cusps. The buccal groove may end on the middle of the buccal surface in a pit (seen in two of the 10 second molars in *Fig. 7-2*). There is *no* distobuccal groove as on the first molar.

3. PROXIMAL CONTACTS OF MANDIBULAR MOLARS FROM THE BUCCAL VIEW

Both types of mandibular molars (in fact, all molars) have their *mesial* contact located more occlusally than the distal, close to the junction of middle and occlusal thirds of the crown. The *distal* contact is located more cervically, in the middle third (near the middle of the tooth cervico-occlusally). This difference in proximal contact height can be seen in most mandibular molars in Figure 7-2.

4. CERVICAL LINES OF MANDIBULAR MOLARS FROM THE BUCCAL VIEW

The cervical lines of both mandibular first and second molars are often nearly straight across the *buccal* surface. On *mandibular first molars,* there is often a ridge of cementum crossing the space in the root bifurcation in a mesiodistal direction,[6] but sometimes there is a point of enamel that dips down

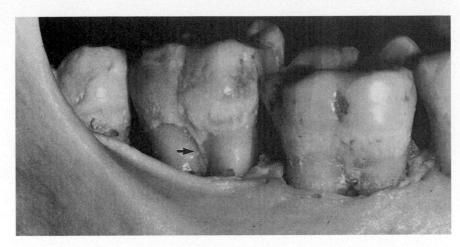

FIGURE 7-4. Enamel extension (*arrow*) downward into the buccal furcation of a mandibular second molar. (Courtesy of Charles Solt, D.D.S., and Todd Needhan, D.D.S.)

nearly into the root bifurcation (*Fig. 7-4*) [This point of enamel is reported to occur in 90% of Mongoloid peoples studied.[1]] Sometimes there is dipping down of enamel on both the buccal and the lingual surfaces, and these extensions may meet in the root bifurcation[1,2] (*Fig. 7-2*, leftmost mandibular second molar). Such enamel extensions may cause periodontal problems because of the deep gingival sulcus in these regions.

5. TAPER OF MANDIBULAR MOLARS FROM THE BUCCAL VIEW

There is proportionally more tapering of the crown from the contact areas to the cervical line on *mandibular first molars* than on *second* molars because of the bulge of the distal cusp (Appendix 8g). The crown of the second molar appears to be wider at the cervix than the first molar because of the absence of a distal cusp (less taper toward the cervix below the contact points). The *mesial* sides of mandibular molar crowns are nearly straight, or slightly concave, from the cervical line to the convex contact area (*Fig. 7-2*). The *distal* sides are straight, or slightly convex, from the cervical line to the contact areas.

Also, the occlusal surface of *both* types of mandibular molars slopes cervically (gets shorter) from mesial to distal, giving the appearance that the crown is tipped distally on its two roots (somewhat less so on first molars, again due partly to the presence of the distal cusp).

6. VARIATIONS IN MANDIBULAR MOLAR CROWNS FROM THE BUCCAL VIEW

The distal cusp of *mandibular first molars* is absent about a fifth of the time (*Fig. 7-5*). [Among 874 dental hygiene students at the Ohio State University College of Dentistry (1971–1983), dental stone casts revealed that 81% of 1327 first molars without restorations had five cusps and 19% had only four cusps. Seventy-seven percent of the females had five-cusp first molars on both sides, 16% had four-cusp first molars on both sides, and 3% had one four-cusp and one five-cusp mandibular first molar.] Consequently, *not all four-cusp molars are second molars*. Almost one-fifth may be *mandibular first molars*.

The mandibular first molar sometimes has an extra cusp on the buccal surface of the mesiobuccal cusp, about in the middle third of the crown. Studies have shown this to occur frequently in the Pima Indians of Arizona[3,14] and in Indian (Asian) populations.[4,5] An extra cusp in the same location has also been found on second and, most frequently, on third molars (see *Fig. 7-6*).

7. ROOTS OF MANDIBULAR MOLARS FROM THE BUCCAL VIEW

Both mandibular first and second molars have *two* roots, one slightly longer mesial root and one distal root (Appendix 8c). [The mesial root averaged only 1 mm longer than the distal root on 281 *first* molars and 0.9 mm longer on 296 *second* molars.] Both roots are nearly twice as long as the crown. [Root-to-crown ratio for first molars is 1.83:1, the highest ratio of any tooth.]

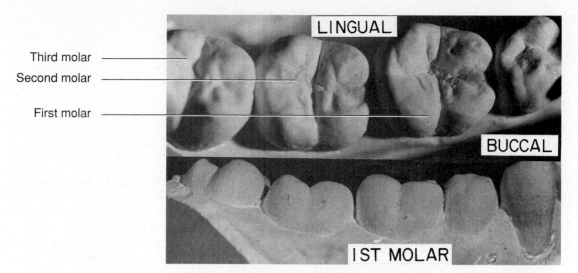

FIGURE 7-5. A mandibular first molar with *only four cusps* (whereas most have five cusps). Buccal view **(below)** and occlusal view **(above).**

The root bifurcation of the **mandibular first molar** is near the cervical line with a depression existing between the bifurcation and cervical line, and its root trunk is relatively short (shorter than on second molars). The roots of the mandibular first molar are widely separated, more so than on the second where they are more parallel (Appendix 8f). Greater root divergence can be seen in most *mandibular first molars* in Figure 7-2.

The *mesial* root of the mandibular first molar bows out mesially, such that the mesial side of this root may extend mesial to the mesial surface of the first molar crown, but the apical half curves distally. The curvature and direction of the roots is enough that the apex of the mesial root may be in line with the mesiobuccal groove of the crown, and the apex of the distal root often lies distal to the distal surface of the crown. (Compare the root spread of the mandibular first molar in Appendix 8c to the spread in a number of actual first molars in Figure 7-2.) From the buccal aspect, it is possible to see the distal surface of the mesial root because of the way it is twisted on the trunk. The *distal* root is straighter than the mesial root and may have a more pointed apex.

The roots of **mandibular second molars** are less widely separated or more parallel (Appendix 8f). The root trunk is slightly longer. There is a depression on the root trunk from the cervical line to the root bifurcation (*Fig. 7-2*). Both roots taper apically and are more pointed than the roots of the first molar. Often the apices of both roots are directed toward the centerline of the tooth, similar in shape to the handle of pliers (2 of the 10 mandibular molars in *Fig. 7-2*; see if you can find them), or both roots may curve distally.

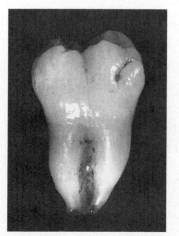

FIGURE 7-6. Unusual extra cusp: four-cusp mandibular right third molar, buccal surface. Note the bulbous crown and the extra cusplet on the buccal surface of the mesiobuccal cusp. This extra cusp or cusplet is *not* called a Carabelli cusp.

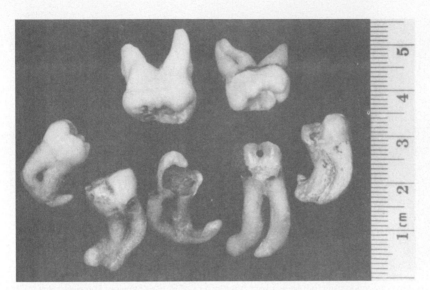

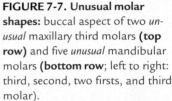

FIGURE 7-7. Unusual molar shapes: buccal aspect of two *unusual* maxillary third molars **(top row)** and five *unusual* mandibular molars **(bottom row**; left to right: third, second, two firsts, and third molar).

8. VARIATIONS IN MANDIBULAR MOLAR ROOTS FROM THE BUCCAL VIEW

Observe the wide variation from the normal in the roots with extreme distal root curvature seen in *Figure 7-7*, lower row. This condition is called **flexion** [FLEK shen].

Occasionally, the mesial root is divided into a mesiobuccal and a mesiolingual root, making three roots on the mandibular first molar. It is reported that this condition is found in 10–20% of the mandibular first permanent molars in Eskimos.[7]

In Mongoloid people, there is usually a longer root trunk.[1] Ten percent of their *mandibular first molars* have an additional distolingual root, and sometimes the mesial root is bifurcated, resulting in a four-rooted first molar.[8] It is reported that in both deciduous and permanent dentitions, three-rooted mandibular molars occur frequently in Mongoloid (Chinese) people but rarely in European groups.[1,9] A small, third root can be seen in *Figure 7-8A*. This peduncular-shaped extra root is approximately 6 mm long. Also, in Figure 7-8B, a right and left bitewing radiograph from a Caucasian male revealed an unusual long third root bilaterally between normal mesial and distal roots.

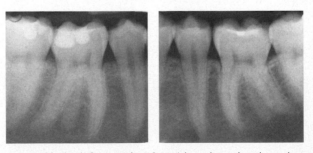

FIGURE 7-8. Unusual roots: A. Mandibular left second molar with peduncular-shaped extra root; buccal view. (Courtesy of Drs. John A. Pike and Lewis J. Claman.) **B.** Radiographs of a right and left mandibular first molar from the mouth of a Caucasian male with unusual, large third roots located between the normal-looking mesial and distal roots. (Brought to the author's attention by Joshua Clark, dental student.)

B. TYPE TRAITS OF MANDIBULAR MOLARS FROM THE LINGUAL VIEW

Refer to *Figure 7-9* for similarities and differences of mandibular molars from the lingual view.

1. CROWN TAPER OF MANDIBULAR MOLARS FROM THE LINGUAL VIEW

As with most teeth, mandibular first and second molar crowns taper from buccal to lingual and thus are narrower on the lingual side; this is more so on first molars where much of the taper is on the distal surface lingual to the distal cusp.

2. RELATIVE SIZE OF MANDIBULAR CUSPS (AND THEIR ASSOCIATED GROOVE) FROM THE LINGUAL VIEW

Since the lingual cusps of *both* types of mandibular molars are both slightly longer and more pointed or conical than the buccal cusps, the buccal cusps are hidden behind them. Therefore, in most cases, only the mesiolingual and distolingual cusps of mandibular molars are visible from the lingual aspect (not true in *Fig. 7-9*, because of the camera angle). The mesiolingual cusp is often the slightly wider and longer of the two (noticeably wider on first molars). [On *mandibular first molars,* the mesiolingual

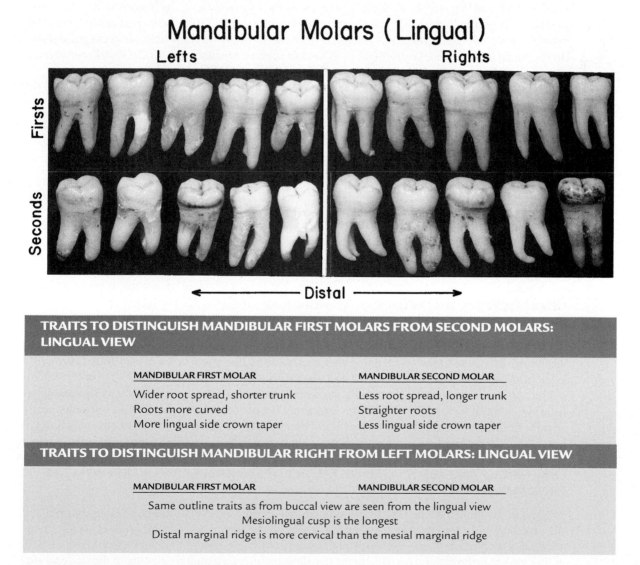

Mandibular Molars (Lingual)
Lefts   Rights

Firsts

Seconds

⟵ Distal ⟶

TRAITS TO DISTINGUISH MANDIBULAR FIRST MOLARS FROM SECOND MOLARS: LINGUAL VIEW	
MANDIBULAR FIRST MOLAR	**MANDIBULAR SECOND MOLAR**
Wider root spread, shorter trunk	Less root spread, longer trunk
Roots more curved	Straighter roots
More lingual side crown taper	Less lingual side crown taper

TRAITS TO DISTINGUISH MANDIBULAR RIGHT FROM LEFT MOLARS: LINGUAL VIEW	
MANDIBULAR FIRST MOLAR	**MANDIBULAR SECOND MOLAR**
Same outline traits as from buccal view are seen from the lingual view	
Mesiolingual cusp is the longest	
Distal marginal ridge is more cervical than the mesial marginal ridge	

FIGURE 7-9. Lingual views of mandibular molars with type traits to distinguish mandibular first from second molars and to help determine rights from lefts.

cusp was wider on 58% of 256 teeth, while on 33% the distolingual cusp was wider. On mandibular *second* molars, the mesiolingual cusp was wider on 65% of 263 of these teeth, compared to only 30% with a wider distolingual cusp.] On cusp sharpness, the lingual cusps were rated about even. [On first molars, 48% of the mesiolingual cusps were more pointed versus 47% distolingual cusps; on second molars, it was 44% versus 51%, respectively.]

The *lingual groove* separates the mesiolingual from the distolingual cusp. It may extend onto the lingual surface but is unlikely to be fissured and form decay on the lingual surface.

3. CERVICAL LINE OF MANDIBULAR MOLARS FROM THE LINGUAL VIEW

The cervical line on the lingual surface is relatively straight (mesiodistally) or irregular but may dip cervically between the roots over the bifurcation as is also sometimes seen on the buccal side of the crown.

4. ROOTS OF MANDIBULAR MOLARS FROM THE LINGUAL VIEW

On *mandibular first molars,* the root trunk appears longer on the lingual than on the buccal side because the cervical line is more occlusal in position on the lingual than on the buccal surface. The roots are narrower on the lingual side than they are on the buccal side. From the lingual aspect, it is often possible to see the mesial surface of the mesial root owing to the way it is twisted on the trunk (seen on five *mandibular first molars* in Fig. 7-9). One can also see the distal side of the distal root because of its taper toward the lingual.

On first and second molars, the short root trunk has a depression between the cervical line and the bifurcation.

C. TYPE TRAITS OF MANDIBULAR MOLARS FROM THE PROXIMAL VIEWS

For proper orientation, as you study each trait, hold the crown so that the root axis line is in a vertical position as seen in *Figure 7-10*.

Recall that *both* types of mandibular molar crowns are relatively shorter cervico-occlusally compared to faciolingually, and that the crowns of *both* types of mandibular molars are tilted lingually from the root base. Remember that this slant is an arch trait characteristic of all mandibular posterior teeth and is nature's way of shaping them to fit beneath and lingual to the maxillary buccal cusps. The buccal outline is convex in the cervical third (over its height of contour), then slightly curved and tapered occlusally in the middle and occlusal thirds.

1. HEIGHT (CREST) OF CONTOUR OF MANDIBULAR MOLARS FROM THE PROXIMAL VIEWS

As with all molars (and premolars), the height of contour or bulge of the *buccal* surface is in the cervical third. It is close to the cervical line on second molars. The buccal crest of curvature is actually a ridge running mesiodistally near the cervical line and is called the *buccal cervical ridge* (or buccal cingulum). It is more prominent on mandibular *second* molars than on first molars (actually seen better from the occlusal view in *Fig. 7-13*). The *lingual* outline of the crown of both molars appears nearly straight in the cervical third with its height of contour in the middle third. This trait is useful to tell buccal from lingual surfaces.

2. CUSP HEIGHT AND ASSOCIATED DISTAL TILT OF MANDIBULAR MOLARS FROM THE PROXIMAL VIEWS

In general, the lingual cusps of both mandibular first and second molars are more conical or pointed than the buccal. In review, the cusp length for mandibular molars is, from longest to shortest, mesiolingual, distolingual, mesiobuccal, distobuccal, and, when present, the smallest cusp found on 81% of first molars is the distal cusp. Due to the distal tilt to the crown and the sloping of the occlusal surface, much of the occlusal surface and all cusps can be seen from the **distal** aspect (as seen on the distal surfaces of all teeth in Fig. 7-10). Subsequently, on both first and second molars, from the distal aspect the tips of the mesiobuccal and mesiolingual cusps can be seen behind the distobuccal and

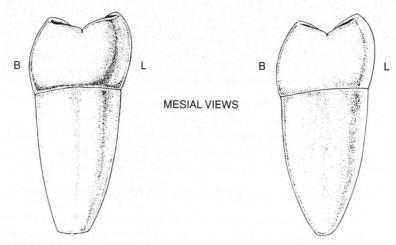

MESIAL VIEWS

Right mandibular first molar   Right mandibular second molar

Mandibular Molars (Proximal)

Rights   Lefts

Firsts

Seconds

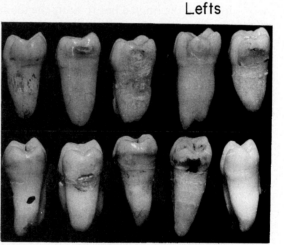

MESIAL SURFACES
←——— Buccal   Lingual ——→

DISTAL SURFACES
←——— Buccal   Lingual ——→

TRAITS TO DISTINGUISH MANDIBULAR FIRST MOLARS FROM SECOND MOLARS: PROXIMAL VIEWS

MANDIBULAR FIRST MOLAR	MANDIBULAR SECOND MOLAR
Mesial root is wide facial to lingual (F–L) with blunt tip	Mesial root less wide F–L with curved tip
Crown is wider faciolingually	Crown is less wide faciolingually

TRAITS TO DISTINGUISH MANDIBULAR RIGHT FROM LEFT MOLARS: PROXIMAL VIEWS

MANDIBULAR FIRST MOLAR	MANDIBULAR SECOND MOLAR
Mesial root broader buccolingually so distal root not seen from mesial view	
Distal marginal ridge is more cervical than mesial marginal ridge	
Distal proximal contact is more cervical than mesial contact	

FIGURE 7-10. PROXIMAL VIEWS of mandibular molars with type traits to distinguish mandibular first from second molars and to help determine rights from lefts.

distolingual cusps. On the first molar, the distobuccal cusp is seen above and somewhat buccal to the smaller, shorter distal cusp.

3. TAPER TO DISTAL OF MANDIBULAR MOLARS FROM THE PROXIMAL VIEWS

On *both* types of molars, the crown is more narrow on the distal side than on the mesial side. Therefore, from the **distal** aspect, some of the lingual and the buccal surfaces can be seen (noted especially on the distal views of mandibular *second* molars in *Fig. 7-10*). The distal contact is centered on the distal surface cervical to the distal cusp on *mandibular first molars*. There may be a wear facet here from proximal wear due to functional movements within the arch.

4. CERVICAL LINES OF THE MANDIBULAR MOLARS WHEN COMPARING PROXIMAL VIEWS

The *mesial* cervical line on *both* first and second molars slopes occlusally from buccal to lingual and curves very slightly toward the occlusal surface [0.5 mm on first molars, 0.2 mm on second molars]. The *distal* cervical line is nearly straight but slants occlusally from buccal to lingual.

5. MARGINAL RIDGES OF MANDIBULAR MOLARS WHEN COMPARING PROXIMAL VIEWS

Differences in mesial and distal marginal ridge heights are apparent on handheld teeth when viewing from the lingual but rotating the tooth first just enough in one direction to see the *mesial* marginal ridge height, and then enough in the opposite direction to compare it to the height of the *distal* marginal ridge. For mandibular molars, as with all posterior teeth (EXCEPT the mandibular first premolar), the *distal* marginal ridges are more cervically located than the mesial marginal ridges. The *mesial* marginal ridge is concave buccolingually, usually longer on the mandibular *first* molar, and often sharply V-shaped on the *second* molar. It is occlusally positioned so that not much of the triangular ridges are visible from the mesial aspect. The *distal* marginal ridge of the *first* molar is short and V-shaped, located just lingual and distal to the distal cusp.

The *mesial* marginal ridges of mandibular molars are often crossed by a marginal ridge groove [68% of 209 first molars and 57% of 233 second molars]. The *distal* marginal ridges of mandibular molars are less likely to have a mesial ridge groove [48% of 215 first molars and 35% of 233 second molars].

6. ROOTS AND ROOT DEPRESSIONS OF MANDIBULAR MOLARS FROM THE PROXIMAL VIEWS

From the **mesial** aspect, the *mesial* root of the **mandibular first molar** is broad buccolingually, hiding the distal root. It has a blunt and wide apex (*Fig. 7-10*, mesial views). It is less broad buccolingually on **mandibular second molars,** narrower in the cervical third, and more pointed at the apex. There is usually a deep depression on the mesial surface of the mesial root on *both* mandibular first and second molars extending from the cervical line to the apex, indicating the likelihood of *two* root canals in this broad root, one buccal and one lingual [as seen in cross-section views in *Fig. 7-11*). Sometimes this root is even divided into a buccal and lingual part[8] (seen in the partially divided mesial root of two mandibular first molars in *Fig. 7-10*). The depressions on the inner surfaces of the mesial and distal roots (that is, the surfaces between the mesial and distal roots) are often deeper than the depressions on the outer surfaces.

The *distal* root of *both* first and second mandibular molars is not quite as broad (buccolingually) nor as long as the mesial root, and it is more pointed at the apex. For this reason, the mesial root is usually visible behind the narrower distal root from the **distal** view (seen most clearly on all but one

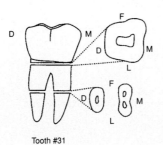

Tooth #31

FIGURE 7-11. Cross sections through the root of a mandibular second molar: the top section is located at the level of the cervical line (showing the shape of the pulp chamber located in the root trunk), and a cross section in the middle third of the bifurcated roots showing the depressions on both sides of the mesial root and two root canals, and the distal root with one canal.

mandibular second molar from the distal view in Fig. 7-10). On some teeth the distal surface of the distal root is convex; on other teeth, there may be a shallow longitudinal depression. The distal root most often has *one* root canal, but a distinct distal root depression may indicate the presence of two root canals in that root.

D. TYPE TRAITS OF MANDIBULAR MOLARS FROM THE OCCLUSAL VIEW

Refer to *Figure 7-12* for similarities and differences of mandibular molars from the occlusal view.

1. LINGUAL INCLINATION OF MANDIBULAR MOLAR CROWNS FROM THE OCCLUSAL VIEW

To follow this description the tooth should be held in such a position that the observer is looking exactly along the root axis line. Because of the inclination lingually of the crown, more of the buccal surface should be visible than the lingual surface when the tooth is properly held in this position, similar to mandibular premolars.

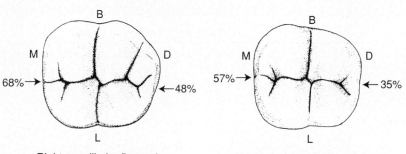

Right mandibular first molar   Right mandibular second molar

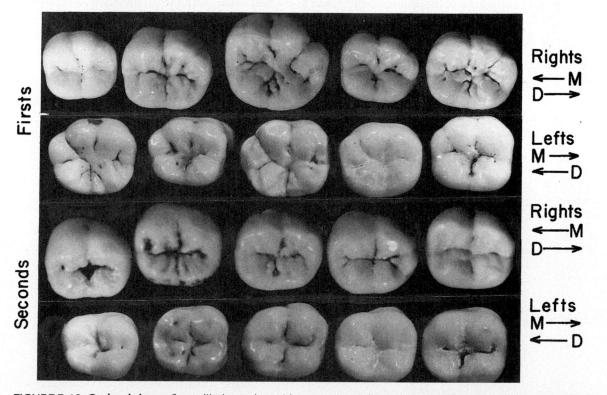

FIGURE 7-12. Occlusal views of mandibular molars with type traits to distinguish mandibular first from second molars and to help determine rights from lefts. Percentages on drawings denote the frequency of occurrence of marginal ridge grooves on more than 400 first and second molars examined by Dr. Woelfel.

TRAITS TO DISTINGUISH MANDIBULAR FIRST MOLARS FROM SECOND MOLARS: OCCLUSAL VIEW

MANDIBULAR FIRST MOLAR	MANDIBULAR SECOND MOLAR
Usually five cusps (three buccal [B] and two lingual [L])	Usually four cusps (two B and two L)
Less prominent buccal cervical ridge	Buccal ridge more prominent (mesially)
Pentagon shape (likely)	More rectangular shape
More crown taper from B to L	Less crown taper from B to L
Fewer secondary grooves	More secondary grooves
Central groove zigzags mesially to distally	Central groove straighter
Mesiobuccal and distobuccal grooves do not align with L groove	B and L grooves align to intersect with central groove like a "+"

TRAITS TO DISTINGUISH MANDIBULAR RIGHT FROM LEFT MOLARS: OCCLUSAL VIEW

MANDIBULAR FIRST MOLAR	MANDIBULAR SECOND MOLAR
Crown tapers to distal	Crown wider on mesial due to buccal cervical ridge
Distal cusp smallest	
	Large mesiolingual and mesiobuccal cusps

FIGURE 7-12. *(continued).*

2. OUTLINE SHAPE AND TAPER OF MANDIBULAR MOLARS FROM THE OCCLUSAL VIEW

As stated previously, *both* types of mandibular molars are wider mesiodistally than faciolingually [by 1.2 mm for 281 first molars and by 0.9 mm for 296 second molars]. The **mandibular second molar** shape is roughly a four-sided rectangle, whereas the **first molar,** with the prominent buccal bulge of the distobuccal cusp and smaller distal cusp, is shaped more like a five-sided pentagon (Appendix 8k). The two major mesial cusps (mesiobuccal and mesiolingual) are larger than the two *major* distal cusps (see *Fig. 7-13*). Recall that the first molar also has a minor distal cusp. There are a couple of exceptions to this among the 10 *mandibular first molars* in Figure 7-12. Can you locate them?

Mandibular molar crowns taper two ways so that they are narrower buccolingually on the distal than mesial half and are narrower mesiodistally on the lingual than on the buccal half (recall Appendix 7b and c). This distal taper is helpful in determining mesial from distal, and thus rights from lefts. This wider buccolingual dimension on the mesial half of the **mandibular second molar** is due primarily to a prominent mesial buccal bulge near the cervix called the **buccal cervical ridge** (Fig. 7-13). The widest

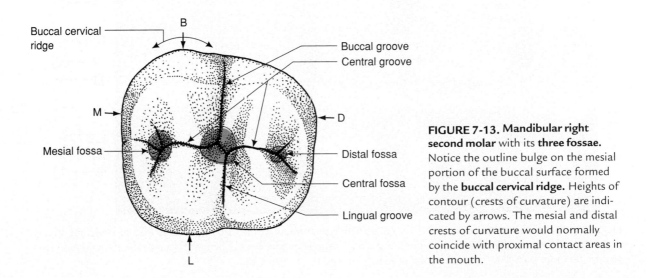

FIGURE 7-13. Mandibular right second molar with its **three fossae.** Notice the outline bulge on the mesial portion of the buccal surface formed by the **buccal cervical ridge.** Heights of contour (crests of curvature) are indicated by arrows. The mesial and distal crests of curvature would normally coincide with proximal contact areas in the mouth.

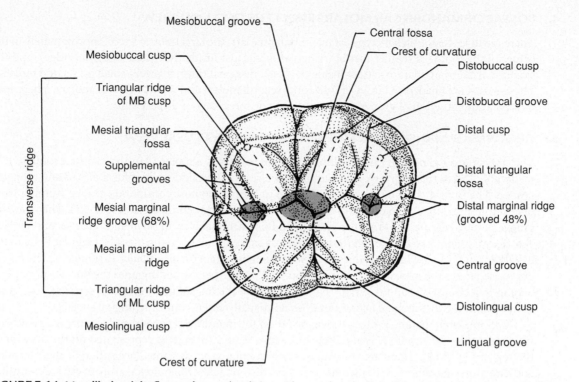

FIGURE 7-14. Mandibular right first molar; occlusal view. Observe that the **buccal crest of contour** is more in the center than on the second molar. There are **three fossae,** with the central fossa largest. Note that the central groove zigzags in its course from mesial to distal pit, and the mesiobuccal and lingual groove are *not* continuous from buccal to lingual. This pattern is quite common on first molars.

buccolingual dimension of the crown is at this bulge, and spotting it should help you locate the mesial side on mandibular second molars (evident on all mandibular second molars in *Fig. 7-12*). However, the widest portion of the crown of the **first molar** (buccolingually) may be located in the middle third of the buccal surface on the distobuccal cusp, thereby giving this tooth a pentagon outline (see crests of curvature in *Fig. 7-14*, and geometric shapes in Appendix 8k).

The outline of the crown on the first molar is convex on the buccal, lingual, mesial, and distal (more so on the buccal). On the second molar, the mesial side outline is more nearly straight compared to the shorter distal side, which is convex.

3. RIDGES OF MANDIBULAR MOLARS FROM THE OCCLUSAL VIEW

On *both* first and second mandibular molars, the triangular ridges of the mesiobuccal and mesiolingual cusps meet to form a transverse ridge, and the triangular ridges of the distobuccal and distolingual cusps form a second transverse ridge (seen on the mandibular first molar in *Fig. 7-15*). Since lingual cusps are higher, the triangular ridges of the lingual cusps of first molars are longer than the triangular ridges of the buccal cusps.

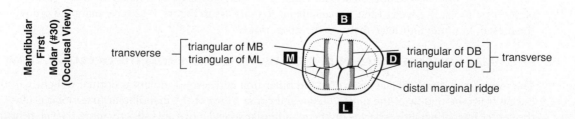

FIGURE 7-15. Mandibular first molar, occlusal view, showing how the triangular ridges of two cusps (mesiobuccal [MB] and mesiolingual [ML]) align to form one **transverse ridge** in the mesial half of the mandibular molar, and another two triangular ridges of the distobuccal (DB) and distolingual (DL) cusps align to form another **transverse ridge** in the distal half.

4. FOSSAE OF MANDIBULAR MOLARS FROM THE OCCLUSAL VIEW

There are three fossae on *both* types of mandibular molars: the large central fossa (approximately in the center of the tooth), a smaller mesial triangular fossa (just inside the mesial marginal ridge), and the smallest distal triangular fossa (just inside the distal marginal ridge; it is very small on second molars). These fossae are shaded red in *Figs. 7-13* (on a second molar) and *7-14* (on a first molar). There may be a pit at the junction of grooves in the deepest portion of any of these fossae.

5. GROOVES OF MANDIBULAR MOLARS FROM THE OCCLUSAL VIEW

The typical groove pattern on **mandibular second molars** is simpler than that on first molars. It is made up of three major grooves: a *central* groove running mesiodistally, plus a *buccal* and a *lingual* groove. The buccal and lingual grooves line up to form an almost continuous groove running from buccal to lingual that intersects with the central groove in the central fossa *(Fig. 7-13)*. The resultant groove pattern resembles a cross (or +) (Appendix 8, occlusal view of the mandibular second molar). The *central groove* passes through the central fossa as it extends from the mesial triangular fossa to the distal triangular fossa. Its mesiodistal course is straighter than on *mandibular first molars*. The *buccal* groove separates the mesiobuccal and distobuccal cusps (often extending onto the buccal surface and ending in a buccal pit) and is usually continuous with the *lingual* groove, which separates the mesiolingual and the distolingual cusps, but does not usually extend onto the lingual surface.

Developmental marginal ridge grooves occur on the **mandibular second molar** more frequently on the mesial than the distal [57% and 35%, respectively, on 233 teeth as represented on the drawing at the top of *Fig. 7-12*]. There are sometimes supplemental grooves named according to their location and direction (mesiobuccal supplemental groove, distolingual supplemental groove, etc.). One author says that mandibular second molars have more secondary grooves and a more rectangular shape than first molars.[10] Supplemental ridges are located between supplemental and major grooves and serve as additional cutting blades. All grooves provide important escapeways for food as it is crushed. Without these ridges and grooves, the teeth would be subject to unfavorable forces during mastication, as well as being inefficient crushers.

The grooves on the **mandibular first molar** separate the five cusps instead of four, so the pattern is slightly more complicated *(Fig. 7-14)*. As on the second molars, there are several main grooves: the *central* groove passes through the central fossa from the mesial triangular to the distal triangular fossa. The central groove is more zigzag or crooked in its mesiodistal course. The *lingual* groove starts in the central fossa and extends lingually between the mesiolingual and the distolingual cusps, but it is rare for a prominent lingual groove to extend onto the lingual surface.

Instead of one buccal groove, the mandibular first molar has two. The *mesiobuccal* groove, like the buccal groove of the second molar, starts from the central groove at or just mesial to the central fossa and extends between the mesiobuccal and the distobuccal cusps onto the buccal surface, possibly ending in a pit. This groove may be nearly continuous with the lingual groove, or it may not join with it. The *distobuccal* groove, unique to the first molar, starts from the central groove between the central fossa and the distal triangular fossa and extends between the distobuccal and the distal cusps, often onto the buccal surface. It may also end in a pit.

The **mandibular first molar** has numerous minor supplemental ridges and grooves (named according to their direction and cusp). The *mesial* marginal ridge is often crossed by a groove [68% of 209 first molars], whereas the *distal* marginal ridge is less often crossed by a marginal ridge groove [48% of 215 first molars]. Seven of the 10 *mandibular first molars* in Figure 7-12 have marginal grooves on the mesial, but only four have them on the distal ridge.

6. PROXIMAL CONTACT AREAS OF MANDIBULAR MOLARS FROM THE OCCLUSAL VIEW

The mesial and distal contact areas of mandibular first and second molars is normally slightly to the buccal from the middle of the tooth. The *mesial* contact area of the mandibular *first* molar is close to the center buccolingually, whereas on the mandibular *second* molar it is slightly more buccal, near the junction of the middle and buccal thirds (second molar contacts are labeled in *Fig. 7-13*). The *distal* contact of the mandibular *first* molar is just lingual to the distal cusp, whereas on the *second* molar, it is more centered buccolingually.

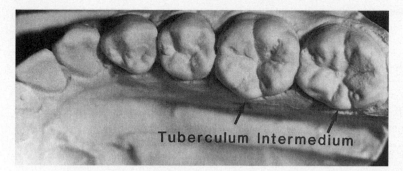

Tuberculum Intermedium

FIGURE 7-16. Mandibular first and second molars with three lingual cusps (**tuberculum intermedium**). When an extra cusp is found on the distal marginal ridge, it is called **tuberculum sextum.**

7. VARIATIONS IN MANDIBULAR MOLARS FROM THE OCCLUSAL VIEW

As mentioned, on 874 casts of dental hygienists' dentitions at Ohio State University, 19% of the 1327 *mandibular first molars* had only four cusps (no distal cusp), so they had only one buccal groove. This *four-cusp* type of mandibular *first* molar does not taper as much from buccal to lingual as a four-cusp mandibular *second* molar (occlusal aspect), but it often tapers from distal to mesial, which is unusual (recall *Fig. 7-5*).

Some *mandibular first molars* have a sixth cusp, which is named **tuberculum sextum** [too BUR kyoo lum SEKS tum] when located on the distal marginal ridge between the distal cusp and distolingual cusp; it is named **tuberculum intermedium** [too BUR kyoo lum in ter MEE di um] *(Fig. 7-16)* when located between the two lingual cusps.[11] A sixth cusp on the lingual aspect (and a third root) are common among the Chinese people.

The pattern of the grooves on the occlusal surface of the **mandibular molars** shows considerable variation. Studies have been made of the occlusal anatomy of these teeth, both in ancient and in modern man. Three principal types of occlusal groove patterns have been described: type Y, in which the zigzag central groove forms a Y figure with the lingual groove (seen in *Fig. 7-14*); type +, in which the central groove forms a + figure with the buccal and the lingual grooves (common in four-cusp type of first molars); and type X, in which the occlusal grooves are somewhat in the form of an X.[12] If you examine a collection of extracted mandibular molar teeth, you will see most of these variations.

It is reported that in the Bantu people in Africa, and sometimes in Eskimos, the mandibular molars often increase in size from first to third so that the third molar is the largest and the first molar is the smallest. This is reported to occur also in Pima Indians.[13] This is not the most frequent order of size found in American and European people.

Five-cusp mandibular second molars (shaped just like five-cusp first molars with a distal cusp) are not uncommon among the Chinese and Negroid populations.[11] In *Figure 7-17*, one is shown from a Caucasian dentition.

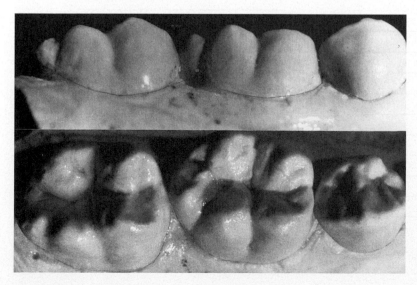

FIGURE 7-17. Unusual number of cusps: mandibular second molar with *three* buccal cusps (buccal view above; occlusal view below with buccal side down).

LEARNING EXERCISE

1. List all 19 ridges that circumscribe or make up the boundary of the occlusal surface of a mandibular first molar as represented in Figure 7-18A.
2. List all 17 ridges that circumscribe or make up the boundary of the occlusal surface of a mandibular second molar as represented in *Figure 7-18*B. In case you wondered, ridge 17 on the second molar is the buccal cervical ridge (sometimes evident, sometimes not).

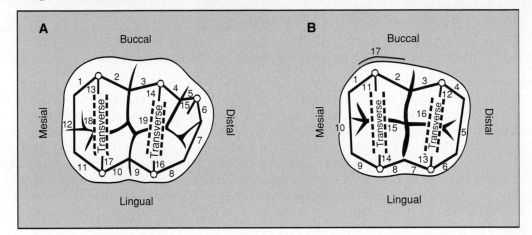

A. Name the ridges		**B.** Name the ridges	
Ridges	Name	Ridges	Name
1. _____		1. _____	
2. _____		2. _____	
3. _____		3. _____	
4. _____		4. _____	
5. _____		5. _____	
6. _____		6. _____	
7. _____		7. _____	
8. _____		8. _____	
9. _____		9. _____	
10. _____		10. _____	
11. _____		11. _____	
12. _____		12. _____	
13. _____		13. _____	
14. _____		14. _____	
15. _____		15. _____	
16. _____		16. _____	
17. _____		17. _____	
18. _____			
19. _____			

FIGURE 7-18. A. Ridges on mandibular first molar with **five cusps** (circles indicate cusp tips). Name all 19 ridges.
B. Ridges on mandibular second molar and on any first molars with **four cusps.** Name all 17 ridges. Answers are on the next page.

16.–transverse ridge (distal); 17.–mesial (mesiobuccal) cervical ridge.

ridge of distolingual cusp; 14.–triangular ridge of mesiolingual cusp; 15.–transverse ridge (mesial);

ridge; 11.–triangular ridge of mesiobuccal cusp; 12.–triangular ridge of distobuccal cusp; 13.–triangular

8.–distal cusp ridge of mesiolingual cusp; 9.–mesial cusp ridge of mesiolingual cusp; 10.–mesial marginal

5.–distal marginal ridge; 6.–distal cusp ridge of distolingual cusp; 7.–mesial cusp ridge of distolingual cusp;

mesiobuccal cusp; 3.–mesial cusp ridge of distobuccal cusp; 4.–distal cusp ridge of distobuccal cusp;

B. Mandibular Second Molar ridges: 1.–mesial cusp ridge of mesiobuccal cusp; 2.–distal cusp ridge of

19.–transverse ridge (distal).

gular ridge of distolingual cusp; 17.–triangular ridge of mesiolingual cusp; 18.–transverse ridge (mesial);

of mesiobuccal cusp; 14.–triangular ridge of distobuccal cusp; 15.–triangular ridge of distal cusp; 16.–trian-

olingual cusp; 11.–mesial cusp ridge of mesiolingual cusp; 12.–mesial marginal ridge; 13.–triangular ridge

tal cusp ridge of distolingual cusp; 9.–mesial cusp ridge of distolingual cusp; 10.–distal cusp ridge of mesi-

cusp; 5.–mesial cusp ridge of distal cusp; 6.–distal cusp ridge of distal cusp; 7.–distal marginal ridge; 8.–dis-

ridge of mesiobuccal cusp; 3.–mesial cusp ridge of distobuccal cusp; 4.–distal cusp ridge of distobuccal

ANSWERS: A. Mandibular First Molar ridges: 1.–mesial cusp ridge of mesiobuccal cusp; 2.–distal cusp

LEARNING EXERCISE

Learning exercise related to mandibular molars:

Examine the mouth of a number of your associates to determine if they have first molars with five cusps and second molars with four cusps. Also, see if their first molars are bigger than their seconds, and seconds are bigger than their thirds.

LEARNING QUESTIONS

Answer the following questions about mandibular molars by circling the best answer(s). More than one answer may be correct.

1. Which of the following grooves radiate out from the central fossa in a mandibular second molar?
   a. central
   b. mesiobuccal
   c. distobuccal
   d. lingual
   e. buccal

2. Which cusp is the largest and longest on a mandibular second molar?
   a. mesiobuccal
   b. distobuccal
   c. mesiolingual
   d. distolingual
   e. distal

3. Which cusp may be absent on a mandibular first or third molar?

    a. mesiobuccal

    b. distobuccal

    c. mesiolingual

    d. distolingual

    e. distal

4. When this cusp is absent in question #3 above, which groove(s) would not be present?

    a. buccal

    b. lingual

    c. mesiobuccal

    d. distobuccal

    e. lingual

5. Which fossae are found on a mandibular first molar?

    a. mesial triangular

    b. distal triangular

    c. buccal

    d. lingual

    e. central

6. Which developmental groove connects with the lingual groove running in the same direction on a mandibular second molar?

    a. mesiobuccal

    b. distobuccal

    c. buccal

    d. mesiolingual

    e. distolingual

7. From which view is only one root visible on a mandibular first molar?

    a. mesial

    b. distal

    c. buccal

    d. lingual

    e. occlusal

8. Which root may occasionally be divided or bifurcated on a mandibular first molar?

    a. buccal

    b. lingual

    c. mesial

    d. distal

    e. mesiobuccal

9. Which cusp triangular ridge does not meet to form a transverse ridge on a five-cusp first molar?

    a. mesiobuccal

    b. distobuccal

    c. mesiolingual

    d. distolingual

    e. distal

10. Which ridges form the boundaries of the mesial triangular fossa of a mandibular molar?
    a. triangular ridge of mesiobuccal cusp
    b. triangular ridge of mesiolingual cusp
    c. mesial marginal ridge
    d. buccal cusp ridge of mesiobuccal cusp
    e. lingual cusp ridge of mesiolingual cusp

11. Which two pairs of cusp triangular ridges make up or join to form the two transverse ridges on a mandibular second molar?

12. List in sequential order the longest to shortest cusps on the mandibular first molar.

SECTION III	TYPE TRAITS THAT DIFFERENTIATE MAXILLARY SECOND MOLARS FROM MAXILLARY FIRST MOLARS

OBJECTIVES

This section prepares the reader to perform the following:
- Describe the type traits that can be used to distinguish the permanent maxillary first molar from the maxillary second molar.
- Describe and identify the buccal, lingual, mesial, distal, and occlusal surfaces for all maxillary molars.
- Assign a Universal number to maxillary molars present in a mouth (or on a model) with complete dentition. If possible, repeat this on a model with one or more maxillary molars missing.
- Holding a maxillary molar, determine whether it is a first or a second and right or left. Then assign a Universal number to it.

A. TYPE TRAITS OF THE MAXILLARY FIRST AND SECOND MOLARS FROM THE BUCCAL VIEW

Examine a maxillary first and second molar as you read. Hold the roots up and the crowns down, with the two somewhat parallel roots toward you.

1. RELATIVE CROWN SIZE AND SHAPE FROM THE BUCCAL VIEW

Refer to *Figure 7-19* for similarities and differences of maxillary molars from the buccal view.

Maxillary first molars are the largest upper teeth (especially mesiodistally), followed closely by the second molars in the same mouth. (Third molars are generally the smallest molar.) [Studies on the variability in the relative size of molars revealed that maxillary *second* molars were larger than first maxillary molars in only 33% of a sample of an Ohio Caucasian population, and in 36% of a Pima Indian population.[23] In contrast, Dr. Woelfel found only two casts of young dental hygienists' mouths, from more than 600 sets of complete dentition casts, in which maxillary second molars were larger than the first molars.]

The crowns of *both* the first and second maxillary molars are broad mesiodistally near the junction of the occlusal and middle thirds and narrower near the cervical line. However, the **maxillary second molar** is less broad mesiodistally than the first molar, and is often tipped distally at the cervix on its root trunk so the occlusal surface slants cervically from mesial to distal. This distal tipping of the

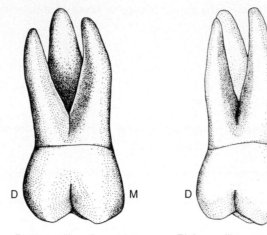

Right maxillary first molar   Right maxillary second molar

Maxillary Molars (Buccal)

Rights   Lefts

Firsts

Seconds

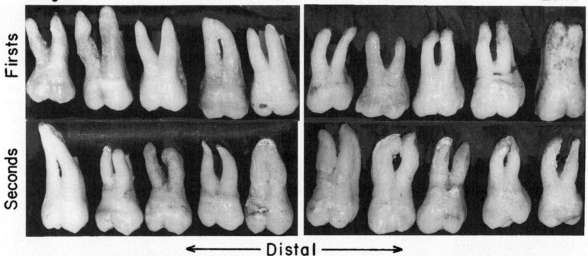

←——— Distal ———→

TRAITS TO DISTINGUISH MAXILLARY FIRST MOLARS FROM SECOND MOLARS: BUCCAL VIEW	
MAXILLARY FIRST MOLAR	**MAXILLARY SECOND MOLAR**
Roots more spread out, shorter trunk	Root less spread out, longer trunk
Roots with less distal bend	Roots with more distal bend
Buccal groove longer, possible pit	Buccal groove shorter, no pit
Buccal cusps almost same size	MB cusp larger than DB

TRAITS TO DISTINGUISH MAXILLARY RIGHT FROM LEFT MOLARS: BUCCAL VIEW	
MAXILLARY FIRST MOLAR	**MAXILLARY SECOND MOLAR**
Distobuccal cusp shorter than wider mesiobuccal cusp	
Crown tilts distally on its root base with the occlusal surface shorter on distal	

FIGURE 7-19. Buccal views of maxillary molars with type traits to distinguish maxillary first from second molars and to help determine rights from lefts.

Maxillary First Molar (#3) (Occlusal View)

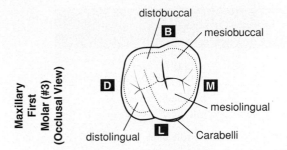

FIGURE 7-20. Maxillary first molar, occlusal view, showing the cusp names and relative sizes of cusps.

crown and the shortness of the distobuccal cusp make the buccal outline of the crown appear to be shorter on the distal than mesial, which is most helpful in determining rights from lefts.

On **maxillary first molars,** from the buccal aspect, the distal side of the crown is nearly flat in the cervical third. Occlusal to this flat region, the surface is convex.

2. NUMBER AND SIZE OF CUSPS ON MAXILLARY MOLARS (AND ASSOCIATED GROOVE) FROM THE BUCCAL VIEW

Both the first and second maxillary molars have four major cusps (seen best on an occlusal view in *Fig. 7-20*), but only two are prominently visible from the buccal view: the mesiobuccal cusp and the distobuccal cusp. The relative heights of the four major cusps of maxillary molars are the longest mesiolingual, followed by the mesiobuccal, distobuccal, and the shortest distolingual (if present). The two lingual cusp tips (mesiolingual and distolingual) may show slightly from the buccal view since the mesiolingual is longest, and both lingual cusps are positioned slightly to the distal of the buccal cusp tips.

Of the two buccal cusps, the mesiobuccal cusp is usually longer and wider than the distobuccal cusp, but not necessarily sharper. [On 1539 maxillary *first* molars, the mesiobuccal cusp was wider 64% of the time; on 1545 *second* molars, this cusp was wider 92% of the time. On 468 *first* molars, the distobuccal cusp was sharper 72% of the time, whereas on 447 *second* molars, the sharpness of buccal cusps was equal.]

The buccal groove lies between the buccal cusps and may extend onto the buccal surface to the middle third of the crown (less on second molars), but are unlikely to be fissured and form decay on the buccal surface.

3. PROXIMAL CONTACTS OF MAXILLARY MOLARS FROM THE BUCCAL VIEW (SAME FOR ALL MOLARS)

For **all** maxillary (and mandibular) first and second molars, the *mesial* contact is located at the junction of occlusal and middle thirds. The *distal* contact is located more cervically in the middle third of the tooth, near the middle. Sometimes you can observe a slightly worn spot (facet) in this location proximally where it contacted the adjacent molar. A summary of the location of the proximal contacts of maxillary and mandibular molars is found in *Table 7-5*, and a review for all teeth discussed so far is presented in *Table 7-6*.

4. ROOTS OF MAXILLARY MOLARS FROM THE BUCCAL VIEW

At the cervical line the crown is attached to a broad, undivided base called the root trunk. Apical to the root trunk, the root separates into *three* parts (three roots): the mesiobuccal root, the distobuccal root, and the lingual root. The area of furcation is often near the junction of the cervical and middle thirds of the roots (seen in most molars in *Fig. 7-19*). This furcation is called a **trifurcation** since three roots come off the trunk. The furcation between the two buccal roots is a greater distance from the cervical line on **second** molars than on the **first** molars since the root trunks of the **second** molars are longer. [In Mongoloid people, the maxillary first molars often have a long root trunk; sometimes there is no furcation at all.[1] See the last maxillary first molar on the upper row, right side, in *Fig. 7-19*.] The three roots are nearly the same length [within 1.5 mm], with the palatal (lingual) root the longest, followed by the mesiobuccal root, then the shortest distobuccal root.

Table 7-5	MOLARS: LOCATION OF PROXIMAL CONTACTS (PROXIMAL HEIGHT OF CONTOUR; SEEN BEST FROM FACIAL)	

		MESIAL SURFACE (WHICH THIRD OR JUNCTION?)	DISTAL SURFACE (WHICH THIRD OR JUNCTION?)
MAXILLARY CROWNS	1st Molar	Occlusal/middle junction	Middle of crown
	2nd Molar	Occlusal/middle junction	Middle of crown
MANDIBULAR CROWNS	1st Molar	Occlusal/middle junction	Middle of crown
	2nd Molar	Occlusal/middle junction	Middle of crown

General Learning Guidelines:
1. For **molars,** the mesial and distal contacts are closer to the middle of the tooth and are more nearly at the same level than on premolars or anterior teeth.
2. Distal proximal contacts are more cervical than mesial contacts.
Source: Brand RW, Isselhard DE: Anatomy of Orofacial Structures. 6th ed. St Louis: C.V. Mosby, 1998.

Table 7-6	SUMMARY OF LOCATION OF PROXIMAL CONTACTS (PROXIMAL HEIGHT OF CONTOUR; SEEN BEST FROM FACIAL VIEW)	

		MESIAL SURFACE (WHICH THIRD OR JUNCTION?)	DISTAL SURFACE (WHICH THIRD OR JUNCTION?)
MAXILLARY CROWNS	Central incisor	Incisal third (near incisal edge)	Incisal/middle junction
	Lateral incisor	Incisal third	Middle third (most cervical of incisor contacts)
	Canine	Incisal/middle junction	Middle third (most cervical of anterior teeth contacts)
	1st Premolar	Middle third or occlusal/middle junction	Middle (but more cervical)
	2nd Premolar	Middle third (near occlusal/middle junction)	Middle (but more cervical)
	1st Molar	Occlusal/middle junction	Middle of crown
	2nd Molar	Occlusal/middle junction	Middle of crown
MANDIBULAR CROWNS	Central incisor	Incisal third (near incisal edge)	Incisal third (near incisal edge; same as mesial)
	Lateral incisor	Incisal third (near incisal edge)	Incisal third (but more cervical)
	Canine	Incisal third (just apical to mesioincisal angle)	Incisal/middle junction
	1st Premolar	Occlusal/middle junction or middle third	Occlusal third (more occlusal than on mesial = EXCEPTION to the rule)
	2nd Premolar	Occlusal/middle junction	Middle third (which is more cervical than on mesial)
	1st Molar	Occlusal/middle junction	Middle of crown
	2nd Molar	Occlusal/middle junction	Middle of crown

General Learning Guidelines:
1. On any single tooth, distal proximal contacts are more cervical than mesial contacts EXCEPT for mandibular central incisors, where the mesial and distal contacts are at the same height, and mandibular first premolars, where the mesial contact is more cervical than the distal.
2. Proximal contacts (heights of contour) become more cervical moving from anterior to posterior teeth.
   a. For **anterior teeth,** most contacts are in the incisal third EXCEPT the *distal* of maxillary lateral incisors and canines, which are more in the middle third.
   b. For **posterior teeth,** the mesial and distal contacts are closer to the middle of the tooth and are more nearly at the same level.
3. No proximal contact (height of contour) is cervical to the middle of the tooth.

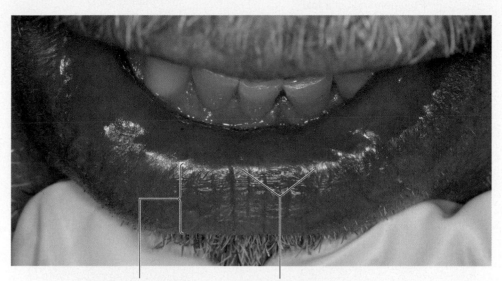

Vermillion border   Wet (wet-dry) line

COLOR PLATE 1. Vermillion border and wet (wet-dry) line.

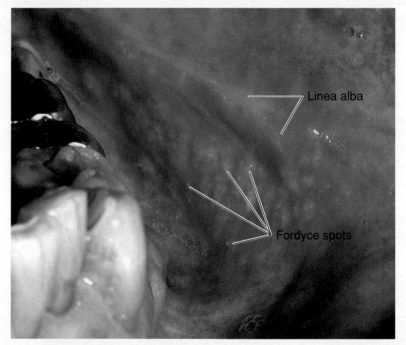

Linea alba

Fordyce spots

COLOR PLATE 2. Buccal mucosa showing a linea alba and Fordyce granules (spots). (Courtesy of Carl Allen, D.D.S., M.S.D.)

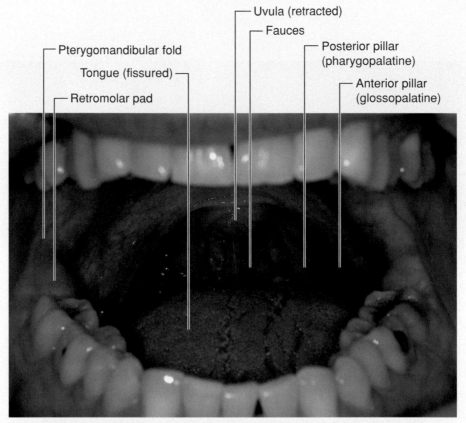

Pterygomandibular fold

Tongue (fissured)

Retromolar pad

Uvula (retracted)

Fauces

Posterior pillar
(pharygopalatine)

Anterior pillar
(glossopalatine)

COLOR PLATE 3. Oropharynx showing the retromolar pad and pterygomandibular fold extending upward from the mandibular second molars, as well as the structures surrounding the fauces: uvula (retracted), anterior pillars (palatoglossal arch), and posterior pillars (palatopharyngeal arch).

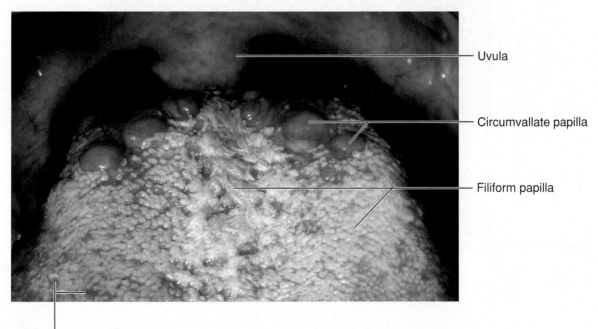

Uvula

Circumvallate papilla

Filiform papilla

Fungiform papillae

COLOR PLATE 4. Dorsal surface of the tongue. Structures include the row of prominent circumvallate papillae, hair-like filiform papillae, and the small, round, red fungiform papillae. The uvula is seen above the tongue. (Courtesy of Carl Allen, D.D.S., M.S.D.)

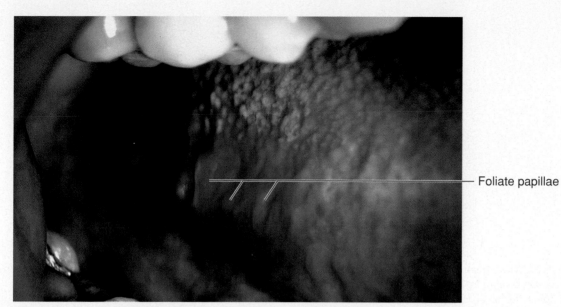

Foliate papillae

COLOR PLATE 5. Lateral surface of the tongue. Prominent fold-like foliate papillae. These must be distinguished from oral cancer that may develop in this area. (Courtesy of Carl Allen, D.D.S., M.S.D.)

Lingual frenum
(broad anteriorly)

Sublingual caruncles

Sublingual fold
(plica sublingualis)

Mandibular torus (large)

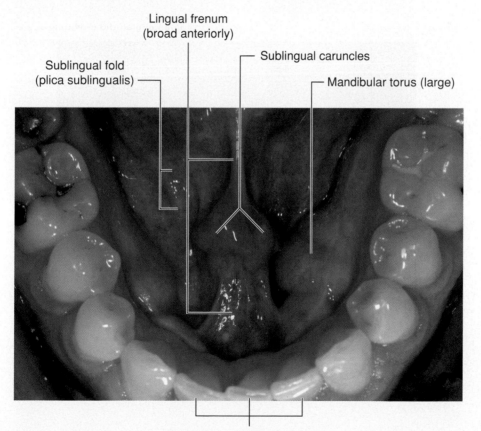

Only three mandibular anteriors

COLOR PLATE 6. Floor of the mouth. The sublingual folds lie over the sublingual glands. The sublingual caruncles are located on either side of the lingual frenum and are where the submandibular glands empty into the mouth (via Wharton's ducts). Also, note the very prominent lingual tori extending off of the lingual bone of the mandible.

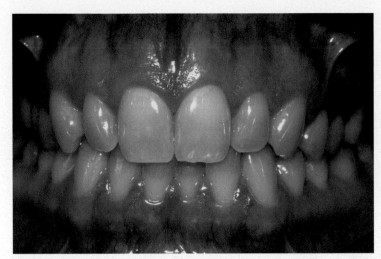

COLOR PLATE 7. Healthy maxillary gingiva showing stippling (orange-peel texture), knife-edge border of the free gingiva that are escalloped in shape, and interproximal papillae that fill the lingual embrasures (interproximal spaces). Also, notice the labial frenum in the midline and the two buccal frenums connecting the mucosa of the cheek to the attached gingiva buccal to the maxillary premolars.

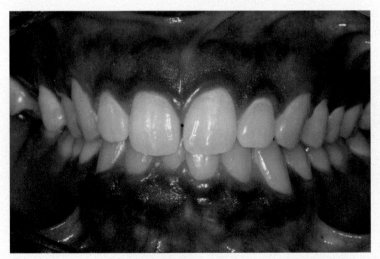

COLOR PLATE 8. Gingiva with heavy melanin (brownish) pigmentation, normal for many ethnic groups. (Note that there is evidence of slight gingival disease.)

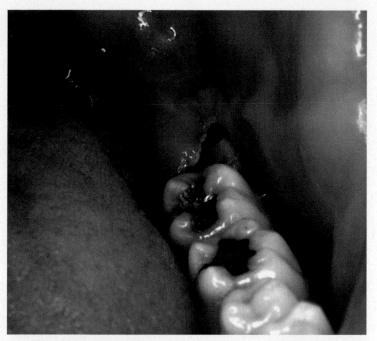

COLOR PLATE 9. Operculum: a flap of tissue over a partially erupted last mandibular molar. This flap is subject to irritation and infection surrounding the crown, known as pericoronitis. (Courtesy of Carl Allen, D.D.S., M.S.D.)

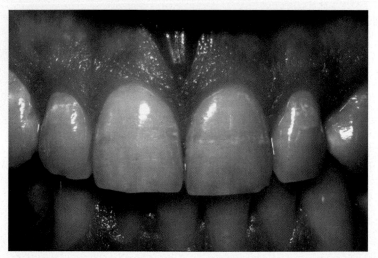

COLOR PLATE 10. Healthy gingiva. Note the ideal scalloped contours, knife edges, and stippled (orange-peel) surface texture that is usually most noticeable on the maxillary labial attached gingiva.

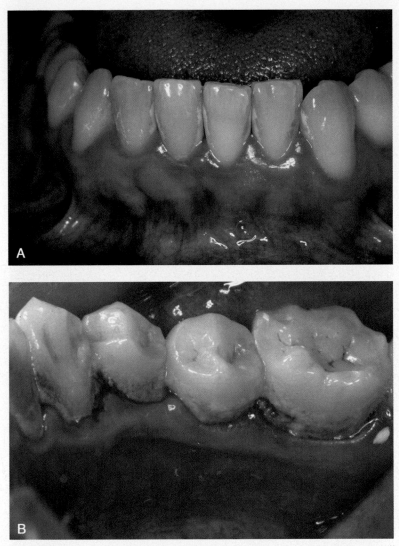

COLOR PLATE 11. Gingivitis. A. Mild to moderate gingivitis with rolled margins and bulbous papilla; smooth, shiny surface texture (loss of stippling); and increased red color. **B. Severe gingivitis** with severely rolled margins and bulbous papilla, no stippling, and spontaneous bleeding (without even probing). Air from the air–water syringe would easily retract this tissue.

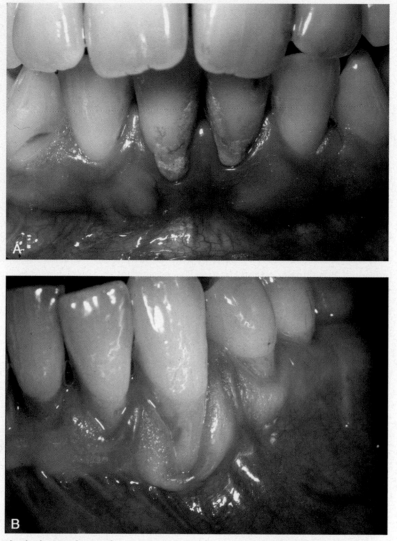

COLOR PLATE 12. Gingival recession and mucogingival defects. A. Areas of gingival recession. The gingiva no longer covers the cementoenamel junction, and the root surface is exposed on teeth #24 and 25. There is no keratinized gingiva on these central incisors compared with lateral incisors. **B.** Severe gingival recession. There is very little keratinized gingiva and no attached gingiva over the canine root. The root prominence, thin tissue, and lack of attached gingiva are factors that may have contributed to the recession. (Courtesy of Alan R. Levy, D.D.S.)

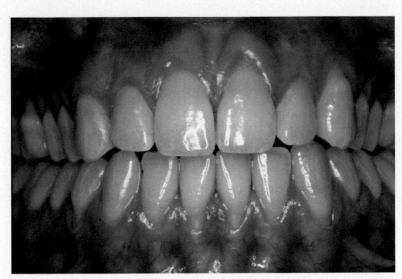

COLOR PLATE 13. Individual with **thin periodontal tissues**. The patient has thin gingival tissues, and a considerable portion of the incisor roots are exposed (recession).

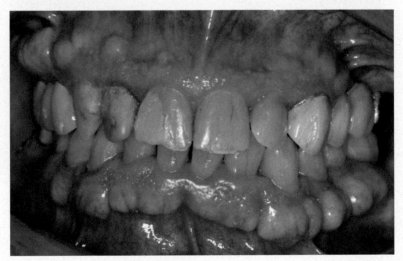

COLOR PLATE 14. Individual with **thick periodontal tissues.** The gingival tissues are generally thick, and there is very thick underlying bone. This thick bone can be called an exostosis.

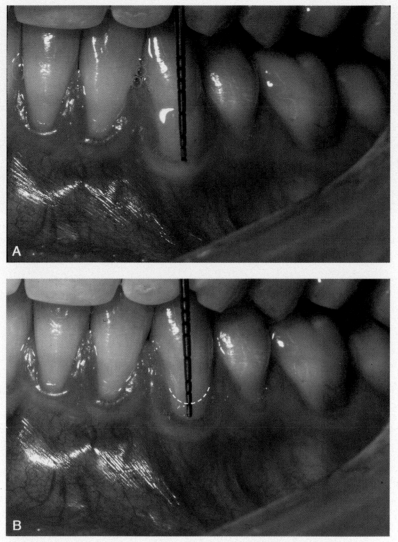

COLOR PLATE 15. Measurements for clinical attachment loss (level). A. First the sulcus is probed (at 1 mm). **B.** Next, the level of the gingiva margin level from the cementoenamel junction is measured at 1 mm. When the two numbers are added together, the amount of attachment loss is determined. In this case, the probing depth of 1 mm and the gingival level of +1 (1 mm recession) results in an attachment loss of 2 mm.

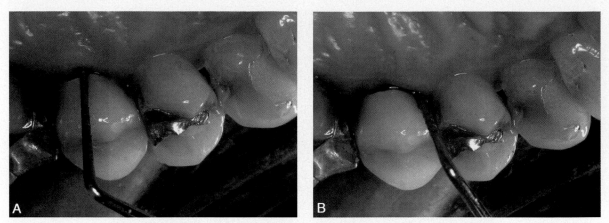

COLOR PLATE 16. Clinical example of probe placement. A. Midlingual probe placement on tooth #13 (showing 3-mm sulcus depth). **B.** Mesial probe placement on tooth #13 probed into the lingual embrasure and angled toward the interproximal. Note the 5-mm pocket at the site, which shows bleeding on probing (BOP).

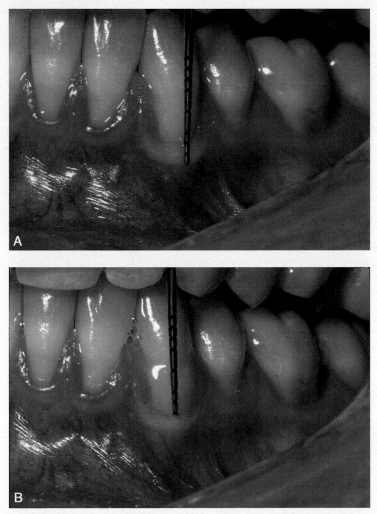

COLOR PLATE 17. Measuring for a mucogingival defect. A. The width of keratinized gingival is measured at 2 mm. **B.** The probe depth is measured at less than 2 mm (only 1 mm), indicating no mucogingival defect. If the probe depth reached or exceeded the mucogingival junction (exceeded the width of keratinized gingiva), there would be no attached gingiva, and a mucogingival defect would be present.

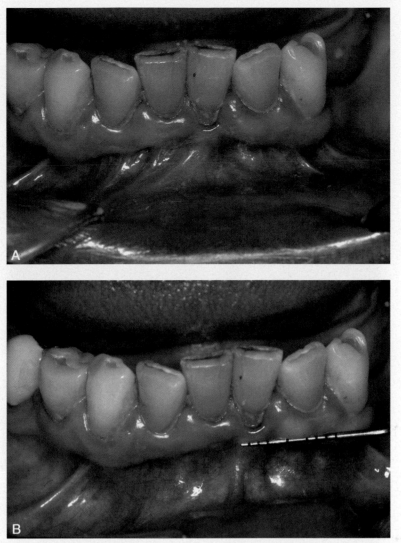

COLOR PLATE 18. Visual test for a mucogingival defect. A. A mucogingival defect is suspected at tooth #24, which has a very narrow zone of keratinized gingiva. **B.** The periodontal probe is positioned at the mucogingival junction and moved incisocervically against the mucosa. Blanching or movement at the gingival margin indicates a mucogingival defect.

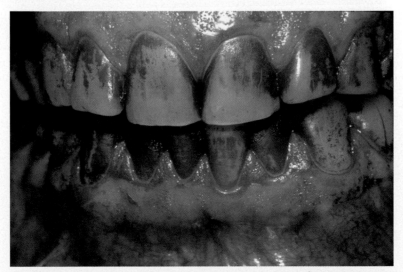

COLOR PLATE 19. Dental plaque. This photograph shows dental plaque after staining with disclosing solution. The patient had voluntarily ceased oral hygiene measures for four days. Plaque is most prominent at interproximal sites and the cervical third of crowns, areas that are **not** self-cleaning (that is, are not easily cleaned by the natural rubbing action of the cheeks, lips, and tongue). Also, note the heavy plaque accumulations on the mandibular anterior teeth, which are slightly malpositioned.

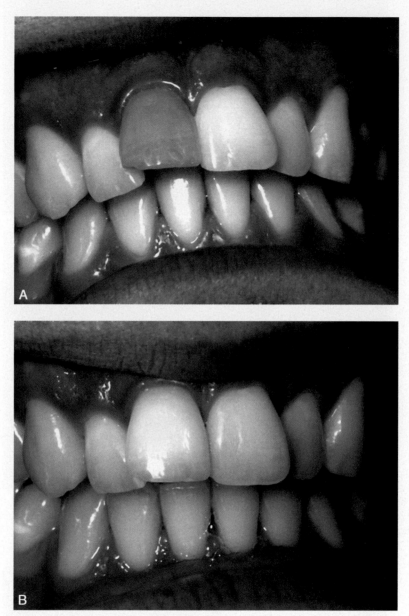

COLOR PLATE 20. Color as an indicator of pulp pathology. A. Discolored devital tooth (#8) after tooth trauma (such as being hit in the mouth with a baseball). **B.** Tooth after bleaching techniques were employed to this devital tooth.

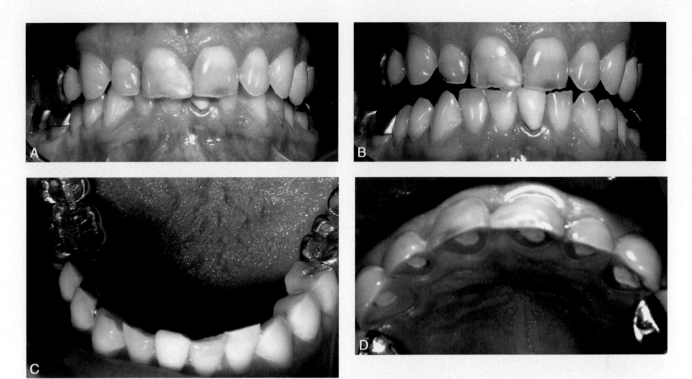

COLOR PLATE 21. Stages of a full mouth rehabilitation. A. Pretreatment: facial surfaces of teeth in maximum inter-cuspal position. Notice the anterior deep overbite. **B.** Pretreatment: facial surfaces of teeth with the mandible pro-truded so the incisors are now in an edge-to-edge position. Notice the translucency of the maxillary central incisors, in-dicating very thin enamel due to severe lingual erosion. Also notice the gingival irritation related to a bulbous existing crown on the mandibular left central incisor (#24). **C.** Pretreatment: incisal/occlusal view of the mandibular teeth. Notice the thinness of the mandibular anterior teeth due to severe lingual erosion. **D.** During treatment: incisal view of maxillary anterior teeth revealing the interim restorations on the lingual surface of each of these teeth. These restora-tions cover the openings that were required to access and remove the pulp from each tooth (endodontic therapy). Figures E, F, G and H on next page. **E.** During treatment: all maxillary anterior teeth (that had been treated with en-dodontic therapy) were prepared for crowns and, due to the reduction of remaining tooth structure, had custom-cast post and cores placed within each tooth. The posts were cemented into spaces prepared by the dentist into the root along the pulp canals, and the core (the metal that shows) provides additional support and retention for the crowns that would be placed over them. **F.** Posttreatment photograph of the mandibular teeth showing complete crowns on both second molars (#18 and 31), metal ceramic crowns on both first molars (#19 and 30), and metal ceramic crowns (metal is not visible) on all premolars (#20, 21, 28, and 29), as well as replacing an old crown on the mandibular left central incisor (#24). All other mandibular anterior teeth were veneered lingually with indirect composite veneers (#22, 23, 25, 26, and 27). **G.** Posttreatment of the maxillary teeth showing porcelain fused to metal crowns on first and sec-ond molars (#2, 3, 14, and 15), metal ceramic crowns (metal is not visible) on the two remaining premolars (#4 and 13 based on patient history), and all-ceramic crowns on the anterior teeth (#6, 7, 8, 9, 10, and 11). **H.** Posttreatment: facial view of all teeth in intercuspal position (which now is the same as centric relation) showing improved esthetics. (Provided by Julie Holloway, D.D.S., M.S.)

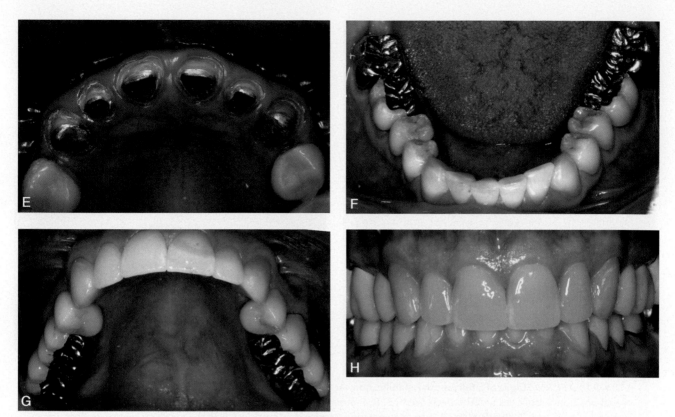

COLOR PLATE 21. Stages of a full mouth rehabilitation. (continued)

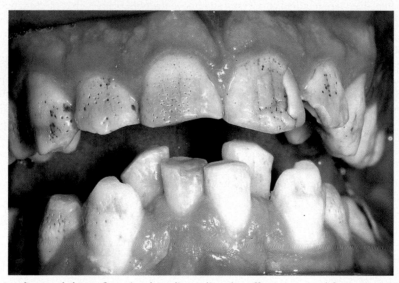

COLOR PLATE 22. Amelogenesis imperfecta is a hereditary disorder affecting enamel formation. (Courtesy of Carl Allen, D.D.S., M.S.D.)

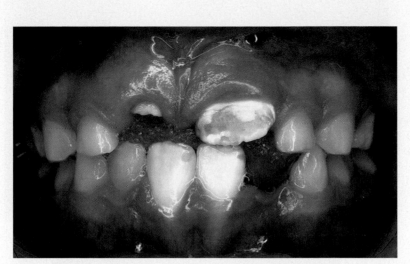

COLOR PLATE 23. Fluorosis. This condition is most evident on the maxillary and mandibular central incisors. It is seen as mottling of color and some pitting (on tooth #9). (Courtesy of Carl Allen, D.D.S., M.S.D.)

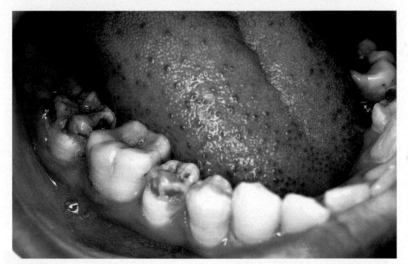

COLOR PLATE 24. Enamel hypoplasia. This tooth damage resulted from disruption of enamel formation on the mandibular second premolar and second molar. (Courtesy of Carl Allen, D.D.S., M.S.D.)

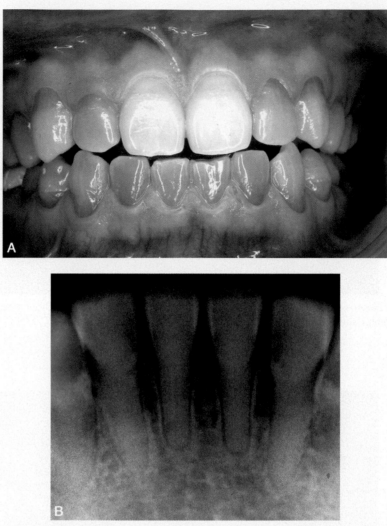

COLOR PLATE 25. Dentinogenesis imperfecta. A. The teeth take on a gray or yellow opalescent appearance.
B. Radiographs reveal the total or partial lack of pulp chambers and canals. (Courtesy of Carl Allen, D.D.S., M.S.D.)

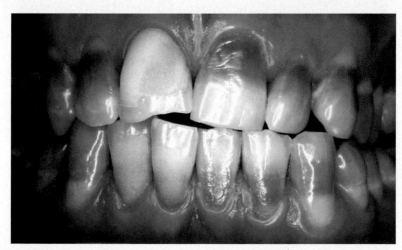

COLOR PLATE 26. Tetracycline staining. These teeth have a yellow to gray-brown color resulting from exposure of the forming teeth to the drug tetracycline, an antibiotic. (Courtesy of Carl Allen, D.D.S., M.S.D.)

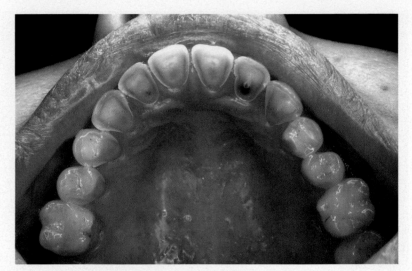

COLOR PLATE 27. Severe erosion is evident on the lingual surfaces of maxillary teeth, especially the anterior teeth. This pattern of tooth destruction is typical of someone with bulimia. Note the exposure of one pulp chamber on tooth #10. (Courtesy of Carl Allen, D.D.S., M.S.D.)

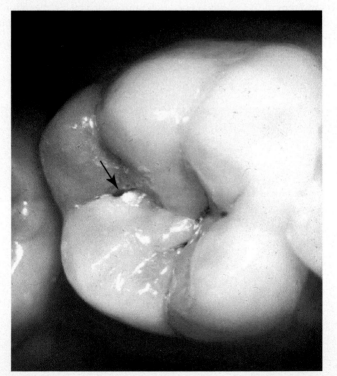

COLOR PLATE 28. Class I caries visible as stained grooves and adjacent demineralization seen as a chalky whiteness surrounding the stained pit.

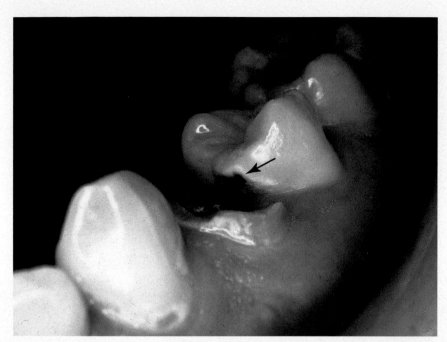

COLOR PLATE 29. Class II caries on the mesial surface of a mandibular second premolar is clearly visible because the adjacent first premolar was broken off at the cervical line. Notice the location of the lesion (just cervical to where the proximal contact had been) and the color: a darkly stained hole surrounded by discoloration and chalkiness. This lesion would have been difficult to detect clinically when the first premolar was intact. Bitewing radiographs are most useful for confirming small class II lesions.

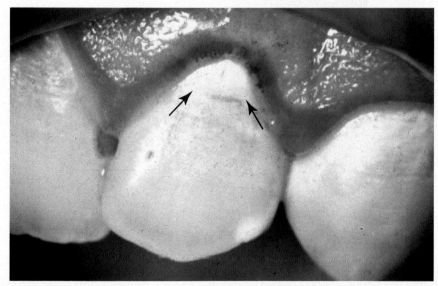

COLOR PLATE 30. Class V demineralization: a chalky white area seen in the cervical third of a maxillary lateral incisor with wear is evidence of the first stages of dental caries. If this demineralization continued and did not reverse itself (through excellent oral hygiene, diet, and use of topical fluoride), this area could develop a cavitation (hole) that would need to be restored. Also notice the inflammation of the adjacent gingiva (gingivitis), which is also caused by bacterial plaque.

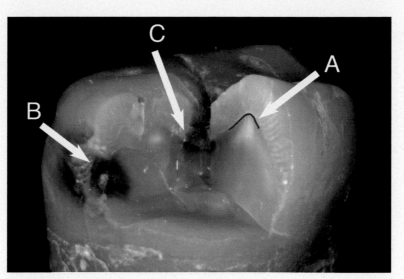

COLOR PLATE 31. Spread pattern of caries in enamel and dentin seen in a partially sectioned tooth. **A.** The red line follows the dentinoenamel junction (DEJ) of one cusp. **B.** The arrow points to caries that began on the smooth proximal surface of the tooth enamel (class II caries) showing that when it reaches dentin, it spreads out along the DEJ. **C.** The arrow points to pit and fissure (class I) caries, which began in the occlusal pit (almost hidden from view clinically) showing that once it reaches dentin, it also spreads out at the DEJ.

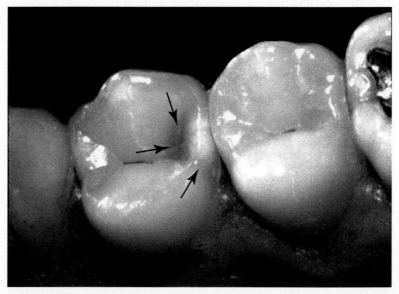

COLOR PLATE 32. Class II caries is suspected when the area of the marginal ridge over the proximal contact of this posterior tooth shows a change in translucency appearing like a brown or gray shadow beneath the surface of the enamel. Inspection of the tooth surrounding the proximal contact and evaluation of bitewing radiographs would be useful to confirm this area of decay.

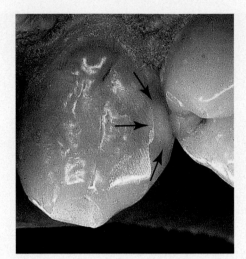

COLOR PLATE 33. Tooth #6 Lingual view. Class III caries is suspected when the area of the marginal ridge lingual to the proximal contact of this anterior tooth shows a change in translucency appearing like a brown or gray shadow beneath the surface of the enamel. Inspection of the tooth surrounding the proximal contact and transillumination or radiographs would be useful to confirm this area of decay.

There is much variation in the shapes of the roots. On **maxillary first molars,** the mesiobuccal and distobuccal roots are often well separated (Appendix 8j, buccal view) and may bend in such a way that they look like the handles on a pair of pliers, or the mesiobuccal and distobuccal roots often are curved distally. The mesiobuccal root bows out mesially in the cervical half before it curves toward the distal. This bend often places the apex of the mesiobuccal root distal to the line of the buccal groove on the crown. Both the mesiobuccal and distobuccal roots taper apically, with the apex of the mesiobuccal root usually more blunt. Characteristically, the spread of the middle third of the two buccal roots is nearly as wide as the crown.

In contrast, the **maxillary second molar** roots are often closer together, less curved, more nearly parallel, and with a longer root trunk. Often both roots bend toward the distal in their apical third. Find the two maxillary second molars in Figure 7-19 that are exceptions.

[In a Japanese study of root formation on 3370 maxillary second molars, 50% had three roots, 49% were split equally between single and double roots, and 1% had four roots. In the three-rooted second molars, 75% had complete separation of roots (no fusion). The tendency to fuse was higher in the roots of teeth extracted from females. Lingual roots were straight in half of the three-rooted teeth.[15]]

B.   TYPE TRAITS OF MAXILLARY MOLARS FROM THE LINGUAL VIEW

Refer to *Figure 7-21* for similarities and differences.

1.   RELATIVE SIZE AND TAPER OF MAXILLARY MOLARS FROM THE LINGUAL VIEW

Little or no mesial or distal surfaces of **maxillary first molar** crowns are visible from the lingual view (except in the cervical third) since these teeth may be as wide or wider on the lingual half than on the buccal half due to a relatively wide distolingual cusp. This is an EXCEPTION, along with the three-cusp mandibular second premolar, to the normal taper towards the lingual for all other posterior teeth. **Second molars** are narrower in the lingual half due to the relatively smaller or nonexistent distolingual cusp. The lingual surface of *both* types of maxillary molars is narrower in the cervical third than in the middle third, since the crown tapers to join the single palatal root (seen clearly in the maxillary molars in *Fig. 7-21*).

2.   NUMBER AND DESCRIPTION OF LINGUAL CUSPS ON A MAXILLARY MOLAR FROM THE LINGUAL VIEW

On the **maxillary first molar,** there are two well-defined cusps on the lingual surface, the larger mesiolingual cusp and the smaller, but still sizeable, distolingual cusp. The mesiolingual cusp is almost always the largest and highest cusp on any maxillary molar (Appendix 8, lingual view of the maxillary molar, and 8i for the cusp of Carabelli). Additionally, on the first molar, there is often a small fifth cusp (or groove or depression) on the lingual surface of the mesiolingual cusp 70% of the time. An actual cusp is evident over 46% of the time. [As data shows in *Table 7-7*, 46.5% of 1558 maxillary first molars had some form of Carabelli cusp (large or small), 24% had a depression in this location, and 29.5% were without any type of Carabelli formation.] This cusp is called the cusp (or tubercle) of Carabelli, after the Austrian dentist Georg von Carabelli (1787–1842), who described it. It is a nonfunctioning cusp, even when large, because it is located about 2 mm short of the mesiolingual cusp tip.

There are two types of **maxillary second molars** based on the number of cusps (four and three). Slightly less than two-thirds of maxillary second molars have *four cusps*: two buccal and *two* lingual cusps, a mesiolingual cusp (which is considerably larger) and a distolingual cusp. About one-third of maxillary second molars have only one lingual cusp. On *both* first and second molars with two lingual cusps, there is a groove extending between the mesiolingual and distolingual cusps that extends onto the lingual surface where it is called the *lingual groove*. This lingual groove may be continuous with the longitudinal depression on the lingual surface of the lingual root.

Over one-third [38% of 1396 unrestored second molars from 808 students' casts examined by Dr. Woelfel] of **maxillary second molars** have three cusps (one lingual and two buccal, called a tricuspid form) where the distolingual cusp is absent, leaving just one lingual cusp, which is large. This type has no lingual groove and no distal (cigar-shaped) fossa on the occlusal surface. See if you can find five of the maxillary second molars with one lingual cusp in Figure 7-21.

Maxillary Molars (Lingual)

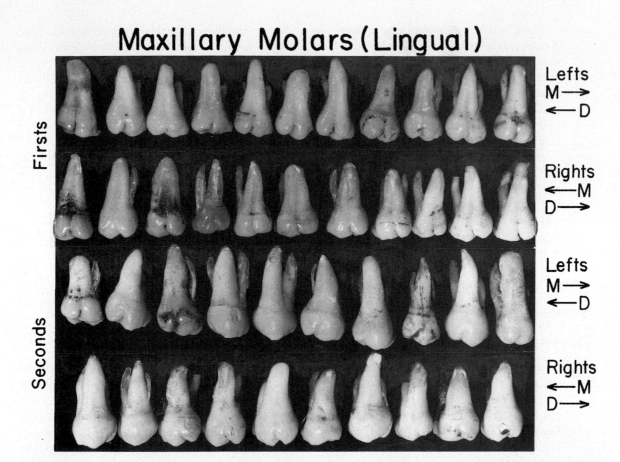

TRAITS TO DISTINGUISH MAXILLARY FIRST MOLARS FROM SECOND MOLARS: LINGUAL VIEW

MAXILLARY FIRST MOLAR	MAXILLARY SECOND MOLAR
Buccal roots spread out behind lingual root	Buccal roots less spread out
Lingual cusps nearly the same length	Distolingual cusp much shorter

TRAITS TO DISTINGUISH MAXILLARY RIGHT FROM LEFT MOLARS: LINGUAL VIEW

MAXILLARY FIRST MOLAR	MAXILLARY SECOND MOLAR
Cusp of Carabelli present on mesiolingual (ML) [46%]	Cusp of Carabelli absent
ML cusp larger than distolingual (DL)	ML even larger relative to smaller DL
The distal half of the crown is shorter than the mesial half	

FIGURE 7-21. Lingual views of maxillary molars with type traits to distinguish maxillary first from second molars and to help determine rights from lefts.

Table 7-7	FREQUENCY OF OCCURRENCE AND TYPE OF CARABELLI CUSP FORMATION ON 1558 MAXILLARY FIRST MOLARS*		
Large Carabelli cusp	19%		
Small Carabelli cusp	27.5%		70.5% some type of Carabelli formation
Slight depression (groove)	24%		
Nothing	29.5%		
Same type on right and left	76%		
Different on each side			
(835 comparisons on casts)	24%		

* Observations from dental stone casts of Ohio dental hygienists made by Dr. Woelfel and his students, 1971–1983.

3. MAXILLARY MOLAR ROOTS FROM THE LINGUAL VIEW

On the **maxillary first molar,** the longest lingual root [averaging 13.7 mm on 308 maxillary first molars] is the third longest root on any maxillary tooth, after the maxillary canine and second premolar roots. The lingual root is not curved when seen from the lingual view, but it does taper apically to a blunt or rounded apex. There is usually a longitudinal depression on the *lingual* side of the lingual root of the first molar (seen in many lingual roots of maxillary first molars in Fig. 7-21). The characteristically wide mesiodistal spread of the curved buccal roots on the first molar is visible from this view.

The lingual root on the **maxillary second molar** is as long as, and resembles, the lingual root of the first molar. However, the buccal roots in the background bend somewhat more distally and are closer together and more parallel than on first molars.

C. TYPE TRAITS OF FIRST AND SECOND MAXILLARY MOLARS FROM THE PROXIMAL VIEWS

Refer to *Figure 7-22* for similarities and differences of maxillary molars from the proximal views.

1. MAXILLARY MOLAR CUSPS FROM THE PROXIMAL VIEWS

Like the crowns of a mandibular molar, **maxillary first molar** crowns appear short occlusocervically and broad faciolingually from the *proximal* view. Recall that the cusps of the first molar, in the usual order of their length occlusocervically, longest to shortest, are mesiolingual, mesiobuccal, distobuccal, and distolingual (if present), followed by the functionless fifth cusp (cusp of Carabelli) when present. Since the mesial two cusps are longer than the distal, four cusps are visible from the *distal* **view:** the distobuccal cusp and smallest distolingual cusp in the foreground, and the cusp tips of the mesiobuccal and largest mesiolingual cusp behind them. When present on first molars, the Carabelli cusp can also usually be seen on the lingual surface from this view.

In contrast, only two (or three) cusps are seen from the *mesial* **view:** the mesiobuccal cusp, the long and large mesiolingual cusp, and, if present, the cusp of Carabelli (2–3 mm cervical to the mesiolingual cusp tip) (Fig. 7-22 drawing). The distobuccal and distolingual cusps are shorter and usually not seen when the tooth is examined from this side. Observe the number of cusps that are visible when comparing the mesial with distal views of maxillary first and second molars seen in Figure 7-22.

From the mesial and distal views, the crown of the **maxillary second molar** looks much like that of the first molar, except that there is no fifth cusp (*Fig. 7-22*). Also, the *distolingual* cusp is absent on more than one-third of these teeth.

2. HEIGHT OF CONTOUR FOR MAXILLARY MOLARS FROM THE PROXIMAL VIEWS (SAME FOR ALL POSTERIOR TEETH)

As on all other posterior teeth, the height of contour of the *buccal* side of *both* first and second maxillary molar crowns is in the cervical third, usually close to the cervical line. The height of contour of

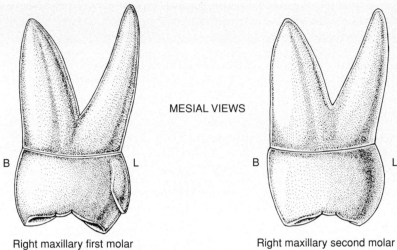

MESIAL VIEWS

Right maxillary first molar   Right maxillary second molar

Maxillary Molars (Proximal)

Lefts   Rights

Firsts

Seconds

DISTAL SURFACES   MESIAL SURFACES

← Facia l   Lingual →

TRAITS TO DISTINGUISH MAXILLARY FIRST MOLARS FROM SECOND MOLARS: PROXIMAL VIEWS

MAXILLARY FIRST MOLAR	MAXILLARY SECOND MOLAR
More mesial (M) marginal ridge tubercles [86%]	Fewer M marginal ridge tubercles [38%]
Parallelogram shape less twisted	Parallelogram shape more twisted
Some root flare beyond crown	Less root flare
Cusp of Carabelli on mesiolingual cusp [46%]	No cusp of Carabelli

TRAITS TO DISTINGUISH MAXILLARY RIGHT FROM LEFT MOLARS: PROXIMAL VIEWS

MAXILLARY FIRST MOLAR	MAXILLARY SECOND MOLAR
Cusp of Carabelli on mesiolingual cusp [46%]	Small or absent distolingual cusp

The distal marginal ridge is located more cervically than the mesial marginal ridge
The distobuccal root is narrow so wider mesiobuccal root is visible from distal view

FIGURE 7-22. Proximal views of maxillary molars with type traits to distinguish maxillary first from second molars and to help determine rights from lefts.

the *lingual* side of the crown is more occlusal, in or near the middle third of the crown. On teeth in which the fifth cusp is large, the lingual crest of curvature is located even more occlusally (*Fig. 7-23*).

3. TAPER TOWARD DISTAL OF MAXILLARY MOLARS FROM THE DISTAL VIEW

On *both* maxillary first and second molars, both the buccal surface and the lingual surface of the crown can be seen because the crown tapers toward the distal and is narrower buccolingually on the distal side than on the mesial side (seen on most distal views in *Fig. 7-22*).

4. MARGINAL RIDGES OF MAXILLARY MOLARS FROM THE PROXIMAL VIEWS

On *both* first and second maxillary molars, the concave *mesial* marginal ridge connects the mesiobuccal cusp and the mesiolingual cusp. It is longer buccolingually and located more occlusally than the distal marginal ridge. Consequently, little of the occlusal surface is visible from the mesial view.

Because the *distal* marginal ridge of these maxillary molars is both short and concave and more cervically positioned than the mesial marginal ridge, more of the occlusal surface (including the triangular ridges) can be seen from the distal view. (Compare mesial and distal views in *Fig. 7-22*.) This marginal ridge height difference is very helpful in determining right from left sides.

In general, **marginal ridge grooves** are more common on the mesial marginal ridge than on the distal, and are more common on first molars than on seconds. [On **first** molars: 78% of 69 teeth had *mesial* marginal grooves, but only 50% of 60 had *distal* marginal grooves; on **second** molars, 67% of 75 teeth had *mesial* marginal grooves, but only 38% of 79 teeth had *distal* marginal ridge grooves.]

On the unworn marginal ridges of the maxillary molars, there may be one or more projections of enamel called **tubercles.** Like marginal ridge grooves, they are more common on mesial marginal ridges than on the distal and more common on first molars than on seconds. [On **first** molars: 86% of 64 teeth had mesial ridge tubercles, but only 18% had distal ridge tubercles; on **second** molars: 38% of 79 teeth had mesial marginal ridge tubercles, but only 9% of 79 teeth had distal ridge tubercles.] These tubercles are seen most clearly on the mesial marginal ridges of the maxillary first and second molars in *Figure 7-24*.

5. CERVICAL LINES OF MAXILLARY MOLARS FROM THE PROXIMAL VIEWS

On *both* types of maxillary molars, the *mesial* cervical line has a slight occlusal curvature [averaging only 0.7 mm on 308 first molars and 0.6 mm on second molars]. There is less curvature of the cervi-

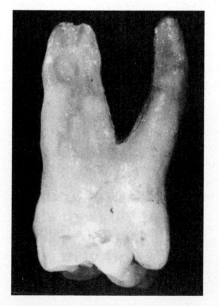

FIGURE 7-23. Maxillary right first molar, mesial view, with an unusually **large cusp of Carabelli** and a lingual height of contour positioned quite occlusally. Also, note that the wide mesiobuccal root hides the narrower distobuccal root.

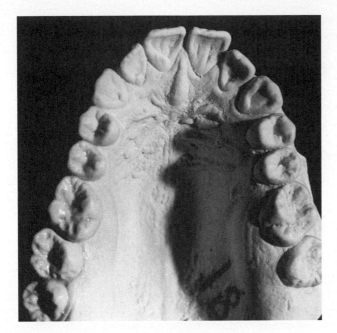

FIGURE 7-24. Dental stone casts of the maxillary dentition demonstrating **decreasing size from first to third molars.** Both *second* molars are *three-cusp types* with only one lingual cusp (tricuspid form). Also note the **tubercles** on the mesial marginal ridges of the first molars. Tooth #16 is missing.

cal line on the *distal* surface than on the mesial surface, but the difference is hardly discernible, since this cementoenamel junction is practically flat buccolingually.

6. ROOTS OF MAXILLARY MOLARS FROM THE PROXIMAL VIEWS

On **maxillary first molars** from the *mesial* view, two roots can be seen: the palatal root and the mesiobuccal root (broad buccolingually) (Appendix 8, mesial views). The breadth of the mesiobuccal root is two-thirds of the faciolingual dimension, so it obscures the third distobuccal root. The apex of this mesiobuccal root is in line with the tip of the mesiobuccal cusp, whereas the convex buccal surface of this root often extends a little buccal to the crown. Observe this characteristic of maxillary first molars from the mesial view in Figure 7-22. The lingual outline of the mesiobuccal root is often more convex and, in the apical third, curves sharply facially toward the apex. The mesial surface of the mesiobuccal root has a longitudinal depression (and although they cannot be seen, there are often *two* root canals in this root).

The lingual root is the longest of the three roots, is bent somewhat like a "banana," and on maxillary first molars extends conspicuously beyond the crown lingually. This feature alone should help you determine maxillary first from second molars. Compare the differences in Figure 7-22. The lingual root tapers apically and is usually curved buccolingually, being concave on its buccal surface. (It has only *one* root canal.)

From the *distal* view of the **maxillary first molar,** the distobuccal root is shorter and more narrow buccolingually than the mesiobuccal root (evident on most distal views in *Fig. 2-22*). Therefore, the mesiobuccal root is visible behind the narrower distobuccal root. The distobuccal root does not extend as far buccally, and its apex is usually more pointed than the mesiobuccal root. The distal surface of the distobuccal root is convex, without a longitudinal depression (and it has only *one* root canal). Other authors describe a slight **concavity on the distal surface of the root trunk** located between the distobuccal root and the cervical line.[10, 6]

On the **maxillary second molars,** the roots are much *less* spread apart than the roots of the first molar (recall Appendix 8j). The banana-shaped lingual root is straighter than on first molars and is usually confined within the crown width from the proximal view, in contrast to first molars (Fig. 7-22). The mesiobuccal root of the maxillary second molar only rarely extends buccally beyond the buccal surface of the crown. From the *distal* view of the maxillary second molar, the mesiobuccal root, which

| Table 7-8 | SUMMARY: PRESENCE AND RELATIVE DEPTH OF LONGITUDINAL ROOT DEPRESSIONS ("ROOT GROOVES") | |

	TOOTH	MESIAL ROOT DEPRESSION?	DISTAL ROOT DEPRESSION?
MAXILLARY TEETH	Maxillary central incisor	No (or slight or flat)	No (convex)
	Maxillary lateral incisor	Yes (sometimes no)	No (convex)
	Maxillary canine	Yes	Yes (deeper)
	Maxillary 1st premolar	Yes (deeper = **UNIQUE,** extends	Yes onto mesial of crown)
	Maxillary 2nd premolar	Yes	Yes (deeper)
	Maxillary 1st and 2nd molars	**Mesiobuccal root:** Yes	Variable
		Distobuccal root: variable	No (convex) but root trunk has concavity between cervical line and distobuccal root[10,27]
		Lingual root: lingual surface depression	
MANDIBULAR TEETH	Mandibular central incisor	Yes	Yes (deeper)
	Mandibular lateral incisor	Yes	Yes (deeper)
	Mandibular canine	Yes	Yes (deeper)
	Mandibular 1st premolar	Yes (or no: about 50%)	Yes (deeper)
	Mandibular 2nd premolar	No (unlikely)	Yes (deeper)
	Mandibular 1st and 2nd molars	**Mesial root:** YES	Yes (deeper)
		Distal root: variable, but deeper	Variable

General Learning Guidelines:
1. **Maxillary incisors** are less likely to have root depressions.
2. **All canines and premolars** (EXCEPT maxillary first premolars) **and mandibular incisors** are likely to have deeper distal surface root depressions.

is wider and longer than the distobuccal root, can be seen behind the distobuccal root. The apex of the lingual root of the second molar is often in line with the tip of the distolingual cusp.

A summary of the presence and relative depth of root depressions for all teeth is presented in *Table 7-8*.

D. TYPE TRAITS OF FIRST AND SECOND MAXILLARY MOLARS FROM THE OCCLUSAL VIEW

Refer to *Figure 7-25* for similarities and differences. To follow the description of traits from the occlusal view, the tooth should be held in such a position that the observer is looking exactly perpendicular to the plane of the occlusal surface. Because of the spread of the first molar roots, some of each of the three roots (particularly the lingual root) may be visible when the tooth is in this position (characteristic of **first** molars as seen in *Fig. 7-26*). In studying these teeth, it must be remembered that the morphology is variable.

1. OUTLINE OF FIRST MOLAR FROM OCCLUSAL VIEW

On the **maxillary first molar,** the outline of the occlusal surface is not quite square, but it gives the general impression of squareness when compared to other teeth. Actually, it is more like a parallelogram, with two acute (sharper) and two obtuse (blunter) angles (Appendix 8k). The acute angles are the mesiobuccal and distolingual. The parallelogram is larger buccolingually than mesiodistally (arch trait for the maxillary molars). The oblique ridge traverses diagonally across the tooth between the obtuse outline angles, that is, from mesiolingual to distobuccal (Appendix 8d). Also, on many maxillary *first*

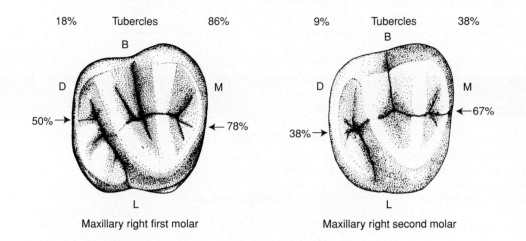

18% Tubercles 86%   9% Tubercles 38%

50% →   ← 78%   38% →   ← 67%

Maxillary right first molar   Maxillary right second molar

Maxillary First Molars (Occlusal)

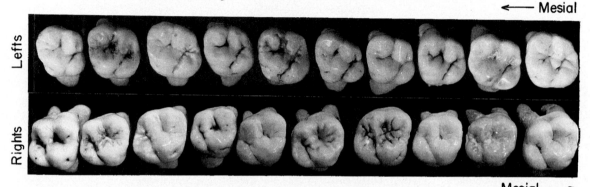

← Mesial

Lefts

Rights

Mesial →

Maxillary Second Molars

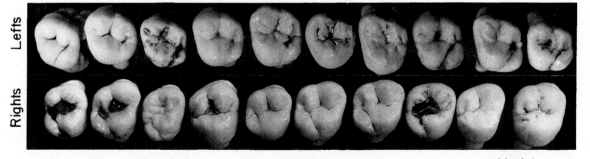

← Mesial

Lefts

Rights

Mesial →

TRAITS TO DISTINGUISH MAXILLARY FIRST MOLARS FROM SECOND MOLARS: OCCUSAL VIEW

MAXILLARY FIRST MOLAR	MAXILLARY SECOND MOLAR
Distolingual cusp slightly smaller than mesiolingual cusp	Distolingual cusp much smaller than mesiolingual or absent
Crowns often wider on lingual half	Crowns narrower on lingual half
Crown outline nearly square	Crown outline more twisted
Crown larger (in same mouth)	Crowns smaller (in same mouth)
More prominent oblique ridge	Smaller oblique ridge
Fewer supplemental grooves	More supplemental grooves (wrinkled)
Less prominent mesiobuccal (MB) cervical ridge	More prominent MB cervical ridge

FIGURE 7-25. Occlusal views of maxillary molars with type traits to distinguish maxillary first from second molars and traits to distinguish rights from lefts. Percentages in drawings indicate the frequency of marginal ridge tubercles and marginal ridge grooves observed by Dr. Woelfel.

TRAITS TO DISTINGUISH MAXILLARY RIGHT FROM LEFT MOLARS: OCCLUSAL VIEW

MAXILLARY FIRST MOLAR	MAXILLARY SECOND MOLAR
Cusp of Carabelli is on mesiolingual (ML) cusp [46%]	Distolingual cusp is smaller than ML

Mesiobuccal and distolingual angles of crown are more acute
Distolingual cusp is smaller than mesiolingual cusp (or absent)
A mesiobuccal cervical ridge is visible
The distal half of the crown is smaller faciolingually
Oblique ridge goes from largest mesiolingual diagonally to distobuccal cusp

FIGURE 7-25. *(continued).*

molars, the mesiodistal dimension of the lingual half of the crown is slightly wider mesiodistally than the buccal half. Try to locate one or two maxillary first molars in Figure 7-25 that are not wider on the lingual than on the buccal sides. They are a minority.

The **maxillary second molar** crown is also wider buccolingually than mesiodistally, but tapers more from buccal to lingual due to the smaller or absent distolingual cusp. There is much variation in the morphology of *maxillary second molars,* particularly in the size of the distolingual cusp. When the distolingual cusp is absent (about one-third of the time), the tooth has only three cusps (six maxillary second molars in *Fig. 7-25* have no distolingual cusps). The three-cusp type is somewhat triangular or heart-shaped, the blunt apex of the triangle being the lingual cusp.

The more common *four-cusp* type of **maxillary second molars** is less square in appearance than the first molar. Even when the distolingual cusp is present, it is not very large. Therefore, second maxillary molars taper to the lingual and so are noticeably narrower mesiodistally on the lingual half than are first molars (Appendix 8h). The fact that the crown of the second molar tapers (gets narrower) from buccal to lingual and from mesial to distal is helpful in differentiating rights from lefts. The parallelogram shape of second molars is twisted more than on first, with the more acute angle at the mesiobuccal corner due in part to a prominent *mesial (or mesiobuccal) cervical ridge* on second molars, visible from this view (all 20 second molars in *Fig. 7-25*). These traits are helpful in differentiating rights from lefts and are vividly apparent on all maxillary second molars in Figure 7-25.

See *Figure 7-27* for a summary of the geometric outlines for all molars.

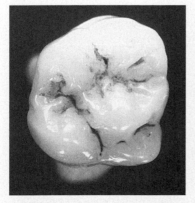 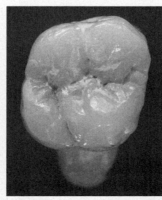

FIGURE 7-26. Two maxillary right first molars comparing the difference in the mesiolingual cusp: one has a very large **cusp of Carabelli,** but the other has a slight depression in the same location. Also, notice the prominent **lingual root** showing from this view due to the large spread of roots on the maxillary first molars.

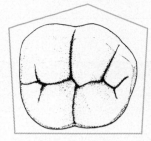

Right mandibular first molar

Pentagon outline:
    Occlusal views of mandibular
    first molar

Right mandibular second molar

Rectangular (tapered) outline:
    Mandibular second molars
"+" shaped groove pattern:
    Mandibular second molars

Maxillary right second molar

Rhomboid-shaped outline:
    Occlusal view of maxillary
    molars; acute angles are on
    mesiobuccal and distolingual
    corners

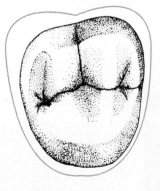

Maxillary right second molar
(Three-cusp type)

Heart-shaped outline:
    Occlusal view of three-cusped
    type maxillary molars

FIGURE 7-27. Geometric outlines of the occlusal surfaces of molars, top to bottom. Mandibular first molars have a **pentagon** outline. Mandibular second molars have a **trapezoid (tapered rectangular)** outline with a **"+"-shaped groove** pattern. Maxillary molars (second shown here) have a **rhomboid or parallelogram** outline with the mesiobuccal and distolingual "corners" forming acute angles. Maxillary molars, three-cusp type, have a **heart-shape** (or somewhat **triangular**) outline.

LEARNING EXERCISE

Match the tooth with the correct geometric shape for its occlusal outline.

 a. Trapezoid (tapered rectangle)
 b. Parallelogram (rhomboid)
 c. Heart shape or triangular
 d. Pentagon

1. Maxillary first molar

2. Maxillary second molar (four-cusp type)

3. Maxillary second molar (three-cusp type)

4. Mandibular first molar

5. Mandibular second molar

ANSWERS: 1-b, 2-b, 3-c, 4-d, 5-a

2. NUMBER AND SIZE OF CUSPS ON MAXILLARY MOLARS FROM THE OCCLUSAL VIEW

Most *first* maxillary molars usually have four larger cusps plus the fifth cusp (cusp of Carabelli), and most *second* molars have four larger cusps (without a cusp of Carabelli) *or* have three cusps (when the distolingual cusp is absent).

Use *Figure 7-28* when comparing the relative size of major cusps for maxillary first and second molars. The cusp size on the *four-cusp* type of *both* maxillary first and second molars are, from largest to smallest, the conspicuous mesiolingual [largest 95% of 1469 first molars on stone casts], mesiobuccal, distobuccal, and distolingual [smallest 72% of the time]. The **first molar** has the smallest fifth (functionless) cusp of Carabelli (or a depression) [present about 70% of the time], whereas the second molar does not have this cusp (see an exception in *Fig. 7-29*.) On **second molars,** there is usually a greater difference in the size of the buccal cusps, with the mesiobuccal noticeably larger (*Fig. 7-28*), and the distolingual cusp either smallest or not present. The triangular shape formed by the three more prominent cusps of a maxillary molar (namely, the mesiolingual, mesiobuccal, and distobuccal cusps) are collectively known as the maxillary molar **primary cusp triangle**.

The cusp of Carabelli varies greatly in shape and size. It may be a conspicuous, well-formed cusp, or, at the other extreme, it may be barely discernible or absent, or there may even be a depression in this location (both extremes are seen in *Fig. 7-26*). Some of the variations in shape and size are seen in the upper two rows of Figure 7-25. The cusp of Carabelli is *rarely* found on **maxillary second mo-**

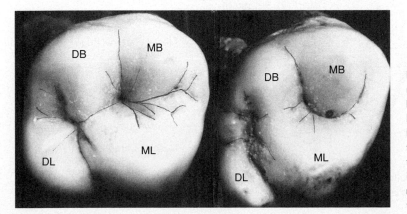

FIGURE 7-28. Left: maxillary right *first* molar (without cusp of Carabelli). **Right:** maxillary right *second* molar. Note how the *first* molar is much wider on the lingual half with a relatively large distolingual cusp, whereas the *second* molar tapers more toward the lingual surface, is twisted slightly, and has more **acute mesiobuccal and distolingual angles** than the first molar.

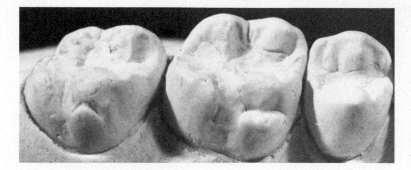

FIGURE 7-29. Unusual cusp of Carabelli: maxillary first and second molars, each with a Carabelli cusp. It is *unusual* to have this Carabelli cusp on the second molar. (Courtesy of Dr. Jeff Warner.)

lars or third maxillary molars. [A number of studies have been done concerning the occurrence and size of the cusp of Carbelli.[16-20] One investigator reports that it is extremely rare in the East Greenland Eskimo. In European people, it is usually present. The Carabelli trait was absent on 35.4% of the teeth in 489 Hindu children.[21] The groove form was more common (35%) than tubercles (26%) on the first molars.[21]]

3. RIDGES OF MAXILLARY MOLARS FROM THE OCCLUSAL VIEW

On the four-cusp type **maxillary first molar,** each of the four major cusps has at least one definite triangular ridge. The largest mesiolingual cusp usually has a *second* triangular ridge mesial to the one that forms the oblique ridge *(Fig. 7-30).* The distal of the two triangular ridges of the mesiolingual cusp aligns with the triangular ridge of the distobuccal cusp to form a diagonal ridge called the *oblique ridge* (an arch trait of most molars in the maxillae) *(Fig. 7-30).* The second, more mesial triangular ridge of the mesiolingual cusp aligns with the triangular ridge of the mesiobuccal cusp to form a *transverse ridge.* The groove between the two triangular ridges on the mesiolingual cusp is called the Stuart groove (named after the late Dr. Charles E. Stuart). Two texts refer to the more distal triangular ridge of the mesiolingual cusp by another name: the distal cusp ridge of the mesiolingual cusp. Subsequently, the oblique ridge is formed by the triangular ridge of the distobuccal cusp and the distal cusp ridge of the mesiolingual cusp.[27, 28]

The oblique ridge is smaller on second molars than on first molars.[22]

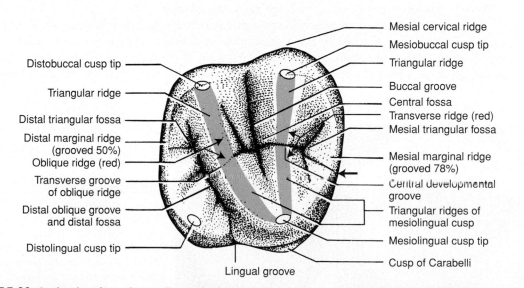

Distobuccal cusp tip

Triangular ridge

Distal triangular fossa

Distal marginal ridge (grooved 50%)

Oblique ridge (red)

Transverse groove of oblique ridge

Distal oblique groove and distal fossa

Distolingual cusp tip

Lingual groove

Mesial cervical ridge

Mesiobuccal cusp tip

Triangular ridge

Buccal groove

Central fossa

Transverse ridge (red)

Mesial triangular fossa

Mesial marginal ridge (grooved 78%)

Central developmental groove

Triangular ridges of mesiolingual cusp

Mesiolingual cusp tip

Cusp of Carabelli

FIGURE 7-30. Occlusal surface of a maxillary right *first* molar (including cusp of Carabelli) with all of the major landmarks named. The landmarks are the same for maxillary four-cusp type maxillary *second* molars, except seconds do not

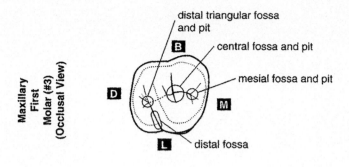

Maxillary
First
Molar (#3)
(Occlusal View)

distal triangular fossa
and pit

B

central fossa and pit

D

mesial fossa and pit

M

L   distal fossa

FIGURE 7-31. Maxillary first molar, occlusal view, showing the relative size and location of the four **fossae.**

4. FOSSAE OF MAXILLARY MOLARS FROM THE OCCLUSAL VIEW

On *four-cusp* type maxillary molars, there are *four* fossae on the occlusal surface *(Fig. 7-31)*. The largest *central* fossa is near the center of the occlusal surface. It is bounded distally by the elevation of the oblique ridge, mesially by the mesial transverse ridge, and buccally by the buccal cusp ridges. The second largest *distal* fossa is an elongated fossa (cigar shaped) extending between the mesiolingual and the distolingual cusps. A smaller, *mesial* triangular fossa is just within the mesial marginal ridge. The fourth minute, *distal triangular fossa* is just mesial to the distal marginal ridge.

On *three-cusp type* maxillary (second) molars, when the distolingual cusp is missing, the distal (cigar-shaped) fossa is also missing and there are only three fossae remaining (one large central and two very small triangular ones).

5. GROOVES ON MAXILLARY MOLARS

Refer to Figure 7-30 while studying these grooves. On the *four-cusp type* of **maxillary first or second** molar, the prominent oblique ridge plays an important role in defining developmental grooves. This type of maxillary molar has five major grooves: the central, buccal, distal oblique, lingual, and sometimes the transverse groove of the oblique ridge. Unlike the mandibular molar where the central groove extends from the mesial fossa to the distal fossa, the *central* groove of the maxillary molar extends from the mesial fossa over the mesial transverse ridge and ends in the central fossa.

Distal to the central groove is the prominent oblique ridge, which usually has no distinct groove crossing it, but when it does, the groove appears to be a continuation of the central groove and is called the *transverse groove of the oblique ridge.* (One author calls these two grooves the mesial and distal groove, respectively, [10] while another combines these grooves and calls them the central groove.[26]) Notice that the groove extending onto the lingual surface on a maxillary molar begins in the distal fossa (and parallels the oblique ridge) compared to the lingual groove on a mandibular molar, which begins in the central fossa (and is more or less at right angles to the central groove).

Distal to the oblique ridge, grooves parallel the direction of the oblique ridge and extend onto the lingual surface of the crown. The *distal oblique groove* extends lingually from the distal triangular fossa between the distolingual cusp and the mesiolingual cusp (along the distal fossa), and continues onto the lingual surface as the *lingual* groove. (One author calls these two grooves combined the distolingual groove.[10]) The *buccal* groove extends buccally from the central fossa and may continue onto the buccal surface of the crown *(Fig. 7-30)*. The *fifth cusp groove* separates the fifth cusp (Carabelli) from the mesiolingual cusp. As on many premolars and mandibular molars, maxillary molars may have two short grooves that extend from the mesial and distal pits toward the corners (facial and lingual line angles) of the tooth. The short grooves off of the mesial pit are called the mesiobuccal and mesiolingual fossa grooves (or sometimes triangular grooves), and the short grooves off of the distal pit are called the distobuccal and distolingual fossa grooves (or sometimes triangular grooves). The groove pattern on **maxillary second molars** may have more supplemental grooves and pits than on the first molar.[22]

On the *three-cusp type* of **second molar,** the distolingual cusp, the oblique ridge, and the cigar-shaped distal fossa are absent, so the grooves normally found within that fossa are also missing: namely, the distal oblique and lingual grooves.

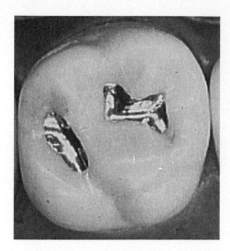

FIGURE 7-32. Occlusal surface of a maxillary right *first* molar with two amalgam restorations prepared separately to avoid crossing over the pronounced oblique ridge that has no fissured groove crossing over it.

All of these grooves are often fissured, so they can become the sites of dental decay. However, since the transverse groove of the oblique ridge is usually *not* fissured, decay on the occlusal surfaces of maxillary molars normally occurs mesially and distally to the oblique ridge. The result is two *separate* occlusal fillings (restorations) similar to two occlusal fillings found on mandibular first premolars where the prominent transverse ridge separates mesial and distal pit decay. An example of a two-part occlusal filling on a maxillary molar is seen in *Figure 7-32*.

6. PROXIMAL CONTACTS OF MAXILLARY MOLARS FROM THE OCCLUSAL VIEW

Mesial and distal contacts of maxillary molars are all slightly to the buccal of the center of the tooth, but are near the center buccolingually. The mesial contact is more buccal than the distal contact on maxillary molars, and the distal contact on maxillary first molars is nearly centered buccolingually.

LEARNING EXERCISE

1. Examine the teeth of your associates and notice the variation in the cusp of Carabelli. This little cusp has intrigued many people. It may be somewhat prominent and pointed, small and blunt, or absent, or you may even see a slight depression in that part of the mesiolingual cusp where the cusp of Carabelli would be found.
2. Name each of the 17 ridges in *Figure 7-33*.

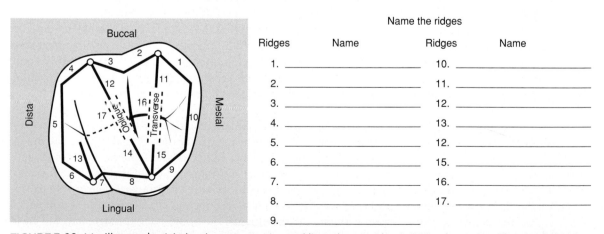

FIGURE 7-33. Maxillary molar (circles denote cusp tips and lines denote ridges). Write the names of each of the 17 ridges next to the number corresponding to its location. Answers are on the next page.

LEARNING QUESTIONS

Maxillary Molars

Circle the correct answer(s) that apply. More than one answer may be correct.

1. Which three grooves radiate out from the central fossa in a maxillary first molar?
   a. central
   b. mesial
   c. transverse groove of oblique ridge (when present)
   d. buccal
   e. lingual

2. Which cusp has two triangular ridges on the maxillary first molar?
   a. mesiobuccal
   b. mesiolingual
   c. distobuccal
   d. distolingual
   e. cusp of Carabelli

3. Which cusp is the largest and longest on a maxillary second molar?
   a. mesiobuccal
   b. mesiolingual
   c. distobuccal
   d. distolingual
   e. cusp of Carabelli

4. Which cusp is most likely to be absent on a maxillary second (or third) molar?
   a. mesiobuccal
   b. mesiolingual
   c. distobuccal
   d. distolingual
   e. distal

5. When the cusp is absent in question 4 above, which groove(s) would not be present?
   a. central
   b. buccal
   c. distal oblique
   d. lingual

6. Of the four fossae on a maxillary first molar, which is the largest?
   a. mesial triangular
   b. distal triangular
   c. central
   d. distal

7. From which view are only two roots visible on a maxillary first molar?
   a. mesial
   b. distal
   c. buccal
   d. lingual

8. Which grooves are likely to radiate out of the mesial triangular fossa on the maxillary first molar?
   a. mesiobuccal fossa groove
   b. mesiolingual fossa groove
   c. mesial marginal ridge groove (when present)
   d. central
   e. buccal

9. Which two cusps have the ridges that make up or join to form the oblique ridge on a maxillary molar?
   a. mesiobuccal
   b. distobuccal
   c. mesiolingual
   d. distolingual
   e. cusp of Carabelli

10. Which two cusps have the triangular ridges that make up or join to form a transverse ridge on most maxillary molars?
   a. mesiobuccal
   b. distobuccal
   c. mesiolingual
   d. distolingual
   e. cusp of Carabelli

11. List in sequential order the largest to smallest cusp area on the maxillary first molar (occlusal view).

ANSWERS: 1-a, c, d; 2-b; 3-b; 4-d; 5-c, d; 6-c; 7-a; 8-a, b, c, d; 9-b, c; 10-a, c; 11-mesiolingual, mesiobuccal, distobuccal, distolingual, cusp of Carabelli (if even present).

SECTION IV MAXILLARY AND MANDIBULAR THIRD MOLAR TYPE TRAITS

OBJECTIVES

After studying this section, the reader should be able to perform the following:
• List the type traits that are unique to all third molars that can be used to distinguish them from first or second molars.

- From a selection of all types of molars, select the mandibular and maxillary third molars and assign each a Universal number.
- In mouths (or casts) of mandibular and maxillary arches with only one or two molars per quadrant, identify which molars are present and which are absent based on crown anatomy and position in the arch. (Remember that second or third molars can drift forward and take up the arch position normally occupied by lost first or second molars, respectively, so arch position should not be the only way to confirm which molars are present.)

A. TYPE TRAITS OF ALL THIRD MOLARS (DIFFERENT FROM FIRST AND SECOND MOLARS)

The mesial surfaces of third molars contact the distal surfaces of second molars, but the distal surfaces of third molars are *not* in proximal contact with any tooth. The *maxillary* third molars occlude with only the mandibular third molars; all other teeth have the potential for occluding with two teeth EXCEPT mandibular central incisors.

Third molars, also known by many as wisdom teeth, have gotten a bad reputation. Due to the posterior location of third molars in the mouth making them more difficult to keep clean and their wrinkled, fissured occlusal surface, these teeth may be more prone to developing decay than other teeth. Further, mandibular third molars often erupt so far distally that they emerge near the vertical mandibular ramus with compromised gingival health, so dentists often suggest that these teeth be removed to prevent future problems. Inflammation of the tissue around these teeth (called pericoronitis) can be a cause of acute pain and spread of infection, resulting in the need for gingival surgery or extraction. This infection is even more likely to occur if the flap of tissue overlying the erupting third molar, called an operculum, becomes irritated as seen in Color Plate #9. However, it is *not* true that third molars have soft enamel, are useless, or should be routinely extracted. If the dental arches are of sufficient length to permit full eruption of third molars and a person's oral hygiene is good, third molars can function for a lifetime without problems. Also, healthy third molars can serve as the posterior attachment (abutment) when replacing lost or missing first or second molars.

Some oral surgeons recommend that when third molars have to be extracted, they be removed at an early age (under 25 years old) to facilitate an easier, less traumatic removal, and a quicker, more comfortable recovery period than when they are extracted later in life.[25] Since many third molars are extracted before the roots are completely formed, you can easily look into the open ends of the root canals at the apices of the roots.

Many third molars never form or develop. [Among 710 Ohio State University dental hygiene students, there were 185 *maxillary* third molars and 198 *mandibular* third molars congenitally absent. Many students were missing more than one third molar, so the percentage of the population missing one or more third molars might be close to 20%.]

Although third molars may resemble first *or* second molars, they all have certain type traits in common that set them apart from the first and second molars in their arches. These third molar traits include the following:

1. Normally, third molars are smaller than first or second molars in the same mouth (*Fig. 7-34*). A common exception is the *five-cusp* third molar, which may have a crown somewhat larger and more bulbous than the second molar.
2. Third molar crowns are bulbous (with fatter contours).
3. Occlusal surfaces of third molars are relatively small compared to first and seconds (that is, the buccal cusp tips are closer to the lingual cusp tips than on first and second molars).
4. Occlusal surfaces of third molars are quite *wrinkled* due to numerous supplemental grooves and ridges (*Fig. 7-35*).
5. A third molar crown may have a number of traits in common with the first *or* second molar within its arch.
6. Third molar roots are short (with small root-to-crown ratio) compared to first and second molars in the same mouth (*Fig. 7-36*).
7. Roots are frequently fused together, subsequently with long root trunks (*Fig. 7-36*).
8. Roots are pointed and frequently curve distally in the apical third.

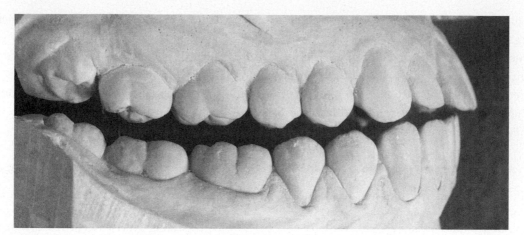

FIGURE 7-34. Dental stone casts of maxillary and mandibular teeth (facial view) showing the decrease in size of molars from first to third molar that is *typical* in most people. (Model courtesy of Ms. Colleen Seto.)

B.   SIZE AND SHAPE OF THIRD MOLARS

Maxillary **third** molars vary considerably in size, but they are usually the *shortest* of the permanent teeth and are therefore smaller than the first or second molar. The roots of maxillary third molars are ordinarily shorter [by 2.0 mm, average of 920 teeth], and the root trunks are proportionally longer than the root trunks of the first and second molars.

Similarly, **mandibular third molars** are usually the shortest of the mandibular teeth [averaging 18.2 mm] although these teeth also vary considerably in size and can be either large or small.

C.   SIMILARITIES AND DIFFERENCES OF THIRD MOLAR CROWNS COMPARED WITH FIRST AND SECOND MOLARS IN THE SAME ARCH

Maxillary **third molars** have the *greatest* morphologic variance of all teeth. The great amount of variation in *maxillary third molars* also makes a general description difficult. The crown may have only one cusp or as many as eight,[24] but it also may resemble a small maxillary first molar (complete with cusp of Carabelli)

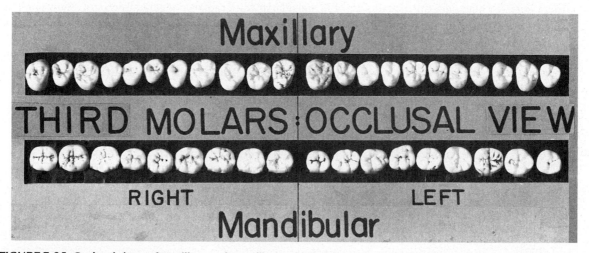

FIGURE 7-35. Occlusal views of maxillary and mandibular third molars. The lingual surfaces of the maxillary teeth face down, and those of the mandibular teeth face up. All mesial surfaces face the centerline. Observe the **wrinkled** occlusal designs in both and try to recognize the similarities to first and second molars in each arch. For example, most of the maxillary third molars are largest faciolingually in contrast to the mandibular third molars, whose greater dimension is mesiodistally.

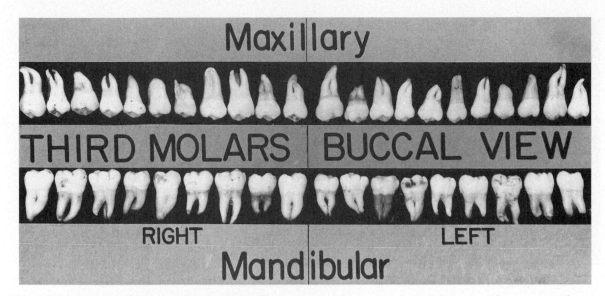

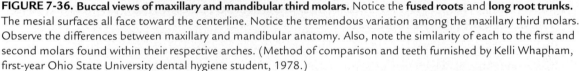

FIGURE 7-36. Buccal views of maxillary and mandibular third molars. Notice the **fused roots** and **long root trunks.** The mesial surfaces all face toward the centerline. Notice the tremendous variation among the maxillary third molars. Observe the differences between maxillary and mandibular anatomy. Also, note the similarity of each to the first and second molars found within their respective arches. (Method of comparison and teeth furnished by Kelli Whapham, first-year Ohio State University dental hygiene student, 1978.)

or second molar (without the cusp of Carabelli, and perhaps without the distolingual cusp). As with the mandibular third molar, the *maxillary third molar* can be distinguished from the first or second molar in its arch because it has more numerous supplemental grooves, a small occlusal surface, and ridges, giving it a *wrinkled* appearance, and its roots are shorter, thin, or often fused.

Sometimes the form of the **maxillary third molar** crown is so irregular that it is difficult to identify the mesiobuccal, the distobuccal, and the lingual cusps. However, the usual relative cusp size from largest to smallest is the same as in the first and second molars: first, the mesiolingual cusp is largest and longest; followed by the mesiobuccal cusp, which is wider and usually longer than the distobuccal cusp; followed by the smallest distolingual cusp (if present). The oblique ridge is poorly developed and often absent (maxillary molars in *Fig. 7-35*).

From the occlusal view, the **maxillary third molar** crown usually tapers from buccal to lingual, being narrower on the lingual side, and tapers from mesial to distal, being considerably larger faciolingually in its mesial half due to a prominent mesiobuccal cervical ridge and large mesiolingual cusp. This latter trait is a great help in identifying rights from lefts from the occlusal view (*Fig. 7-35*). Also, the buccal surface can be distinguished from the lingual because it is relatively more flat.

The **mandibular third molar** also exhibits great variance in size and shape as seen in *Figure 7-37*. However, quite often, its crown resembles the crown of the mandibular second molar (with four cusps) or the crown of the mandibular first molar (with five cusps), or it may bear little resemblance to either. As with mandibular first and second molars, the crown may appear tipped distally on the root base, so from the buccal aspect, the distal half of the crown is usually noticeably shorter than the mesial half.

The lingual cusps of the **mandibular third molar** are often larger and longer than the buccal cusps, with the mesiolingual cusp being the largest of all. The mesiobuccal cusp is often the widest and usually highest of the two or three buccal cusps. This difference in cusp height aids in determining mesial from distal sides and, therefore, rights from lefts.

The occlusal outline of a **mandibular third molar** crown is rectangular or oval and wider mesiodistally than buccolingually. The crown of the *four-cusp* type tapers from mesial to distal, but only slightly from buccal to lingual (occlusal aspect). [It was wider mesiodistally than faciolingually by 1.2 mm on 262 teeth.] The buccal crown outline is often relatively flat compared to the more curved lingual outline (occlusal view).

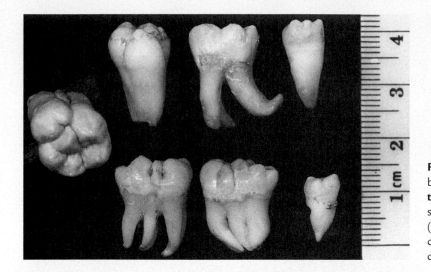

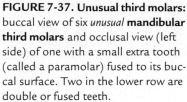

FIGURE 7-37. Unusual third molars: buccal view of six *unusual* **mandibular third molars** and occlusal view (left side) of one with a small extra tooth (called a paramolar) fused to its buccal surface. Two in the lower row are double or fused teeth.

D. SIMILARITIES AND DIFFERENCES OF THIRD MOLAR ROOTS COMPARED WITH FIRST AND SECOND MOLARS IN THE SAME ARCH

As on maxillary first and second molars, **maxillary third molars** usually have three roots: mesiobuccal, distobuccal, and lingual, which may be separated, as in the first and second molars, but more commonly are *fused* most of their length. This results in a *long root trunk* with the furcation located only a short distance from the apices of the roots. Often the roots are entirely fused from the cervix to the apices as seen in 10 maxillary teeth in Figure 7-36. The roots are noticeably *shorter* than on the first and second molars [303 teeth averaged 2 mm shorter on their buccal roots and 2.5 mm shorter on their lingual roots]. The roots, fused or not, are often very crooked, and the majority of them curve distally in their apical third.

As with first and second mandibular molars, **mandibular third molars** have two roots, mesial and distal, but often these are fused together. If the roots are separate, the root trunk is long and the roots are usually more pointed at the apex than on the other molars (*Fig. 7-36*). Often they curve more distally than the roots of first and second molars. They may have one or more extra roots. The mandibular third molar roots are normally significantly shorter than those on the second molar [averaging over 2 mm shorter on 839 mandibular molars]. The roots on mandibular third molars are only about one and a half times as long as the crown, and the root-to-crown ratio is noticeably different from that of mandibular first and second molars [1.6:1 compared to 1.8:1 on 839 teeth].

LEARNING EXERCISE

Learning exercises for all molars:

1. First, review all arch traits that differentiate the maxillary from the mandibular molars in Table 7-4. Then review the summary tables in this chapter of type traits that differentiate the maxillary first from second molars, maxillary right from left molars, mandibular first from second molars, and mandibular right from left molars.
2. Assign a Universal number to a handheld molar.

Suppose a patient just had all of his or her permanent teeth extracted. Imagine being asked to find tooth #14 from among a pile of 32 extracted teeth on the oral surgeon's tray because you wanted to evaluate a lesion seen on the radiograph on a root of that molar. How might you go about it? Try the following steps:

*   From a selection of all permanent teeth (extracted teeth or tooth models) select only the molars (based on class traits).
*   Determine whether each molar is maxillary or mandibular. You should never rely on only one characteristic difference between teeth to name them; rather, make a list of many traits that suggest the tooth is a

maxillary molar as opposed to only one trait that makes you think it belongs in the mandible. This way you can play detective and become an expert at recognition at the same time.

- If you determine that the tooth is maxillary, position the roots up; if it is mandibular, position the roots down.
- Next, using type traits, determine the type of molar you are holding (first, second, or third).
- Use characteristic traits for each surface to identify the buccal surface. This will permit you to view the tooth as though you were looking into a patient's mouth.
- Finally, determine which surface is the mesial. While viewing the molar from the facial and picturing it within the appropriate arch (upper or lower), the mesial surface can be positioned toward the midline in only one quadrant, the right or left.
- Once you have determined the quadrant, assign the appropriate universal number for the molar in that quadrant. For example, the first molar in the upper left quadrant would be tooth #14.

REFERENCES

1. Tratman EK. A comparison of the teeth of people. Indo-European racial stock with Mongoloid racial stock. Dent Record 1950;70:31–53, 63–88.
2. Masters DH, Hoskins SW. Projection of cervical enamel into molar furcations. J Periodontol 1964;35:49–53.
3. Dahlberg AA. The evolutionary significance of the protostylid. Am J Phys Anthropol 1950;8:NS:15.
4. Dahlberg AA. Geographic distribution and origin of dentitions. In Dent J 1965;15:348–355.
5. Hellman M. Racial characters of human dentition. Proc Am Philosoph Soc 1928;67:No.2.
6. Everett FG, Jump EG, Holder TD, et al. The intermediate bifurcation ridge: a study of the morphology of the bifurcation of the lower first molar. J Dent Res 1958;37:162.
7. Scott JH, Symons NBB. Introduction to dental anatomy. London: E & S Livingstone, Ltd., 1958.
8. Tratman EK. Three-rooted lower molars in man and their racial distribution. Br Dent J 1938;64:264–274.
9. Turner CG. Three-rooted mandibular first permanent molars and question of American Indian origin. Am J Phys Anthropol 1971;34:239–242.
10. Brand RW, Isselhard DE. Anatomy of orofacial structures. 6th ed. St. Louis: C.V. Mosby, 1998:438.
11. Jordan R, Abrams L. Kraus's dental anatomy and occlusion. St. Louis: Mosby Year Book, 1992.
12. Jorgensen KD. The Dryopithecus pattern in recent Danes and Dutchmen. J Dent Res 1955;34:195.
13. Garn SM, Lewis AB, Kerewsky RS. Molar size sequence and fossil taxonomy. Science 1963;142:1060.
14. Dahlberg AA. The dentition of the American Indian. In: Laughlin WS, ed. The physical anthropology of the American Indian. New York: The Viking Fund, 1949.
15. Matsumoto Y. Morphological studies on the roots of the Japanese maxillary second molars. Shikwa Gukuho 1986;86:249–276.
16. Carbonelli VM. The tubercle of Carabelli in the Kish dentition, Mesopotamia, 3000 B.C. J Dent Res 1960;39:124.
17. Garn SM, Lewis AB, Kerewsky RS, et al. Genetic independence of Carabelli's trait from tooth size or crown morphology. Arch Oral Biol 1966;11:745–747.
18. Kraus BS. Carabelli's anomaly of the maxillary molar teeth. Observations on Mexican and Papago Indians and an interpretation of the inheritance. Am J Hum Genet 1951;3:348.
19. Kraus BS. Occurrence of the Carabelli trait in the Southwest ethnic groups. Am J Phys Anthropol 1959;17:117.
20. Meredith HV, Hixon EH. Frequency, size, and bilateralism of Carabelli's tubercle. J Dent Res 1954;33:435.
21. Joshi MR, Godiawala RN, Dutia A. Carabelli trait in Hindu children from Gujarat. J Dent Res 1972;51:706–711.
22. Brand RW, Isselhard DE. Anatomy of the orofacial structures. St. Louis: C.V. Mosby, 1982;159:163.
23. Garn SM, Lewis AB, Kerewsky RS. Molar size sequence and fossil taxonomy. Science 1963;142:1060.
24. Jordan R, Abrams L. Kraus's dental anatomy and occlusion. St. Louis: Mosby Year Book, 1992.
25. Chiles DG, Cosentino BJ. Third molar question: report of 522 cases. J Am Dent Assoc 1987;115:575–576.
26. Bath-Balogh M, Fehrenbach MJ. Illustrated dental embryology, histology, and anatomy. Philadelphia: W.B. Saunders, 1997.
27. Ash MM, Nelson SJ. Wheeler's dental anatomy, physiology and occlusion. Philadelphia: Saunders 2003.
28. Lundeen HC. Introduction to Occlusal Anatomy. Gainesville, FL: L&J Press, 1973.

GENERAL REFERENCES

Oregon State System of Higher Education. Dental anatomy. A self-instructional program. East Norwalk: Appleton-Century-Crofts, 1982:403–414.
Proskaves C, Witt F. Pictorial history of dentistry. (Cave P, trans.) Koln: Verlag M. Dumont Schauberg, 1962.
Renner RP. An introduction to dental anatomy and esthetics. Chicago: Quintessence Publishing, 1985.
Ring ME. Dentistry: an illustrated history. St. Louis: C.V. Mosby, 1985.

8 Periodontal Considerations Related to External Morphology and Surrounding Structures

CONTRIBUTED BY LEWIS CLAMAN, D.D.S., M.S., ASSOCIATE PROFESSOR, SECTION OF PERIODONTOLOGY, THE OHIO STATE UNIVERSITY

The periodontal considerations related to external morphology and surrounding structures are presented in eight sections:

A. Definitions of basic periodontal terms
B. The healthy periodontium
C. Anatomy of diseased periodontium
D. Periodontal measurements: indicators of disease and conditions
E. Relationship of periodontal disease and restorations (fillings)
F. Relationship of tooth support and root morphology
G. Influence of root anatomy and anomalies on periodontal disease
H. Periodontal therapy

OBJECTIVES

This chapter is designed to prepare the learner to perform the following:

• List the functions of gingiva, the periodontal ligament, alveolar bone, and cementum.
• Describe and recognize the signs of gingivitis, periodontitis, and gingival recession.
• Describe the periodontal measurements that can be used to differentiate periodontal diseases from the healthy periodontium and be able to *record* these findings on a dental chart.
• Describe the relationship of periodontal disease with restorations placed close to the gingival attachment.
• Describe the relationship of tooth support with root morphology.
• List contemporary methods of periodontal therapy.

While the anatomy of the crown is significant to tooth function from an occlusal standpoint, the root morphology and healthy surrounding structures determine the actual support for the teeth. This section focuses on how external root morphology affects the progression of disease of the periodontium, and why the periodontium, which seems so perfect in health, may be challenged when periodontal disease affects tooth support and stability. An emphasis is placed on periodontal disease initiation, the measurements and descriptions that can be used to differentiate periodontal health from disease, and the therapies that can be used to stop or prevent the disease. As this is a basic text on dental anatomy, the important relationship of periodontal disease relative to sound restorative dentistry involving the placement of fillings and crowns is also introduced. Before reading this chapter, you should review the descriptions of the normal periodontium presented in Chapter 2.

A. DEFINITIONS OF BASIC PERIODONTAL TERMS

The following definitions are important to the understanding of periodontal disease and related therapy:

1. **Periodontium**: The tissues that invest (surround, envelop, or embed) the teeth—that is, the gingiva, cementum (covering the tooth root), periodontal ligament, the alveolar and supporting bone, and the alveolar mucosa (Refer to *Fig. 8-1* to locate these surrounding structures.)
2. **Gingivitis**: Inflammation (disease) of the gingiva
3. **Periodontitis**: Inflammation (disease) of the supporting tissues of the teeth; a spread of inflammation of the gingiva into the adjacent periodontium (bone and periodontal ligament) usually resulting in a progressively destructive change involving loss of bone and periodontal ligament

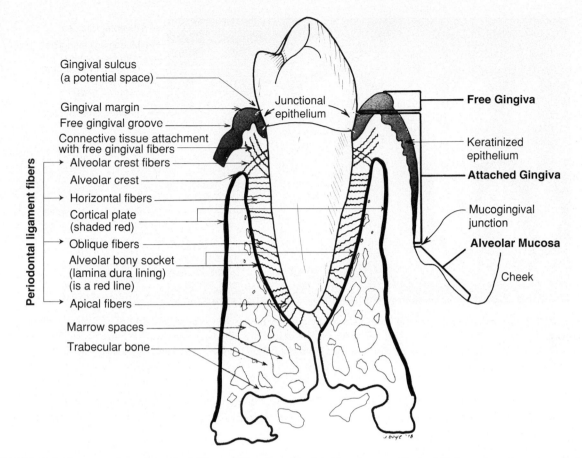

FIGURE 8-1. Cross section of tooth within periodontium. Mesial side of a mandibular left first premolar suspended in its alveolus by groups of fibers of the periodontal ligament. Periodontal ligament fibers include the apical, oblique, horizontal, and alveolar crest fibers. Other fibers include free gingival fibers, and a sixth group (not visible in this view) called transseptal fibers that run directly from the cementum of one tooth to the cementum of the adjacent tooth at a level between the free gingival and alveolar crest fibers. The fibers of the periodontal ligament are *much* shorter than depicted here, averaging only 0.2 mm long (about the thickness of a human hair).

4. **Periodontal diseases**: Those pathologic processes affecting the periodontium, most often gingivitis and periodontitis

5. **Dental plaque (currently known as biofilm)**: A layer containing microorganisms that adheres to teeth and contributes to the development of gingival and periodontal diseases, as well as to tooth decay (dental caries)

6. **Dental calculus (tartar)**: A hard concretion that forms on teeth or dental prostheses through calcification of bacterial plaque

7. **Periodontics**: That specialty of dentistry that encompasses the prevention, diagnosis, and treatment of diseases of the supporting tissues of the teeth or their substitutes; the maintenance of the health, function, and esthetics of these structures and tissues; and the replacement of lost teeth and supporting structures by grafting or implantation of natural and synthetic devices and materials

8. **Periodontist**: A dental practitioner who by virtue of special knowledge and training limits his or her practice or activities to periodontics

B. THE HEALTHY PERIODONTIUM

1. ZONES (AND MARGINS) OF GINGIVA

The zones of gingiva, as described in Chapter 2, are summarized here in *Fig. 8-2*. Beginning at the free gingival margin, the zones include the free gingiva and interdental papilla (with periodontal probe

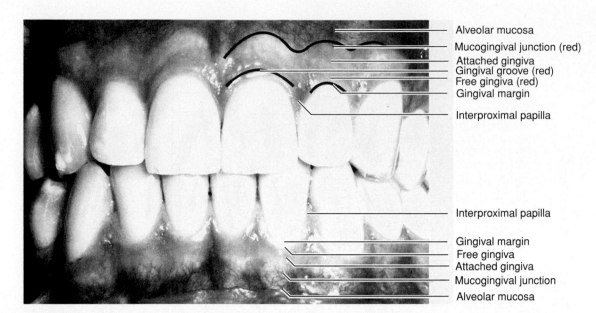

Alveolar mucosa
Mucogingival junction (red)
Attached gingiva
Gingival groove (red)
Free gingiva (red)
Gingival margin

Interproximal papilla

Interproximal papilla

Gingival margin
Free gingiva
Attached gingiva
Mucogingival junction
Alveolar mucosa

FIGURE 8-2. Clinical zones of the gingiva. Note that the interdental papillae should, but do not completely, fill the interproximal spaces between the mandibular incisors. The tissues are otherwise healthy. The more heavily keratinized, lighter (pinker) attached gingiva can be distinguished from the darker (redder), less keratinized alveolar mucosa (best seen in the Color Plate 7).

depths in health that range from 1 to 3 mm), the free gingival groove (when present), attached gingiva (highly keratinized and rich in collagen), the mucogingival junction, and the alveolar mucosa (movable tissue rich in blood vessels).

2. FUNCTIONS OF HEALTHY GINGIVA

In health, the gingiva provides support, protection, and esthetics to the dentition.

a. Support

The gingiva somewhat *supports* the tooth by means of attachment coronal to the crest of the alveolar bone that forms a dentogingival junction near the cementoenamel junction from tooth to gingiva. It includes the **junctional epithelium** [average width = 0.97 mm] and the **connective tissue attachment** [average = 1.07 mm] (Fig. 8-1). The more coronal band (junctional epithelium) attaches gingiva to the tooth by cell junctions [called hemidesmosomes, or half desmosomes], while the more apical band (connective tissue) attaches gingiva to cementum by several gingival fiber groups made up of connective tissue called collagen.

b. Esthetics

In health, gingiva covers the roots of teeth, and the gingival papillae normally fill the gingival embrasure areas between adjacent teeth (see Color Plate 10 and *Fig. 8-3*). The shape of healthy gingiva contributes to what we consider to be an esthetic smile. For the anterior teeth, the gingival margin of each tooth is almost parabolic in shape with the gingival line for the maxillary

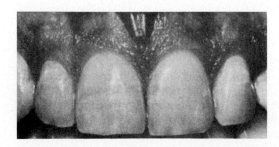

FIGURE 8-3. Healthy gingiva, close up. Note the ideal scalloped contours, knife edges, and stippled (orange-peel) surface texture that is usually most noticeable on the maxillary labial attached gingiva. *(Also see Color Plate 10.)*

central incisors and canines at about the same level, but the gingival line for the lateral incisors is about 1 mm coronal (more gingiva is visible). Symmetry, especially between the maxillary central incisors, is essential. When the patient smiles, the upper lip should be at about the level of the free gingival margin of the central incisors and canines and the lower lip should just cover the incisal edges. In health, the gingiva is pink (or has masking pigmentation), is firm in consistency with knife-edged margins, has a stippled (orange-peel) or matte surface texture, and does not bleed, even when probed. (See Color Plate 10.) This chapter contains many illustrations of healthy and nonhealthy gingiva.

c. Protection

The gingiva generally protects underlying tissue because it is composed of dense fibrous connective tissue covered by a relatively tough tissue layer called **keratinized epithelium**. It is resistant to bacterial, chemical, thermal, and mechanical irritants. Keratinized gingiva helps prevent the spread of inflammation to deeper underlying periodontal tissues. However, the sulcular lining (epithelium) and junctional epithelium of the marginal gingiva and interdental papillae provide less protection. Since these areas are *not* keratinized, they are more permeable to bacterial products, providing only a weak barrier to bacterial irritants, and may even allow bacterial penetration in aggressive forms of periodontal diseases.

Healthy gingiva is somewhat protected by ideally positioned and contoured natural teeth and well-contoured restorations. The protection provided by ideal tooth contours, including appropriate heights of contour, helps to minimize injury from food during mastication (chewing) since food is diverted away from the thin gingival margin and the nonkeratinized sulcus. However, poor tooth or restoration contours, especially overcontoured restorations, contribute to the retention of bacteria-laden dental plaque that may predispose to gingival and periodontal diseases, and will be described in more depth later. Ideal *proximal* tooth contours and contacts help prevent food from impacting between teeth and damaging the interdental papilla or contributing to periodontal disease interproximally. Be aware, however, that even ideal tooth contours *do not prevent* the formation of bacterial plaque and development of periodontal disease.

d. Phonetics

Phonetics pertains to the articulation of sounds and speech. Gingival tissues should cover the roots of the teeth, but if exposure of the roots occurs, especially interproximally, speech may be affected as air passes through the open embrasure spaces. *Figure 8-4* shows a patient who has had past periodontal disease with severe tissue loss that contributes to poor phonetics as well as poor esthetics.

3. FUNCTIONS OF THE HEALTHY PERIODONTAL LIGAMENT, ALVEOLAR BONE, AND CEMENTUM

The entire periodontal ligament consists of numerous collagen fiber bundles, which attach the cementum of the tooth root to the alveolar bony sockets. In that sense the periodontal ligament is

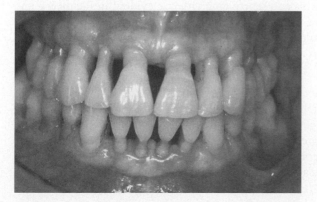

FIGURE 8-4. Severe gingival recession on a patient with previous periodontal disease. The gingival margin no longer covers the cementoenamel junction, and there is severe root exposure. Interproximally, the interdental papillae no longer fill the interdental embrasures. Recession may result in tooth sensitivity and alterations in speech (phonetics).

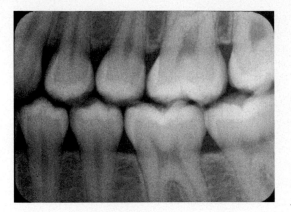

FIGURE 8-5. Radiograph of healthy bone levels showing interproximal bone about 1 to 2 mm apical to the cementoenamel junctions of adjacent teeth.

analogous to a ligament, which attaches one bone to another. These fibers, from apex to free gingiva, include apical, oblique, horizontal, and alveolar crest fibers (refer back to Fig. 8-1). Transseptal and free gingival fibers attach the free gingiva to the cementum. The periodontal ligament, with its insertion into bone, provides the majority of *support* for the teeth and resistance to forces such as those encountered during chewing (mastication). It is a viable structure that, in health, is capable of adaptation and remodeling. Healthy bone levels can be best appreciated on radiographs. Observe in *Figure 8-5* that, in health, the level of the interproximal alveolar bone is 1 to 2 mm apical to the level of the cementoenamel junctions of the adjacent teeth.

C. ANATOMY OF DISEASED PERIODONTIUM

1. GINGIVITIS

Traditionally, periodontal disease (the inflammation in the periodontium) begins as **gingivitis**, an inflammatory condition confined to and altering the gingival tissues. Alterations in the gingiva may reflect gingivitis alone, active slight periodontitis, more advanced disease, or evidence of previous disease that has been arrested. Gingival inflammation results over time from the metabolic products of bacterial colonies within dental plaque that are in close proximity to gingival tissues. The earliest indication of gingivitis on a *microscopic* level involves an increase in inflammatory cells and breakdown of the connective tissue (collagen) in the gingiva. This leads to an increase in tissue fluids (edema, that is, swelling), proliferation of small blood vessels (redness), and some loss of the integrity of the epithelium (ulceration). As this breakdown progresses, changes in the tissues can be clinically observed.

Clinically, gingival characteristics that should be evaluated as indicators of gingival health (versus disease) include its shape and size, color, consistency, and surface texture, and the presence or absence of bleeding and/or suppuration (purulence or pus). Visually, the inflammation and edema of **mild gingivitis** is seen as slight redness; rolled, swollen margins; smooth and shiny surface texture (loss of stippling); and loss of resiliency (tissues can be depressed or free gingiva can be deflected from the tooth when a stream of air is directed toward it). In **moderate or severe gingivitis**, these changes become more pronounced and the proliferation of small blood vessels and ulcerations results in bleeding upon probing. Slight gingivitis and severe gingivitis are evident in *Figure 8-6* and Color Plate 11A and B. Additionally, in severe inflammation, especially with periodontitis, *suppuration*, or expressing of pus (also known as purulent exudate), may occur. See *Table 8-1* for normal gingival characteristics compared to descriptions of tissue exhibiting gingivitis.

2. PERIODONTITIS

As with the gingiva, the periodontal ligament, bone, and cementum are at risk for breakdown during inflammation with resultant loss of bone height and periodontal ligament. In the classic progression of disease, gingivitis, if untreated, may progress to **periodontitis**. This occurs when inflammatory breakdown extends from the gingiva to the periodontal ligament and bone and when the junctional epithelium (which normally attaches to tooth at the cementoenamel junction) migrates apically onto

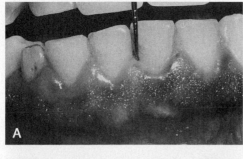

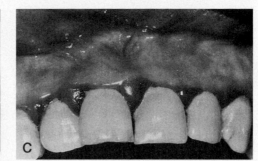

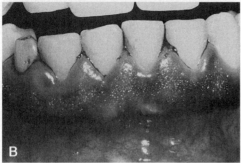

FIGURE 8-6. Gingivitis. A. A periodontal probe is inserted into the gingival sulcus and gently "walked" around the tooth. **B.** The examiner looks for **gingival bleeding** that occurs within 30 seconds. (Note the generalized physiologic melanin pigmentation [dark regions] on the attached gingiva common in persons with some ethnic heritages.) **C. Inflamed gingiva:** Note the contour changes (bulbous papillae, rolled margins); increased size; and glazed (not stippled) surface texture. Clinically, the papillae and margins are red and bleed easily when probed. The gingiva separates (retracts) from the teeth easily when air is directed at it.

the root because the connective tissue attachment has broken down. Periodontitis associated with alveolar bone loss is best appreciated in dental radiographs (*Fig 8-7A* compared to *B*). The bone height (crestal bone) is no longer at predisease levels. Although the immune system protects the periodontium, bone resorption occurs when **osteoclasts** (bone-resorbing cells) are stimulated by the host and by bacterial products. **Chronic periodontitis** is the most common form of periodontal disease. It usually progresses slowly, is usually most prevalent in adults, and is associated with plaque and dental calculus. A second form of periodontal disease is **aggressive periodontitis** that usually has an earlier age of onset. Features may include rapid attachment loss and bone destruction, a familial pattern, and abnormalities in the immune system. Both forms of periodontitis can result in exposure of the cemen-

Table 8-1	CHARACTERISTICS OF NORMAL GINGIVA COMPARED TO DISEASED GINGIVA	
GINGIVAL CHARACTERISTICS	**NORMAL (EXAMPLES)**	**NOT NORMAL/DISEASE (EXAMPLES)**
SIZE AND SHAPE:		
Papillae	Fill embrasures, thin	Blunted; bulbous; cratered
Margins	Knife edged in profile	Rolled (thickened) in profile
Scallops	Present and normal, parabolic	Flattened; exaggerated; reversed; clefted
COLOR	Coral pink, or pink with masking melanin pigmentation	Red, bluish-red cyanotic
CONSISTENCY	Resilient, firm, nonretractable with air	Soft and spongy, air retractable
SURFACE TEXTURE	Stippled (orange peel); matte (dull)	Smooth and shiny (glazed); pebbled (coarse texture)
BLEEDING	None	Upon probing or spontaneous
MUCOGINGIVAL DEFECT	None (adequate zone of keratinized gingiva)	Pockets traverse mucogingival junction; lack of keratinized gingiva; frenum inserts on marginal gingiva
SUPPURATION (PURULENT EXUDATE OR PUS)	None	Exudate is expressed when the gingival pocket wall is compressed; exudate streams out of the pocket after probing

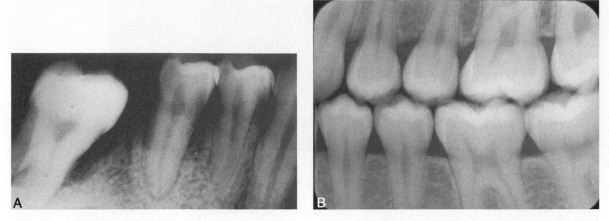

FIGURE 8-7. Radiographic bone loss. A. This radiograph shows advanced periodontal disease as indicated by loss of bone (especially around teeth #29 and 31; note tooth #30 is missing), which would normally be surrounding all teeth to a level much closer (within 2 mm) to the cementoenamel junction. **B.** Radiograph showing **normal bone levels** relative to the cementoenamel junction.

tum on the root surface, which is less mineralized than enamel, making it more susceptible to the effects of pathogenic bacteria and their products, which contribute to root caries (decay) formation.

Factors Contributing to Periodontitis

In addition to the primary role of bacteria in the pathogenesis, there are many factors that contribute to periodontal disease development and progression. To date, the only two risk factors that are proven to increase the odds of periodontal disease progression and tooth loss are smoking and diabetes. Other factors that may contribute to this disease include specific bacterial pathogens, alterations in the tooth form and surface that influence the accumulation and retention of dental plaque, systemic illnesses or conditions (including genetics and emotional stress) that modify or impair the immune response, and injury to the periodontium resulting from heavy forces during tooth function (occlusion).

Breakdown of the periodontium resulting in attachment loss and bone loss usually begins in an inaccessible area (such as adjacent to a root concavity or an exposed furcation) that is neither self-cleansing nor easy for a patient to reach with oral hygiene aids. Therefore, it is paramount that both the dentist and the dental hygienist be thoroughly familiar with root anatomy as they perform a periodontal examination in order to detect periodontal disease at these inaccessible locations that are at greatest risk to breakdown. Further, an essential objective in treating periodontal disease involves using special instruments to remove deposits (plaque and calculus) and smooth or remove cementum on root surfaces that have become affected by periodontal disease. Knowledge of root morphology also helps when identifying sites that are difficult or impossible to reach, or ones that have not responded to treatment during root cleaning (debridement, which includes root planing), and when providing instructions to patients for the appropriate use of oral hygiene aids.

Periodontitis itself *may* be a contributing factor for several systemic diseases including cardiovascular disease, stroke, and the control of diabetes, as well as contributing to low birth weight and preterm babies when the pregnant mother has periodontal disease.

3. GINGIVAL RECESSION

Gingival recession is a loss of gingival tissue (usually with underlying loss of bone) resulting in the exposure of more root surface (*Fig. 8-8* and Color Plate 12A and B). In gingival recession, the gingival margin is apical to the cementoenamel junction, and the papillae may be blunted or rounded, and no longer fill the interproximal embrasure. Gingival recession is often seen in older individuals, hence the reference to an older person as being "long in the tooth." It may be part of an active process of periodontal disease or may reflect previous disease that is now under control. However,

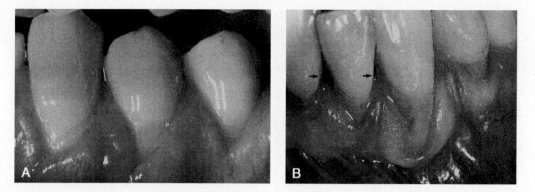

FIGURE 8-8. Gingival recession and mucogingival defects. A. Area of gingival recession (clefting). The gingiva no longer covers the cementoenamel junction, and the root surface is exposed. **B.** Severe gingival recession. The prominent canine root and lack of attached gingiva are factors that may have contributed to the recession. Note the blunted papillae (*arrows*). Both figures show marginal depths where there is a diminished zone of keratinized gingiva, and probe depths reach or transverse the mucogingival junction indicating a mucogingival defect. (Courtesy of Alan R. Levy, D.D.S.)

destruction of the periodontium (including gingival recession) should *not* be regarded as a natural consequence of aging.[1]

Conditions that contribute to gingival recession around individual teeth, especially in the presence of plaque, are poorly aligned teeth within an arch resulting in abnormal tooth and root prominence (*Figs. 8-8B* and *8-9*), a lack of attached gingiva,[2] or aggressive tooth brushing. Abnormal tooth positions do not necessarily indicate disease, but they do contribute to other tissue alterations such as flattened or exaggerated contours, and variations in tissue thickness. Additionally, patients may exhibit thin or thick periodontal tissues (overlying bone and gingiva). Patients with thin periodontal tissues (thin periodontal biotype) may have prominent roots that are not completely covered with bone (Color Plate 13). Patients with thick periodontal tissues have thicker plates of bone or gingival tissues. The very thick ledges of bone in Color Plate 14 are called **exostoses**. Patients with thin periodontal tissues are more at risk for gingival recession. The risk for gingival recession is more apparent when viewing alveolar bone of a skull. Normally, the bone is 1 to 2 mm apical to the cementoenamel junction (*Fig. 8-10*). In prominent teeth, such as canines, there may be no bone covering much of the root, although the patient may not have signs of periodontal disease or gingival recession. An

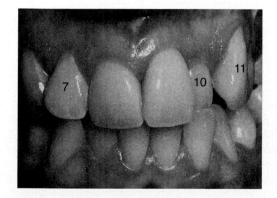

FIGURE 8-9. Effects of tooth position (alignment) within the arch on gingival shape: Examples of contour variations caused by tooth malpositions. Tooth #11 is too labial, showing exaggerated scalloping and thin gingiva. Tooth #10, which is in lingual version, has flattened gingival contours and thicker tissue. Rotated tooth #7 shows V-shaped gingival margin contour on the labial gingiva.

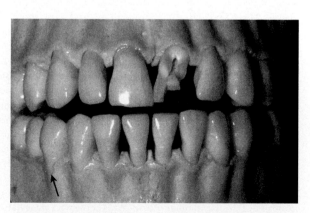

FIGURE 8-10. Normal bony architecture. The alveolar crest is normally between 1 and 2 mm apical to the cementoenamel junction. The only obvious exception is tooth #28 (mandibular right first bicuspid), which shows a slight bony dehiscence.

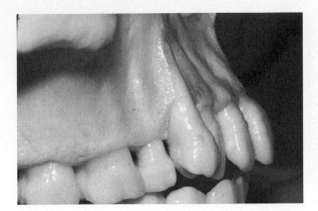

FIGURE 8-11. Example of root dehiscence. The maxillary first bicuspid is buccal to the alveolar process. There is no bone over most of the buccal aspect of the root, although the bone over the other tooth surfaces is at a normal level. Teeth with prominent roots are prone to gingival recession.

isolated area of tooth root denuded of its bony covering is called root **dehiscence** [dee HISS enss] (seen on the first premolar in *Fig. 8-11*). Root dehiscence may or may not be covered with soft tissue.

D. PERIODONTAL MEASUREMENTS: INDICATORS OF DISEASE AND CONDITIONS

Several clinical measurements are critical when evaluating overall periodontal status. These measurements can be used to describe a tooth's stability and loss of support and a patient's degree of inflammation and pattern of disease. They help to establish a diagnosis, guide the development of a treatment plan, and document changes following active therapy. Throughout this discussion, references will be made to documenting this information using the clinical chart obtained from the Ohio State University College of Dentistry (*Fig. 8-12*).

1. TOOTH MOBILITY

Tooth mobility is the movement of a tooth in response to applied forces. Teeth may become mobile due to repeated excessive occlusal forces, inflammation, and weakened periodontal support (often associated with a widened periodontal ligament as noted on radiographs). The healthy periodontal

FIGURE 8-12. Charting periodontal findings (on a partial reproduction of the form used at the Ohio State University College of Dentistry). This form provides a logical method for documenting periodontal findings (as well as other findings). **A.** The left column provides the key for recording the following: **Fremitus** is recorded as **F** as on tooth #5; **mobility** is denoted by **1** for tooth #2, **2** for tooth #5, and **0** (no mobility) for teeth #3 and 4. **Probe depths** (six per tooth) are recorded during the initial examination (initial probe depths) in the three boxes for three facial depth locations on each facial surface and three boxes for three lingual depth locations. After initial periodontal therapy has been completed, they should be recorded again (as postinitial preparation [PIP] probe depths). This permits easy comparison to identify sites that respond to treatment and those that do not respond. **Bleeding on probing (BOP)** is denoted by a red dot over the probe depth readings as on the *facial* surfaces of teeth #2 (mesial, midfacial, and distal), #3 (distal), and #5 (mesial and distal); and *lingually* on all mesial, midlingual, and distal surfaces. **Gingival margin position** is recorded as numbers in red on the root of teeth as follows: +1 (1 mm *apical* to the cementoenamel junction) on the facial of teeth #2 and #3; +2 on the facial of tooth #5; −1 (1 mm *occlusal* to the cementoenamel junction) on the lingual of teeth #3 and #4; and 0 (located at the level of the cementoenamel) on all other surfaces. **Furcation classes** are seen as red triangular shapes (incomplete, outlined, or solid). Class I involvement is evident on the midfacial of tooth #3. Class II involvement is noted midfacial on #2, as well as on the mesial (from the lingual) on #2, and the distal (from the lingual) on #3. Class III involvement is noted on a mandibular molar discussed below. A **mucogingival defect** is recorded as a red wavy line seen on the facial of tooth #5. **B.** A mandibular molar (#30) showing a **class III furcation** evident from the facial and lingual views. Note that the triangle point is directed *up* toward the furcation in the mandibular arch but was directed *down* toward the furcation in the maxillary arch as shown in **A. C. Calculation of plaque index %** and **BOP %.** The **plaque index %** can be calculated by dividing the number of surfaces with plaque by the total number of surfaces (four per tooth). When considering only the four teeth in this figure, nine surfaces had plaque divided by 16 possible surfaces = 56%. The **BOP %** is the number of tooth surfaces that bleed on probing divided by the total number of surfaces (six per tooth). When considering only the four teeth in this figure, 14 surfaces bled divided by 24 total surfaces = 58%.

ligament (PDL) is about 0.2 mm wide, decreasing to only 0.1 mm with advanced age. Tipping movements are minimal at the rotational middle of the tooth root (cervicoapically) and greater at either the cervical or apical end of the root. Thus, there is a functional difference in the width of the periodontal ligament in these three regions. At any age, it is wider around both the cervix and the apex than around the middle of the root, depending upon the amount of rotational movements to which the tooth is subjected. Further, the periodontal ligament of a natural tooth in occlusal function is

FIGURE 8-12. (continued) Legend is on previous page.

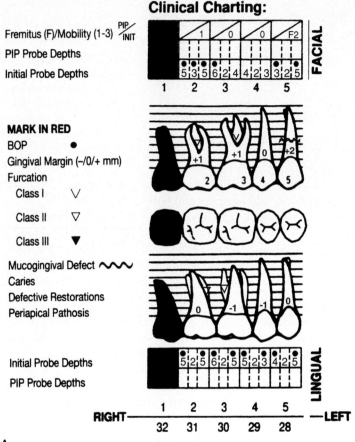

Clinical Charting:

MARK IN RED
BOP   ●
Gingival Margin (–/0/+ mm)
Furcation
   Class I   ∨
   Class II   ▽
   Class III   ▼
Mucogingival Defect ∿∿
Caries
Defective Restorations
Periapical Pathosis

A

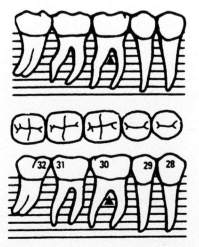

B

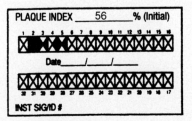

Init BOP _____ 58 ___%
PIP BOP _____%

PLAQUE INDEX _____ 56 _____% (Initial)

C

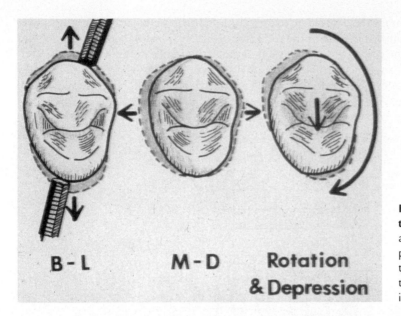

FIGURE 8-13. Method for determining **tooth mobility**. Two rigid instruments are applied to the tooth to see if it can be displaced either buccolingually or mesiodistally. For teeth with severe mobility, the tooth can be depressed or rotated (which is category 3 mobility).

slightly wider than in a nonfunctional tooth because the nonfunctional tooth does not have an antagonist to stimulate the periodontal ligament and bone cells to remodel.[3]

Injury to the periodontium from occlusal forces is known as **occlusal trauma**. It may contribute to destructive changes in the bone, widening of the periodontal ligament, and root shortening (resorption), all of which may contribute to increased tooth mobility. Many of the changes are reversible, meaning that the periodontium can accommodate.[4] Occlusal trauma is a disorder that does *not* initiate, but can influence the course of, inflammatory periodontal disease under specific circumstances.[5]

Technique to Determine Tooth Movement

To determine tooth **mobility**, first, the patient's head should be stabilized to minimize movement. Next, view the occlusal surfaces and observe movement of the marginal ridges of the tooth being tested relative to adjacent teeth as you use two rigid instruments (such as the mirror and probe handles) to apply reciprocating forces first one way, then another. The forces should be fairly light and alternate (reciprocate fairly rapidly). Observe the tooth for movement in a buccolingual or mesiodistal direction, as well as for vertical "depressibility." *Figures 8-13* and *8-14* illustrate the technique to determine tooth mobility. Numbers assigned to denote the extent of mobility are presented in *Table 8-2*. Tooth mobility can be

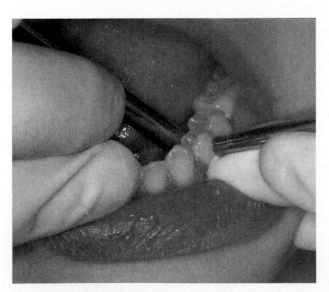

FIGURE 8-14. Technique for determining buccolingual mobility. Light, alternating (reciprocating) buccolingual forces are applied and movement observed relative to adjacent teeth.

Table 8-2	NUMBERS ASSIGNED TO MOBILITY CATEGORIES	
MOBILITY CATEGORY	CLINICAL OBSERVATION	MAGNITUDE
0	No observed movement	
1	Slight movement	Less than 1 mm
2	Moderate movement	Greater than 1 mm
3	Extreme movement	Depressible

recorded as "0" for no mobility, "1" for slight mobility, "2" for moderate mobility, or "3" for extreme mobility that includes depressing the tooth. See Figure 8-12 for charting examples of mobility (categories 0, 1, 2, or 3).

Fremitus is the vibration of a tooth during occlusal contact. It is determined by placing the nail of the gloved index finger at right angles to the facial crown surface using a light force. The patient is asked to tap his or her teeth or clench and move the mandible from right to left (excursive movements). If definite vibration is felt, fremitus is confirmed and could be noted as an "F" on a patient's chart for that tooth (as seen in Fig. 8-12). If tooth displacement is detected, **functional mobility** is confirmed. Functional mobility (biting stress mobility) occurs when teeth move other teeth during occlusal function.

2. PROBE DEPTHS

Determining (probing) the depth of the potential space between the tooth and gingiva (called the **gingival sulcus or crevice**) is a critical periodontal finding that is routinely performed in dental offices and may indicate the presence of periodontal disease. A blunt-tipped instrument with millimeter markings called a **periodontal probe** (*Fig. 8-15*) is inserted into the gingival sulcus (*Figs. 8-16* and *8-17*). In the presence of periodontal disease, this gingival sulcus may be called a **periodontal pocket**. **Probing depth** (referred to as *pocket* depth if periodontal disease is present) is the distance from the gingival margin to the apical portion of the gingival sulcus. Probing depths in healthy gingival sulci normally range from 1 to 3 mm. A depth of *greater than 3 mm* is a possible cause for concern. However, if gingival tissues are overgrown (as may result as a side effect from some medications), a pocket depth reading of 4 mm or greater (called a **pseudopocket**) may be present even in the absence of periodontitis. On the other hand, if there is gingival recession (described below), there may be shallow probing depths in the presence of true periodontal disease. Therefore, the critical determinant of whether periodontitis has occurred is the presence of **attachment loss** (to be described later).

Probing Technique

The probe should be "walked around" the tooth with a light force to ensure a tactile sense and to minimize probing beyond the base of the pocket. The probe should be directed

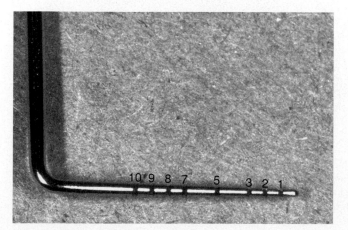

FIGURE 8-15. A standard, frequently used **periodontal probe**. To make measurements easier, there are dark bands at 1, 2, 3, 5, 7, 8, 9, and 10 mm.

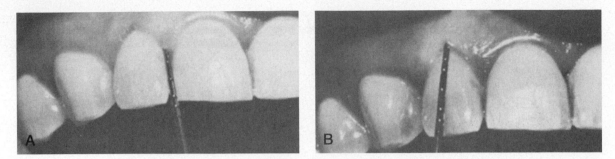

FIGURE 8-16. Periodontal probe in place in the gingival sulcus. **A.** Interproximal probing. **B.** Midfacial probing. In health, the area probed is the gingival sulcus. If periodontal disease is present, it is called a pocket.

apically within the sulcus along the root surface (to prevent it from engaging or being impeded by the pocket wall) (Fig. 8-17A). The intent is to probe apically within the sulcus just to the attachment, although in reality the probe usually broaches (impinges on) some of the attachment even in health. When the depth of the sulcus/pocket has been reached, resilient resistance is encountered. Probing depths are generally recorded as the deepest measurement for each of the six areas around each tooth. Three areas are recorded while moving in very small steps within the sulcus on the buccal surface (starting in the mesial interproximal, stepping around to the midbuccal, and finally stepping around to the distal interproximal). Interproximally, when the teeth are in proximal contact, the probe should progress toward the contact until it touches both adjacent teeth before angling it approximately 10° to 15° buccal (or lingual) to the tooth axis line (Fig. 8-17B). The three buccal readings to record are the deepest readings for mesial interproximal, midbuccal, and distal interproximal. Similarly, three areas are recorded while probing around the lingual of the tooth.

3. GINGIVAL MARGIN LEVEL (GINGIVAL RECESSION OR NONRECESSION)

Before any periodontal disease has occurred, the gingival margin level of a young healthy person is slightly coronal to the cementoenamel junction, which is the reference point. If the gingival margin is apical to the cementoenamel junction, there has been gingival recession, and the root is exposed (seen in Figs. 8-4 and 8-8, and Color Plate 12).

By convention, the following denotes the gingival margin level:

- Negative (−) numbers denote that gingiva is coronal to the cementoenamel junction.
- Zero (0) denotes that the gingiva is at the cementoenamel junction.
- Positive (+) numbers denote recession (the gingival level is apical to the cementoenamel junction).

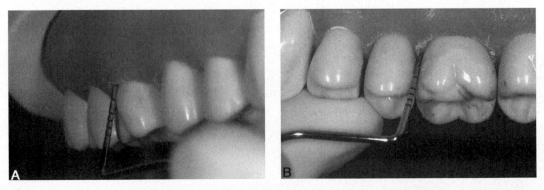

FIGURE 8-17. Probe placement technique on models. **A.** Technique for facial (or lingual) probe placement. The probe is guided along the tooth surface, and care is taken not to engage the sulcular gingival tissues. **B.** Interproximal probe placement. The probe is angled slightly distally on the mesial surface of tooth #3 as it is guided along the tooth surface and is not impeded by the interproximal papilla. Although not easily appreciated from this view, it is also angled 10° to 15° to reach the most direct proximal area.

Technique to Determine the Gingival Margin Level

If recession has occurred, the distance between the cementoenamel junction and the gingival margin can be visually measured with the periodontal probe. If the gingival margin covers the cementoenamel junction, the distance from the gingival margin to the cementoenamel junction may be estimated by inserting the probe in the sulcus and feeling for the cementoenamel junction. If this junction is difficult to detect or is subgingival, the probe should be at a 45° angle. The overlap between enamel and cementum will stop the probe at their junction. Gingival margin levels are charted as "0", or a + or − number, in red on the roots near the cementoenamel junction as seen in Figure 8-12.

4. CLINICAL ATTACHMENT LOSS (SAME AS CLINICAL ATTACHMENT LEVEL)

Clinical attachment level refers to the distance from the cementoenamel junction to the apical extent (depth) of the periodontal sulcus. It is a measurement that indicates how much support has been lost and is therefore a critical determinant of whether periodontal disease has occurred.

Technique to Determine Clinical Attachment Loss

Add the probing depth and the gingival margin level measurements together to obtain the clinical attachment level. A patient with a 3-mm pocket and a gingival level of +2 (2 mm of recession) has 5 mm of attachment loss. A patient with a 3-mm pocket and a gingival level of −2 mm (the gingiva covers the cementoenamel junction by 2 mm) has only 1 mm of attachment loss. See an example of clinical attachment calculation on a tooth in Color Plate 15 (A and B). Clinical attachment loss may be severe with minimal pocket depths if there is considerable gingival recession. There may be no attachment loss with deep pockets if **pseudopockets** are present (that is, pockets formed by an overgrowth of gingiva, possibly as a response to certain medications). Periodontists also make interproximal measurements of the gingival margin level, which is a more challenging task. The severity of periodontal disease can therefore be accurately determined at the six sites around each tooth by measurements.

5. BLEEDING ON PROBING

Bleeding on probing occurs when bacterial plaque affects the gingival sulcular epithelium, resulting in inflammation in the underlying connective tissue. Bleeding visible from the gingival margin when probing is an important indicator of inflammation (Fig. 8-6B and Color Plate 16A and B).

Technique to Document Bleeding on Probing

When bleeding is noted after probing several teeth, teeth that exhibit bleeding can be recorded at each probing site on the chart as a red dot above the probe depth. The percentage of sites that bleed can be calculated by dividing the number of bleeding sites by the number of total sites (where total sites equal the number of teeth present times six probe sites per tooth). Bleeding sites are charted in Figure 8-12, and a percentage has been calculated for four teeth.

6. FURCATION INVOLVEMENT

A furcation is the branching point between roots on a multirooted tooth. Normally, furcations cannot be clinically probed because they are filled in with bone and periodontal attachment. With advancing periodontal disease, however, attachment loss and bone loss may reach a furcation area resulting in a **furcation involvement**. Pockets that extend into the furcation create areas with difficult access for the dentist and dental hygienist to clean during regular office visits and are a real challenge for patients to reach and clean during their normal home care. Therefore, these areas of furcation involvement readily accumulate soft plaque deposits and mineralized calculus (seen on extracted teeth in *Fig. 8-18*). These deposits frequently become impossible to remove and may provide a pathway for periodontal disease to continue to progress.

With advancing periodontal disease, attachment loss and bone loss may reach the furcation area. Initially, there may be an incipient (initial or beginning) furcation involvement. As disease progresses

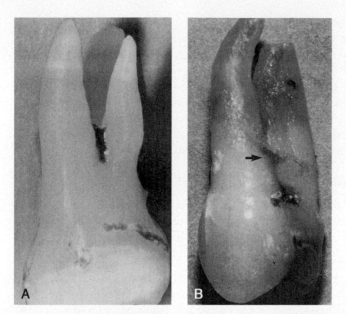

FIGURE 8-18. Calculus in the furcation area and root depressions. A. Extracted molar with mineralized deposits (calculus) extending into the furcation. Once disease progresses into the furcation area, access for removal by the dentist or hygienist becomes exceedingly difficult. **B.** Calculus deposit (*arrow*) in the longitudinal depression on the mesial side of the root of a maxillary first premolar.

into the interradicular (furcation) area, attachment loss and bone loss will change directions and begin to progress horizontally between the roots. At that point, a furcation probe (like a Nabor's probe with a blunt end and curved design) can probe into a subgingival furcation area. It can be used to detect the concavity between roots *(Fig. 8-19A and B)*. The first sign of detectable furcation involvement is termed grade I and can progress to a grade II involvement when the probe can hook the furcation roof (the part of the root forming the most coronal portion of the furcal area) as demonstrated in *Figure 8-20A*. In the most extreme circumstances, the furcation probe may actually extend from the furcation of one tooth aspect to the furcation on another tooth aspect. This is referred to as a through-and-through (grade III) furcation involvement *(Fig. 8-20B)*. (A summary of the grades of furcation involvement is presented in *Table 8-4*.)

The location of the furcation is an important consideration (summarized in *Table 8-3*). Recall that *mandibular* molar furcations are located between mesial and distal roots near the midbuccal and midlingual (as illustrated in *Fig. 8-21A and B*). *Maxillary* molar furcations are identified by probing midbuccal (between mesiobuccal and distobuccal roots seen as in *Fig. 8-22A*), mesially (between lingual and mesiobuccal roots as in *Fig 8-22B*), and distally (between lingual and distobuccal roots as seen in *Fig. 8-22C*). Clinically, more coronal furcations will become involved with periodontal disease

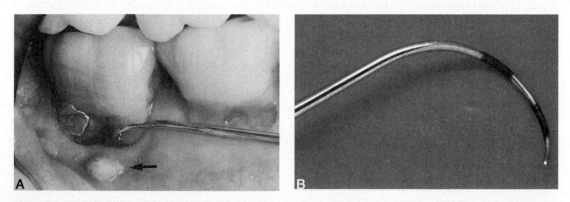

FIGURE 8-19. Probing to check for furcation involvement. A. Severe buccal furcation involvement on a mandibular second molar. The furcation probe is able to engage far into the interradicular area because of periodontal destruction. (Note the arrow pointing to an abscessed area indicating infection.). **B.** The furcation (Nabor's) probe has a rounded point, is curved to allow negotiation of furcations, and frequently has markings at 3-mm intervals (as shown here). This allows the estimation of how far the probe horizontally penetrates into the furcation.

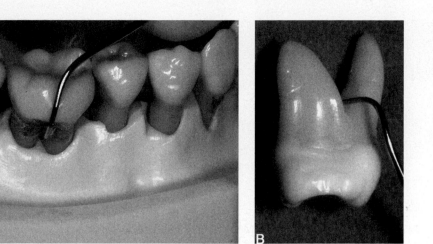

FIGURE 8-20. Confirming furcation involvement. A. The furcation probe is engaging the roof of a furcation and does not completely penetrate to the lingual entrance of the furcation. This would represent a grade 2 furcation involvement. **B.** The furcation probe engages the mesial furcation on an extracted maxillary first molar. Note how close the furcation is to the mesiolingual line angle of the tooth due to the wide mesiobuccal root.

Table 8-3	NORMAL LOCATION OF FURCATIONS
TOOTH TYPE	**POTENTIAL FURCATIONS**
MAXILLARY MOLARS	Midbuccal
	Mesial (accessed from the lingual)
	.Distal (accessed from the lingual)
MANDIBULAR MOLARS	Midbuccal
	Midlingual
MAXILLARY PREMOLARS (with buccal and lingual roots)	Middle of mesial
	Middle of distal

Table 8-4	NOTATIONS FOR THREE CATEGORIES OF FURCATION INVOLVEMENT			
FURCATION GRADE	**NOTATION**	**BONE/ATTACHMENT LOSS**	**CLINICAL FINDING**	**CLINICAL EXPLANATION**
Grade I: incipient	Caret: ∨ or ^	No real bone loss No attachment loss in furcation	Probe engages concavity	Probe locks horizontally; does not catch furcation roof
Grade II: moderate	Open triangle: △ or ▽	Definite bone loss or attachment loss	Probe catches furcation roof	Probe hooks onto roof of furcation and must be rotated to disengage, but probe cannot be passed to another tooth aspect
Grade III: (through and through)	Solid triangle: ▲ or ▼	Complete bone loss with clinical attachment loss under the furcation roof	Probe can pass from one tooth aspect to another	

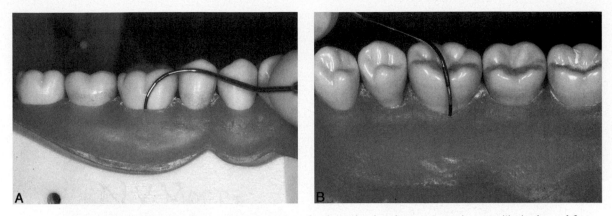

FIGURE 8-21. Location used to confirm MANDIBULAR molar furcation involvement. A. The mandibular **buccal** furcation is probed midbuccally. The probe is shown at the apical and horizontal extent of the penetration into the facial furcation. **B.** The mandibular **lingual** furcation is probed near the midlingual.

more readily than more apically positioned furcations since less bone destruction is required to expose the more cervical furcation. However, more coronally positioned furcations are more easily treated by traditional periodontal therapy due in part to improved access. Recall that the furcation is closer to the cementoenamel junction on first molars (since their root trunks are shorter) than on second molars, and closer to the cementoenamel junction on second molars than on thirds (*Fig. 8-23*). The more apical the furcation, the more complex the treatment will become. The maxillary first premolar provides a good example of a furcation that is located nearer to the apex (Fig. 8-18B). *Proximal* furcations, once they are involved with disease, are particularly difficult to gain access to because of vertical longitudinal depressions coronal to the furcation and close approximation to adjacent teeth (seen in the radiograph in *Fig. 8-24*).

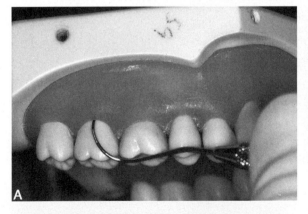

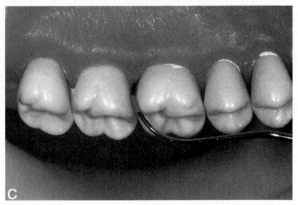

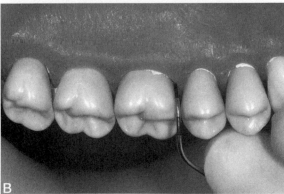

FIGURE 8-22. Location used to confirm MAXILLARY molar furcation involvement. A. Buccal furcation is probed midbuccal. The furcation probe is shown as it enters the potential furcation near the middle of the facial surface of this maxillary molar. **B.** The maxillary **mesial** furcation is probed near the mesiolingual line angle (through the lingual embrasure since the mesiolingual root is wider than the palatal root). **C.** The maxillary molar **distal** furcation is probed at the most interproximal point (through either the facial or lingual embrasure since the distolingual root is about as wide as the palatal root).

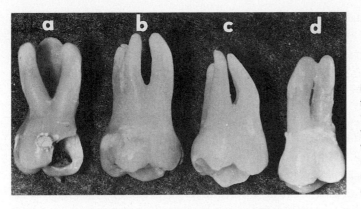

FIGURE 8-23. Variations in furcation location for maxillary molars. A. Divergent roots with the furcation in the coronal one-third of the root with a short root trunk. **B.** Convergent roots with the furcation in the middle one-half of the root with a longer root trunk. **C.** Very convergent roots. **D.** Fused roots with the furcation in the coronal one-third of the root.

Technique to Document Furcation Involvement

When probing into a potential furcation area, the furcation probe should be positioned at the gingival margin at the location around the tooth where the furcation is suspected. The probe should first be directed apically. When the bottom of the pocket is reached, the probe should be directed toward the tooth to engage the roof of the furcation. Figure 8-20A shows a probe engaging a furcation area. Deep horizontal penetration of the furcation probe is indicative of severe periodontal disease. The notation used to record each grade of furcation is summarized in Table 8-4, and examples of charting the degree of furcation involvement are presented in Figure 8-12 (using a caret [∨ or ∧] for incipient involvement, open triangle [△ or ▽] for moderate involvement, or a solid triangle [▲ or ▼] over the areas of the root where a through-and-through furcation is detected).

7. MUCOGINGIVAL DEFECTS:

A width of **keratinized gingiva** (recall Fig. 8-2) normally surrounds each tooth, extending from the gingival line to the mucogingival line. Mucosa apical to the mucogingival junction is more moveable, more vascular (redder), less firm, and nonkeratinized. In health, a width of **attached gingiva** is that portion of the keratinized gingiva that is firmly bound to the underlying tooth and/or bone.

A **mucogingival defect** is present in the following three circumstances:

1. Keratinized gingiva is present, but there is a lack of *attached* gingiva. This condition is confirmed when the periodontal probe depth of the gingival sulcus reaches or exceeds (traverses) the external mucogingival junction indicating an absence of attached gingiva (Color Plate 17A and B). In this case, keratinized gingiva may form part of the pocket wall, but it is not attached to the underlying structures as confirmed by the sulcus depth.
2. There is a lack of keratinized gingiva.

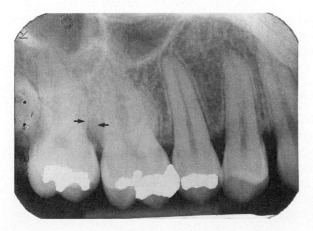

FIGURE 8-24. Radiograph showing close root approximation between the distal root surface of the maxillary first molar and the mesial root surface of the second molar (*arrows*). Furcations and concavities like these are virtually inaccessible when destruction occurs at those locations.

3. A frenum inserts into the marginal tissues so that when tension is applied there is movement or blanching at the gingival margins (a possible contributing factor in Color Plate 8-18B).

Mucogingival defects are most likely to be present on the aspects of teeth where the normal keratinized attached gingiva is adjacent to the movable alveolar mucosa, in other words, on the facial aspects of maxillary teeth and the facial and lingual aspects of mandibular teeth (examples are presented in Fig. 8-8A and B). It is very unusual for mucogingival defects to be present on the palatal aspects of maxillary teeth where the entire palate is keratinized. The only exception is when teeth are positioned so far posteriorly that they are near the *soft* palate. Mucogingival defects may place a tooth at risk for progressive gingival recession.

Technique for Determining Mucogingival Defects

Both visual observations and measurements are required for detecting mucogingival defects. In the visual method, a periodontal probe can be moved incisocervically or occlusocervically as it is pressed gently against the tissue surface at the mucogingival line. Movement or blanching at the margin is indicative of a mucogingival defect (Color Plate 8-18A and B). The width of keratinized gingiva should first be measured. If the periodontal probe depth reaches or exceeds the mucogingival junction, a mucogingival defect is confirmed and can be charted as a horizontal wavy line placed over the root apical to recession readings (seen in the chart in Fig. 8-12). See a clinical example for measuring to confirm a mucogingival defect in Color Plate 17A and B.

8. THE PLAQUE SCORE (INDEX)

Bacterial dental plaque biofilm is a thin layer containing organized microorganisms that loosely adheres to teeth, but can be removed with proper tooth brushing and flossing. It is an almost *invisible* layer that accumulates on teeth in the absence of excellent oral hygiene. Therefore, applying a mechanism to identify the location of this nearly invisible plaque can be helpful when teaching plaque removal techniques and when monitoring a person's success using specific oral hygiene techniques designed to reduce and eliminate his or her plaque.

The metabolism of these attached, organized colonies of microorganisms contributes to the inflammation of gingival tissue associated with gingivitis, the destruction of bone and periodontal ligament associated with periodontitis, and the destruction of mineralized tooth structure during the formation of dental decay (dental caries). Many factors contribute to plaque retention, including tooth malpositions and malformations, the irregular surface of advancing dental caries (decay), defective restorations, and accumulation of calculus (tartar).

Technique to Determine (Calculate) a Plaque Score (Index)

Plaque can be stained with *disclosing solution*, a dye that is absorbed by bacterial plaque (Color Plate 8-19). When this solution is swished in the mouth, four tooth surfaces of each tooth are usually evaluated for the presence of the stained plaque: mesial, facial, distal, and lingual. The **plaque index** is calculated as the percentage of sites with plaque divided by the total sites (number of teeth times four). Note: Disclosing solutions should not be used until periodontal measurements and the oral physical exam have been made and reviewed since the color change to oral tissues from the solution may influence the ability to observe the initial findings. A charting example of plaque score calculation is presented for four teeth in Figure 8-12.

E. RELATIONSHIP OF PERIODONTAL DISEASE AND RESTORATIONS (FILLINGS)

A healthy **biologic width** of attached gingiva (known as the dentogingival junction) includes the junctional epithelium (about 1 mm wide), as well as a band of connective tissue fibers (about 1 mm wide) attaching the gingiva to the cementum. Care must be taken when restoring teeth to protect this biologic width of attachment. If a restoration encroaches into the attachment, it could be a factor in initiating periodontal disease (periodontitis/bone loss/attachment loss), gingival recession, or chronically inflamed gingival tissue. Therefore, if a restoration is to be placed to restore an area of decay that has destroyed tooth structure very close to bone, it is advisable to perform a surgical procedure called **crown lengthening** to ensure the restoration does not encroach on the biologic width. Crown lengthening is a procedure that increases the extent of supragingival tooth structure by causing surgical recession through removal of gingival tissue, or apical positioning gingival tissue and usually removing supporting bone.

Further, a defective restoration, especially one that is overcontoured or is not flush with the tooth structure, may retain bacterial plaque more readily, so it could be an initiating factor for periodontal disease. Therefore, it is always important to keep in mind that when teeth must be restored, ideal tooth contours, as have been discussed in the earlier chapters of this text, should be reproduced.

F. RELATIONSHIPS OF TOOTH SUPPORT AND ROOT MORPHOLOGY

The area of root attachment is of primary importance to the stability and health of a tooth. Root attachment area depends on root length, the number of roots, and the cross-sectional diameter of the root from the cementoenamel junction to the apex (*Fig. 8-25*). It also depends on the presence or absence of concavities and other root curvatures. These features greatly influence the resistance of a tooth to occlusal and other forces, particularly when they are applied in a lateral (buccolingual) direction.

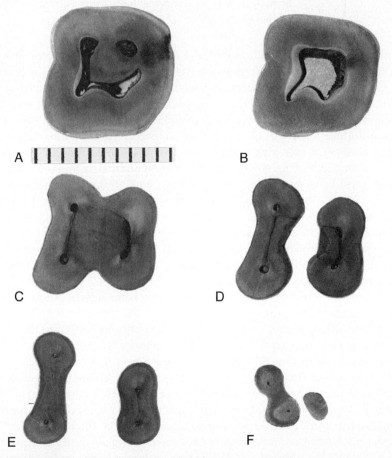

FIGURE 8-25. Series of stained cross sections of a root of a lower first molar from crown to near apices. For each section, the mesial aspect is left, the lingual aspect is above, the distal aspect is right, and the buccal aspect is below. There is a 10-mm scale between the top and the middle section on the left. **A.** Cross section through the crown showing enamel, dentin, and pulp. (Caries is evident distally—on the right.) **B.** Cross section near the cementoenamel junction. Note the shape of the pulp chamber. **C.** Cross section of the root trunk slightly coronal to the bifurcation (furcation). Buccal and lingual depressions are coronal to the entrances to the bifurcation. **D.** Cross section of mesial and distal roots slightly apical to the bifurcation. Note the root canals. Thickened cementum (darkly stained) is apparent on the furcal aspect (between the roots). **E.** Cross section of roots 4 mm apical to the bifurcation. There are pronounced concavities on the mesial aspect of the mesial root and the furcal aspects of both roots. **F.** Cross section of the roots near the apex. The mesial (left) root is longer. The complex shape of molar roots helps provide a greater surface area of attachment and greater tooth stability, but becomes a problem to treat during progressive periodontal disease.

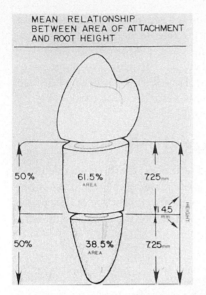

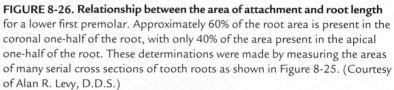

FIGURE 8-26. Relationship between the area of attachment and root length for a lower first premolar. Approximately 60% of the root area is present in the coronal one-half of the root, with only 40% of the area present in the apical one-half of the root. These determinations were made by measuring the areas of many serial cross sections of tooth roots as shown in Figure 8-25. (Courtesy of Alan R. Levy, D.D.S.)

In health, prior to periodontal disease, connective tissue fibers insert into cementum on the entire root surface. This attachment represents insertion of the *gingival fibers* (coronal to the bone level) near the cementoenamel junction, and *periodontal ligament fiber* insertions for the majority of the root. Long roots and wide cross-sectional tooth diameters increase support. Concavities and other root curvatures increase periodontal support in two ways. First, they augment the total surface area. Second, the concave configuration provides multidirectional fiber orientation, which makes the tooth more stable and resistant to occlusal forces. For example, a root with a mesial concavity is more resistant to buccolingual forces than a tooth that is conical or convex (Fig. 8-25). Vertical and longitudinal depressions and concave areas occur commonly on the mesial and distal root surfaces of many anterior and most posterior teeth (as described in earlier chapters). More coronally located root depressions are also found on the mesial surface of maxillary first premolars (both on the root and crown) and on molar root surfaces just coronal to furcations.

Likewise, multirooted teeth have increased support and resistance to applied forces. For those teeth, the location of the furcation is important; the more coronal it is, the more stability is afforded. Additionally, convergence or divergence of roots influences support. Divergent roots increase stability and allow for more interradicular bone support (Fig. 8-23).

Another important factor for determining tooth stability is the degree of root taper. Teeth with conical roots, such as mandibular first premolars, tend to have the majority of their root area (greater than 60%) in the coronal half of the root, and much less area (only about 40%) in the apical half of the root (Fig. 8-26).[6] The degree of root taper influences the support once periodontal disease has occurred. *A conical root may have lost more than 60% of the periodontal ligament, even though it has lost only 50% of the bone height.* This is because a small proportion of the root area is present near the apex. For severely conical roots, the apical half of the root may account for even less attachment area than seen in Figure 8-26.

Based on root area alone, one would generally expect to find the maxillary canine to be the most stable single-rooted tooth, and the mandibular central incisors to be the least stable. For posterior teeth, one would expect maxillary first molars, with their three divergent roots, to be more stable than third molars, which frequently have fused roots. While these rules generally apply, additional factors, such as the presence or absence of inflammatory periodontal disease and excessive occlusal forces, may greatly influence tooth stability. Also, the density and structure of the supporting bone have an influence on tooth stability.

G. INFLUENCE OF ROOT ANATOMY AND ANOMALIES ON PERIODONTAL DISEASE

Although furcations, concavities, vertical grooves, and other root curvatures tend to increase the area of attachment, making the tooth resistant to occlusal forces, these root anatomy features may also become locations (foci) where forces are concentrated. These foci occur because the root curvature and the corresponding bone and periodontal ligaments that conform to it permit the tooth to compress against

3. Which one *maxillary* tooth has its furcation closest to the cervical line of the tooth?
   a. first premolar
   b. second premolar
   c. first molar
   d. second molar
   e. third molar

4. What is the clinical attachment loss of a tooth with +2 mm of gingival recession and a 4-mm pocket?
   a. +2 mm
   b. +6 mm
   c. −6 mm
   d. −2 mm

5. Which of the following periodontal fibers attach to cementum *and* alveolar bone?
   a. horizontal
   b. oblique
   c. transseptal
   d. apical
   e. alveolar crest

6. Which of the following are possible indications of periodontal disease?
   a. bleeding gums
   b. loss of bone
   c. type IV mobility
   d. mucogingival stress
   e. gingival sulcus readings of 3 mm

7. The furcations are likely to be farthest away from the cervical portion of the tooth in which ONE of the following teeth?
   a. mandibular first molar
   b. mandibular second molar
   c. mandibular third molar
   d. maxillary first molar
   e. maxillary second molar

ANSWERS: 1–a, b, c, e; 2–a, b, c, e; 3–c; 4–b; 5–a, b, d, e; 6–a, b, c, d; 7–c

REFERENCES

1. Burt BA. Periodontitis and aging: reviewing recent evidence. JADA 1994;125(Mar):273–279.
2. Kennedy J, Bird W, Palcanis K, et al. A longitudinal evaluation of varying widths of attached gingiva. J Clin Periodontol 1985;12:667.
3. Renner RP. An introduction to dental anatomy and esthetics. Chicago: Quintessence Publishing, 1985:162.
4. Zander H, Polson A. Present status of occlusion and occlusal therapy in periodontics. J Periodontol 1977;48:540.
5. Ericsson I, Lindhe J. Effect of long-standing jiggling on experimental marginal periodontitis in the beagle dog. J Clin Periodontol 1982;9:497.
6. Levy A, Wright W. The relationship between attachment height and attachment area of teeth using a digitizer and digital computer. J Periodontol 1978;49:483.
7. Ramfjord SP, Nissie R. The modified Widman flap. J Periodontol 1974;45:601.
8. Zakariasen KL. New and emerging techniques: promise, achievement and deception. JADA 1995;126(Feb):163.
9. Basaraba N. Root amputation and tooth hemisection. Dent Clin North Am 1969;13:121.
10. Oschenbein C. Current status of osseous surgery. J Periodontol 1977;48:577.

11. Langer B, Langer L. Subepithelial connective tissue flap for root coverage. J Periodontol 1985;56:15.
12. Esthetics and plastic surgery in periodontics. Periodontal 2000 1996;11:1–111.
13. Allen E. Surgical crown lengthening for function and esthetics. Dent Clin North Am 1993;37:163–179.

RESOURCES AND AUTHORITIES FOR PERIODONTICS

The American Academy of Periodontology, Suite 800, 737 North Michigan Avenue, Chicago, Illinois 60611-2690. Website: http://www.perio.org

The American Dental Association, 211 East Chicago Avenue, Chicago, Illinois. 60611. Website: www.ada.org

RESOURCE FOR PERIODONTAL TERMS

Glossary of periodontal terms. 4th ed. Chicago: The American Academy of Periodontology, 2001.

BASIC TEXTBOOKS

Carranza F, Newman M. Clinical periodontology. 9th ed. Philadelphia: W.B. Saunders Company, 2002.

Lindhe J. Clinical periodontology and implant dentistry. 4th ed. Blackwell Munksgaard, Malden, MA, 2003.

RESOURCES FOR THE PATHOGENESIS, DIAGNOSIS, AND RISK FACTORS FOR PERIODONTAL DISEASES AND PERIODONTAL THERAPY

Proceedings of the 1996 World Workshop in Periodontics, 1996. The Annals of Periodontology. Chicago: The American Academy of Periodontology.

Periodontal literature reviews: a summary of current knowledge. Chicago: The American Academy of Periodontology, 1996.

RESOURCE FOR PERIODONTAL DISEASE CLASSIFICATION

1999 International workshop for a classification of periodontal diseases and conditions. The Annals of Periodontology. Chicago: The American Academy of Periodontology.

Application of Root and Pulp Morphology Related to Endodontic Therapy

9

CONTRIBUTED BY JOHN M. NUSSTEIN, D.D.S., M.S., ASSOCIATE PROFESSOR, SECTION OF ENDODONTICS, THE OHIO STATE UNIVERSITY

OBJECTIVES

This chapter is designed to prepare the learner to perform the following:

- Describe the four types of root canal configurations I to IV.
- Describe the normal shape and location of the pulp chamber for each class of tooth.
- Identify the number of pulp horns normally found within each type of secondary (adult) tooth.
- Identify the number of canals most likely to be found within the roots of each type of secondary (adult) tooth.
- Describe the scope of responsibility for an endodontist.
- Describe endodontic therapy.

SECTION I. INTERNAL PULP CAVITY MORPHOLOGY RELATED TO ENDODONTIC AND RESTORATIVE THERAPY

A. THE SHAPE OF PULP CAVITIES AND CONFIGURATION OF PULP CANALS

The **pulp cavity** is the cavity in the central portion of the tooth containing the nerves and blood supply to the tooth. It is divided into the pulp chamber (more coronal) and the root canals (in the roots).

1. PULP CHAMBER AND PULP HORNS

The **pulp chamber** is the most occlusal or incisal portion of the pulp cavity. There is one pulp chamber in each tooth. It may be located partly in the crown of anterior teeth, but in posterior

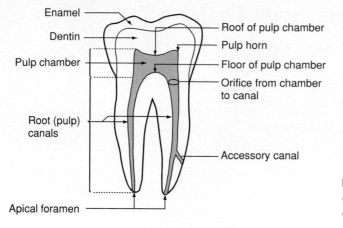

Enamel
Dentin
Pulp chamber
Root (pulp) canals
Apical foramen

Roof of pulp chamber
Pulp horn
Floor of pulp chamber
Orifice from chamber to canal
Accessory canal

FIGURE 9-1. Parts of a pulp cavity. The pulp cavity of this mandibular second molar is made up of a coronal pulp chamber and two root (pulp) canals.

teeth, it is mostly in the cervical part of the root. Its walls are the innermost surface of the dentin. Each pulp chamber has a *roof* at its incisal or occlusal border often with projections called **pulp horns**, and the pulp chambers of multirooted teeth have a *floor* at the cervical portion with an opening (orifice) for each root canal (*Fig. 9-1*). The number of pulp horns found within each cusped tooth (molars, premolars, and canines) is normally one horn per functional cusp, and in young incisors, it is three (one horn per facial lobe, which is the same as one lobe per mamelon). An **exception** is one type of maxillary lateral incisor (called a peg lateral with an incisal edge that somewhat resembles one cusp) that forms from one lobe so has only one pulp horn. Refer to *Table 9-1* for a summary of the number of pulp horns related to the number of cusps normally found within different tooth types.

2. ROOT CANALS (PULP CANALS)

Root canals (pulp canals) are the portions of the pulp cavity located within the root(s) of a tooth. Root canals connect to the pulp chamber through **canal orifices** on the floor of the pulp chamber and open to the outside of the tooth through openings called **apical foramina** (singular foramen) most commonly located at or near the root apex (Fig. 9-1). The shape and number of root canals in any one root

Table 9-1	GUIDELINES FOR NUMBER OF PULP HORNS IN ADULT TEETH:	
	# CUSPS	# PULP HORNS
Maxillary central incisor	—	3
Maxillary lateral incisor	—	1–3 (variable)
Maxillary canine	1	1
Maxillary 1 premolar	2	2
Maxillary 2 premolar	2	2
Maxillary 1 molar	4 (or 5 if Carabelli)	4 (Carabelli is functionless)
Maxillary 2 molar	4	4
Mandibular central incisor	—	3
Mandibular lateral incisor	—	3
Mandibular canine	1	1
Mandibular 1 premolar	2	1 or 2 (lingual cusp may be functionless)
Mandibular 2 premolar	2–3	2–3
Mandibular 1 molar	5	5
Mandibular 2 molar	4	4

General Learning Guidelines
INCISORS: 3 (Except maxillary lateral, which could be peg = 1)
CUSPED TEETH: 1 pulp horn under each functional cusp

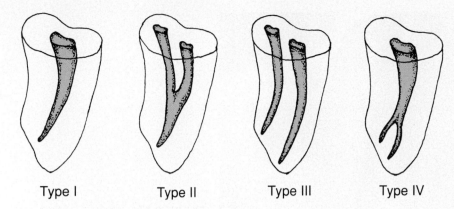

| Type I | Type II | Type III | Type IV |

FIGURE 9-2. Types of canal configurations occurring in one root.

have been divided into four major, anatomic configurations (*Fig. 9-2*). The type I configuration has one canal, whereas types II, III, and IV have either *two* canals or one canal that is spilt into *two* for part of the root. The four canal types are defined as follows:

Type I—*one canal* extends from the pulp chamber to the apex.
Type II—*two separate canals* leave the pulp chamber, but they join short of the apex to form one canal apically and one apical foramen.
Type III—*two separate canals* leave the pulp chamber and remain separate, exiting the root apically as two separate apical foramina.
Type IV—one canal leaves the pulp chamber but divides in the apical third of the root into *two separate canals* with two separate apical foramina.

Accessory (or lateral) canals also occur, located most commonly in the apical third of the root (*Fig. 9-3A and B*) and, in maxillary and mandibular molars, in the furcation area [64% of the time[1]].

B.   SHAPE OF PULP CAVITIES IN SOUND YOUNG TEETH

LEARNING EXERCISE

Section extracted teeth to expose the pulp cavity: the size, shape, and variations of pulp cavities are best studied by the interesting operation of grinding off one side of an extracted tooth. Wearing a mask and gloves, you can use a dental lathe equipped with a fine-grained abrasive wheel about 3 inches in diameter and 3/8-inch thick to remove any part of the tooth. Simply decide which surface is to be removed, hold the tooth securely in your fingers, and apply this surface firmly to the flat surface of the abrasive wheel. Operating the lathe at a fairly high speed is less apt to flip the specimen from your fingers than operating it at a low speed. If you can devise an arrangement by which a small stream of water is run onto the surface of the wheel as the tooth is ground, you will eliminate flying tooth dust and the bad odor of hot tooth tissue. If such an arrangement is not feasible, keep the tooth moist by frequently dipping the surface being ground in water or by dripping water onto the wheel with a medicine dropper. Look often at the tooth surface you are cutting and adjust your applied pressure to attain the plane in which you wish the tooth to be cut. A high-speed dental handpiece and bur will greatly facilitate your exploration of the insides of teeth.

Extracted teeth should always be sterilized as described in the introduction of this text, and kept moist. As you remove different sides of each kind of tooth, notice how the external contours of the pulp chamber are similar to the external morphology of the tooth. On incisors and canines, remove either the facial or

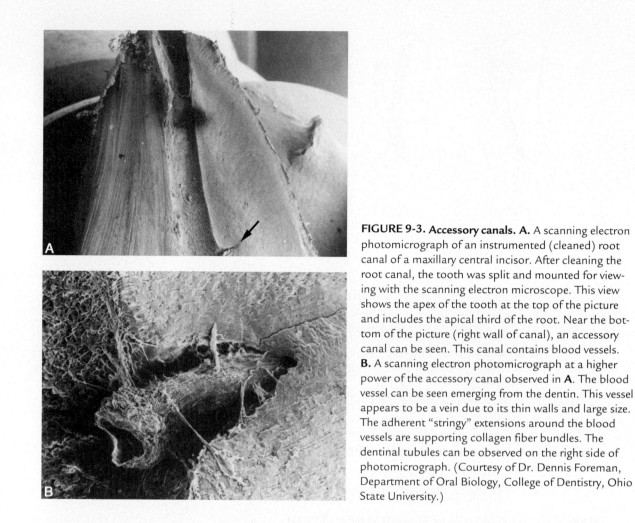

FIGURE 9-3. Accessory canals. A. A scanning electron photomicrograph of an instrumented (cleaned) root canal of a maxillary central incisor. After cleaning the root canal, the tooth was split and mounted for viewing with the scanning electron microscope. This view shows the apex of the tooth at the top of the picture and includes the apical third of the root. Near the bottom of the picture (right wall of canal), an accessory canal can be seen. This canal contains blood vessels. **B.** A scanning electron photomicrograph at a higher power of the accessory canal observed in **A**. The blood vessel can be seen emerging from the dentin. This vessel appears to be a vein due to its thin walls and large size. The adherent "stringy" extensions around the blood vessels are supporting collagen fiber bundles. The dentinal tubules can be observed on the right side of photomicrograph. (Courtesy of Dr. Dennis Foreman, Department of Oral Biology, College of Dentistry, Ohio State University.)

lingual side from some teeth to view the mesiodistal plane (as seen in *Fig. 9-4A and E*), and remove the mesial or distal side from others to view the faciolingual plane (as seen in *Fig. 9-4B, C, and D*).

On premolars and molars, the removal of either the mesial or distal side will expose the outline of the roof of the pulp chamber where pulp horns can be seen extending beneath the cusps (as seen in premolars in Fig. 9-4C and D). When the buccal or lingual sides are removed to the level of the buccal and lingual cusp tips, pulp cavities can be seen in a mesiodistal plane (as seen in Fig. 9-4E), the view similar to that seen on a dental radiograph. Finally, on molars, the removal of the occlusal surface will reveal the openings (orifices) to the root canals on the floor of the pulp chamber (as seen later in the diagram in *Fig. 9-9* and the close-up view in Fig. 9-13).

1. PULP SHAPE IN ANTERIOR TEETH (INCISORS AND CANINES)

a. Pulp Chamber and Pulp Horns of Anterior Teeth

When cut mesiodistally and viewed from the *facial* (or lingual) (similar to the view on dental radiographs), the pulp chambers of incisors are broad and may have a suggestion of multiple pulp horns. (Only two horns can be seen in the maxillary central incisors in *Fig. 9-5*.) However, the incisal border of the pulp wall (roof of chamber) of a young tooth may show the configuration of three mamelons (that is, has developed with three pulp horns: located mesially, centrally, and distally). Also, recall that the unusual peg lateral incisor only has one pulp horn. Knowing the number and location of these pulp horns becomes important when the tooth is fractured or badly decayed and must be prepared for an incisal restoration. When cut labiolingually and viewed

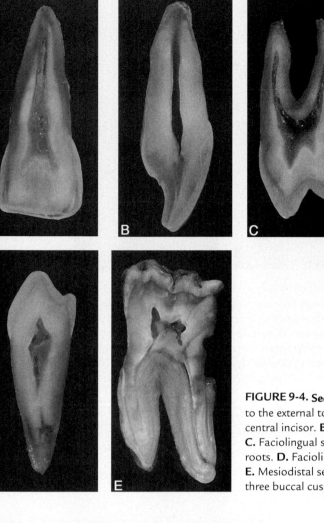

FIGURE 9-4. Sectioned teeth showing pulp cavity shape relative to the external tooth surface. A. Mesiodistal section of a maxillary central incisor. B. Faciolingual section of a maxillary canine. C. Faciolingual section of a maxillary first premolar with two roots. D. Faciolingual section of mandibular first premolar. E. Mesiodistal section of a mandibular first molar through its three buccal cusps.

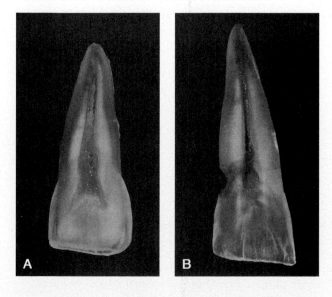

FIGURE 9-5. Maxillary central incisors sectioned mesiodistally. A. Maxillary central incisor (young tooth), facial side removed. The high pulp horns (only two are visible in this tooth section) and the broad root canal indicate that this is a young tooth. This outline of the pulp cavity may be seen on a dental radiograph. B. Maxillary central incisor (old tooth), facial side removed. The pulp chamber of this older tooth is partially filled with secondary dentin and the root canal is narrower than in the tooth shown in A. Also, the incisal edge is worn to a straight line. (The damage to the cervical part of the root on the distal [left] side of the tooth has been there for some time because the underlying dentin has been altered by a defense mechanism of the pulp tissues.)

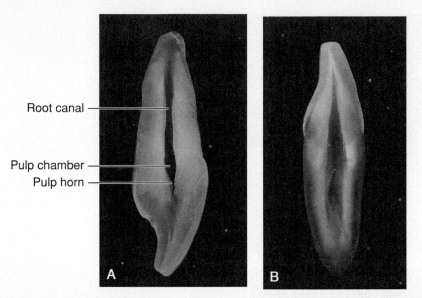

Root canal

Pulp chamber

Pulp horn

FIGURE 9-6. Incisors sectioned faciolingually. A. Maxillary central incisor, mesial side removed. There is wear (attrition) on the incisal edge, and secondary dentin has begun to fill in the incisal part of the pulp chamber. The root canal is moderately wide. As commonly occurs, much of the pulp chamber is located in the cervical third of the root. It is *not* possible to see this view of the pulp cavity on a dental radiograph. **B.** Mandibular lateral incisor, mesial side removed (young tooth). Curvature of the root prevented cutting the pulp cavity in one plane, so that the apical portion was lost. Notice how the pulp cavity extends in a narrow point toward the incisal edge. Even extensive attrition on the incisal edge would not likely to expose the pulp since secondary dentin would form in the incisal part of the pulp chamber and the pulp would be additionally protected.

from the *proximal*, the pulp chambers of anterior teeth taper to a point toward the incisal edge *(Fig. 9-6)*. In maxillary and mandibular canines, the incisal wall or roof of the pulp chamber is often rounded, having only one pulp horn *(Fig. 9-7)*.

b. Root Canal(s) of Anterior Teeth

Recall that all anterior teeth are most likely to have one root. *The number of root canals in each type of anterior tooth is also most frequently one. Maxillary* central incisors, lateral incisors, and canines *almost always* have one canal (type I), whereas *mandibular* anterior teeth, although *most likely* to

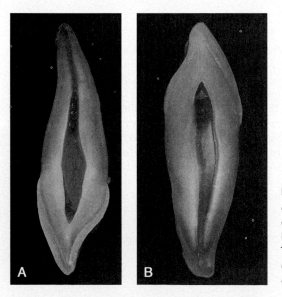

FIGURE 9-7. Canines sectioned faciolingually. A. Maxillary canine, mesial side removed (young tooth). There is no attrition evident on the incisal edge, and the pulp cavity is still large. **B.** Mandibular canine, mesial side removed (young tooth). The pulp cavity is large. Only at the incisal tip is there a little evidence of secondary dentin formation. The roof of the chamber is slightly more rounded than on incisors.

have one canal (60% of the time), may have two canals (one facial and one lingual) with the frequency varying depending on the study cited.[2–4] [For example, **mandibular central incisors** may have two canals with two separate apical foramina (type III) 3% of the time, and two canals converging to one foramen (type II) from 17 to 43% of the time. **Mandibular lateral incisors** may have two canals from 20 to 45% of the time (usually type II with one foramen or type III with two separate foramina about 3% of the time).] **Mandibular canines** may have two canals from 4 to 22% of the time. When two canals are present, one is facial, and one is lingual [often with type IV formation]. (Recall that the mandibular canine is the anterior tooth most likely to have two *roots*: one facial and one lingual.)

2. PULP SHAPE IN PREMOLARS

a. Pulp Chambers and Pulp Horns in Premolars

When premolars are cut mesiodistally and viewed from the facial (or lingual) similar to the view on dental radiographs, the occlusal border or roof of the pulp chamber is curved beneath the cusp similarly to the curvature of the occlusal surface (*Fig. 9-8A*). When cut buccolingually and viewed from the proximal, the pulp chamber often has the general outline of the tooth surface, sometimes including a constriction near or apical to the cervix (seen in *Fig. 9-8B*). The pulp horns on the roof are visible beneath each cusp, and their relative lengths are similar to the relative heights of the cusps. Thus, the buccal horn is longer than the lingual horn.

In general, premolars have one pulp horn per functional cusp. Therefore, the premolars that are the two-cusp type most often have two pulp horns, but mandibular second premolars that are the three-cusp type have three pulp horns, and the mandibular first premolars that have a functionless lingual cusp may have only one pulp horn, similar to a canine.

b. Root Canal(s) and Orifices of Premolars

Maxillary first premolars *most often have two roots* (one buccal and one lingual) *and two canals* (one in each root). Approximately 57% of these first premolars have two roots, but only 39% have one root.[5] The average incidence of two canals, one in the buccal root and one in the lingual root, is 90%. [When two roots are present, the canals in both roots exhibit a type I configuration, and, when one root is present, the canal configuration is either a type II or type III.[5]] The incidence of

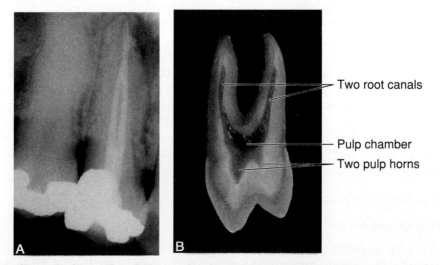

Two root canals

Pulp chamber

Two pulp horns

FIGURE 9-8. A. Radiograph of a maxillary first premolar reveals the two root canals (filled with a filling material that makes the canals appear whiter). This is a similar view as a premolar sectioned mesiodistally. **B. Maxillary first premolar sectioned faciolingually,** mesial side removed (young tooth). The curvature of the tips of the roots prevented cutting the root canals in one plane. The pulp horns are sharp; there is little, if any, secondary dentin; and the floor of the pulp chamber is rounded. The buccal pulp horn is considerably longer than the lingual horn. Notice the floor of the pulp chamber, which has two openings, one for each canal. Also, note the constriction of the pulp chamber near the cervix.

Endodontic access openings

Maxillary teeth | Mandibular teeth

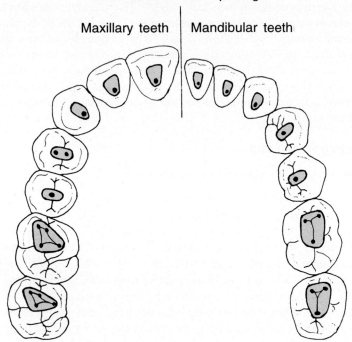

FIGURE 9-9. Access preparations into pulp chambers showing orifices to canals. Ideally shaped openings provide access into the pulp chamber for endodontic treatment. Pulp canal orifices on the floor of each pulp chamber correspond with the number and location of pulp canals in each tooth. The left half of the arch shows maxillary teeth; the right half shows mandibular teeth.

three roots is approximately 4%.[5] The dentist must know the location of each canal opening on the pulp chamber floor in order to remove diseased pulpal tissue from the *entire* pulp cavity. The buccal canal orifice in the maxillary first premolar (viewed through the prepared access opening and the roof of the pulp chamber removed in *Fig. 9-9*) is located just lingual to the buccal cusp tip. The lingual canal orifice is located just lingual to the central groove.

Maxillary second premolars most often have *one root* but may have one or two canals. According to one researcher, the average incidence of two canals is about 59% [type II or type III].[6] Three canals occur about 1% of the time.[6] When there is one canal, its orifice on the pulp chamber floor is located in the exact center of the tooth (Fig. 9-9). If the orifice is located toward the buccal or the lingual, it probably means that there are two canals in the root.

Mandibular first and second premolars most frequently have *one root* and *one root canal* (type I) about 70% of the time in first premolars (*Fig. 9-10A*) and 98% in second premolars. Mandibular first premolars may have two canals (type IV) 24% of the time (*Fig. 9-10B*), but mandibular second premolars have two canals only 2.5% of the time.[7] The single canal orifice is located on the floor of the pulp chamber just buccal to the center of the occlusal surface (see Fig. 9-9).

3. PULP SHAPE IN MOLARS

a. Pulp Chambers and Pulp Horns in Molars

The pulp chamber of **maxillary first and second molars** is broader buccolingually than mesiodistally (like the crown) and is often constricted near the floor of the chamber (seen best in *Fig. 9-11A and B*). On **mandibular first and second molars**, the chamber is broader mesiodistally than buccolingually (like the overall crown shape). This difference in shape of pulp chambers for maxillary versus mandibular molars can be appreciated by studying the openings used to access the pulp chambers for molars in Figure 9-9. As in all cusped teeth, molars have one pulp horn per functional cusp, and they are located in the roof of the pulp chamber well be-

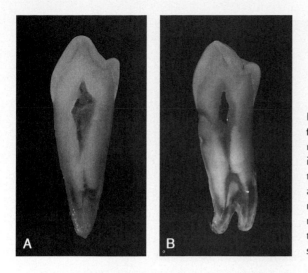

FIGURE 9-10. Mandibular first premolars sectioned faciolingually. A. Mandibular first premolar, distal side removed. Root curvature prevented cutting the root canal in one plane. The pulp horn in the buccal cusp is large; in the lingual cusp, it is small. It is unusual to observe much of a pulp horn beneath the nonfunctional lingual cusp on mandibular first premolars. B. Mandibular first premolar, mesial side removed, with root and root canal divided near the apex (type IV). Only one pulp horn is evident in this sectioned tooth.

neath each cusp. Therefore, if we consider the cusps of Carabelli to be functionless, all four-cusp types of molars have four pulp horns, and the mandibular first molar with five cusps is the only type of molar to have five pulp horns. (Notice the three pulp horns under the three buccal cusps in Figure 9-12A.) The pulp chamber is normally deep to, or some distance from, the occlusal surface, actually located within the cervical part of the root trunk *(Fig. 9-12)*. Surprisingly, the pulp chamber on a maxillary molar often is not penetrated by the dentist until the drill reaches the level of the gum line. One exception might be the pulp horn of the prominent mesiolingual cusp of the maxillary molars (Fig. 9-11A). The *floor* of the pulp chamber is considerably apical to the cervical line; it is located in the root trunk. The pulp floor has multiple openings (orifices), one for each root canal. The floor is level or flat in young teeth. It may become convex in older teeth with the deposition of additional dentin over time.

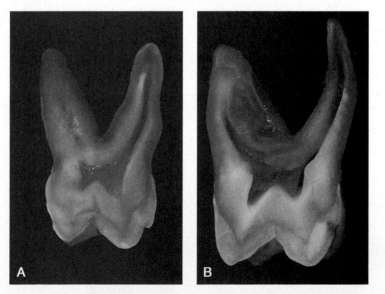

FIGURE 9-11. Maxillary first molars sectioned buccolingually. A. Young tooth with mesial side removed; lingual side (with cusp of Carabelli) is on the right. The tooth is sectioned through the center of the lingual root canal, but not through the center of the mesiobuccal canal. The pulp chamber is seen to open into the lingual root canal. The floor of the pulp chamber is relatively flat as it often is on young teeth. B. Young tooth with mesial side removed; lingual side is on the right. There is an area of dental decay (caries) appearing darker in the groove where the small cusp of Carabelli is attached to the mesiolingual cusp. The tooth is sectioned through the mesiobuccal and lingual root canals. The pulp chamber is mostly in the root trunk. Only mesiobuccal and mesiolingual pulp horns extend a little into the part of tooth we define as the anatomic crown (covered with enamel).

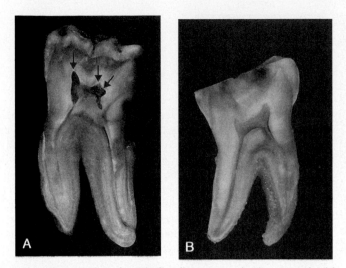

FIGURE 9-12. Mandibular first molars sectioned mesiodistally. A. Buccal side removed (old tooth). The apical foramen of the distal root is on the distal side of the root, not at the root tip. Notice the three pulp horns (at arrows) under the three buccal cusps shown in this section. The unusual thickening of cementum on the roots is hypercementosis. **B.** Old tooth (exhibiting occlusal wear) with lingual side removed. Again, notice that the roof of the pulp chamber is about at the level of the cervical line. Two pulp horns extend occlusal to the cervical line. The rest of the pulp chamber is in the root trunk. The floor of the pulp chamber is convex (a condition founded in older teeth) because of the deposition of secondary dentin. (There appears to be caries in the enamel above the mesiolingual pulp horn, but it has penetrated only slightly into the dentin.)

b. Root Canal(s) and Orifices of Molars

Maxillary first molars most frequently have *three roots* (mesiobuccal, distobuccal, and palatal), *but four canals*: one each in the distobuccal and palatal root, but two in the mesiobuccal root. In the **palatal root**, the canal is larger and more easily accessible from the floor of the pulp chamber than for the other two roots, but this root and its canal often curve toward the buccal in the *apical* third, requiring skillful procedures to clean and treat it. The **mesiobuccal root** of the maxillary first molar has two canals 90% of the time [one located more buccally within this root called *mesiobuccal canal*, and one located more lingually within this root called the *mesiolingual canal*.[8] Type III canal systems have been reported to occur 33–60% of the time.[8]] The distobuccal root most often has one canal.

On maxillary first molars, there are four orifices on the floor of the pulp chamber: one for each canal *(Fig. 9-13)*. Opening into the palatal root canal, the palatal orifice on the floor of the pulp chamber is located beneath the mesiolingual cusp (Fig. 9-9). Opening into the mesiobuccal root, the mesiobuccal orifice is located slightly mesial to and beneath the mesiobuccal cusp tip. The mesiolingual orifice is located slightly to the palatal aspect of the mesiobuccal orifice. Usually, this orifice is difficult to locate because of an overhanging dentin shelf. Opening into the distobuccal root, the distobuccal canal orifice is located on a line between the palatal orifice

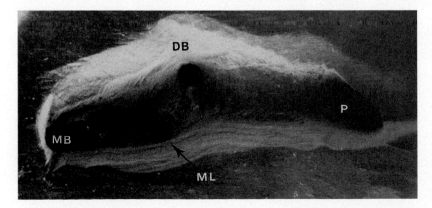

FIGURE 9-13. Scanning electron photomicrograph of the pulp chamber floor of a maxillary molar with four canal orifices. The palatal (P), mesiobuccal (MB), distobuccal (DB), and mesiolingual (ML, *arrow*) orifices are identified for orientation. (Original magnification ×20.) (Courtesy of Dr. James Gilles and Dr. Al Reader.)

and the buccal developmental groove at a point just short of the angle formed by the buccal and distal walls of the pulp chamber.

Maxillary second molars, like maxillary first molars, most frequently have *three roots and four canals*. The distobuccal and palatal roots each have one canal. The mesiobuccal root has two canals 70% of the time.[8] The location of the orifices in the maxillary second molar is similar to the maxillary first molar, except that they are closer together (Fig. 9-9).

Both mandibular first and second molars most frequently have *two roots* (mesial and distal) and *three canals* (two in the wider mesial root and one in the distal root). The roof of the pulp chamber is often at the same level as the cervical border of the enamel, with only the pulp horns extending into the anatomic crown (Fig. 9-12). Most of the pulp chamber is located within the root trunk. The **mesial root** usually has two canals: *mesiobuccal* and *mesiolingual*. [The mesial roots of mandibular *first* molars have two canals virtually all of the time: a type III canal system is present 60% of the time and a type II canal system is present 40% of the time.[9] The mesial roots of mandibular *second* molars have two canals 64% of the time: a type II canal system 38% of the time and a type III canal system 26% of the time, but one canal 27% of the time.[7]] The **distal roots** of mandibular first and second molars usually have one canal [but, on mandibular first molars, there are two canals approximately 35% of the time, usually type II configuration,[10] whereas the distal roots of mandibular second molars have one canal 92% of the time[7]].

In both **mandibular first and second molars**, the mesiobuccal canal orifice on the chamber floor is located slightly mesial but close to the *mesiobuccal* cusp tip (Fig. 9-9). The *mesiolingual* canal orifice is just lingual to the mesial developmental groove of the mesial marginal ridge. It is not under the mesiolingual cusp tip but is in a more central location. If the distal root has one canal, the *distal canal orifice* is large and located just distal to the center of the crown. When two canals are present, the distolingual orifice is small and is located centrally just lingual to the central fossa. Careful inspection of the chamber floor toward the buccal will successfully locate the distobuccal orifice.

Maxillary third molars usually have three root canals and **mandibular third molars** usually have two. However, they do vary considerably in form with some teeth having only two root canals. Third molars are 9–11 years younger biologically than first molars, completing their development later in life than first and second molars. Therefore, on radiographs (x-ray films), their pulp chambers and root canals are generally larger than in the other molars in the same mouth, especially for patients between the ages of 15 and 35 years.

Refer to *Table 9-2* for a summary of the number of root canals related to the number of roots normally found within different tooth types.

Table 9-2	MOST COMMON NUMBER OF ROOTS AND CANALS IN ADULT TEETH	
TOOTH NAME	**# ROOTS**	**# ROOT CANALS**
Maxillary central incisor	1	**1**
Maxillary lateral incisor	1	**1**
Maxillary canine	1	**1**
Maxillary 1st premolar	2 (buccal and lingual) or 1	**2** (even if 1 root)
Maxillary 2nd premolar	1	**1**
Maxillary 1st molar	3 (mesiobuccal, distobuccal, and lingual)	**4** (2 in mesiobuccal root)
Maxillary 2nd molar	3 (mesiobuccal, distobuccal, and lingual)	**4** (2 in mesiobuccal root)
Mandibular central incisor	1	**1**
Mandibular lateral incisor	1	**1**
Mandibular canine	1 (but has 2 roots more often than other anterior teeth: buccal and lingual)	**1**
Mandibular 1st premolar	1	**1**
Mandibular 2nd premolar	1	**1**
Mandibular 1st molar	2 (mesial and distal)	**3** (2 in mesial)
Mandibular 2nd molar	2 (mesial and distal)	**3** (2 in mesial)

4. PULP SHAPE IN PRIMARY TEETH

The shape of the pulp chamber in **primary** (deciduous) **teeth** will be discussed in Chapter 10. Briefly, these teeth generally have thinner amounts of dentin and enamel, so their pulp cavities are proportionally much larger than on secondary teeth, and their pulp horns are closer to the occlusal surface.

C. WHY PULP CAVITIES GET SMALLER IN OLDER TEETH

In a young tooth, the pulp chamber is large and resembles the shape of the crown surface. It has projections called horns extending beneath the cusps or mamelons in the roof of the chamber and is usually constricted somewhat at the cervix. In old teeth, the pulp chamber becomes smaller and is more apically located because of deposits of **secondary** (additional) **dentin** produced by specialized cells called odontoblasts lining the pulp chamber. Dentin formation normally continues as long as the pulp is intact or vital. Dentin forms on the wall of the pulp cavity, thickening the dentin and making the pulp chamber and canals smaller. Dentin formation over a lifetime may be stimulated to occur *more rapidly* or in greater quantity when the tooth is subjected to attrition (wear), trauma, or caries (that is, tooth decay), or when calcium hydroxide dental cement is applied on the pulp. A **pulp cap** is a term describing a procedure where the dentist places calcium hydroxide next to the pulp (an indirect pulp cap) or over a small bit of exposed healthy pulp (a direct pulp cap) at the depth of a very deep cavity preparation in order to stimulate the formation of a new layer of dentin to help the tooth heal.

The deposition of dentin over time results in reduction in size of the pulp chamber. In some cases, it may become entirely filled. Reduction in size makes finding and accessing the pulp chamber more difficult in an older patient than in the younger patient where the teeth still have larger chambers. The floor of the pulp chamber is nearly flat in young teeth, later becoming convex. [In a radiographic study of 259 children in England, from their 11th to 14th birthdays, the mesiodistal and roof-to-floor pulp dimensions were recorded with a Lysta-Dent Digitizer. Mesiodistal reduction in size in mandibular first molars over 3 years was minimal (1–3.5%) compared to a considerable height reduction (15%) of the pulp chambers. This was mostly the result of secondary dentin deposition on the floor, not the roof, of the chamber.[11]]

The diameter of the root canal also decreases in size with age, getting small in older teeth because of the gradual addition of dentin of the internal wall over the years. The canal may be round, flat, or ribbon shaped. Teeth, other than third molars, exhibiting unusually large pulp chambers on dental radiographs are immediately suspected of having **necrotic pulps** (that is, pulps that no longer have vital nerve or blood supply), which can be a possible source of infection. Without vital pulp tissue, dentin formation ceases, and the pulp chamber size remains constant (once the pulp died) rather than continuing to decrease in size as is normal for vital teeth.

D. CLINICAL APPLICATION OF PULP MORPHOLOGY RELATED TO RESTORATIVE DENTISTRY

The dentist's knowledge of normal pulp shape, size and depth beneath the enamel is important to the dentist when preparing teeth that have deep decay. When the dentist determines that the tooth can be restored without the need to remove the pulp, he or she prepares the tooth in such a way to avoid disturbing or injuring the pulpal tissues. Whenever possible, the goal is to leave some sound (undecayed) dentin on the floor of the cavity preparation to provide support for the restoration (such as a filling using composite resin or amalgam), and to avoid exposing any part of the pulp cavity with a cutting bur or hand instrument. This is accomplished through a knowledge of the shape of the pulp chamber and canals, and a careful evaluation of the patient's radiographs to determine the location of the pulp relative to the decay and external surface of the tooth. An example of deep decay relative to the pulp is seen in Figure 9-14. Also, the dentist must avoid overheating or drying out (desiccating) the tooth during preparation by using water to reduce the heat that is generated by the cutting burs used in a high-speed handpiece.

Sometimes, however, signs (what is seen), symptoms (what the patient feels), and diagnostic tests may indicate that a pulp inflammation (**pulpitis**) is *irreversible*, and cannot be resolved without removing the pulp tissue. When these signs, symptoms, and diagnostic test results indicate a pulp is not likely to respond well by placing just a filling (dental restoration of amalgam or composite), the pulp tissue must be removed and a root canal filling placed (endodontic therapy must be performed). The implications of dental anatomy on restorative dentistry are discussed in more detail in Chapter 13.

E. CLINICAL APPLICATION OF PULP MORPHOLOGY RELATED TO ENDODONTICS

1. ENDODONTICS DEFINED

Endodontics is a specialty branch of dentistry concerned with the morphology, physiology, and pathology of human dental pulp and periapical tissues. Its study and practice encompasses the related basic and clinical sciences, including biology of the normal pulp; the etiology, diagnosis, prevention, and treatment of diseases and injuries of the pulp; and resultant pathologic **periradicular** conditions (that is, pathosis around the root).[12]

An **endodontist** is a dentist who specializes in endodontics (root canal therapy). An endodontist is specially trained to provide root canal therapy, including treating patients with more difficult and complex endodontic situations that may be referred from a general dentist. Treatment may involve difficult root canal anatomy, medically compromised patients, and/or surgical treatments of periapical pathosis and infection.

2. DIAGNOSIS OF PULPAL AND PERIAPICAL DISEASE

Irreversible pulpitis (inflammation of the pulp that cannot be healed) is a condition of the pulp tissue where the pulp will not heal and root canal treatment is indicated. The tooth is unusually sensitive to cold or hot, and sometimes either stimulus may cause an exaggerated response (prolonged pain). The patient may also experience *spontaneous* pain in the tooth (that is, pain felt without provocation of such stimuli as heavy chewing, or exposure to hot or cold). The usual cause of irreversible pulpitis is deep caries (decay), although deep or poorly adapted restorations may also contribute. The proximity of caries to the pulp can often be evaluated best using dental radiographs (*Fig. 9-14*). As the caries approaches the pulp, a normal defense reaction will occur involving inflammation and formation of reparative dentin. However, when the caries reaches (exposes) the pulp, bacteria will overwhelm the defenses, and the tooth usually becomes painful. This prompts the patient to seek emergency dental treatment. Access to, and removal of, affected pulp tissue will provide relief from the pain. The pulp tissue *cannot* be successfully treated with medications alone once the pulp is *irreversibly* damaged.

Periapical disease occurs when the pulp has died (becomes **necrotic**). When the pulp has been overwhelmed by the disease process in the crown, the pulp tissue in the root canals gradually dies. The bacteria and products of pulpal breakdown contained within the root canals cause the periapical tissue around the tooth to react to this insult. A chronic inflammatory response ensues in the bone with the formation of a **granuloma** (that is, a mass of chronic inflammatory tissue enclosed within a fibrous capsule). Since a granuloma is less dense than bone, a radiograph will usually reveal

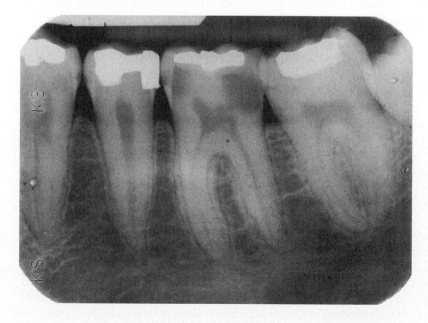

FIGURE 9-14. Dental decay (caries) exposing the pulp. Radiograph of a lower left first molar with a distal carious lesion (seen as an area of lost enamel and darkened dentin) that has reached (exposed) the pulp. There is also mesial caries on this tooth that does not appear to have reached the pulp.

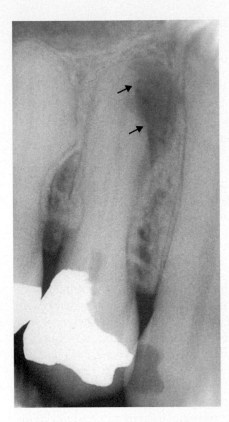

FIGURE 9-15. Periapical radiolucency. Radiograph of a maxillary first premolar with the dark surrounding the root apices indicating the pulp has become necrotic and a granuloma or cyst has developed in the bone, probably as a result of the exposure of the pulp to deep caries that was removed and restored with a large amalgam filling (seen as a white outline) that covers the distal and occlusal surfaces of this tooth.

a radiolucency (**periapical radiolucency** is the dark area at end of the root; *Fig. 9-15*). In some cases, the granuloma undergoes degeneration and a **cyst** is formed. A cyst is an epithelium-lined sac filled with liquid or semiliquid material. The difference between a granuloma and a cyst cannot be determined on a radiograph.

When the bacteria from the root canal overwhelm the defenses of the periapical tissues or the patient's immune system is compromised, bacteria invade the surrounding bone and soft tissue, resulting in severe pain and/or facial swelling. Cleaning the root canals and draining the area of infection will usually provide relief within 2 to 3 days.

Another sequela to pulpal trauma (like being hit in the mouth with a baseball) is the discoloration of the tooth crown to a gray or brownish color, which indicates the need to evaluate the tooth for possible endodontic treatment. After the root canal, the discoloration can be greatly reduced by using an intracoronal bleaching technique where the bleach is placed within the access opening to the pulp chamber for a period of time. See the change on tooth color in Color Plate 20A and B.

3. ENDODONTIC THERAPY

The *goal* of endodontic therapy is to relieve pain, control infection, and preserve the tooth so it may function normally during mastication. Endodontic treatment is normally preferred to extraction because if the tooth was extracted, the patient would be without the tooth throughout the healing process and during the time required to construct and place the replacement tooth. Further, endodontic therapy is less expensive than having a tooth extracted and subsequently replaced with a dental prosthesis (bridge) or an implant.

The first step of the endodontic procedure is for the dentist to gain access to the pulp chamber and the root canals of teeth through an **access opening** in the crown of the tooth. On anterior teeth, the opening is made on the lingual surface and on posterior teeth through the occlusal surface. These access openings vary considerably from cavity preparations used in operative dentistry. The shape (outline form), size, and position of the access opening are determined by studying ideal openings of maxillary and mandibular teeth shown in Figure 9-9, and then modifying them to conform to what is present on the initial radiograph of the tooth. Finding the pulp may be difficult in older teeth or teeth that have large or deep restorations since the formation of secondary or reparative dentin may

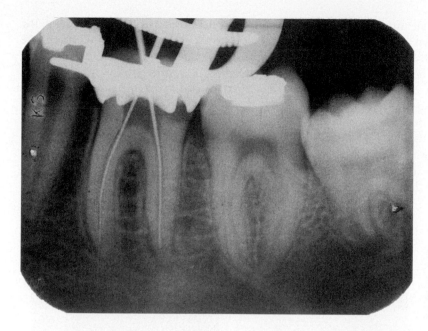

FIGURE 9-16. Endodontic files seen on radiograph. Radiograph of a lower left first molar where endodontic files have been placed within the root canals to the cementodentinal junction apically.

obliterate the pulp chamber, making endodontic access difficult. Further, if the tooth is covered with a metal crown, the pulp chamber will not be visible on the radiograph.

Once the access opening is complete, the dentist locates the root canal orifices on the floor of the pulp chamber. A knowledge of the number of root canals present in teeth is *critically important* to successful endodontic treatment. Not locating and cleaning all the canals may result in continued discomfort for the patient or unsuccessful endodontic treatment with ensuing periapical disease. When the canal orifices have been located, endodontic files are used to remove the diseased pulp tissue, and to clean and refine the canals. The files are carefully inserted into the root canals after the file length is approximated by measuring the length of the corresponding root and crown on the preoperative radiograph. A radiograph is then made with the files in the root *(Fig. 9-16)*. The positions and length of the files are adjusted to extend to approximately 1 mm short of the radiographic apex of the root (which corresponds to the natural constriction of the canal at the cementodentinal junction). The canals are then cleaned and shaped at this length with incrementally larger diameter files until the root canal system is ready to be filled.

Following this cleaning procedure, the root canals may be filled with **gutta percha** (a rubber-type material) and a sealer *(Fig. 9-17)*. Examples of sealers used today include resin, glass ionomer, zinc

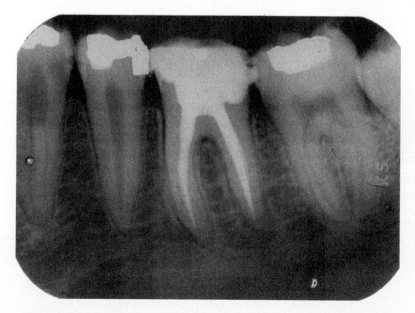

FIGURE 9-17. Radiograph of completed endodontic treatment. A lower left first molar where the root canals have been filled with gutta percha and sealer. The part of the crown that was lost has also been restored with a temporary filling. Both the gutta percha and the temporary filling appear whiter than enamel or dentin on the radiograph.

oxide and eugenol, and calcium hydroxide. When there is sufficient tooth structure remaining, the opening through the crown used to access the pulp may be restored with a tooth-colored composite or silver amalgam restorative material. Since teeth requiring endodontic treatment usually have large restorations or are weakened by extensive decay, tooth structure may be restored with a crown. In some instances, a post placed into the prepared root canal space is used in order to provide sufficient retention for the prosthetic (artificial) crown (*Fig. 9-18*).

Once a tooth has had endodontic therapy and the pulp has been removed, it should not be considered a "dead tooth" even though it no longer has a vital pulp. Although it cannot respond to stimuli like hot or cold, and cannot form reparative dentin, the periodontal support is the same as if it never had endodontic treatment. Therefore, if the periodontium remains healthy, the treated tooth generally can last for the lifetime of the patient.

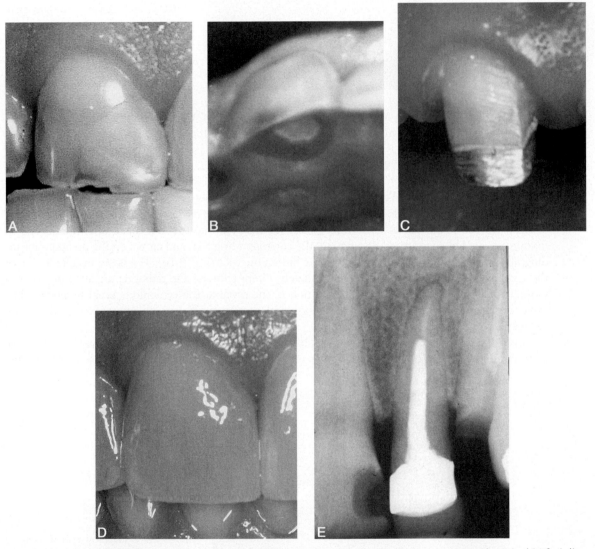

FIGURE 9-18. Tooth #8 treated with a root canal, post and core, and all-ceramic crown. A. Tooth #8 is thin faciolingually due to gastric acid reflux and is fractured incisally. **B.** The lingual access opening (used to reach and remove the pulp tissue) is filled with a provisional (temporary) restoration. **C.** The tooth is prepared for a crown with the post and core cemented in place to provide additional crown support and retention. The core is the part of the metal that reproduces lost tooth crown. The attached post fits within the preparation in the center of the tooth root. **D.** An all-ceramic crown has been cemented over the tooth and post and core. (**A, B, C,** and **D** courtesy of Julie Holloway, D.D.S., M.S., Ohio State University.) **E.** Radiograph of a post and core with a metal ceramic crown showing the post fitting over halfway into the endodontically treated root.

SECTION II.   LOCATION OF ROOT AND CERVICAL CROWN CONCAVITIES, FURCATIONS, DEPRESSIONS, AND CANALS

OBJECTIVES

The purpose of this section is to summarize the shape of the external root surface and the internal pulp shape at the level of the cementoenamel junction and halfway down the root toward the apex. The following tooth drawings are labeled:

M = Mesial, D = Distal, F = Facial, and L = Lingual

A.   MAXILLARY CENTRAL INCISORS

- The cross section of the root at the cervix is somewhat triangular with the mesial side longer than the distal side, consistent with the slight distal placement of the cingulum.
- There are no prominent root grooves (depressions) on this incisor, though the *mesial* surface may be flattened or have a *slight* longitudinal depression. The *distal* root surface is convex.
- It has one root canal close to 100% of the time.

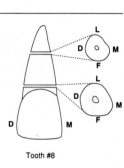

Tooth #8

B.   MAXILLARY LATERAL INCISORS

- The cross section of the root at the cervix is "egg shaped" or ovoid, with the widest mesiodistal portion on the labial.
- A shallow longitudinal root depression is often found on the middle of the *mesial* root surface extending about half of the root length, but *not* on the distal surface.
- There is one root canal close to 100% of the time.

Tooth #7

C.   MANDIBULAR CENTRAL AND LATERAL INCISORS

- In cross section, the cervical portion of the root is ovoid, considerably broader labiolingually than mesiodistally [by about 2 mm].
- Longitudinal root depressions are present on *both* proximal sides with the distal depression more distinct than the mesial.
- Most commonly there is one root canal [about 70% of the time for centrals and 55% for laterals].

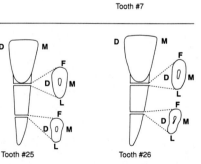

Tooth #25   Tooth #26

D.   MAXILLARY CANINES

- The cervical cross section is broad labiolingually and appears ovoid.
- Developmental grooves (depressions) are present on *both* the mesial and distal sides providing better anchorage. The groove may be more distinct on the distal.
- As in other maxillary anterior teeth, there is one root canal almost 100% of the time.

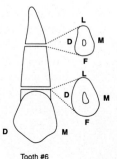

Tooth #6

E. MANDIBULAR CANINES

- Roots are wide labiolingually in the cervical half.
- Longitudinal root depressions are present on *both* sides, often deeper on the distal.
- Variations in double-root depressions include clearly separated roots (one labial and one lingual) to deep proximal grooves.
- There is most often one root canal [70% of the time].

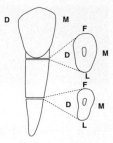

Tooth #27

F. MAXILLARY FIRST PREMOLARS

- There are most often two canals [90% of the time].
- Most have two roots (one buccal and one lingual) and two canals, or when one root is present, two pulp canals are usually found.
- *Mesial* and *distal* root depressions occur on both one- and two-rooted first premolars.
- The prominent *mesial* developmental depression of the *crown* continues across the cervical line to join the deep mesial root depression (between the buccal and lingual roots or between the buccal and lingual halves of a single root).
- When considering all premolars, it has the only root where the *mesial root depression is deeper* than a distal root depression.
- When two roots are present, the bifurcation occurs in the apical third to half of the root.

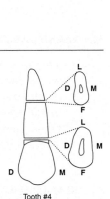

Tooth #5

G. MAXILLARY SECOND PREMOLARS

- Although there is normally only one root, there may be two roots 11% of the time.
- There may be a shallow developmental groove on the *mesial* side of the root, but it does not extend onto the crown, as was seen on the maxillary first premolar. A root depression can usually be found on the *distal* side, often deeper than on the mesial.
- There is most often one root canal [over 59% of the time].

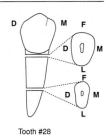

Tooth #4

H. MANDIBULAR FIRST PREMOLARS

- In cross section, the cervical portion of the root is ovoid and is widest buccolingually.
- Longitudinal depressions are often present on *both* sides, deeper on the distal. Sometimes these depressions may be quite deep and end in a buccolingual apical bifurcation.
- There is usually one root canal [70% of the time].

Tooth #28

I. MANDIBULAR SECOND PREMOLARS

- The cross section of the cervical portion of the root is ovoid buccolingually.
- Longitudinal depressions are *not* common on the mesial root surface but are frequent on the *distal* surface in the middle third.
- The cervical cross section of the root of the three-cusp premolars is particularly wide on the lingual, more so than on two-cusp types.
- The root is rarely bifurcated and normally has one root canal [96% of the time].

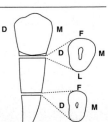

Tooth #29

J. MANDIBULAR FIRST AND SECOND MOLARS

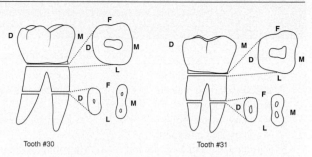

Tooth #30   Tooth #31

- Mandibular molars normally have two roots: mesial (broader and longer) and distal. Both roots are broad buccolingually.
- Mandibular first *and* second molars normally have three root canals, two in the mesial root and one in the distal root.
- The *mesial root* of both molars commonly has prominent root depressions on the mesial and distal surfaces, and there are usually two root canals [nearly 100% of the time]. This root may even be divided into a buccal and lingual part. The *distal root* surface contours are more variable but may be convex.
- The *distal roots* in the mandibular first and second molars usually have one canal [65% of the time in the first molar and 92% of the time in the second molar.]
- Access to the root bifurcations is located near the midbuccal and midlingual root surfaces.
- The root trunk is shorter on first molars than on second molars; the furcation is nearest to the cervical line on the buccal of first molars. The cervical line is more occlusal on the lingual of first molars. Buccal and lingual depressions are seen on the relatively short root trunk, extending from the cervical lines to buccal and lingual furcations. (Recall that enamel at the buccal and lingual cementoenamel junction may extend into the bifurcation.)
- First molar roots are broader and more widely separated than second molar roots, which may exhibit a distal inclination.

K. MAXILLARY FIRST AND SECOND MOLARS

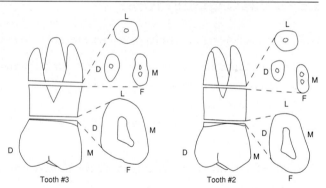

Tooth #3   Tooth #2

- There are normally three roots: mesiobuccal, distobuccal (shortest), and lingual (longest).
- Maxillary first *and* second molars usually have four root canals: two in the wide mesiobuccal root and one each in the distobuccal and lingual roots.
- The *mesiobuccal root* has mesial and distal side root depressions (and usually has *two root canals*).
- The distal contour of the *distobuccal root* varies but is normally convex (and normally has *one canal*).
- There is usually a slight longitudinal depression on the lingual side on the *lingual root* (which has *one canal*).
- Access to furcations between the roots is located in the cervical third of the root: on the buccal surface near the center mesiodistally and on the mesial and distal surfaces, located slightly lingual to the center buccolingually.
- Often a depression extends from the trifurcation to the cervical line and sometimes into the enamel of the crown on first molars. A distal crown depression is often noted on the distal surfaces of maxillary first molars.
- Separation between roots is more pronounced on first molars than on second molars; on second molars, the buccal roots are more nearly parallel and inclined distally in their apical third.
- The root trunk is broader (longer) than on mandibular molars, so the furcation between the mesiobuccal and distobuccal root may be at the junction of the cervical and middle thirds of the mesiobuccal root, especially on second molars.

A summary of the presence and relative depth of longitudinal root depressions is presented in *Table 9-3.*

Table 9-3	SUMMARY: PRESENCE AND RELATIVE DEPTH OF LONGITUDINAL ROOT DEPRESSIONS ("ROOT GROOVES")	
TOOTH	**MESIAL ROOT DEPRESSION?**	**DISTAL ROOT DEPRESSION?**
MAXILLARY TEETH		
Maxillary central incisor	No (or slight or flat)	No (convex)
Maxillary lateral incisor	Yes (sometimes no)	No (convex)
Maxillary canine	Yes	Yes (deeper)
Maxillary 1st premolar	Yes (deeper, extends onto mesial of crown)	Yes
Maxillary 2nd premolar	Yes	Yes (deeper)
Maxillary 1st and 2nd molars	**Mesiobuccal root**: Yes	Variable
	Distobuccal root: variable	No (convex)
	Lingual root: lingual surface depression	
MANDIBULAR TEETH		
Mandibular central incisor	Yes	Yes (deeper)
Mandibular lateral incisor	Yes	Yes (deeper)
Mandibular canine	Yes	Yes (deeper)
Mandibular 1st premolar	Yes (or no: about 50%)	Yes (deeper)
Mandibular 2nd premolar	No (unlikely)	Yes (deeper)
Mandibular 1st and 2nd molars	**Mesial root**: Yes	Yes (deeper)
	Distal root: variable	(variable, but *deeper)

General Learning Guidelines:
1. Maxillary incisors are less likely to have root depressions.
2. All canines and premolars (EXCEPT maxillary first premolars) and mandibular incisors are likely to have deeper distal surface root depressions.

LEARNING QUESTIONS

Each of the following questions may have more than one correct answer.

1. Which teeth are NOT likely to have root depressions on both the mesial and distal root surface?
   a. maxillary central and lateral incisor
   b. maxillary canine
   c. maxillary second premolar
   d. mandibular second premolar

2. Maxillary anterior teeth are most likely to have how many root canals?
   a. one
   b. two
   c. three
   d. one or two

3. Maxillary first molars are most likely to have _____ roots and _____ root canals?
   a. two, two
   b. two, three
   c. two, four
   d. three, three
   e. three, four

4. The one premolar most likely to have two roots (and two root canals) is the:
   a. maxillary first premolar
   b. maxillary second premolar
   c. mandibular first premolar
   d. mandibular second premolar

5. The two roots of a maxillary first premolar are called:

a. mesial and lingual

b. mesial and distal

c. buccal and mesial

d. buccal and lingual

e. mesiobuccal and distobuccal

6. A root depression associated with a furcation between roots on a maxillary first molar might be detectable on which of the following surfaces?

a. buccal surface

b. lingual surface

c. mesial surface

d. distal surface

ANSWERS: 1–a, d; 2–a; 3–e; 4–e; 5–d; 6–a, c, d

REFERENCES

1. Perlich MA, Reader A, Foreman DW. A scanning electron microscopic investigation of accessory foramens on the pulpal floor of human molars. J Endodontics 1981;7:402–406.
2. Benjamin KA, Dowson J. Incidence of two root canals in human mandibular incisor teeth. Oral Surg 1974;38:123–126.
3. Rankine-Wilson RW, Henry P. The bifurcated root canal in lower anterior teeth. JADA 1965;70:1162–1165.
4. Bellizzi R, Hartwell G. Clinical investigation of in vivo endodontically treated mandibular anterior teeth. J Endodontics 1983;9:246–248.
5. Vertucci FJ, Gegauff A. Root canal morphology of the maxillary first premolar. JADA 1979;99:194–198.
6. Bellizzi R, Hartwell G. Radiographic evaluation of root canal anatomy of in vivo endodontically treated maxillary premolars. J Endodontics 1985;11:37–39.
7. Vertucci FJ. Root canal anatomy of the human permanent teeth. Oral Surg 1984;58:589–599.
8. Gilles J, Reader A. An SEM investigation of mesiolingual canal in human maxillary first and second molars. Oral Surg Oral Med Oral Path 1990;70:638–643.
9. Neaverth EJ, Kotler LM, Kaltenbach RF. Clinical investigation (in vivo) of endodontically treated maxillary first molars. J Endodontics 1987;13:506–512.
10. Skidmore AE, Bjorndal AM. Root canal morphology of the human mandibular first molar. Oral Surg 1971;32:778–784.
11. Shaw L, Jones AD. Morphological considerations of the dental pulp chamber from radiographs of molar and premolar teeth. J Dent 1984;12:139–145.
12. The American Association of Endodontists. http://www.aae.org/media/index.html

OTHER GENERAL REFERENCES

Estrela C, Pereira HL, Pecora JD. Radicular grooves in maxillary lateral incisor: case report. Braz Dent J 1995;6(2):143–146.

Pecora JD, Saquy PC, Sousa Neto MD, et al. Root form and canal anatomy of maxillary first premolars. Braz Dent J 1991;2(2):87–94.

Pecora JD, Sousa Neto MD, Saquy PC, et al. In vitro study of root canal anatomy of maxillary second premolars. Braz Dent J 1992;3(2):81–85.

Pecora JD, Woelfel JB, Sousa Neto MD. Morphologic study of the maxillary molars. Part I: external anatomy. Braz Dent J 1991;2(1):45–50.

Pecora JD, Woelfel JB, Sousa Neto MD, et al. Morphologic study of the maxillary molars. Part II: internal anatomy. Braz Dent J 1992;3(1):53–57.

Walton RE, Torabinejad M. Principles and practice of endodontics. 3rd ed. Philadelphia: W.B. Saunders Company, 2002.

Web site: American Association of Endodontists (with information for the professional and for media/public). http://www.aae.org/media/index.html

10 Primary (and Mixed) Dentition

OBJECTIVES

This chapter is designed to prepare the learner to perform the following:
- Describe the important functions of the primary dentition and the problems that can occur from premature loss of primary teeth.
- List the time ranges for primary and secondary tooth eruption.
- List the time ranges for crown and root formation for primary and secondary teeth.
- Give the order of eruption of primary and secondary teeth.
- Describe the dentition (set) traits that differentiate primary from secondary teeth.
- Describe class and type traits that distinguish the primary incisors, canines, and molars from all views.
- Describe the size and shape of primary tooth pulp chambers.
- Using the Universal Identification System, identify permanent and primary teeth present in the mouth with mixed dentition.
- Establish the expected "dental age" of a person by studying their mixed dentition.

SECTION I. BACKGROUND INFORMATION

A. DEFINITIONS

Primary teeth are often called **deciduous** [dee SIJ oo es] **teeth**. Deciduous comes from the Latin word meaning to fall off. Deciduous teeth fall off or are shed (like leaves from a deciduous tree) and are replaced by the adult teeth that succeed them. Common nicknames for them are "milk teeth," or "temporary teeth," which, unfortunately, denote a lack of importance. The dentition that follows the primary teeth may be called the **permanent dentition**, but since many of the so-called permanent teeth are lost due to disease, trauma, or other causes, the authors have chosen to call it the **secondary dentition** (or **adult dentition**). [There are millions of people in the United States who have lost all of their "permanent teeth" (are edentulous).]

B. DENTAL FORMULAE

As stated in Chapter 1, the number and type of primary teeth in each half of the mouth is represented by this formula:

$$\text{Incisors } \frac{2}{2} \qquad \text{Canines } \frac{1}{1} \qquad \text{Molars } \frac{2}{2} = \frac{5 \text{ maxillary teeth per side}}{5 \text{ mandibular teeth per side}}$$

Compare this formula to that for the secondary dentition, and you will be able to draw some interesting conclusions:

Incisors $\dfrac{2}{2}$ Canines $\dfrac{1}{1}$ Premolars $\dfrac{2}{2}$ Molars $\dfrac{3}{3} = \dfrac{8 \text{ maxillary teeth per side}}{8 \text{ mandibular teeth per side}}$

Notice that there are no primary premolars. When primary teeth are replaced by teeth of the secondary dentition, the *primary molars* are replaced by *premolars*. The 20 secondary teeth that succeed their primary tooth predecessors are called **succedaneous** [suck si DAY nee ous] **teeth**. The 12 secondary molars, however, have no predecessors in the primary dentition and erupt distal to the primary molars. Therefore, in the strict sense, secondary molars are *not* succedaneous teeth.

Primary teeth exhibit an arch form similar to permanent teeth (*Fig. 10-1*). Recall from Chapter 3 that the 20 primary teeth can be identified using the universal identification system by assigning letters A (for the primary right maxillary second molar) through T (for the primary right mandibular second molar). Another method that can be used to identify these teeth uses a "D" to denote deciduous preceded by numbers 1 (1D for the primary right maxillary second molar) through 20 (20D for the primary right mandibular second molar). Both of these systems are seen in Figure 10-1. (Two other methods for numbering deciduous teeth were presented in Table 3-1.)

C. FUNCTIONS OF THE PRIMARY DENTITION

Some parents do not consider the care of the primary teeth of their children to be a priority since they consider them as "temporary" or "baby" teeth, but it is important to remember that primary teeth are the *only* teeth that children have until approximately their sixth birthday, and some remain functioning until

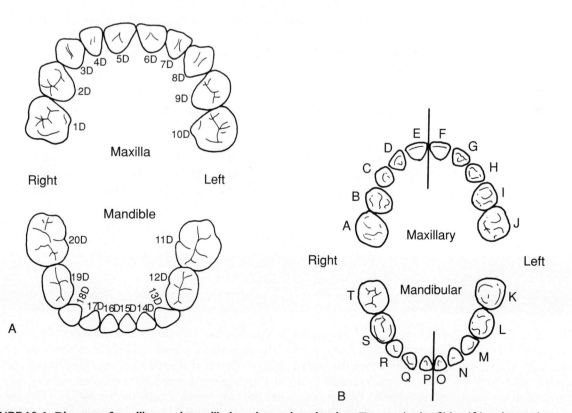

Primary dentition

FIGURE 10-1. Diagram of maxillary and mandibular primary dental arches. Two methods of identifying these primary teeth are shown. On the right diagram, the Universal System of assigning letters to each tooth is shown, while on the left diagram, a numbering system 1 through 20 followed by "D" for deciduous is shown.

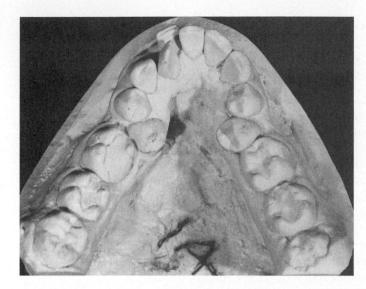

FIGURE 10-2. A crowded mandibular secondary dentition caused by the premature loss of deciduous molars. Notice that the left lateral incisor almost contacts the right central incisor and that the left first premolar is only 2.5 mm from contacting the first molar.

age 12. Primary teeth are actually in the mouth functioning for almost 6 years for mandibular central incisors to almost 10 years for maxillary canines [the average being 8 years for maxillary teeth and 7.6 years for mandibular teeth[1]]. When people live to be 70 years of age, they will have spent 6% of their life chewing (masticating) solely with primary teeth. This small proportion of time should not infer a lack of importance of primary teeth, however, because they play a very important role in "reserving" space for the permanent teeth, which ensures proper alignment, spacing, and occlusion of the permanent teeth. Consider the following functions of primary teeth in order to confirm the importance of keeping them healthy:

- Primary teeth are needed for efficient chewing (mastication) of food.
- They provide support for the cheeks and lips maintaining a normal facial appearance and smile.
- They are necessary for the formulation of clear speech.
- They are critical for maintaining the space and arch continuity required to provide room for the eruption of secondary teeth.

When primary teeth are lost prematurely, or are not shed as succedaneous teeth emerge, the results on tooth alignment can be devastating (*Figs. 10-2 and 10-3*). Correction of tooth alignment and deformities in these children would require extensive orthodontic therapy (involving placement of orthodontic appliances, or braces, which can be used to improve tooth alignment). Further, maintenance of a proper diet and good oral hygiene are necessary to avoid dental decay of primary teeth, which can cause infection with concomitant pain, possibly making the child reject foods that are difficult to chew. Finally, an abscess from the infection of the pulp of a primary tooth can cause dark spots (Turner's spots) on the developing secondary tooth beneath it (seen later in Fig. 12-43).

SECTION II.   DEVELOPMENTAL DATA FOR PRIMARY AND SECONDARY TEETH

Dental students and dental hygiene students should become familiar with the emergence dates of primary and secondary teeth in order to adequately and correctly inform worried parents and patients about the normal times when teeth emerge or erupt above the gingiva (gums). Expected eruption patterns for primary and secondary teeth from one study are presented in Table 10-1A; eruption patterns from another study of only primary teeth are presented in Table 10-1B. An emergence time for *primary* teeth can be within 4 to 5 months (early or late) of the dates in Table 10-1A and still be considered normal. *Secondary* tooth emergence can be within 12 to 18 months (early or late) of those dates and still be of no real concern. Early emergence of these teeth usually presents no problems other than a concern about instituting oral hygiene measures.

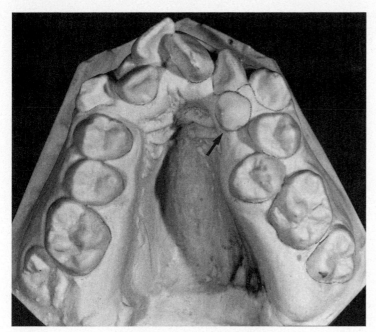

FIGURE 10-3. Extreme crowding of a maxillary permanent dentition in a 12-year-old child. The left deciduous canine (*arrow*) was not shed because its successor emerged labially to it. Both 12-year molars (three-cusp type) are in the process of emerging.

Dental radiographs (x-ray films) are the best means for determining what is covered up (unerupted) or missing in a dentition when the expected teeth have not emerged, particularly when they are considerably overdue. (See Fig. 10-7 later in this chapter.)

A. IMPORTANT TIMES FOR TOOTH EMERGENCE

Instead of memorizing the specific times of eruption of each tooth (which would be a daunting task), first consider this overview of the development of permanent and primary teeth based on their normal eruption patterns. If you learn the following time ranges, you will be well on your way to understanding the schedule of tooth eruption for both dentitions.

- **Birth–6 (or 8) months old**: there are no teeth visible within the mouth.

PRIMARY DENTITION ONLY
- **6 (or 8) months–2 (or 2 ½) old**: all 20 primary teeth emerge into the child's mouth over this period.
- **2 (or 2 ½)–6 (or 5 ¾) years old**: all primary teeth are present; no permanent teeth are yet visible in the mouth.

MIXED DENTITION
- **6 (or 5 ¾) years old**: secondary teeth start to appear, beginning with the first molars (also called **6-year molars**) just distal to the primary second molars. This is followed closely by the loss of the primary mandibular central incisors, which are quickly replaced by the secondary mandibular central incisors.
- **6–9 years old**: all eight secondary incisors replace primary incisors that are exfoliated (shed).
- **9–12 years old**: all eight premolars and four canines replace primary molars and canines.
- **12 years old**: second molars (also called **12-year molars**) emerge distal to the permanent first molars.

ADULT DENTITION ONLY (after 12 years)
- **17–21 years old**: third molars (if present) emerge.

B. CROWN AND ROOT DEVELOPMENT

With these basic time periods in mind, one must not forget that much more is taking place during the development of these teeth than just their eruption and/or exfoliation. Prior to eruption, tooth crowns are forming from lobes and are calcifying within the jawbones. After **crown calcification** is completed, the tooth

Table 10-1A DECIDUOUS AND SECONDARY TOOTH FORMATION AND EMERGENCE TIMES

		TOOTH	HARD TISSUE FORMATION BEGINS	CROWN COMPLETED	EMERGENCE	ROOT COMPLETED
DECIDUOUS DENTITION	Maxillary teeth	Central incisor	**4 mo in utero (first primary to begin)**	4 mo	$7^1/_2$ mo	$1^1/_2$ yr
		Lateral incisor	$4^1/_2$ mo in utero	5 mo	9 mo	2 yr
		Canine	5 mo in utero	9 mo	18 mo	$3^1/_4$ yr
		First molar	5 mo in utero	6 mo	14 mo	$2^1/_2$ yr
		Second molar	6 mo in utero	11 mo	24 mo	3 yr
	Mandibular teeth	Central incisor	$4^1/_2$ mo in utero	$3^1/_2$ mo	6 mo	$1^1/_2$ yr
		Lateral incisor	$4^1/_2$ mo in utero	4 mo	7 mo	$1^1/_2$ yr
		Canine	5 mo in utero	9 mo	16 mo	3 yr
		First molar	5 mo in utero	$5^1/_2$ mo	12 mo	$2^1/_4$ yr
		Second molar	6 mo in utero	10 mo	20 mo	3 yr
PERMANENT DENTITION	Maxillary teeth	Central incisor	3–4 mo	4–5 yr	7–8 yr	10 yr
		Lateral incisor	10–12 mo	4–5 yr	8–9 yr	11 yr
		Canine	4–5 mo	6–7 yr	11–12 yr	13–15 yr
		First premolar	$1^1/_2$–$1^3/_4$ yr	5–6 yr	10–11 yr	12–13 yr
		Second premolar	2–$2^1/_4$ yr	6–7 yr	10–12 yr	12–14 yr
		First molar	**Birth (first secondary to begin)**	$2^1/_2$–3 yr	6–7 yr	9–10 yr
		Second molar	$2^1/_2$–3 yr	7–8 yr	12–15 yr	14–16 yr
		Third molar	7–9 yr	12–16 yr	17–21 yr	18–25 yr
	Mandibular teeth	Central incisor	3–4 mo	4–5 yr	6–7 yr	9 yr
		Lateral incisor	3–4 mo	4–5 yr	7–8 yr	10 yr
		Canine	4–5 mo	6–7 yr	9–10 yr	12–14 yr
		First premolar	$1^3/_4$–2 yr	5–6 yr	10–12 yr	12–13 yr
		Second premolar	$2^1/_4$–$2^1/_2$ yr	6–7 yr	11–12 yr	13–14 yr
		First molar	**Birth**	$2^1/_2$–3 yr	6–7 yr	9–10 yr
		Second molar	$2^1/_2$–3 yr	7–8 yr	11–13 yr	14–15 yr
		Third molar	8–10 yr	12–16 yr	17–21 yr	18–25 yr

Chart based on Logan WH and Kronfield R. Development of the human jaws and surrounding structures from birth to age fifteen. J.A.D.A., 20:379–424, 1933 or 35. Modified by McCall and Schour: Schour I, McCall JO. Chronology of the Human Dentition. In: Orban B: Oral Histology and Embryology, St. Louis, C.V. Mosby, 1944, p240.

Table 10-1B	TOOTH DEVELOPMENT AND ERUPTION: PRIMARY TEETH				
		HARD TISSUE FORMATION BEGINS (WEEKS IN UTERO)	ENAMEL COMPLETED (MONTHS AFTER BIRTH)	ERUPTION (MONTHS)	ROOT COMPLETED (YEAR)
Maxillary	Central incisor	14	$1^1/_2$	10 (8–12)	$1^1/_2$
	Lateral incisor	16	$2^1/_2$	11 (9–13)	2
	Canine	17	9	19 (16–22)	$3^1/_4$
	First molar	$15^1/_2$	6	16 (13–19 boys) (14–18 girls)	$2^1/_2$
	Second molar	19	11	29 (25–33)	3
Mandibular	Central incisor	14	$2^1/_2$	8 (6–10)	$1^1/_2$
	Lateral incisor	16	3	13 (10–16)	$1^1/_2$
	Canine	17	9	20 (17–23)	$3^1/_4$
	First molar	$15^1/_2$	$5^1/_2$	16 (14–18)	$2^1/_4$
	Second molar	18	10	27 (23–31 boys) (24–30 girls)	3

From Lunt RC, Law DB. A review of the chronology of deciduous teeth. J Am Dent Assoc 1974;89:872.

root starts to form, which results in the movement of the tooth through bone toward the surface (**eruption process**) and eventually through the oral mucosa into the oral cavity (**emergence**). After emergence, the root continues to form until **root formation** is completed.

The process of *primary* tooth formation and eruption is followed by the development, calcification, and eruption of the *succedaneous* teeth apical to their roots. The eruption of these succedaneous teeth results in **resorption** of the roots of the primary teeth (that is, the gradual physiologic destruction or dissolution of the primary tooth root by the underlying erupting permanent tooth). When the secondary tooth is close to emergence, the primary tooth roots are resorbed so much that they can no longer support the remaining primary tooth crown. The primary tooth becomes loose and is eventually **exfoliated** (shed or lost). The exfoliation of the primary tooth is followed closely by the emergence of the succedaneous tooth just beneath the surface.

Now let us look at this entire process in more detail, discussing it step by step. All of the following information is derived from Table 10-1A.

1. CROWN CALCIFICATION OF PRIMARY TEETH

The crowns of all 20 primary teeth *begin* to calcify between *4 and 6 months in utero* (seen developing in *Fig. 10-4*). *Crown completion* of all primary teeth occurs within the first year after birth, taking an average of 10 months from the beginning of tooth calcification. [The time from beginning hard tissue formation until complete enamel calcification ranges from a minimum of 9 months for incisors to a maximum of 13 months for primary second molars.]

2. ROOT FORMATION AND EMERGENCE OF PRIMARY TEETH

Root formation for primary (and permanent) teeth begins immediately after the enamel on the crown is completely formed, and at this time, the tooth starts its occlusal movement toward the oral cavity. This tooth movement is called **eruption**. In the process of eruption, the primary tooth crowns finally **emerge** into the oral cavity from age 6 months to 2 years (24 months). [The time of emergence of primary teeth after crown calcification is complete ranges from about 3 months for mandibular central incisors to about 13 months after calcification for maxillary second molars.] The eruptive movement continues after emergence, until eventually the tooth comes into occlusion with teeth in the opposite arch. Even then these teeth continue to erupt to compensate for wear (attrition) on the incisal or occlusal surface and/or when there are no opposing teeth.

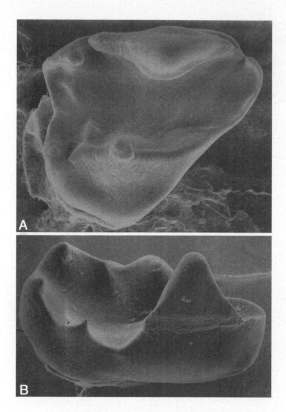

FIGURE 10-4. Developing human primary molars. A. Occlusal view of a 19-week in utero maxillary right first molar. Note the large, well-developed, mesiobuccal cusp, which is covered with a mineralized enamel cap and is the first formed and largest cusp of the trigon, the early molar form that has three cusps. (Original magnification ×36.) **B.** Buccal view of a 20-week in utero mandibular right first molar. Note the strongly elevated mesiobuccal cusp that dominates the mesial portion of the tooth. The mesiolingual cusp is the second to differentiate and shows incipient mineralization. (Original magnification ×36.) These two examples illustrate that the mesiobuccal cusps of both the maxillary and mandibular molars are the first to form and mineralize.

3. ORDER OF EMERGENCE OF PRIMARY TEETH (FROM 6 MONTHS TO ABOUT 2 YEARS OLD)

The sequence of emergence for primary teeth presented in *Table 10-2* shows that the first primary teeth to emerge are the mandibular central incisors, at about 6 months of age, followed by the mandibular laterals and then the maxillary incisors (centrals before laterals). (Note the difference in eruption patterns in Table 10-1B, where data showed that mandibular central incisors emerge first, but are followed by maxillary central incisors, maxillary lateral incisors, and finally mandibular lateral incisors.) Next to emerge are the first molars, canines, then second molars. Thus, the last primary teeth to emerge, thereby completing the primary dentition, are the maxillary second molars, at about 2 years (24 months) of age.

As primary teeth erupt, developmental spaces often occur between anterior teeth, especially as the maxillae and the mandible bones grow larger. Spaces that occur mesial to the maxillary canines and distal to the mandibular canines are called **primate** spaces.[11] These spaces frequently concern parents but are perfectly natural and even beneficial since they provide room for the secondary incisors and canines, which are considerably wider than their predecessors. Refer to *Table 10-3* for differences in sizes between primary and adult teeth.

4. ROOT COMPLETION OF PRIMARY TEETH

The primary tooth roots are completed between the ages of 1½ to 3 years. [The time from tooth emergence until the completion of the root ranges from about 10.5 months for maxillary central incisors to

Table 10-2	CHART REPRESENTING ORDER OF PRIMARY TOOTH EMERGENCE. (1 = FIRST TOOTH TO ERUPT, 2 = SECOND, ETC.) BASED ON DATA IN TABLE 10-1A				
	CENTRAL INCISOR	**LATERAL INCISOR**	**CANINE**	**FIRST MOLAR**	**SECOND MOLAR**
Maxillary	3rd (7¹/₂ mo)	4th (9 mo)	8th (18 mo)	6th (14 mo)	10th (24 mo)
Mandibular	1st (6 mo)	2nd (7 mo)	7th (16 mo)	5th (12 mo)	9th (20 mo)

Table 10-3 — DECIDUOUS TOOTH SIZE COMPARED TO THEIR SUCCESSORS

		CROWN LENGTH		ROOT LENGTH		OVERALL LENGTH		MESIODISTAL CROWN		FACIOLINGUAL CROWN		MESIODISTAL CERVIX		FACIOLINGUAL CERVIX		AVERAGE OF ALL MEASUREMENTS
		mm	%	mm	%	mm	%	mm	%*	mm	%	mm	%	mm	%	%
Maxillary teeth	Central incisor	6.4	57	11.3	82	17.2	73	7.4	86	5.0	70	5.7	89	4.4	70	75.3
	Lateral incisor	7.4	76	10.9	81	16.8	75	5.8	88	4.9	79	4.0	85	4.5	78	80.3
	Canine	7.6	72	13.5	78	20.2	80	7.4	97	5.4	67	5.3	95	5.0	66	78.8
	First molar	6.0	70	12.5	93	17.1	80	8.1	*114	9.5	103	5.9	123	8.9	108	98.7
	Second molar	6.4	83	10.4	74	15.9	75	9.7	*147	10.3	114	7.1	151	9.6	118	108.8
Mandibular teeth	Central incisor	6.1	69	10.5	83	16.0	77	4.5	85	4.5	79	3.5	100	4.2	78	81.6
	Lateral incisor	7.3	78	10.6	78	16.5	75	4.9	86	4.8	79	3.7	94	4.5	78	81.4
	Canine	8.2	74	11.7	74	18.7	72	6.1	90	5.7	74	4.2	81	5.0	67	76.0
	First molar	7.1	81	9.7	67	15.9	71	8.7	*124	7.4	96	7.2	150	5.3	78	95.3
	Second molar	6.6	80	10.8	68	15.5	70	10.3	*145	9.2	112	7.6	152	7.1	97	103.4

Measurements are derived from 2392 maxillary and 2180 mandibular secondary tooth specimens compared to plastic model replicas of primary teeth made by the Shofu Dental Manufacturing Company (Kyoto, Japan) reflecting the size of Japanese primary teeth. In most instances, these measurements on the plastic model teeth were 0.5–1 mm larger than measurements made by G.V. Black at the turn of the century (deciduous teeth).

Percentages are based on the average size for the secondary dentition successor as equaling 100%. In instances in which the deciduous tooth dimension is greater than its successor, the percentage is over 100, even as high as 152% on the mandibular second molar mesiodistal cervix dimension, indicating that this part of the deciduous molar is 1.5 times larger than the corresponding region on its successor, the mandibular second premolar.

* Denotes percentages where primary crown measurements are wider mesiodistally than succedaneous teeth.

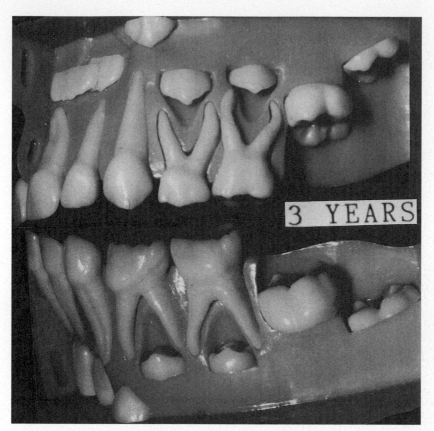

FIGURE 10-5. Models depicting the stage of development of the dentitions of a 3-year-old child. All primary teeth have emerged into the oral cavity, and they have full roots, prior to resorption. Notice the various amounts of crown development and locations of the partially formed crowns of the secondary dentition. (Models courtesy of 3M Unitek, Monrovia, CA.)

about 21 months for upper canines.] The *complete* primary dentition (with 20 teeth) is in the mouth from about 2 years of age to 5¾ or 6 years, during which no permanent teeth are present.

5. EXFOLIATION (SHEDDING) OF PRIMARY TEETH WITH THE SIMULTANEOUS ERUPTION AND EVENTUAL EMERGENCE OF THE SECONDARY (ADULT) TEETH

The roots of primary teeth are complete for a short period of time (as seen in *Fig. 10-5*). Only about 3 years after completion, primary tooth roots begin to **resorb**, usually at the apex or on one side near the apex. Resorption of the primary tooth root occurs as the crown of the succedaneous tooth that is to replace it begins its occlusal migration, thus infringing upon the primary root. Increasing loss of root attachment from root resorption results in the eventual loosening of the deciduous teeth so they "fall off" the jaw. This process of shedding is called **exfoliation**. As the primary teeth are shed, the crowns of the succedaneous teeth are close to the surface, ready to emerge shortly (as seen in *Fig. 10-6*).

6. MIXED DENTITION (PRESENT FROM 5 ¾ OR 6 YEARS TO 12 YEARS OLD)

During the time when *both* primary and secondary teeth are present in the mouth, the dentition is known as a **mixed dentition**. The mixed dentition begins at age 5¾ or 6 years old when the first (6-year) molars emerge. Next, the first primary incisors are gradually replaced by their larger successors. The mixed dentition ends at about age 12 when all primary teeth have been replaced. Usually, 24 teeth are seen in the mouth throughout the mixed dentition (all 20 primary teeth OR their successors, *plus* the four 6-year first molars). At 12 years old, all succedaneous teeth have replaced their primary predecessors (marking the end of mixed dentition). When the 12-year second molars erupt, 28 teeth are present. The full complement of 32 permanent teeth is not reached until the third molars erupt during the late teenage years or early 20s.

Soon after the 6-year first molars emerge, their eruptive forces, along with their tendency to drift toward the mesial, push the primary teeth forward. If this were to continue, there would be insufficient

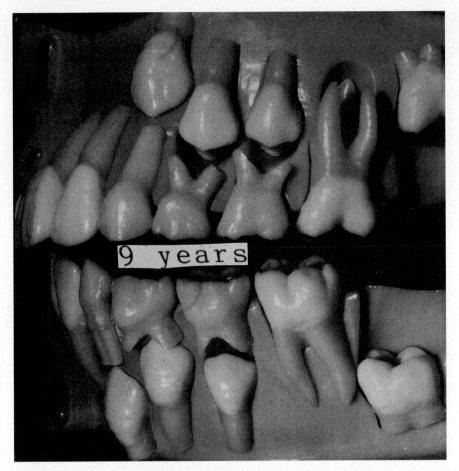

FIGURE 10-6. Tooth development of a 9-year-old child with mixed dentition. The secondary central and lateral incisors and first molars have emerged into a functional level. The deciduous canines and molars are still functioning, although much of their roots have resorbed. You can appreciate by the position within the bone of the maxillary canine why it is often the last permanent tooth to erupt except for the third molars (not shown). (Models courtesy of 3M Unitek, Monrovia, CA.)

space for the premolars to come in. The flared roots of the primary molars, however, resist the mesial displacement (seen in Fig. 10-5). This, along with the fact that the primary molar crowns are wider mesiodistally than their premolar successors and primate spaces develop, helps to preserve sufficient space for the premolars and secondary canines.[2]

7. CROWN FORMATION OF SECONDARY TEETH

The first *secondary* tooth crowns to begin forming (*at birth*) are the first molars. Crowns of the secondary dentition continue to form up to age 16 when crowns of third molars are completed. On average for the adult dentition, there is a *3- to 4-year span* from completion of crown calcification until the tooth emerges into the mouth [with a range of from 2.7 years for the lower anterior teeth to 4.7 years for the lower posterior teeth].

8. ORDER OF EMERGENCE FOR SECONDARY TEETH

Table 10-4 includes the sequence of emergence for secondary teeth. After the 6-year molars erupt just prior to the child's sixth birthday, the order of emergence for the succedaneous teeth is essentially the same as for the order of exfoliation of the primary teeth they replace. If you know the time *range* (for emergence of incisors, or for canines and premolars) and sequence of eruption within that time range, you can estimate the emergence time for any succedaneous tooth.

Table 10-4	CHART REPRESENTING THE USUAL ORDER OF SECONDARY DENTITION TOOTH EMERGENCE BASED ON DATA FROM TABLE 10-1A							
	CENT INC	LAT INC	CANINE	1st PREMOLAR	2nd PREMOLAR	1st MOLAR	2nd MOLAR	3rd MOLAR
Age Range	6–9 yr			9–12 yr		6 yr	12 yr	
Maxillary	2nd (t) (7–8 yr)	3rd (8–9 yr)	6th (t) (11–12 yr)	5th (t) (10–11 yr)	5th (t) (10–12 yr)	1st (t) (6–7 yr)	7th (t) (12–15 yr)	8th (t) (17–21 yr)
Mandibular	1st (t) (6–7 yr)	2nd (t) (7–8 yr)	4th (9–10 yr)	5th (t) (10–12 yr)	6th (t) (11–12 yr)	1st (t) (6–7 yr)	7th (t) (11–13 yr)	8th (t) (17–21 yr)

1st = first tooth to erupt, 2nd = second, etc., same number with a "(t)" denotes essentially a tie in eruption time. Mandibular teeth often precede their maxillary counterpart within the time ranges given except for second premolars. (Mandibular first molars are often the first secondary teeth to erupt.)

Recall that as the secondary 6-year molars erupt, the mandibular central incisors erupt almost at the same time, followed closely by the other six secondary incisors between 6 and 9 years of age. The specific sequence within this range is secondary incisors begin to replace primary incisors (centrals preceding laterals), and mandibular incisors precede maxillary incisors. Since the mandibular central incisors erupt first in this time range, they emerge closer to 6 years old, whereas maxillary lateral incisors erupt closer to the end of that time range, that is, closer to 8 or 9 years old.

Next, the adult canines and premolars erupt between ages 9 and 12. The eruption sequence during this range is as follows: *mandibular* canines replace primary mandibular canines, and then premolars replace primary molars. Note in Table 10-4 that in the adult dentition, most teeth in the lower arch usually emerge slightly earlier than their maxillary counterparts; the ONLY maxillary tooth to emerge before its mandibular counterpart is the *maxillary* second premolar, which precedes the *mandibular* second premolar. Finally, *maxillary canines are the last primary teeth to be replaced*. Knowing the range and sequence, you can estimate the emergence time of the *mandibular* canine as close to 9 years, while the *maxillary* canine emerges last within this range, or at about 11½ to 12½ years of age.

Roots of secondary teeth are completed *about 3 years after their emergence* into the oral cavity.

SECTION III. DENTITION TRAITS OF ALL PRIMARY TEETH

Your best specimens for the study of crown morphology of primary teeth can be found in the mouth of a 2 to 6 year old who is willing to open his or her mouth wide, long, and often enough to permit your examination. Extracted or exfoliated primary teeth with complete roots and crowns are difficult to find since most of these have resorbed roots and severe attrition (occlusal wear). Plastic tooth models, if available, are most helpful and have the added advantage of complete roots.

General Traits of All Primary Teeth Compared to Secondary Teeth

First, consider the general traits of *all* primary teeth that set them apart from the secondary teeth:

- Primary teeth are smaller in size than the analogous secondary teeth (that is, primary incisors and canines are smaller than secondary incisors and canines, respectively, and primary first and second molars are smaller than secondary first and second molars, respectively).
- Primary teeth are whiter in color.
- The crowns and roots of primary teeth have a marked constriction at the cervix, appearing as if they are being squeezed with a rubber band. Thus, the enamel (especially on the facial and lingual surfaces) seems to bulge close to the cervical line forming labial

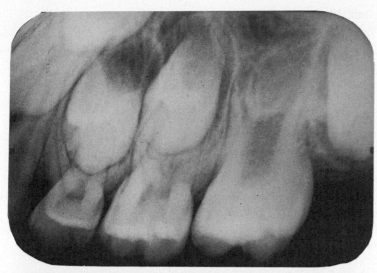

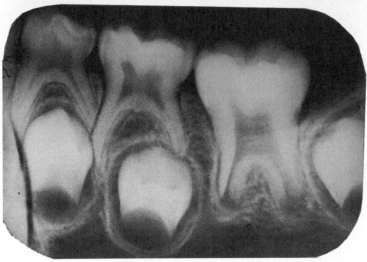

FIGURE 10-7. Radiographs made of an 8-year-old child showing the first and second deciduous molars and first adult molars in the mouth. The top radiograph shows maxillary teeth, and the lower radiograph shows mandibular teeth. Notice the premolar crowns between the partially resorbed roots of the maxillary and mandibular deciduous molars. Part of the 12-year second molar crown is seen on the far right of each radiograph. The lesser size, lesser enamel thickness, and larger pulp cavities are evident in the deciduous molars compared to the larger secondary molars just distal to them. (Courtesy of Professor Donald Bowers, Ohio State University.)

cervical ridges and lingual cingula[3] rather than gradually tapering toward the occlusal surface as in secondary teeth. This is seen best from the proximal view in Appendix 9a and Appendix 10e.

- Primary teeth have relatively longer roots compared to their crowns.
- The layers of enamel and dentin of primary teeth are thinner than on secondary teeth, but the pulp cavities are proportionally larger and are therefore *closer to the surface* (seen in the radiographs in *Fig. 10-7* where the outer layer of enamel is whiter, dentin is more gray, and the pulp, in the center of the tooth, is nearly black). Therefore, decay can progress to the pulp more quickly through this thinner enamel and dentin than through the thicker adult enamel and dentin, and the dentist must take care not to expose the tooth pulp when preparing primary teeth for fillings since the pulp is closer to the surface.
- Primary teeth are less mineralized so become very worn.[3,4] These teeth are prone to considerable **attrition** [at TRISH en] (tooth wear from tooth-to-tooth contact), which is made worse by the shifting relationship of the upper and lower teeth due to expanding growth of the jaws in young children. Attrition therefore is not really a dentition trait, but a fact of life or normal occurrence.[4]
- Primary teeth have more consistent shapes than the secondary dentition (fewer anomalies).[3]

Traits of All Primary Anterior Teeth

Next, consider the unique traits of the **primary anterior teeth** (refer to Appendix page 9 while studying these traits):

- The cervical ridges on facial surfaces are prominent (running mesiodistally in the cervical third) (Appendix 9a, facial surfaces).
- The lingual cingula are prominent or seem to bulge and occupy about one-third of the cervicoincisal length (Appendix 9a, lingual surfaces).
- Usually, there are no depressions, mamelons, or perikymata on the labial surface of the crowns of the primary incisors. These surfaces are smoother than their successors.

Root Traits of Primary Anterior Teeth

- The roots of primary anterior teeth are long in proportion to crown length (Appendix 9f) and are relatively narrow mesiodistally (Appendix 9b).
- The roots of primary anterior teeth bend labially in their apical one-third to one-half by as much as 10° (Appendix 9c).

Traits of All Primary Posterior Teeth

Now consider the unique traits of the **primary posterior teeth** (refer to Appendix page 10 while studying these traits):

- The prominent *mesial cervical ridge* or bulge on the buccal surface is exaggerated by the curve of the cervical line apically (best seen when viewed from the buccal) and by the constriction at the cervical line (best viewed from the proximal, Appendix 10e). This mesial cervical bulge makes it easy to distinguish rights from lefts.
- Due to the taper of the crown from the cervical bulges toward the occlusal surface, the molar crowns have a narrow **occlusal table** (Appendix 10c). (The occlusal table is the chewing surface inside the line formed by the continuous mesial and distal cusp ridges for all cusps and the mesial and distal marginal ridges). In other words, the occlusal table is considerably smaller than the entire outline of the tooth from the occlusal view.
- From the buccal view, all molar crowns are wide mesiodistally relative to the height cervico-occlusally (Appendix 10a).
- The primary molar occlusal anatomy is shallow. In other words, the cusps are short (not pointed or sharp, almost flat) (Appendix 10d), the occlusal ridges are not pronounced, and the fossae and sulci are correspondingly not as deep as on secondary molars.
- There are few grooves or depressions in the crowns.
- Primary second molars are decidedly larger than primary first molars, different than in the secondary dentition (Appendix page 10, compare firsts to seconds).
- Microscopically, the enamel rods at the cervix slope occlusally, unlike in permanent teeth where these rods slope cervically.

Root Traits of Primary Posterior Teeth

- The root furcations are near the crown, with little or no root trunk (Appendix 10f).
- The roots are thin and slender, and spread beyond the outlines of the crown, more widely on primary second molars than the first molars (the opposite of the adult molars)[5] (Appendix 10g). This root divergence makes room for the development of the succedaneous premolars. Extraction of a deciduous molar when roots are complete and before they have started to resorb may cause the developing portion of the premolar to be removed along with the deciduous molar.[7]
- The roots of the primary molars are similar to those of the secondary molars in relative size and number. Primary maxillary molars have three roots (mesiobuccal, distobuccal, and palatal), while primary mandibular molars have two roots (mesial and distal).

SECTION IV.   CLASS AND TYPE TRAITS OF PRIMARY TEETH

A.   PRIMARY INCISOR TRAITS

1.   PRIMARY INCISORS FROM THE LABIAL VIEW

a.   Outline Shape of Primary Incisor Crowns from the Labial View

Incisal edges of primary **maxillary central incisors** are relatively straight except for some rounding at the distoincisal angle. Mesial sides of maxillary central incisor crowns are fairly flat, whereas the distal sides are more convex. The crowns of **primary maxillary central incisors** are the ONLY incisor crowns (primary or secondary) that are wider mesiodistally than they are long incisocervically (Appendix 9e).

The **maxillary lateral incisor** crowns are similar in shape to the central incisor, but are longer incisocervically than wide mesiodistally, and are less symmetrical. Distoincisal angles of lateral incisors are even more rounded. Note this difference between the shapes of primary maxillary incisors in Figures 10-8 and 10-9. Laterals are smaller than central incisors in the same dentition.

The crowns of the **mandibular incisors** resemble their replacement incisor crowns, but are much smaller. As with secondary mandibular incisors, primary **mandibular lateral incisor** crowns are a little larger than the crowns of central incisors and less symmetrical (with more rounded distoincisal angles) than the central incisors of the same dentition (*Fig. 10-8*).

The locations of proximal contact areas on primary incisors are comparable to those of their successors.

b.   Surface Morphology of Primary Incisors from the Labial View

Labial surfaces of maxillary central incisors are smooth; usually there are no depressions. Mandibular incisors are also relatively smooth but may have shallow depressions on their labial surfaces in the incisal third.

c.   Root-to-Crown Proportion of Primary Incisors from the Labial View

Prior to root resorption, primary incisor roots are much longer relative to the crown length than on secondary incisors (Appendix 9f). Primary incisor roots are about twice the length of the crown. The roots of **maxillary lateral incisors** appear proportionally even longer. On primary

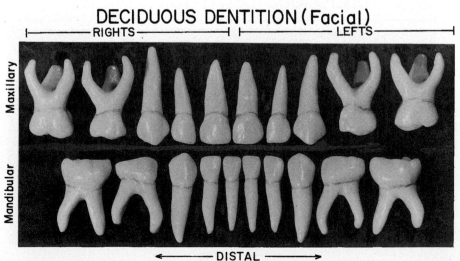

FIGURE 10-8. Deciduous dentition, facial views.

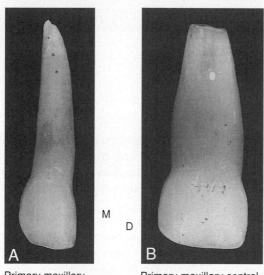

D A M
Primary maxillary
lateral incisor (right)

D B M
Primary maxillary central
incisor (right)

FIGURE 10-9. Primary maxillary incisors. A. The maxillary right lateral incisor crown is less symmetrical and is longer (incisocervically) than it is wide. **B.** The maxillary right central incisor crown is wider (mesiodistally) than it is high (incisocervically). There has been some resorption of the root tips on both teeth (more so on the central incisor), but even so, the roots are twice as long as the crowns.

extracted or shed teeth, there is usually some root resorption (evident in *Fig. 10-9B*). Often the entire root is gone.

2. PRIMARY INCISORS FROM THE LINGUAL VIEW

Refer to *Figure 10-10*.

a. Cingula of Primary Incisors from the Lingual View

The cingula of primary **maxillary central incisors** are often proportionally large, so that lingual fossae are in only the incisal and middle thirds of the lingual surface. The lingual surface of **mandibular incisors** also has a cingulum and a slight lingual fossa.

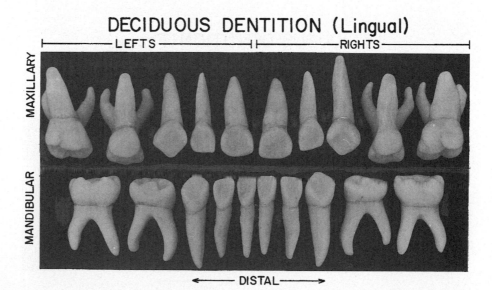

DECIDUOUS DENTITION (Lingual)
LEFTS — RIGHTS
MAXILLARY
MANDIBULAR
← DISTAL →

FIGURE 10-10. Deciduous dentition, lingual views. Notice on maxillary molars that the lingual cusps are not as long as the mesiobuccal cusps.

DECIDUOUS DENTITION (Proximal)

⊢————— Mesial Surfaces —————⊣⊢———— Distal Surfaces ————⊣

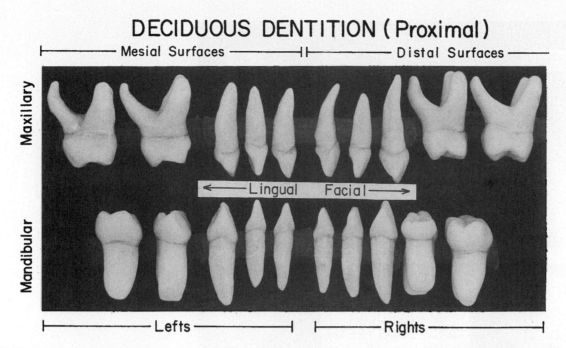

←—— Lingual   Facial ——→

⊢————— Lefts —————⊣ ⊢———— Rights ————⊣

FIGURE 10-11. Deciduous dentition, proximal views. Notice on the molars that more of the occlusal surfaces are visible from the distal view than from the mesial view. Also notice that the apical third of roots of anterior teeth bend labially, especially in the maxillary dentition.

b. Marginal Ridges of Primary Incisors from the Lingual View

On maxillary central incisors, marginal ridges are often distinct and prominent (like shovel-shaped incisors). On mandibular incisors, marginal ridges are more faint (*Fig. 10-10*).

3. PRIMARY INCISORS FROM THE PROXIMAL VIEWS (MESIAL AND DISTAL)

a. Primary Incisor Crown Outlines from the Proximal Views

Although the faciolingual dimension of these crowns appears small from these aspects, crowns are wide labiolingually in their cervical one-third because of prominent, convex labial cervical ridges and lingual cingula. Similar to their successors, incisal ridges of primary maxillary central incisors are located labial to the root axis line, whereas incisal ridges of mandibular incisors are located on the root axis line (*Fig. 10-11*).

b. Cervical Line of Primary Incisors from the Proximal Views

As on secondary incisors, the curve of the cervical line toward the incisal is greater on the mesial than on the distal. The cervical line is positioned more apically on the lingual than on the labial side.

c. Root Shape of Primary Incisors from the Proximal Views

The roots of **maxillary incisors** are curved from this view, bending lingually in the cervical third to half (Appendix 9d), and labially by as much as 10° in the apical half (Appendix 9c).[5] Roots of the **mandibular incisors**, in contrast, are straight in their cervical half, but then bend labially about 10° in their apical half (Appendix 9c).[5] This bend helps make space for the developing succedaneous incisors, which should be in a *lingual and apical position*.

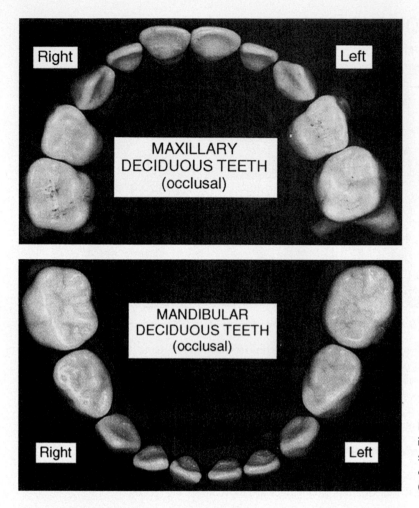

FIGURE 10-12. Deciduous dentition, incisal and occlusal views. Notice the striking resemblance of the second deciduous molars to secondary first (6-year) molars.

4. PRIMARY INCISORS FROM THE INCISAL VIEW

Incisor crowns have a smoothly convex labial outline. The 1-mm thick incisal ridge is slightly curved mesiodistally. The crowns have lingual surfaces that become narrower toward the lingual, at the cingulum.

Crowns of primary **maxillary central incisors** are *much* wider mesiodistally than faciolingually [by 2.4 mm] compared to maxillary lateral incisors, which are only 0.9 mm wider mesiodistally. These proportions are evident in Figure 10-12. Both **mandibular incisor crowns** have mesiodistal and faciolingual dimensions that are essentially equal.

B. PRIMARY CANINE TRAITS

1. PRIMARY CANINES FROM THE LABIAL VIEW

a. Outline Shape of Primary Canines from the Labial View

Maxillary canine crowns may be as wide as they are long. They are constricted at the cervix. They have convex mesial and distal outlines, with distal contours more broadly rounded than mesial contours, which are somewhat angular *(Fig. 10-13).* **Mandibular canine crowns** are longer incisocervically than wide mesiodistally [by 2.1 mm] and are 1.3 mm narrower mesiodistally than maxillary canine crowns (Appendix 9g).

1. Cusp Ridge Outlines
Maxillary canine cusps are often very sharp (pointed) with two cusp ridges meeting at an acute angle. The mesial cusp ridges of these maxillary canines are UNIQUE in that they are

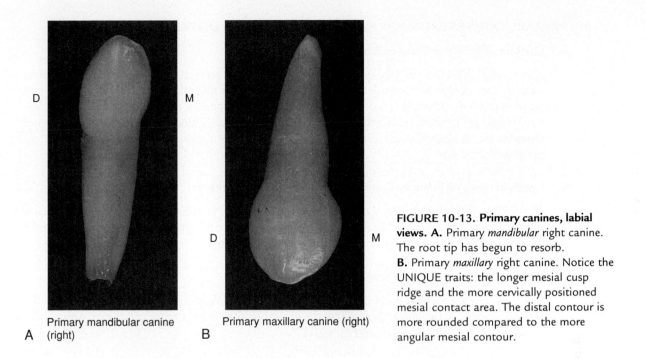

D   M

D   M

Primary mandibular canine
A   (right)

B   Primary maxillary canine (right)

FIGURE 10-13. Primary canines, labial views. A. Primary *mandibular* right canine. The root tip has begun to resorb. **B.** Primary *maxillary* right canine. Notice the UNIQUE traits: the longer mesial cusp ridge and the more cervically positioned mesial contact area. The distal contour is more rounded compared to the more angular mesial contour.

longer than the distal cusp ridges (similar to only the secondary maxillary first premolars, but just the *opposite* of all other premolars and canines, secondary and primary) (Appendix 9h, maxillary canine, and Fig. 10-13B). These mesial cusp ridges are flat to concave and less steeply inclined[6] than the shorter distal ridges, which are more convex. **Mandibular canines** have sharp cusp tips pointed like an arrow (Fig. 10-13A). As on the secondary mandibular canines, the mesial cusp slope is shorter than the distal cusp slope (Appendix 9h, mandibular canine).

2. Contact Areas

Distal contact areas of primary canines rest against the mesial surfaces of primary first molars since there are no primary premolars. Mesial and distal contact areas of **primary maxillary canines** are near the center of the crown cervicoincisally, with *the mesial contact more cervically located* (a condition UNIQUE to this tooth and the mandibular first premolar) (Appendix 9i).

b. Cervical Lines of Primary Canines from the Labial View

Cervical lines on maxillary canines are nearly flat on the labial surface.

c. Roots of Primary Canines from the Labial View

Maxillary canine roots prior to resorption are the longest of the primary teeth [13.5 mm] tapering to a blunt apex. The roots of mandibular canines are more tapered and pointed, and shorter than maxillary canine roots [by 1.8 mm].

2. PRIMARY CANINES FROM THE LINGUAL VIEW

The cingulum on a maxillary canine crown is bulky with well-developed mesial and distal marginal ridges that are, however, less prominent than on the secondary canines (Fig. 10-10).

A lingual ridge, with an adjacent mesial and distal fossa, is located on a maxillary canine crown somewhat distal to the middle of the crown. Distal fossae on these teeth are narrower and deeper than mesial fossae, which are broader and shallower.[5,6] In contrast, lingual ridges are barely discernible on mandibular canines, with faint marginal ridges and usually a single concavity or fossa (Fig. 10-10).[7]

3. PRIMARY CANINES FROM THE PROXIMAL (MESIAL AND DISTAL) VIEWS

a. Outline of Primary Canines from the Proximal Views

The cervical third of a primary canine is much thicker than on an incisor. On **maxillary** canines, cusp tips are positioned considerably labial to the root axis line (Fig. 10-11), whereas the cusp tip of **mandibular** canines is most often located slightly lingual to the root axis line. Labial cervical ridges are prominent on *both* maxillary and mandibular canines, bulging similar to lingual cingula. The S-shaped lingual crown outline of **maxillary** canines is more concave than on permanent canines.

b. Cervical Lines of Primary Canines from the Proximal Views

Cervical lines of both maxillary and mandibular canines curve incisally more on the mesial side than on the distal side, just like all other anterior teeth. Like primary incisors, the cervical lines are positioned more apical on the lingual than on the labial.

c. Roots of Primary Canines from the Proximal Views

The roots of *both* maxillary and mandibular canines are bulky in the cervical and middle thirds, tapering mostly in the apical third where the apex is bent labially, similar to primary central and lateral incisors (Appendix 9c and Fig. 10-11).

4. PRIMARY CANINES FROM THE INCISAL VIEW

a. Crown Outline of Primary Canines from the Incisal View

The crown outline of **maxillary canines** taper noticeably toward the cingulum, which is centered mesiodistally. The *mesial* half of these crowns is thicker faciolingually than the distal half (similar to secondary maxillary canines). From the incisal aspect, **mandibular canine** crowns have a *diamond shape* and are nearly symmetrical, except for the mesial position of the cusp tips, and they appear to have slightly more bulk in the distal half (Fig. 10-12). Cingula are centered or just distal to the center.

b. Crown Proportions and Size of Primary Canines from the Incisal View

Primary **maxillary canine** crowns are broader faciolingually than incisor crowns, but are still wider mesiodistally than faciolingually [by 2 mm]. The 1.5-mm thick mesial and distal cusp ridges curve toward the lingual at both ends. **Mandibular canine** crowns are only slightly wider mesiodistally than faciolingually [by 0.4 mm]. The smallness of these teeth, compared to their replacement counterparts, is quite noticeable.

C. PRIMARY MOLAR TRAITS

As stated earlier, primary molar roots are thin and widely spread to make room for the developing premolar crowns that are forming beneath them *(Fig. 10-14)*. Recall that primary *first molars* form over the crowns of developing *first premolars* and erupt just distal to primary canines and just mesial to primary second molars. Primary *second molars* form over the crowns of developing *second premolars*, just distal to primary first molars and, after age 6, just mesial to 6-year first molars. It could be said that these primary molars are saving a place in the arch for the teeth that will succeed them, namely, the first and second premolars, respectively.

Primary **second molars** have considerable similarities to *secondary first molars* in their respective arches. Since these teeth are adjacent to one another during the time of mixed dentition (or longer in the case of retained primary teeth), it is important to distinguish between the primary second molars and the 6-year first molars that erupt just distal to them. One obvious difference between primary and secondary molar crowns is the presence of a prominent mesial cervical ridge on the buccal surface of primary molars. This bulge is sometimes called a buccal cingulum.[4] Also, primary second molars are smaller than 6-year first molars in the same dentition. Tooth position from the midline is also an

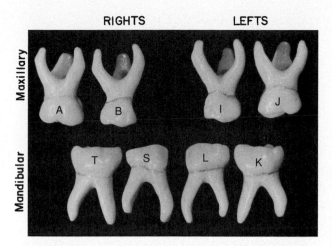

RIGHTS   LEFTS

Maxillary

Mandibular

FIGURE 10-14. All eight primary molars, buccal views. Each tooth is identified with its Universal letter.

important clue for tooth identification. Primary second molars are normally the fifth tooth from the midline, whereas secondary first molars are sixth from the midline. The differences in size and position between the primary maxillary second molar and the secondary maxillary first molar are evident in Figures 10-15 and 10-16.

Primary first molars are more unique in their shape. One author feels that primary *maxillary* first molars are the most atypical of human molars,[8] while another author feels that the crowns somewhat resemble premolars (from the occlusal view).[9] It is agreed that primary *mandibular* first molars resemble no other tooth in either dentition.

When considering **arch traits** of all primary molars, consider the number of roots. **Primary maxillary molars** generally have three roots (mesiobuccal, distobuccal, and palatal, as on secondary maxillary

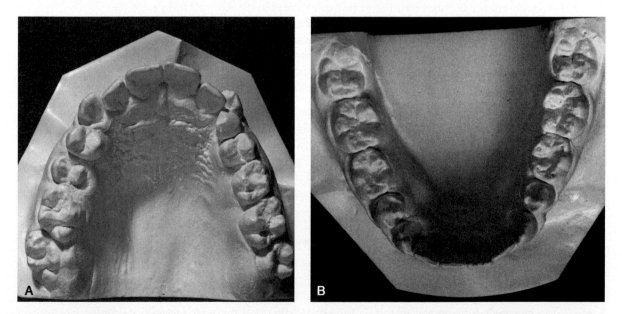

FIGURE 10-15. Mixed dentition. A. In the maxillary arch, the fifth tooth from the midline on the left side of the photograph is a second premolar, but the fifth tooth on the right side is a primary second molar. Notice the similarity of the primary second molar with the larger 6-year molar just distal to it. Also notice the position of the secondary maxillary canine, which is normally the last succedaneous tooth to erupt (positioned just labial to the primary canine which is still present). B. In the mandibular arch, the fifth tooth from the midline on both the right and left sides is the primary second molar. Notice the similarity in morphology with the larger 6-year molar just distal to it (sixth from the midline). (Models courtesy of Dr. Brad Woodford, Ohio State University.)

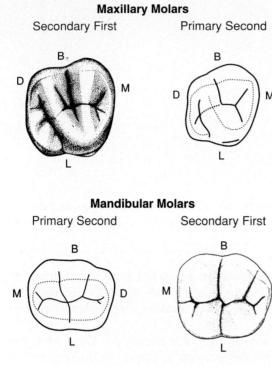

Maxillary Molars

Secondary First   Primary Second

Mandibular Molars

Primary Second   Secondary First

FIGURE 10-16. Comparison of occlusal morphology of primary second molars compared to secondary first molars. The secondary first molars are located just distal to primary second molars from about age 6 through 11 or 12 years old. **Top:** The secondary **maxillary** first molar is larger but otherwise similar to the primary maxillary second molar in overall shape, number of cusps (maybe even a cusp of Carabelli), grooves, ridges (including oblique), and fossae. **Bottom:** The secondary **mandibular** first molar is larger but otherwise similar to primary mandibular second molars in overall shape, number of cusps, grooves, ridges, and fossae. The three buccal cusps, however, are more equal is size on the primary mandibular molars, whereas the distal cusp on the secondary first molar is the smallest.

molars), whereas **primary mandibular molars** have only two roots (mesial and distal, as on secondary mandibular molars). Also, like secondary molars, *maxillary* primary molars tend to be wider buccolingually than mesiodistally, whereas *mandibular* molars tend to be wider mesiodistally than buccolingually. Compare the occlusal outlines of primary molars in the Appendix on page 10.

Each type of primary molar will be discussed in detail at this time, emphasizing the traits that further differentiate each type. Discussion begins with primary *second* molars since they are similar to the secondary first (6-year) molars discussed previously in Chapter 7.

1.   TYPE TRAITS OF THE PRIMARY MAXILLARY SECOND MOLAR

Primary maxillary second molars *resemble the 6-year (adult) maxillary first molars*, which erupt just distal to them (as evident on the right side of the photograph in *Fig. 10-15A*), but are smaller [by 13.2% when all dimensions are averaged]. They are similar in most respects, with the cusp ridges and fossae corresponding to those of permanent first molars. Maxillary primary second molars may even have a cusp of Carabelli (*Fig. 10-17B and C*). Primary maxillary second molar crowns are wider [mesiodistally by 47%] than the maxillary second premolars that will replace them.

a.   Crown Morphology of the Primary Maxillary Second Molar

Due to the prominent mesiobuccal cervical ridge and small occlusal table, these primary molars, when viewed from the proximal aspect (*Fig. 10-18*), appear to taper narrower considerably toward the occlusal (Appendix 10c and e).[5] From the occlusal aspect, the crown also tapers considerably narrower from mesial to distal, accentuated by the prominent mesiobuccal bulge (seen in the Appendix page 10, occlusal view).

Further, the mesiolingual corner of the occlusal surface is flattened as though it were compressed toward the distal[5] (Appendix 10h), displacing the mesiolingual cusp more distally than on the permanent first molars. This results in more taper from buccal to lingual, an oblique ridge that is straighter in its course buccolingually,[5] and a smaller, oblong distal fossa buccolingually (Fig. 10-17C).

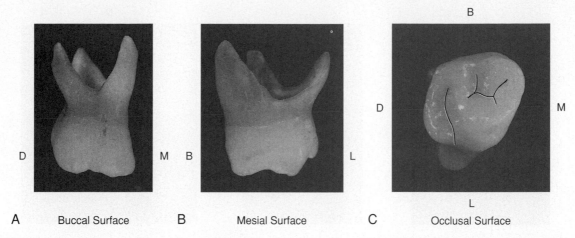

| A | Buccal Surface | B | Mesial Surface | C | Occlusal Surface |

FIGURE 10-17. Primary maxillary right second molar. A. Buccal surface. **B.** Mesial surface. Notice the spread of the roots. The crown of the maxillary second premolar develops in the space bounded by these roots. Some root resorption has occurred (especially on the lingual root). **C.** Occlusal surface. From this aspect, the primary maxillary second molar resembles a miniature 6-year first molar (even with a Carabelli cusp).

The mesiobuccal cusp is almost equal in size or slightly larger than the mesiolingual cusp (Appendix 10i). (Recall that the mesiolingual cusp is largest on permanent maxillary first molars.)

b. Roots of Primary Maxillary Second Molar

The three roots (mesiobuccal, distobuccal, and palatal) are thin and slender and widely spread apart, with the root furcation very close to the cervical line so there is very little root trunk.

2. TYPE TRAITS OF THE PRIMARY MANDIBULAR SECOND MOLAR

The primary mandibular second molars *resemble the 6-year (adult) mandibular first molars*, which erupt just distal to them (Fig. 10-16B), but are smaller [by 17.3% when all dimensions are averaged]. They are similar in most respects, with the cusp ridges and fossae corresponding to those of

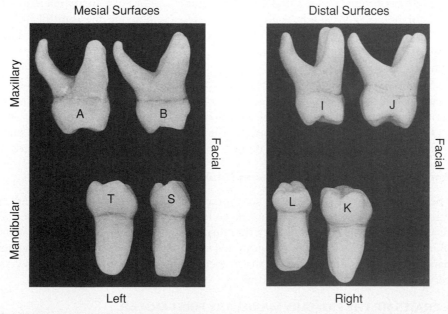

FIGURE 10-18. All eight primary molars, proximal views. Each tooth is identified with its Universal letter. Notice on mesial views that the wider mesiobuccal root of the maxillary molars hides the narrower distobuccal root, just as in adult maxillary molars.

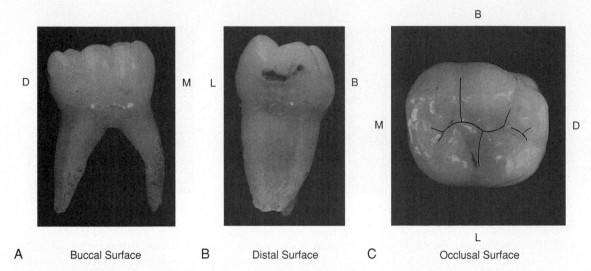

A   Buccal Surface   **B**   Distal Surface   **C**   Occlusal Surface

FIGURE 10-19. Primary mandibular second molar (right). A. Buccal surface. The short root trunk and the widespread roots, as well as the small size, distinguish this tooth from the secondary mandibular first molar. The mesiobuccal, distobuccal, and distal cusps are often about the same size. **B.** Distal surface. **C.** Occlusal surface.

secondary first molars *(Fig. 10-19)*. Primary mandibular second molar crowns are wider [mesiodistally by 45%] than the mandibular second premolars that will replace them.

a. Crown Morphology of the Primary Mandibular Second Molar

Compared to *secondary* mandibular *first* molars, *primary* mandibular *second* molars have a more prominent mesial cervical ridge, the roots are more slender and more widely spread, and the three buccal cusps (mesiobuccal, distobuccal, and distal) are of *nearly equal size* (Appendix 10j). The middle buccal cusp (called the distobuccal) is the widest (largest). As on the 6-year mandibular molars, these cusps are separated by mesiobuccal and distobuccal grooves. The mesiolingual and distolingual cusps are about the same size and height, slightly shorter than the buccal cusps.[5] A lingual groove separates these two lingual cusps.

From the proximal views, the mesial marginal ridge of the primary mandibular second molar is high and is crossed by a groove that may extend about one-third of the way down the mesial surface.[9] This mesial surface is generally convex but flattens cervically. The contact area with the primary first molar is in the shape of an inverted crescent just below the notch of the marginal ridge.[9]

Since the crown is shorter on the distal side and the distal marginal ridge is lower (more cervical) than the mesial marginal ridge, all five cusps can be seen from the distal aspect. The distal contact with the mesial side of the 6-year first molar is round in shape and is located just buccal and cervical to the distal marginal groove (furrow) (Fig. 10-19B).[9] The cervical line is almost flat on both the mesial and distal sides of the crown but slopes occlusally toward the lingual.

b. Roots of Primary Mandibular Second Molar

The two roots (mesial and distal) are thin and slender and widely spread apart, with the root furcation very close to the cervical line so there is very little root trunk. The roots are about twice as long as the crowns and are thin mesiodistally. The *mesial* root is broad and flat with a blunt apex, and has a shallow longitudinal depression. The *distal* root is broad and flat and is narrower and less blunt at the apex than the mesial root. The root furcation is very close to the cervical line with very little root trunk.

3. TYPE TRAITS OF THE PRIMARY MAXILLARY FIRST MOLAR

Primary maxillary first molars are quite unique in appearance *(Fig. 10-20)*. According to one author, they do not resemble any other molars.[8] According to another author, from the occlusal view they resemble maxillary first premolars that replace them (Appendix page 10, occlusal view).[9]

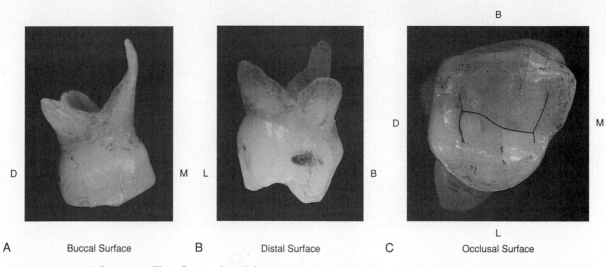

A   Buccal Surface   B   Distal Surface   C   Occlusal Surface

FIGURE 10-20. Primary maxillary first molar (right). A. Buccal surface. The mesiobuccal root is less resorbed than the distobuccal and lingual roots. The lingual root is barely discernible. **B.** Distal surface. **C.** Occlusal surface. The prominent cervical ridge below the mesiobuccal cusp gives the tooth an angular appearance. Notice the "H"-shaped groove pattern, somewhat resembling the occlusal view of a maxillary premolar.

The crowns are slightly wider than the premolars that will replace them [mesiodistally by 14%]. From the buccal aspect, these crowns appear very wide relative to their height, and are noticeably shorter occlusocervically toward the distal. The mesiobuccal cusp has a buccal ridge (running occlusocervically) that extends to the cervical line.

When the buccal surface is viewed from the proximal, the prominent mesial buccal cervical ridge and adjacent flat buccal outline from cervical ridge toward the occlusal surface results in a considerable taper from the wide cervical third to the narrow occlusal third (Appendix 10c and e, proximal views). The *lingual* outline from the proximal view is more gradually convex in the cervical and middle third and flat in the occlusal third.

a. Crown Morphology of Primary Maxillary First Molars

The occlusal outline is basically rectangular (wider faciolingually than mesiodistally [by 1.4 mm]) (Appendix 10m and *Fig. 10-21*, teeth B and I). Further, the prominent mesiobuccal cervical ridge (running mesiodistally in the cervical third) results in a wider dimension buccolingually in the mesial half, and a taper toward the distal. This tooth also tapers toward the lingual due to the mesial marginal ridge, which does not run straight toward the lingual, but rather runs obliquely in a distolingual direction. This taper is similar to that on the mesiolingual corner in the primary maxillary second molar (Appendix 10n). In contrast, the *distal* marginal ridge runs in a straight direction buccolingually, joining both the buccal and lingual borders at right angles,[7] best seen in Figure 10-20, occlusal view.

The mesial contact is flat where it contacts the canine in the occlusal third. The distal crown outline is decidedly more convex than the mesial, and contacts the primary second molar in the middle third.

Primary maxillary first molars, like secondary maxillary molars, usually have four cusps, but they may appear somewhat like maxillary premolars from the occlusal view since they have only *two prominent* cusps (a wide mesiobuccal cusp and a narrower, slightly more distinct, mesiolingual cusp). The other two cusps, the distobuccal and distolingual, are relatively indistinct and may blend into the distal marginal ridge. When a distolingual cusp is present (four-cusp type), it is inconspicuous and it is often only a small nodule on the lingual half of the distal marginal ridge. Sometimes, the distolingual cusp is absent (three-cusp type), and the triangular ridge of the narrow distobuccal cusp actually becomes the distal marginal ridge.

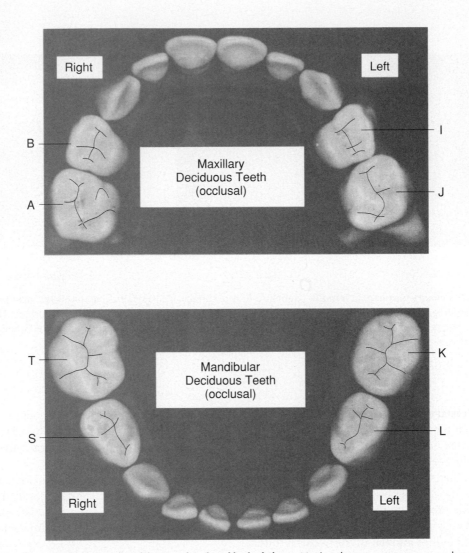

FIGURE 10-21. Complete primary dentition, occlusal and incisal views. Notice the groove patterns and outlines of the primary molars from this view.

The mesiobuccal cusp is the longest (but second sharpest) cusp.[5] The mesiolingual cusp is the second longest, but sharpest, cusp. In the four-cusp type, the triangular ridges of the distobuccal cusp join the more distal of the two triangular ridges from the mesiolingual cusp as a barely discernible transverse ridge.[9] There is no buccal groove on the buccal surface, just a slight notch that divides the large mesiobuccal cusp from the indistinct distobuccal cusp (Appendix 10l). This notch is distal to center. A groove between the two lingual cusps is present only when the distolingual cusp is definite.

There are three fossae on these maxillary first molars: a medium-size central fossa, a large and deep mesial triangular fossa, and a minute distal triangular fossa, each with a pit: central, mesial, and distal, respectively (Appendix 10o).

The occlusal grooves of the four-cusp type primary maxillary first molar teeth usually form an "H" pattern (seen in Fig. 10-20). The crossbar of the "H" is the central groove that connects the central and mesial triangular fossae. [Some textbooks say there is no central groove and that the crossbar is made up of a mesial and distal groove instead.[9]] Supplemental grooves running buccolingually just inside of the mesial marginal ridge form the mesial side of the "H," and the buccal groove (dividing the buccal cusps) combined with the distolingual groove (between the large mesiolingual and minute distolingual cusps on four-cusp type molars only) form the distal side of the "H." The mesial marginal ridge may be crossed by a marginal groove.

b. Roots of Primary Maxillary First Molar

The three roots (mesiobuccal, distobuccal, and palatal) are thin and slender and widely spread apart, with the root furcation very close to the cervical line so there is very little root trunk (Appendix 10f).

4. TYPE TRAITS OF THE PRIMARY MANDIBULAR FIRST MOLARS

These mandibular first molars do *not* resemble any other primary or secondary tooth (Fig. 10-21, teeth L and S, and *Fig. 10-22*). According to one author, the chief differentiating characteristic may be an overdeveloped mesial marginal ridge (Appendix 10q).[9] The mesial marginal ridge is so well developed that it resembles a cusp.[2] This longer, prominent mesial marginal ridge is positioned more occlusally than the short (buccolingual), less prominent distal marginal ridge. (Compare mesial and distal views in Fig. 10-18 for marginal ridge heights and lengths.)

Primary mandibular first molar crowns are wider [mesiodistally by 24%] than the mandibular first premolars that will replace them.

a. Crown Morphology of the Primary Mandibular First Molar

From the *facial* (and *lingual*) views, the crowns of these first molars are wider mesiodistally than high cervico-occlusally [by 1.6 mm] (Fig. 10-22A). Facially, they are longer (occlusocervically) on the mesial, due in part to the slope of the cervical line gingivally toward the mesial, separating the very prominent mesiobuccal cervical ridge from the root, and also due to the cervical slope of the occlusal border from mesial to distal. The mesial contact area with the canine is located more cervically than the distal contact area, which is in the middle of the crown.

The cervical line on the mesial, although it arcs toward the occlusal, also slopes gingivally toward the buccal (where the mesiobuccal cervical ridge meets the root, Fig. 10-22B). On the distal or lingual surface, the cervical line is practically flat or horizontal from buccal to lingual or from mesial to distal, respectively.

Recall that the crowns of all *mandibular* posterior teeth, primary and secondary, appear to lean lingually, even more so with primary teeth. This primary mandibular first molar crown appears to lean decidedly toward the lingual (accentuated by the prominent mesiobuccal cervical ridge), placing the buccal cusp tips well over the root base.[6] The lingual cusp tip may even be outside the lingual margin of the root (Fig. 10-22B). From the proximal views, the buccal crown contour is nearly (but not quite) flat from the buccal crest of curvature to the occlusal surface and cervico-occlusally. The lingual surface is more convex cervico-occlusally.

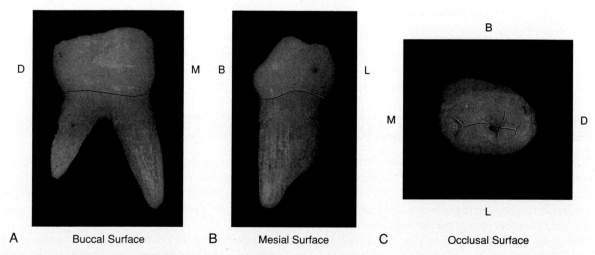

A	Buccal Surface	B	Mesial Surface	C	Occlusal Surface

FIGURE 10-22. Primary mandibular first molar (right). A. Buccal surface. The distal root has been considerably shortened by resorption. Notice that the crown is longer mesially (right side) than distally. **B.** Mesial surface. Again, the buccal cervical ridge is outstanding. Notice the very narrow occlusal surface and how the crown appears to tilt lingually. If the root apex was not partially resorbed, the root would appear to taper to a more blunt end. **C.** Occlusal surface. The buccal cervical ridge on the mesiobuccal cusp is conspicuous.

The general shape of the *entire* occlusal outline is somewhat oval or rectangular (wider mesiodistally than buccolingually, as seen in Figs. 10-21 and 10-22C). As with the primary maxillary molars, these teeth taper narrower toward the lingual but do so primarily due to the taper of the mesial surface (Appendix 10s), and not of the distal side.[2] Subsequently, the mesiobuccal angle is acute, whereas the distobuccal angle is obtuse. The mesial crown contour is nearly flat buccolingually, whereas the distal surface is convex; the lingual surface is convex mesiodistally.

The shape of the *occlusal table* is wider mesiodistally than buccolingually (Appendix 10r).[9] There is a *prominent transverse ridge* between the mesiobuccal and mesiolingual cusps (Appendix 10u and Fig. 10-21, teeth L and S). Even though the *entire tooth outline* from the occlusal view appears to be wider on the mesial half due to the prominent mesial cervical ridge, the *occlusal table width* distal to the transverse ridge is larger than that portion mesial to the transverse ridge (Appendix 10v). Subsequently, the mesial triangular fossa and pit are relatively small, and the *distal fossa* is larger, extending almost into the center of the occlusal surfaces (Appendix 10v). In the large *distal fossa*, there is a central pit and a small distal pit near the distal marginal ridge. There is no *central fossa*.

This tooth has *four cusps*. The cusps are often difficult to distinguish, but careful examination of an unworn tooth will reveal (in order of diminishing size) a mesiobuccal, mesiolingual, distobuccal, and the smallest (also shortest) distolingual cusp. The *mesiobuccal cusp* of the mandibular first molar is always the largest and longest cusp, occupying nearly two-thirds of the buccal surface (Appendix 10t; Fig. 10-22A). This cusp is characteristically *compressed buccolingually*, and its two long cusp ridges extend mesially and distally, serving as a blade when occluding with the maxillary canine.[5] The smaller *distobuccal cusp* is separated from the mesiobuccal cusp by a depression rather than a distinct groove. The *mesiolingual cusp* is larger, longer, and sharper than the distolingual cusp, and there is a slight groove between these two lingual cusps that ends in a depression near the cervix of the crown. The distal spur of the *distolingual cusp* forms the lingual third of the distal marginal ridge ending in a furrow.[5]

A central groove separates the mesiobuccal and mesiolingual cusps and connects with a mesial marginal groove (furrow). There is a short buccal groove and a short lingual groove on the occlusal surface. The buccal groove does not extend onto the buccal surface, and the lingual groove becomes a shallow depression on the lingual surface. Both marginal ridges have furrows or grooves between them and cusp ridges of lingual cusps[6] similar to the supplemental grooves in the triangular fossae of other posterior teeth. These grooves serve as escapeways during mastication.

b. Roots of Primary Mandibular First Molars

The two roots (mesial and distal) are thin and slender and widely spread apart, with the root furcation very close to the cervical line, so there is very little root trunk (Appendix 10f). The mesial root is wider (square and flat) and longer than the distal root. The distal root is more rounded, less broad, thinner, and shorter than the mesial root.

SECTION V.   PULP CAVITIES OF PRIMARY TEETH

Primary anterior teeth have pulp cavities that are similar in shape to the pulp cavities of the secondary teeth, but are much larger in proportion because of the thinner, more uniform enamel covering, and the thinner portion of dentin in the deciduous teeth. On anterior primary teeth, there are slight projections on the incisal border corresponding to the lobes, and there is usually no demarcation or constriction between the single canal and pulp chamber except on the mandibular central incisor.[9]

Primary molar teeth, when compared with secondary molars, have pulp chambers much less elongated vertically relative to the size of the tooth. In primary molars there is little or almost no root trunk, so the pulp chambers are mostly in the tooth crown (*Fig. 10-23A*). Compare this to secondary molars, where much of the pulp chamber is located in the root trunk. The pulp chambers of primary molars have long and often very narrow pulp horns extending beneath the cusps. The mesiobuccal pulp horn (and cusp) of the primary maxillary second molar is longest in that tooth, compared to the mesiolingual horn (and cusp) in the

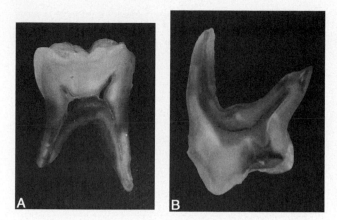

FIGURE 10-23. **Cross section of primary molars.**
A. Primary *mandibular* right second molar, **cross section** (buccal side ground off to expose pulp cavity). An interesting feature is the long narrow shape of the pulp horns, which often extend more into the crown, even higher or closer to the occlusal surface than seen in this cross section. **B.** Primary *maxillary* first molar, **cross section** (mesial side removed). The root canals of the mesiobuccal root and of the lingual root (right side of picture) are exposed. An extensive area of decay beneath the enamel of the lingual cusp has reached the prominent pulp horn.

secondary maxillary first molar. Great care must be taken when preparing primary teeth for restorations to avoid cutting into (exposing) the pulp horns during cavity preparation *(Fig. 10.23B).*

LEARNING EXERCISES

1. If you are fortunate to have a collection of primary teeth, study the morphology for variations. Observe differences in the amount of root resorption, examine the occlusal surface for wear facets due to attrition, and evaluate the interior pulp chamber (after sectioning) for size, pulp horns, and thickness of enamel and dentin. Use the distinguishing characteristics in *Table 10-5* and 10-6 to identify each tooth within your collection of deciduous teeth. If you do not have any teeth to study, try to recognize these traits as seen in the figures in this chapter.

2. In the four cases that follow, identify each tooth in a mixed dentition, and estimate "expected dental age" based on average eruption dates as follows: If you have learned the important range of dates for tooth eruption and the sequence of eruption within those ranges, you should be able to estimate the "expected dental age" of a child based on what teeth are present in the mouth.

   CASE 1: For example, look at *Figure 10-24* and estimate the expected age of the child based on the teeth visible in the mouth and those developing within the bone and still not erupted.

   Answer: Let us look at the facts. First, all primary teeth have erupted (which can be deduced based on their relatively small size, thin roots, and the fact that all permanent succedaneous teeth are forming apical to their primary tooth predecessors). Therefore, the child is at least 2 years old. Next, the first permanent molars are not even close to emerging, so the child must be considerably younger than 6 years old. Finally, no resorption has begun on the primary tooth roots, so we can conclude that the child is closer to 3 or 4 years old, rather than to 5 or 6, since primary teeth roots begin to resorb about 3 years after eruption, which for the mandibular central incisors would be about 3½ years old.

   CASE 2: Next, estimate the dental age of the child based on the shapes of teeth in the radiographs in *Figure 10-25.*

   Answer: We see two *mandibular* premolar-shaped crowns (with no roots) forming under the roots of two primary molars (evidenced by their divergent roots). Distal to the primary second molars are the larger, erupted 6-year molars with incomplete roots. The secondary maxillary canine and

Table 10-5	ARCH TRAITS THAT DISTINGUISH PRIMARY MAXILLARY FROM MANDIBULAR TEETH

Maxillary Central Incisor	Mandibular Central Incisor
Short, wide, symmetrical crown	Long, narrow, symmetrical, very small
Root bends facially in apical one-third	Root straighter but still bends facially in apical one-third
Root long and bulky	Root long and thin
Large, elevated cingulum	Smaller, less prominent cingulum
Maxillary Lateral Incisor	**Mandibular Lateral Incisor**
Crown narrow and oblong	Smaller cingulum
Root bends facially in apical one-third	Root bends facially in apical one-third
Maxillary Canine	**Mandibular Canine**
Wide crown mesiodistally	Crown longer, narrower, less symmetrical
Cusp tip sharp and centered	Cusp tip toward mesial
Mesial cusp ridge longer, steeper than distal	Mesial cusp ridge shorter than distal
Cingulum centered	Cingulum distally located
Mesial contact more cervical than distal	Distal contact more cervical than mesial
Root bends facially in apical one-third	Root with less facial bend in apical one-third
Flat labial cervical line	
Maxillary First Molar	**Mandibular First Molar**
3 roots (if intact): mesiobuccal (MB), distobuccal (DB), and lingual	2 roots (if intact): mesial and distal
3–4 cusps: MB largest, DB, mesiolingual (ML), and distolingual (DL) may be absent	4 cusps: MB, DB, ML, and DL
Crown wider faciolingually than mesiodistally; tapers to lingual	Crown much wider mesiodistally than faciolingually
Crown wider faciolingually on mesial than distal; tapers to distal	Occlusal table has small mesial triangular fossa; large distal fossa
H-shaped occlusal grooves	Well-developed mesial marginal ridge
Unique crown shape (or premolar-like)	Unique crown shape
Maxillary Second Molar	**Mandibular Second Molar**
3 roots (if intact): MB, DB, and lingual	2 roots (if intact): mesial and distal
Crown resembles small secondary maxillary first molar	Crown resembles small secondary mandibular first molar

maxillary second molar crowns (only partially visible) are still within the bone. By deduction, the child should be over 6 but not yet 12. Since the primary molars' roots are partially resorbed, the succedaneous premolars are close to emerging, making the child closer to 8 or 9 years old. *If you could confirm that the succedaneous incisors were all erupted, you could estimate the age at just over 9 years old.*

CASE 3: Using the logic of deduction, look at the cutaway model in *Figure 10-26* and see if you can estimate the expected dental age before reading the answer here.

Answer: The secondary first molars have emerged into the mouth, making the child at least 6 years old. The relatively large size of the anterior incisor crowns and lack of succedaneous teeth apical to the roots indicate that the erupted incisors are succedaneous, which places the age at 9 years old or older. The 12-year molar has not emerged, so the child is between 9 and 12 years old. Since none of the succedaneous canines or premolars has yet emerged, the dental age is around 9.

CASE 4: Finally, examine the unique dentition in *Figure 10-27* to determine which teeth are present and which teeth are absent. *Use the position from the midline as a guide to look for each tooth you expect to occupy that*

Table 10-6	HOW TO TELL RIGHT FROM LEFT PRIMARY TEETH

Maxillary Central Incisor	Mandibular Central Incisor
90° mesioincisal angle Distal contact more cervical than mesial Distoincisal angle more rounded Crown outline flat on mesial More cervical line curvature on mesial	Difficult to discern
Maxillary Lateral Incisor	**Mandibular Lateral Incisor**
Flat mesial and rounded distal outline Distal contact more cervical than mesial More rounded distoincisal angle More cervical line curvature on mesial	More rounded distoincisal angle and distal crown bulge Distal contact more cervical than mesial More rounded distoincisal angle
Maxillary Canine	**Mandibular Canine**
Longer mesial cusp ridge Deeper and narrower distal than mesial fossa Mesial contact more cervical than distal Flat mesial crown outline More cervical line curvature on mesial	Shorter mesial cusp ridge Distal contact more cervical than mesial More cervical line curvature on mesial
Maxillary First Molar	**Mandibular First Molar**
Crown longer on mesial than distal (facial) Crown wider (faciolingually) on mesial than distal Mesial cervical crown bulge Distal marginal ridge more cervical than mesial Distobuccal root (if intact) is smallest; shortest Mesiolingual cusp pointed	Crown longer on mesial than distal (facial) Occlusal table has small mesial triangular fossa; large distal fossa Mesial cervical crown bulge Distal marginal ridge more cervical than mesial Mesial root (if intact) longer and wider (faciolingually)
Maxillary Second Molar	**Mandibular Second Molar**
Mesial cervical crown bulge Crown longer on mesial than distal (facial view) Large mesiolingual cusp Distal marginal ridge more cervical than mesial Distobuccal root shortest and smallest	Mesial cervical crown bulge Crown longer on mesial than distal (facial view) Has fifth (distal) cusp Distal marginal ridge more cervical than mesial Mesial root (if intact) longer and wider (faciolingually)

position, but always remember that the space could be occupied by the primary tooth OR its succedaneous tooth. Also, realize that spaces are not always present when a tooth is missing. The teeth on either side of the space may move together and close the space either through orthodontic treatment or due to a common tendency for teeth distal to a space to move (drift) into, and close, the space. Therefore, if a space is not occupied by the *expected* primary *or* secondary tooth, it may be because the tooth has been extracted or is missing, and you will have to adjust your positioning from the midline accordingly.

Answer: In this case, beginning at the midline, the large incisors appear to be adult central incisors, but the next teeth from the midline do not resemble lateral incisors. Instead, these teeth look like secondary canines, followed distally by first premolars. We therefore need to suspect that the lateral incisors are missing *or* still unerupted (impacted) within the maxillae. The teeth distal to the first premolars, which in an adult dentition should be the second premolars, instead resemble small maxillary first molars, followed by larger maxillary first molars. This leads us to conclude that the smaller molars, in the place of the maxillary second premolars, could be *primary* second molars (resembling the larger emerged 6-year first molars just distal to them). Since the 12-year second molars are also present (though partially cut off in the photo), the patient would be at least 12 years old. If that is true, we need to ask why there are no secondary lateral incisors or second premolars,

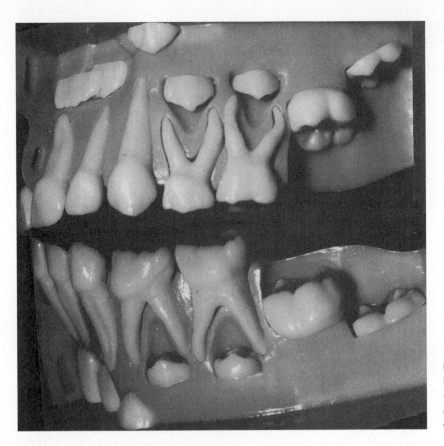

FIGURE 10-24. Learning Case 1: Using the guidelines presented in this chapter, estimate the expected dental age of the child with this mixed dentition.

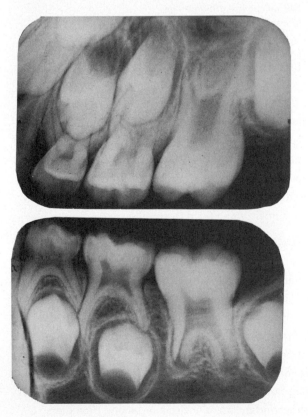

FIGURE 10-25. Learning Case 2: Based on these radiographs of mixed dentition, estimate the expected dental age of this child. (Radiographs courtesy of Professor Donald Bowers, Ohio State University.)

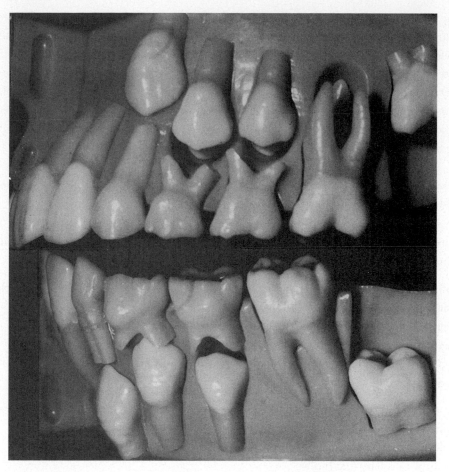

FIGURE 10-26. Learning Case 3: Estimate the expected dental age of the child with this mixed dentition.

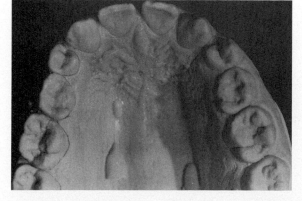

Expected Teeth Based on Normal Position from the Midline	
Position from midline:	Teeth expected in that position (if there are no missing or extra teeth):
1st tooth from midline	Primary central incisor
	OR
	secondary central incisor
2nd tooth from midline	Primary lateral incisor
	OR
	secondary lateral incisor
3rd tooth from midline	Primary canine
	OR
	secondary canine
4th tooth from midline	Primary first molar
	OR
	first premolar (adult)
5th tooth from midline	Primary second molar
	OR
	second premolar (adult)
6th tooth from midline	Secondary (6-year) first molar
7th tooth from midline	Secondary (12-year) second molar
8th tooth from midline	Secondary third molar

FIGURE 10-27. Learning Case 4: Identify each visible tooth in the unique dentition of this 15 year old. Use the **chart** to guide your decision, but notice that some teeth are missing with the spaces filled in by adjacent teeth.

and why the primary second molars are still present. A good history (to determine which teeth have been extracted or have been confirmed as missing) along with excellent radiographs are needed to see whether the secondary lateral incisors or second premolars are still unerupted within the bone (impacted). If the lateral incisors are not present and never formed, they would be considered **congenitally absent** (that is, as a result of factors existing at birth). If the primary second molars were maintained into the adult dentition (usually because the second premolars were congenitally absent), the primary teeth in an adult would be called **retained deciduous teeth**. More on the topic of missing teeth will be presented in the chapter on dental anomalies.

LEARNING QUESTIONS

Circle the correct answer(s). More than one answer may be correct. Unless otherwise stated, teeth are identified using the Universal Identification System.

1. Which primary teeth have crowns that are wider mesiodistally than they are long inciso- or occluso-cervically?
   a. maxillary central incisor
   b. maxillary first molar
   c. mandibular lateral incisor
   d. mandibular first molar
   e. mandibular canine

2. Which one tooth is adjacent and distal to the primary maxillary second molar in a 7 year old?
   a. maxillary first premolar
   b. maxillary second premolar
   c. secondary maxillary first molar
   d. secondary maxillary second molar
   e. primary maxillary first molar

3. How many teeth should be visible in the mouth of a 3 year old?
   a. none
   b. 10
   c. 20
   d. 24
   e. 28

4. How many teeth should be present in the mouth of a 13 year old?
   a. 10
   b. 20
   c. 24
   d. 28
   e. 32

5. Which primary molar most resembles a secondary maxillary right first molar?
   a. tooth A
   b. tooth E
   c. tooth F
   d. tooth T
   e. tooth B

6. What would you estimate to be the dental age of a child with the following teeth: all primary maxillary incisors, canines, and molars; secondary mandibular incisors and first molars.
   a. 2–4 years
   b. 5–7 years
   c. 8–9 years
   d. 10–11 years
   e. over 12 years

7. Which teeth (primary or secondary) have the mesial proximal contact positioned more cervically than the distal proximal contact?
   a. mandibular first premolar
   b. maxillary first premolar
   c. primary maxillary canine
   d. primary mandibular canine
   e. mandibular second premolar

8. Which teeth (secondary or primary) have the mesial cusp ridge of the facial cusp longer than the distal cusp ridge of the facial cusp?
   a. mandibular first premolar
   b. maxillary first premolar
   c. primary maxillary canine
   d. primary mandibular canine
   e. mandibular second premolar

9. Which succedaneous tooth erupts beneath tooth J?
   a. #1
   b. #5
   c. #10
   d. #13
   e. #16

10. Which of the following traits can be used to differentiate primary teeth from secondary teeth?
    a. Primary teeth have greater facial cervical bulges.
    b. Primary teeth have relatively thinner and longer roots.
    c. Primary teeth are whiter.
    d. Primary anterior teeth are larger than their successors.
    e. Primary teeth have relatively larger pulps.

11. Which of the following secondary teeth would you expect to be erupted in the average 9 to 10 year old?
    a. maxillary lateral incisor
    b. maxillary central incisor
    c. mandibular canine
    d. maxillary canine
    e. mandibular second molar

12. Which traits apply to a primary mandibular first molar?

   a. Its roots are resorbed by the eruption of the 6-year mandibular first molar.

   b. It resembles a mandibular 6-year first molar.

   c. It has a prominent buccal cervical bulge.

   d. It has a prominent mesial marginal ridge.

   e. It has a prominent transverse ridge.

   f. It has an occlusal table larger in the mesial half than in the distal half.

ANSWERS: 1–a, b, d; 2–c; 3–c; 4–d; 5–a; 6–b; 7–a, c; 8–b, c; 9–d; 10–a, b, c; 11–a, b, c, e; 12–c, d, e

REFERENCES

1. Hellman M. Nutrition, growth and dentition. Dental Cosmos 1923;Dec.
2. Brand RW, Isselhard DE. Anatomy of orofacial structures. St. Louis: C.V. Mosby, 1998:462–490.
3. Osborn JW, ed. Dental anatomy and embryology. Oxford: Blackwell Scientific Publications, 1981:144–151.
4. Huang L, Machida Y. A longitudinal study of clinical crowns on deciduous anterior teeth. Bull Tokyo Med Dent Univ 1987;28:75–81.
5. Jorgensen KD. The deciduous dentition—a descriptive and comparative anatomical study. Acta Odontol Scand 1956;14(Suppl 20):1–192.
6. Pagano JL. Anatomia dentaria. Buenos Aires: Editorial Mundi S.A., 1965:471–540.
7. DuBrul EL. Sicher's oral anatomy. 7th ed. St. Louis: C.V. Mosby, 1980:238–244.
8. Kraus B, Jordan R, Abrams L. Dental anatomy and occlusion. Baltimore: Williams & Wilkins, 1969:115–131.
9. Finn S. Clinical pedodontics. Philadelphia: W.B. Saunders, 1957:54–80.
10. Paulson RB, Gottlieb LJ, Sciulli PW, et al. Double-rooted maxillary primary canines. ASDC J Dent Child 1985;52:195–198.
11. Pinkham JR, Casamassino PS, Fields HW Jr. Pediatric dentistry, infancy through adolescence. 4th ed. St. Louis: Elsevier Saunders, 2005:191.

Functional Occlusion and Malocclusion

11

I. Ideal occlusion versus malocclusion
   A. Ideal class I occlusion
   B. Dental malocclusions (including class I)
   C. Class II malocclusion (including division 1 and division 2)
   D. Class III malocclusion
II. Jaw relationships of the mandible to the maxillae
   A. Maximal intercuspal position (centric occlusion)
   B. Centric jaw relation (retruded contact position)
   C. Occlusal vertical dimension
   D. Jaw relations during horizontal movements of the mandible
III. Normal movements within the temporomandibular joint
   A. Movements within the lower joint space
   B. Movements within the upper joint space
   C. Total joint movement
IV. Functional movements: chewing and swallowing
   A. Incising
   B. Masticating (chewing)
   C. Swallowing (deglutition)
V. Parafunctional movements and contacts, signs and symptoms
VI. Treatment modalities related to malocclusion
VII. Dislocation of the mandible (luxation or condylar subluxation)
VIII. Accurate recording of the centric relation jaw position

An introduction to ideal *static* occlusion was discussed earlier in Chapter 3, Section VI. In this chapter, the more advanced aspects of tooth and jaw relationships *during function* are discussed, as well as the terminology and concepts associated with malocclusion (which literally means "bad" occlusion).

OBJECTIVES

This chapter is designed to prepare the learner to perform the following:

- Define Angle's class I, II, and III relationships.
- List and describe types of tooth and jaw malocclusions.
- List and describe signs or symptoms of malocclusion (including the possible effects of premature contacts and parafunctional movements).
- Describe and recognize the following jaw relationships: maximal intercuspal position, centric jaw relation (retruded contact position), and occlusal vertical dimension.
- Describe and recognize the following horizontal eccentric movements: protrusive movement (including the effect of horizontal and vertical overlap on incisal guidance) and lateral movement (including the effect of canine overlap on canine-protected occlusion).
- Define and recognize tooth relationships during lateral movements on the working and nonworking (balancing) articulation.
- Describe and demonstrate mandibular movement within the lower joint space (rotation) and within the upper joint space (translation).

- Describe the relationship of teeth and adjacent oral structures during eating.
- Describe (and sketch) an ideal envelope of motion from the facial and sagittal views and label mandibular tooth positions or movements for each segment of the envelope.
- Define and provide examples of parafunctional movements.
- Describe mandibular dislocation (luxation) and demonstrate how to alleviate this problem with appropriate mandibular manipulation.
- List and describe possible methods of treatment for bruxing, myofunctional trigger points (pain), and temporomandibular disorders including the steps for construction of an occlusal device (bite guard).
- Describe a method for accurately recording a centric relation position of the mandiblle.
- Sketch, from memory, the tooth crown outlines on one side of the mouth in ideal class I occlusion.

SECTION I.   IDEAL OCCLUSION VERSUS MALOCCLUSION

Ideal occlusion is the relationship of teeth and jaws that dentists and dental specialists would like to reproduce when restoring a patient's entire mouth to form and function. **Malocclusion**, on the other hand, is literally a "bad" occlusion that can result from a poor occlusal relationship acquired naturally or from incomplete orthodontic treatment. Examples of malocclusion include poor tooth alignment within an arch, interferences of tooth ridges or cusps during jaw movement that result from discrepencies in tooth height relative to other teeth within an arch, or from differences in the relative sizes of the dental arches affecting tooth alignment between arches. Malocclusions include tooth or *dental* malocclusions, *skeletal* relationships that adversely affect the occlusion (that is, discrepencies beween the size and/or alignment of the maxillae with the mandible), or a combination of both.

Three classes of *skeletal* relationships are recognized. They were first classified by Dr. Edward H. Angle in 1887. The ideal *skeletal occlusal* relationship is called class I occlusion. In contrast, class II and class III relationships are considered to be *skeletal mal*occlusions because of the considerable difference in size, or the abnormal positional relationship, of the maxillae and the mandible. Skeletal malocclusions are often obvious when observing a person's profile *(Fig. 11-1)*. The anterior profile of a person with class I occlusion tends to be a rather straight line from the top half of the face to the anterior border of the mandible and is called **orthognathic** [OR thog NA thik], where "gnathic" pertains to the jaw and "ortho" means a straight or normal jaw profile. (Compare the word orthognathic to orthodontics, which means tooth straightening.) (This profile may also be called **mesognathic** [not mesiognathic].) A person with class II occlusion has a mandible that is too small (or maxillae that are too large), resulting in a mandible that appears behind (retruded from) where it should normally be located (that is, the mandible is in **disto-occlusion**). This profile is convex, and is called **retrognathic** [ret rog NATH ik] (Fig. 11-1). A person with class III occlusion has

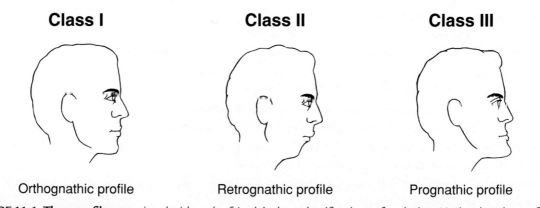

Class I   **Class II**   **Class III**

Orthognathic profile   Retrognathic profile   Prognathic profile

FIGURE 11-1. Three profiles associated with each of Angle's three classifications of occlusion. Notice that the profile associated with the person with class I occlusion is normal in appearance, whereas the person with class II occlusion often has a relatively small mandible and the person with class III occlusion often has a relatively large mandible.

Class I (72%)

Normal   Normal   Orthognathic profile

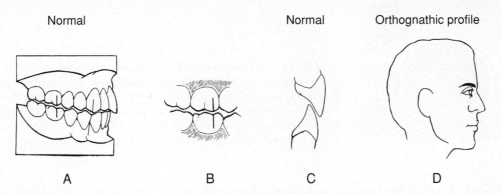

A   B   C   D

FIGURE 11-2. **Angle's class I occlusion:** occurs in approximately 72% of the population. **A.** Lateral view of tooth models with the teeth aligned in class I occlusion. **B.** The first molar relationship showing the mesiobuccal cusp of the maxillary first molar aligned with the mesiobuccal groove of the mandibular first molar. **C.** Normal anterior relationship of incisors. **D.** The normal, orthognathic profile of a person having class I tooth relationships.

a mandible that is too large, resulting in a mandible that appears to be jutting forward to where it should be normally (that is, the mandible is in **mesio-occlusion**). This profile is concave and is called **prognathic** [prog NA thik] (where the mandible appears to <u>pro</u>trude or be "in front of" where it should be) (Fig. 11-1). Each class of skeletal relationship is defined by describing the occlusion of the first teeth to erupt in the adult dentition, namely, the maxillary and mandibular first molars, or by the relationship between the maxillary and mandibular canines, as described in the following sections.

A. *IDEAL* CLASS I (SKELETAL) OCCLUSION (ALSO CALLED NORMAL OCCLUSION OR NEUTROCCLUSION)

The profile of a person with class I occlusion is called **orthognathic** [or thog NA thik], characterized by a lack of obvious protrusion *or* retrusion of the resting mandible relative to the maxillae. Recall from Chapter 3 that class I occlusion is defined by the relationship of the first permanent molars: the tip of the mesiobuccal cusp of the maxillary first molar is aligned directly over the mesiobuccal groove on the mandibular first molar *(Fig. 11-2A and B)* and the maxillary canine fits into the facial embrasure between the mandibular canine and first premolar (Fig. 11-2A).

The static *tooth* relationships considered to be normal or ideal include the following:

- The incisal edges of maxillary teeth are labial to the incisal edges of mandibular teeth (known as normal **horizontal overlap** or **overjet**, as shown in *Fig. 11-3A*).
- The incisal edges of mandibular incisors are hidden from view by the overlapping maxillary incisors (known as normal **vertical overlap** or **overbite**, as shown in *Fig. 11-3B*).

Normal

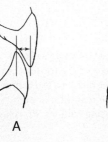

A   B

FIGURE 11-3. **Angle's class I occlusion: incisor relationship. A.** Normal *horizontal* alignment has the incisal edge of the maxillary incisors anterior to the incisal edge of the mandibular incisors, also known as **normal overjet** (denoted by the horizontal arrow). **B.** Normal vertical alignment has the incisal edge of the maxillary incisors overlapping (hiding from view) the incisal third of the mandibular incisor, also known as **normal overbite** (denoted by the vertical arrow).

Normal

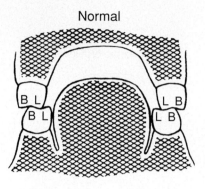

FIGURE 11-4. Normal molar relationship in cross section. Notice that the buccal cusps of maxillary molars are facial to the buccal cusps of the mandibular molars, and the lingual cusps of the mandibular molars are lingual to the lingual cusps of the maxillary molars. Also notice that the lingual cusps of maxillary molars occlude with the fossae in mandibular molars, and the buccal cusps of mandibular molars occlude with fossae in maxillary molars.

- Buccal cusps and buccal surfaces of the *maxillary* posterior teeth are buccal to those in the mandibular arch, whereas the lingual cusps and lingual surfaces of the *mandibular* posterior teeth are lingual to those in the maxillary arch (*Fig. 11-4*).
- Lingual cusps of *maxillary* teeth rest in occlusal fossae of the mandibular teeth, whereas the buccal cusps of the *mandibular* teeth rest in occlusal fossae of the maxillary teeth (Fig. 11-4).
- The vertical (long) axis midline of each maxillary tooth is positioned slightly distal to the vertical axis of the corresponding mandibular tooth. For example, in *Figure 11-5*, the center of the maxillary canine (#6) is distal to the mandibular canine (#27), the center of the maxillary first premolar (#5) is distal to the mandibular first premolar (#28), and so forth.
- Normal occlusion is an absence of individual tooth malocclusions, although they may occur even in class I relationships.[15]

During function, *ideal* or normal occlusion exists when only the canines touch as the mandible moves laterally (without molar and premolar contacts), known as canine-protected articulation; no tooth contacts occur on the side opposite of the direction the mandible is moving (that is, no contacts on the nonworking side); and the anterior teeth occlude (couple) together to disocclude (separate) the posterior teeth during protrusive movements (known as anterior guidance or anterior protected articulation). These concepts will be discussed in depth in next section of this chapter.

B. *DENTAL* MALOCCLUSIONS (INCLUDING CLASS I)

Malocclusion can be detrimental to oral health if it adversely affects appearance, comfort, or function. Dental malocclusions of individual teeth can occur in mouths with a class I, II, or III skeletal relationship. When individual teeth or groups of teeth are malaligned relative to the *ideal* parabolic arch form and level occlusal plane, the type of malocclusion includes the following variations. A tooth that is out of alignment to the labial or buccal compared to the ideal arch form of other teeth is said to be in **labial**

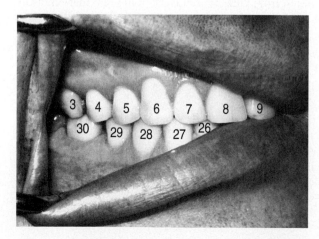

FIGURE 11-5. Ideal tooth alignment in Angle's class I occlusion. Notice that the center axis of the tooth types in the maxillary arch are aligned just distal to the center axis of the same type of tooth in the mandibular arch. For example, look at the two opposing canines: #6 is just distal to #27.

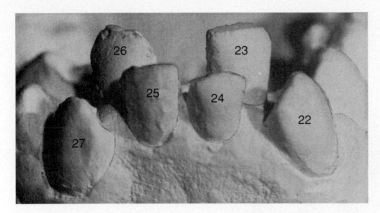

FIGURE 11-6. Crowding of anterior teeth.
Notice that the mandibular right canine (#27) is in **labial version** (positioned labial to the normal arch form), whereas the lateral incisors (#23 and #26) are in **lingual version**.

version (also **labioversion**) a term used for an *anterior* tooth like tooth #27 in Figure 11-6, or **buccal version** (also **buccoversion**) if referring to a posterior tooth. A tooth that is out of alignment to the lingual compared to other teeth in the arch is said to be in **lingual version** (also **linguoversion**), a term used to describe teeth #23 and #26 in *Figure 11-6*. A tooth that is twisted (rotated) around its tooth axis is described as **torsiversion**, a term used to describe tooth #8 in *Figure 11-7*. If a tooth is overerupted so it is abnormally elongated relative the rest of the occlusal plane, it is called **supraerupted**, or **extruded**, or it is in **supraversion**, a term used to describe the maxillary third molar in *Figure 11-8*. If a tooth is abnormally short relative to the rest of the occlusal plane, it is in **infraversion**. This may occur when a short primary tooth is retained into adulthood or may be due to **ankylosis** [ANG ki lo sis] of a primary or secondary tooth, which is defined as the loss of its periodontal ligament and the subsequent fusion of alveolar bone and cementum.

Malaligned teeth may occlude before other teeth in the mouth (said to be **premature contacts** or in heavy occlusion). These teeth can be subject to heavier forces than other teeth (especially persons who brux or grind their teeth), which could ultimately contribute to the wearing away of enamel forming a **facet** or flat spot, clearly evident on the occlusal surfaces of the mandibular premolars and first molar in Figure 11-8. Other evidence of heavy occlusion on only one or two teeth was discussed earlier in Chapter 8, and includes widening of the periodontal ligament, loosening of the tooth, and, in the presence of factors that contribute to the formation of periodontal disease, a worsening of that disease process. These premature contacts could also be called **deflective occlusal contacts** if, upon closing in a posterior position with muscles (called centric relation), the teeth do not close directly into best or tightest fit, but instead hit the prematurity that then deflects the mandible (changes direction of the mandible) before it can reach its tightest fit. The result may be an imbalance in the way the relaxed muscles and articular fossa and emminence directs the mandible to comfortably close, versus the way

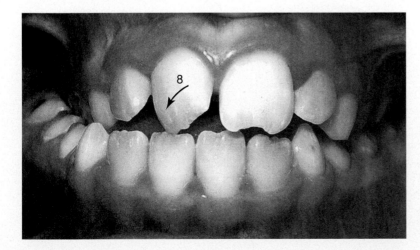

FIGURE 11-7. Torsiversion (twisting) of tooth #8, the maxillary right central incisor. Also notice that the posterior teeth on the patient's right side (left side of photo) are in **crossbite**, and on the patient's left side, the premolars in the shadows appear to be in an **end-to-end** relationship.

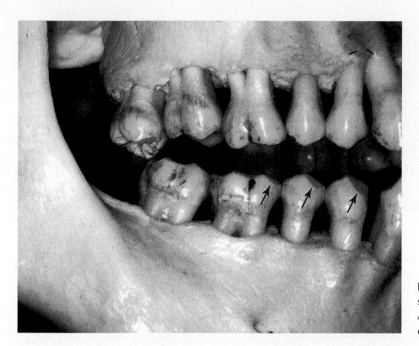

FIGURE 11-8. Supereruption (extrusion) of the maxillary third molar, #1. Arrows point to facets (flattened areas) caused by heavy tooth contacts.

the ridges of malaligned teeth direct the mandible to close. Under certain circumstances, this imbalance can cause muscle pain.

When mandibular teeth do not align themselves ideally relative to maxillary teeth, the following variations can occur. When one or more maxillary or mandibular teeth are either too facial or too lingual to teeth in the opposing arch, the relationship is called a **posterior crossbite**. This can occur when a mandibular posterior tooth is aligned *considerably* to the buccal (as in buccal version) relative to the ideal interarch relationship, and the lingual cusps of mandibular teeth are positioned in the central fossae of the maxillary teeth, also know as **reverse articulation** (seen between the posterior molars in the left side of the photograph in Fig. 11-7 and Fig. 11-9C). It may also possible for mandibular posterior teeth to be in crossbite if they are entirely to the lingual (in complete lingual version) relative to the maxillary teeth. This is almost the case in *Figure 11-9B*. where the maxillary molars are in buccal version. When mandibular *incisors* are facial to maxillary incisors, this is called an **anterior crossbite**. (Compare the incisor rela-

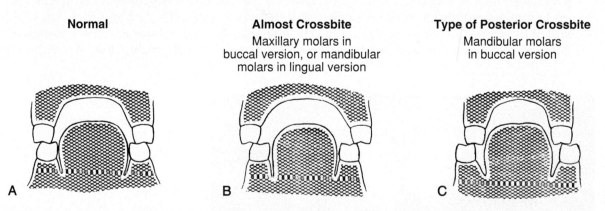

FIGURE 11-9. Molar relationships in cross section. A. Views of the **normal** occlusion with the buccal surfaces of maxillary molars facial to mandibular molars. **B.** Maxillary molars in **buccoversion** or more buccal than normal. If these maxillary molars were completely to the buccal of the mandibular molars, this would be a type of posterior crossbite (with mandibular molars in lingual version). This condition is common in persons with class II malocclusion where the mandible is small relative to the maxillae. **C. Posterior crossbite** (reverse articulation) with the **buccal** cusps of maxillary molars and **lingual** cusps of mandibular molars occluding into opposing fossae; mandibular molars are in buccal version. This condition is common in persons with class III malocclusion, where the mandible is large relative to the maxillae.

Anterior crossbite

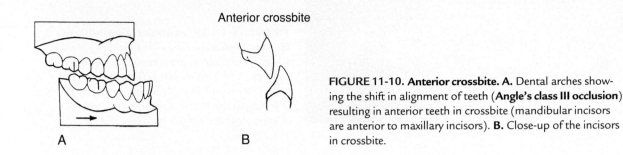

FIGURE 11-10. Anterior crossbite. A. Dental arches showing the shift in alignment of teeth (**Angle's class III occlusion**) resulting in anterior teeth in crossbite (mandibular incisors are anterior to maxillary incisors). **B.** Close-up of the incisors in crossbite.

A   B

tionship in anterior crossbite in *Fig. 11-10* to ideal anterior relationships where the maxillary incisors are labial to the mandibular incisors.)

Normally, when viewed from the facial, approximately the incisal thirds of mandibular incisors are covered by the **vertical overlap** of maxillary incisors (recall Fig. 11-3). The amount of *vertical* overlap is called **overbite**. When this overbite is severe (**severe overbite**, as seen in *Fig. 11-11A*) where the maxillary incisors overlap the mandibular incisors down to the level of the cervical lines of the mandibular teeth, the ability of the mandible to freely move into protrusion is compromised since the mandible must drop down considerably before it can move forward. With a severe overbite, the mandibular incisors may actually impinge upon the incisive papilla of the hard palate and result in a visible imprint in that keratinized tissue. When the incisors have no vertical overlap, the result may be an **edge-to-edge** relationship (Fig. 11-11B), or an anterior **openbite** or **open occlusal relationship** of anterior teeth (Fig. 11-11C) where there is a space between the incisal edges. In patients with this relationship, the posterior teeth occlude as the mandibular moves forward, and not the anterior teeth. If posterior teeth line up with maxillary buccal cusps aligned over mandibular buccal cusps, the relationship is called an **end-to-end** occlusion. (An end-to-end occlusal relationship is seen for the premolars in the shadows on the right side of the photograph in Fig. 11-7.)

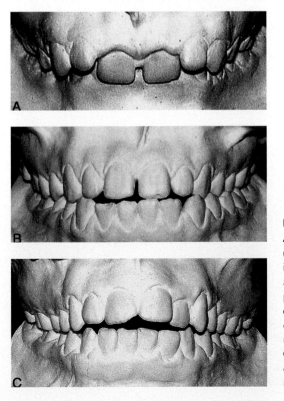

FIGURE 11-11. Three types of anterior tooth relationships. A. Severe overbite with maxillary incisors completely overlapping (covering up) the mandibular incisors. Note that the maxillary incisors are tipped inward relative to the lateral incisors, which are flared normally outward. This is a common relationship in patients with **Angle's class II, division 2 occlusion. B. Edge-to-edge bite** where the incisal edges of the maxillary incisors line up directly over the incisal edges of mandibular incisors. This anterior relationship is common in persons with class III occlusion. **C. Anterior open bite** where the incisal edges of the maxillary incisors neither overlap vertically nor touch the incisal edges of mandibular incisors.

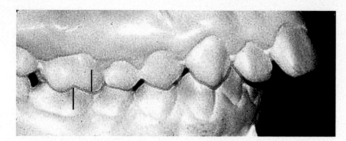

FIGURE 11-12. Severe overjet relationship of incisors. Notice the flare of the maxillary incisors, which is common in persons with **division 2** anterior relationship of **class II occlusion**. Class II occlusion is confirmed since the mesiobuccal groove of the mandibular first molar is distal to the mesiobuccal cusp of the maxillary first molar.

Also, it is normal for the incisal edge of the mandibular incisors to occlude with the lingual surface of maxillary incisors. The amount of **horizontal overlap** between these teeth is called the **overjet**. A **severe overjet** is seen in *Figure 11-12* where the maxillary incisors are *considerably* anterior to the mandibular incisors. This figure also shows the anterior relationship that occurs in division 2 of class II occlusion where maxillary incisors flare labially. Some evidence indicates that people with this type of malocclusion have more crepitus because of the frequent necessity to protrude the jaw considerably forward in order to properly enunciate and to incise.

C. CLASS II MALOCCLUSION (INCLUDING DIVISION 1 AND DIVISION 2)

This is a skeletal type of malocclusion with a *small mandible* relative to the maxillae (*Fig. 11-13A*). This could involve a very small mandible, very large protruding maxillae, or both. The mandibular teeth are in a distal and sometimes lingual relationship to their normal maxillary opponents (buccoversion of maxillary teeth as seen in Fig. 11-9B). For persons with a class II molar relationship, the mesiobuccal groove of the mandibular first molar is *distal* to the mesiobucccal cusp of the maxillary first molar (Fig. 11-13A and B). That is, the mandible is *distal* to where it would be located in a person with class I occlusion by at least the width of a premolar. If the alignment differs by less distance than the width of a premolar, it is called a **tendency toward** class II occlusion. The patient's curved **retrognathic** (convex) facial profile appears to have a receded chin (Fig. 11-13D). Often there is an abnormally large horizontal overlap of anterior teeth with the maxillary incisors 5–10 mm labial to the mandibular incisors. There are two subdivisions of this type of skeletal malocclusion based on the inclination of the maxillary incisors. They are known as division 1 and division 2 (as seen in Fig. 11-13C).

- **Class II, division 1** is the *incisor* relationship where all maxillary incisors have a *labial* inclination or tip similar to that found in normal class I occlusion (seen in Fig. 11-12). People with this subdivision of anterior malocclusion often have a long face, a tapered arch with high palate, a severe *horizontal*

Class II (22%)

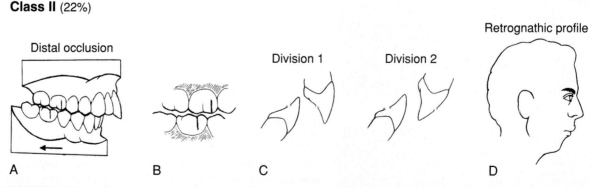

FIGURE 11-13. Angle's class II occlusal relationship. A. Lateral view of tooth models with the teeth aligned in class II occlusion. **B.** The first molar relationship showing the mesiobuccal groove of the mandibular first molar *distal to* the mesiobuccal cusp of the maxillary first molar. **C.** Two divisions of anterior relationship of incisors: Division 1 is where maxillary and mandibular incisors flare labially. Division 2 is where the maxillary incisors (especially central incisors) are flared (tipped) to the lingual. **D.** The retrognathic profile associated with a person having class II tooth relationships.

overlap or overjet of maxillary incisors labial to mandibular incisors, supereruption of mandibular incisors, diminished muscle tone in the upper lip, and an overactive lower lip.[26]

- **Class II, division II** is the *incisor* relationship where one or more maxillary incisors have a *lingual* inclination or tip. This is evident in Figure 11-11A where maxillary central incisors tilt quite a bit to the lingual, especially relative to the adjacent labially flared lateral incisors. Also, these people have a short, wide face, square arch, less horizontal overlap than in division 1, a severe *vertical* overlap or overbite, severe anteroposterior curve (of Spee), anterior crowding, and well-developed chin musculature.[26]

D. CLASS III MALOCCLUSION (ALSO CALLED MESIAL OCCLUSION, MESIO-OCCLUSION, OR MANDIBULAR PROGNATHISM)

This is a skeletal type of malocclusion with a relatively *large mandible* compared to the maxillae, and with the mandibular teeth in a mesial, and often facial, relationship to their upper counterparts (*Fig. 11-14A and B*). The patient's facial profile is concave with a very prominent chin (or **prognathic** profile) (Fig. 11-14D). For persons with a class III molar relationship, the mesiobuccal groove of the mandibular first molar is *mesial* to the mesiobuccal cusp of the maxillary first molar by at least the width of a premolar (Fig. 11-14A and B). If the difference in alignment is less distance than the width of a premolar, it is called a **tendency toward** class III occlusion. That is, the mandible is *mesial* to where it is located in a person with class I occlusion. In addition to a massive mandible, people with this class of malocclusion have a long narrow face, a tapered upper arch with a high vaulted palate, increased activity of their upper lip, and decreased activity of their lower lip. The anterior teeth may be in an edge-to-edge or crossbite relationship (lowers are facial to uppers) (edge-to-edge relationship is seen in Fig. 11-11B, and anterior crossbite is seen in Fig. 11-10B). Other terms for this anterior tooth relationship in persons with class III occlusion are underbite, anterior crossbite, or reverse articulation. Crepitus is not common with class III malocclusion since little, if any, protrusion is required to clearly enunciate or to incise.

From eight unrelated surveys of the prevalence of malocclusion treated by orthodontists on 21,328 children, ages 6–18, in the United States between 1951 and 1971, Dr. Woelfel averaged the results and derived the following information:

- 71.7% had malocclusion (range: 31–95%)
- 28.3% had acceptable occlusion
- 72.3% had Angle's class I malocclusion (range: 62–88%)
- 22.0% had Angle's class II malocclusion (range: 8–32%)
- 5.7% had Angle's class III malocclusion (range: 2–12%)

It is possible that the classification of occlusion for a patient may be described as one class on the right side and a different class on the left side.

Class III (6%)

Mesial occlusion

Anterior crossbite

Prognathic profile

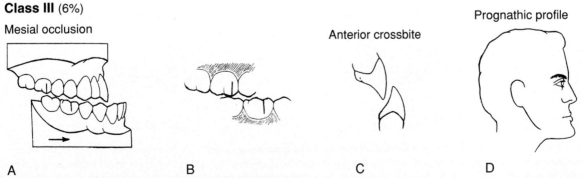

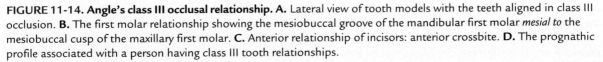

A   B   C   D

FIGURE 11-14. Angle's class III occlusal relationship. A. Lateral view of tooth models with the teeth aligned in class III occlusion. **B.** The first molar relationship showing the mesiobuccal groove of the mandibular first molar *mesial to* the mesiobuccal cusp of the maxillary first molar. **C.** Anterior relationship of incisors: anterior crossbite. **D.** The prognathic profile associated with a person having class III tooth relationships.

SECTION II. JAW RELATIONSHIPS OF THE MANDIBLE TO THE MAXILLAE

The maxillae (right and left) are firmly and immovably attached at suture lines to each other and to other bones of the facial skeleton. The maxillae move only as the head moves, not independently as does the mandible. The mandible articulates with the skull at the temporomandibular joints; it moves and changes its position in relation to the relatively stable maxillae and cranium. **Jaw relation** refers to the position of the mandible relative to the maxillae and could be thought of as a tooth-to-tooth relationship between maxillary and mandibular teeth, as well as a bone-to-bone (mandible-to-maxillae) relationship between the maxillae and mandible.

A. MAXIMAL INTERCUSPAL POSITION (CENTRIC OCCLUSION)

Maximal intercuspal position (MIP) is a relationship between teeth. It is the tightest or best fit between maxillary and mandibular posterior teeth (*Fig. 11-15B*). Other names for this are complete intercuspation, most occlusal position, acquired or habitual occlusion, centric occlusion, and natural bite. One can fit two casts of a person's upper and lower teeth together in the maximal intercuspal position without looking into the mouth (*Fig. 11-16B*).

B. CENTRIC JAW RELATION (RETRUDED CONTACT POSITION)

The most posterior position of the mandible relative to the maxillae with the mandible retruded maximally is called the **centric jaw relation** or **centric relation**. It is a bone-to-bone relationship between the upper and lower jaws *without tooth contact* (or with one or only a few teeth *initially* contacting but not yet closing more tightly together into maximal intercuspal position).[1–3] It is most often behind (distal to) the maximal intercuspal position by 1–2 mm.[1,4,5] (In Fig. 11-16, compare the short vertical pencil lines on two pairs of opposing maxillary and mandibular teeth that line up when the teeth are in the maximal intercuspal position but reveal how distally the mandible is positioned when in centric jaw

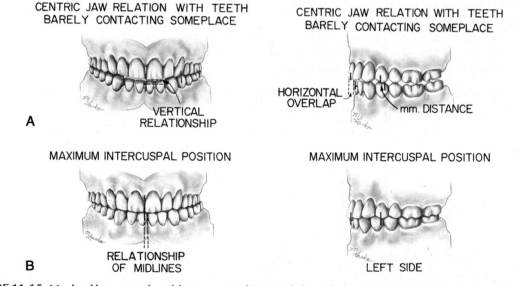

FIGURE 11-15. Maximal intercuspal position compared to centric jaw relation. A. Mandible has closed in the most retruded arc or **centric jaw relation** until the first tooth contact between any upper and lower teeth (indicating a prematurity or deflective contact). **B.** The mandible has continued to close from the first tooth contact into **maximal intercuspal position,** and as a result, the mandible has deviated (deflected) forward (as seen in the shift of the relationship of the vertical lines placed on the maxillary and mandibular first premolars) and laterally to the left (as seen in the shift of the alignment of the midlines of the maxillary and mandibular dentition). The deviation of the mandible was caused by deflective tooth interferences, which guided the terminal (most upward) portion of jaw closure.

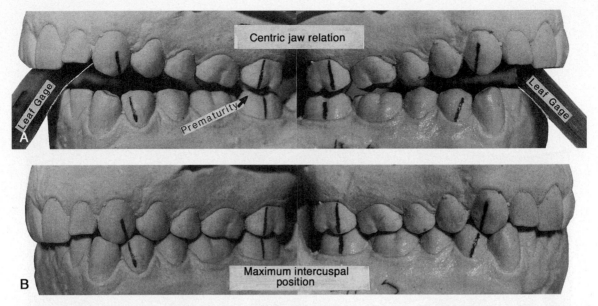

FIGURE 11-16. Maximal intercuspal position compared to centric jaw relation on a patient with severe deflective tooth contacts. A. Patient's casts (left side and right side) mounted in **centric jaw relation**. An articulator mounting of these casts in centric jaw relation using a leaf gauge revealed the *severe* deflective left second molar contact that is impossible to correct by an equilibration. This person's mandible would deflect forward 2 mm and to the right 1 mm as the teeth closed into maximal intercuspal position. **B.** Same patient's casts (left side and right side) mounted in **maximal intercuspal position**.

relation.) [Posselt found the distance between centric relation and maximal intercuspal position to average 1.25 ± 1 mm with a range of 0.25–2.55 mm.[4]] Centric jaw relation also includes the *range of positions* with the mandible *retruded maximally* while rotating open *without bodily moving forward*. This relation can be obtained by tipping the head back with the mandible retruded or by using an upward sloping gauge of variable thickness inserted between overlapping incisors to help guide a retracted closure of the mandible (a technique discussed later in this chapter).

In centric jaw relation, the condyles articulate with the thinnest avascular portion of their respective discs, and the condyle/disc complex is in an anterior-superior position against the posterior slopes of the articular eminence (*Fig. 11-17*). The presence or absence of teeth, or the type of occlusion or malocclusion, does not change this relationship.

It is a relatively rare but ideal occurrence when centric relation coincides with the maximal intercuspal position. This occurs when there is simultaneous, even contact between maxillary and mandibular teeth in maximum interdigitation as the mandible closes in its most retruded centric relation position.[2–4,6,7] This type of ideal occlusal relationship results from a balance between the guidance afforded by jaw muscles, condyle position, and fitting together of the teeth. This condition does not occur in most people unless they have just had a well-executed **occlusal equilibration** where small amounts of interfering occlusal enamel are removed by the dentist to equalize occlual stress,[6] had a well-made removable denture, or had a complete dental arch rehabilitation replacing or reorienting all occlusal surfaces (described later in this chapter).

When centric relation does *not* coincide with maximal intercuspal position, premature or deflective tooth contacts exist. **Premature** or **deflective occlusal contacts** refer to the teeth that contact first as the jaw closes in centric relation (most retruded position). Deflective occlusal contacts of opposing teeth are those which guide or direct the mandible away from centric relation, either forward or to one side or both, as the teeth slide together into maximal intercuspal position.

Mandibular deviation refers to the direction and movement of the mandible from the first slight premature tooth contact with the jaw in centric relation to the maximal intercuspal position. The direction of the deviation of the mandible is usually forward and upward with or without simultaneous lateral movement.[3,5,8] This is illustrated in Figure 11-15, where premature contacts deflect the mandible forward and to the left as the teeth move from centric jaw relation into maximal intercuspal position

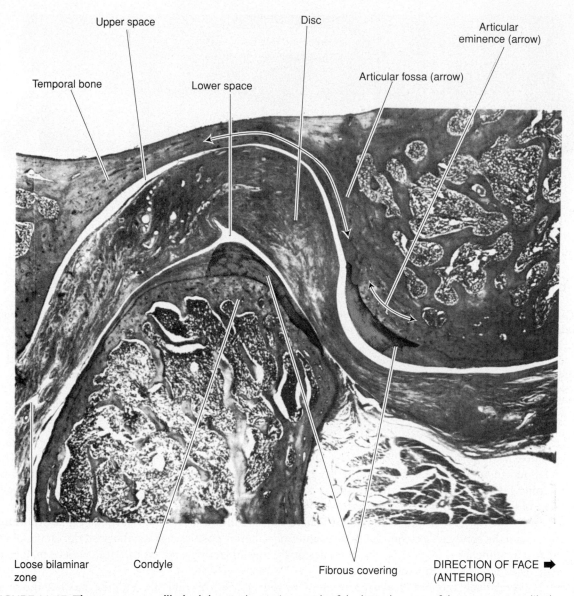

Upper space

Disc

Articular eminence (arrow)

Temporal bone

Lower space

Articular fossa (arrow)

Loose bilaminar zone

Condyle

Fibrous covering

DIRECTION OF FACE ➡ (ANTERIOR)

FIGURE 11-17. The temporomandibular joint. A photomicrograph of the lateral aspect of the temporomandibular joint showing the close proximity of the anterior head of the condyle against the thinnest (avascular) part of the disc, which is next to the posterior slope of the articular eminence. (Courtesy of Dr. Rudy Melfi.)

(from A to B), and in Figure 11-16, where the mandible is deflected forward 2 mm and to the right 1 mm (from A to B). It is also obvious on the skull in *Figure 11-18* that the supererupted maxillary third molar occludes before any other teeth when the mandible closes in its most posterior centric relation (this tooth has a **deflective occlusal contact**), and for the mandible to close into maximal intercuspal position, the mandible must move forward and superiorly.

Most people have deflective malocclusion to some degree. See *Table 11-1*, which gives information on deflective contacts for 811 dental hygienists.[6] Less than 1% of this group had maximal intercuspal position coincide with centric relation, yet most were asymptomatic. **Fremitus** is the palpable or visible movement of a tooth when subjected to heavy occlusal forces. Fremitus is not necessarily an unhealthy condition but may be an indication of a premature centric relation tooth contact or an interference during lateral excursions.

Edentulous people (with no teeth) who wear complete dentures or false teeth are provided with centric relation that coincides with maximal intercuspal position because they can learn to pull the mandible back and close into a *stable and repeatable position* of centric relation during jaw closure. This enables the

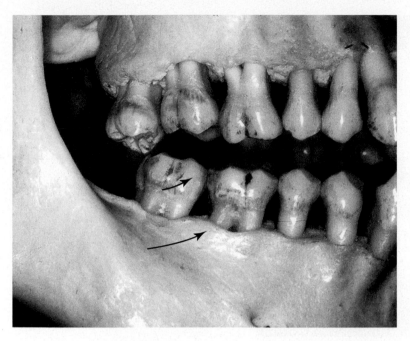

FIGURE 11-18. Centric prematurity contact of a supererupted maxillary third molar. When the mandible is positioned posteriorly as it closes (as in centric relation), the first tooth to contact in this dentition is the third molar. The mandible must then shift forward and upward in order for all teeth to come together in the maximal intercuspal position.

tight occlusion of denture teeth to coincide with the repeatable closed-jaw position, so the dentures will remain tightly secured against the mucosa and not rock loose when functioning. Dentists who make dentures attempt to duplicate and improve upon the patient's jaw relationships when teeth were present.

An **articulator** is a mechanical device that holds casts of the two arches, permitting a close duplication of the patient's open and closing centric jaw relations (*Fig. 11-19*). Notice the fit of the ball of the lower (mandibular) part fitting into a concavity on the upper (maxillary) part. This design somewhat simulates the heads of the condyles fitting into the articular fossae. It is easier to study these relationships with the patient's dental arches (dental stone casts) on the articulator in your hands, rather than with your hands in the patient's mouth. What better way is there to determine whether or not the maxillary and mandibular lingual cusps fit together tightly or properly in the maximal intercuspal relationship?

Table 11-1	DEFLECTIVE CENTRIC RELATION TOOTH CONTACT DATA FROM 811 DENTAL HYGIENISTS		
LOCATION OF FIRST CENTRIC RELATION TOOTH CONTACT		**NUMBER OF HYGIENISTS**	**PERCENT**
Premolars one side		232	28.6
Premolars both sides		90	11.1
Molars one side		328	40.5
Molars both sides		113	13.9
Molar one side; premolar one side		38	4.7
Canine		4	0.5
Maximal intercuspal position = centric jaw relation (no prematurities)		6*	0.7
TYPE AND PLACE OF DEFLECTIVE CONTACT		**PERCENT**	
Premolars only		39.7	
Molars only		54.4	
Unilateral prematurity		69.2	
Bilateral prematurity: same tooth		25.8	
Bilateral prematurity; premolar–molar		4.7	

* Three of the six recently had an equilibration by their dentists.
Research conducted by Dr. Woelfel at the Ohio State University, 1974–1986.

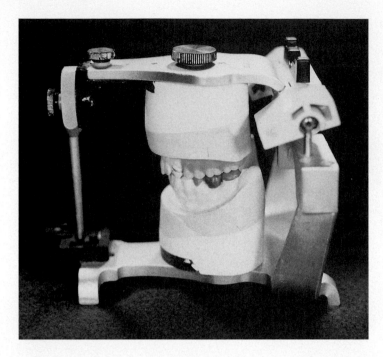

FIGURE 11-19. Casts mounted on an articulator. This articulator (Denar, Anaheim, CA) can be used to mount casts of the patient's dentition in order to reproduce the position and movements of mandibular teeth relative to maxillary teeth. This mounting was used to design the tooth anatomy and occlusion for a fixed dental prosthesis (bridge) from tooth 18 to 20 (replacing tooth 19) and a removable partial dental prosthesis replacing teeth 12 through 15. (Mounting courtesy of Dr. Lisa Knobloch, Ohio State University.)

LEARNING EXERCISE

Tip your head way back with the teeth *slightly* apart, consciously retrude (pull back) your mandible, and close very slowly in a hinge motion (without sliding the jaw forward) until the first teeth initially touch gently. The relationship of your jaws prior to your first gentle tooth contact or contacts with the mandible retruded is your *centric jaw relation*. The relation of this retracted, pure hinge opening is a most important one to record when making extensive dental restorations for a patient. If your mandible is guided (hits and slides) forward as you continue to close your teeth together into their maximal intercuspal position where they fit together most tightly, you are experiencing *deflective* or premature occlusal contacts, and you are among the majority of people whose centric relation does *not* coincide with the maximal intercuspal position. The mandible will almost always slide forward from centric relation into maximal intercuspal position, either straight forward or to one side. More than likely, your own deflective tooth contacts will not be as severe as that shown in Figure 11-16. Can you determine which direction your premature tooth contacts deflect your mandible? Compare the location of your first (premature) tooth contact in centric relation with those in Table 11-1.

C. OCCLUSAL VERTICAL DIMENSION

Occlusal vertical dimension refers to the distance between a selected point on the mandible and a selected point on the maxillae. This dimension can be measured with the jaws positioned in centric relation or in maximal intercuspal position. **Vertical dimension of rest position** (or the **physiologic rest position**) is the position of the mandible when all of its supporting muscles (eight muscles of mastication plus the supra- and infrahyoids) are in their resting posture.[9] Physiologic rest position is further defined as the mandibular position when the person's head is upright, the muscles of mandibular movement are in equilibrium, and the condyles are in an unstrained position. Unless we are nervous, eating, talking, yawning, or using our muscles to perform other less natural functions, such as playing a clarinet, the mandible is in this comfortable resting position most of the time (over 23 hours each day).

When a person with an erect posture makes no conscious effort to open or close the mouth and the mandible is in its physiologic rest position, there is a space between the occlusal surfaces of the maxillary and mandibular teeth called the **interocclusal rest space** or **freeway space**. This space is normally

2–6 mm between the incisal surfaces and between the occlusal surfaces of the maxillary and mandibular teeth. Of course, when the teeth are missing (in an edentulous person), there would be a 1-cm or more distance between the residual toothless ridges when the mandible is resting.[10]

A simple change in posture, such as looking up at the sky or stretching the neck back in the reclined dental chair, will change the resting position of the jaw, separating the teeth farther than when in a comfortable upright position (*Fig. 11-20*). This change is due to the pull on the mandible by stretching skin and underlying fascia. Therefore, when a dentist places a restoration (filling) for a patient who is reclined in the dental chair, a final assessment and possible adjustment of the occlusion on this new restoration should take place with the patient in a relaxed *upright* position.

D. JAW RELATIONSHIPS DURING HORIZONTAL MOVEMENTS OF THE MANDIBLE

Relationships of the mandible relative to the maxillae can be documented as the mandible moves *horizontally* out of the centric relationship into other positions. **Eccentric** jaw relationships are any deviation of the mandible from the centric relation position. These relationships occur when the lower jaw moves anteriorly **(protrusion)**, laterally (**mandibular lateral translation** or excursion), or any combination thereof.

1. PROTRUSIVE JAW RELATION AND OCCLUSION

When pulled forward simultaneously by the lateral pterygoid muscles, the mandibular condyles and discs can slide forward down under the articular eminences in a movement known as **protrusion**. When pulled simultaneously by the posterior fibers of the temporalis muscles and assisted by the infra- and suprahyoid muscles, the mandible can move backward in a movement known as **retrusion (retraction)**. As protrusion occurs, the movement of the mandible is influenced by the amount of overlap of the anterior teeth. When teeth are positioned in normal maximal intercuspal position, upper incisors and canines overlap lower incisors and canines (*Fig. 11-21*). As stated earlier in this chapter, this overlap can be described in terms of a **horizontal overlap** where maxillary incisal edges are labial to the mandibular incisal edges, and a **vertical overlap** where maxillary incisal edges overlap (and facially hide from view) part of the mandibular incisor crowns. (See *Table 11-2* for the average and range of variations for these relationships.)

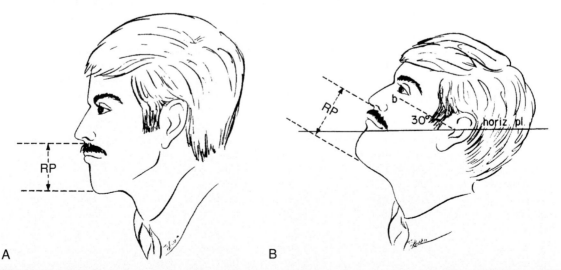

FIGURE 11-20. Physiologic rest position: effects of posture. A. This man assumes a normal posture with his mandible in physiologic rest position (RP). Posterior teeth, though not visible, are separated by an interocclusal distance. **B.** Now the man is looking up and his mandible is again in physiologic rest position with his posterior teeth separated, but more so than in **A** because of the stretch of fascia, skin, and the supra- and infrahyoid muscles. The resting position of the mandible varies with such factors as body posture, fatigue, and stress.

MAXIMUM INTERCUSPATION

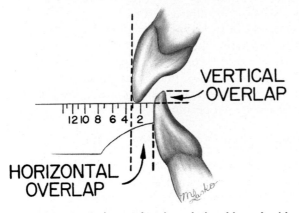

VERTICAL OVERLAP

HORIZONTAL OVERLAP

12 10 8 6 4 2

INCISAL AND CANINE GUIDANCE ANGLE ON 1114 STUDENTS			
	Incisal Angle (Central Incisors)	Canine Rise Angle	
		Right Side	Left Side
Average	50°	56°	57°
Low	minus 26° (open bite)	0°	0°
High	86°	84.2°	83°

FIGURE 11-21. Incisor and canine relationship and guidance. Lateral view of maxillary and mandibular incisors showing the normal vertical and horizontal overlap of incisors when the posterior teeth are in maximum intercuspation. The incisal guidance angle is the angle formed between the occlusal plane (horizontal numbered line on illustration) and a line connecting the upper and lower incisal edges. It is only 37° in this illustration, which is less steep than in many dentitions. A canine guidance (rise) angle of 60° or more is necessary to provide **canine-protected articulation** (or canine guidance). **Chart**: Incisal and canine guidance angles of 1114 students.

Protrusive movement occurs when the mandible moves anteriorly (as when incising food between the anterior teeth), so that both mandibular condyles *and* discs are forward in their articular (or glenoid) fossae, functioning against and beneath the articular eminences whose sloping morphology guides the mandible downward as it moves forward. Also, when a person with an *ideal* occlusal relationship moves the mandible forward, the incisal edges of the mandibular anterior teeth glide against the lingual surfaces of the maxillary anterior teeth, also guiding the mandible downward when protruding (*Fig. 11-22*). This is known as **incisal guidance**, which is a type of anterior guidance, or **anterior protected articulation**. It is influenced by the amount of movement and the angle at which the lower incisor and mandible must move downward and forward from the normally overlapping position of anterior teeth in maximal intercuspal position, to reach the edge-to-edge relationship of the mandibular and maxillary incisors. **Anterior guidance** (coupling) is a tightly overlapping relationship of the opposing maxillary and mandibular incisors and canines that produces disocclusion (separation) of the posterior teeth when the mandible protrudes or moves to either side from 1 to 4 mm.[11,12] [The average incisal guidance angle for 1114 dental hygiene and dental students was 50° as shown in the chart in Figure 11-21. Many of these people did not have ideal class I occlusion.]

Table 11-2	INCISOR AND CANINE OVERLAP OF 1114 STUDENTS					
				CANINE OVERLAP		
		INCISOR OVERLAP		HORIZONTAL		VERTICAL
		Horizontal (mm)	Vertical (mm)	Right (mm)	Left (mm)	Right (mm)	Left (mm)
DENTAL HYGIENE STUDENTS (796)	Average	2.78	3.27	2.01	2.02	3.23	3.19
	Low	minus 2.5	minus 1.0	minus 1.0	minus 1.0	minus 1.0	minus 1.0
	High	9.0	13.0	6.2	6.2	11.0	9.0
DENTAL STUDENTS (318)	Average	2.88	3.60	4.05	4.25	—	—
	Low	minus 6.5 (prognathic)	minus 2.0 (open bite)	0.0	0.0	—	—
	High	10.0	8.0	8.5	9.0	—	—

Research conducted by Dr. Woelfel at the Ohio State University, 1974–1986.

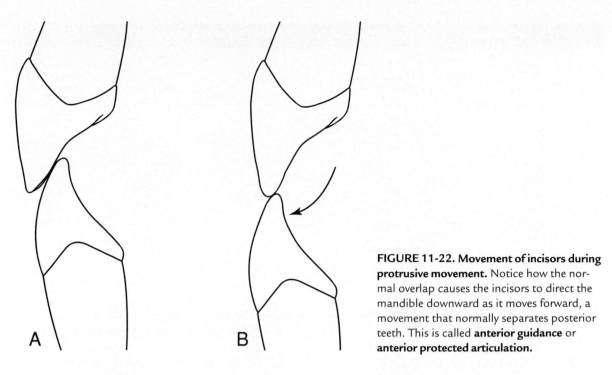

FIGURE 11-22. Movement of incisors during protrusive movement. Notice how the normal overlap causes the incisors to direct the mandible downward as it moves forward, a movement that normally separates posterior teeth. This is called **anterior guidance** or **anterior protected articulation.**

When the mandible is *fully* protruded, the incisal edges of the mandibular incisors are in front of the maxillary anterior teeth (*Fig. 11-23*). [The average maximum forward protrusion for 1114 young men and women was 8.3 mm with a range from 2.5 to 16.0 mm (*Table 11-3*). These extremes included a very tight temporomandibular joint compartment that exhibited the smallest protrusion, and a very large jaw with loose ligament attachments that exhibited 16 mm protrusion.]

2. LATERAL MANDIBULAR RELATION AND OCCLUSION

During **mandibular lateral translation**, the mandible is moved to the right or left side and slightly downward as when masticating (chewing) food. When the mandible moves to one side, both condyles do not move equally toward that side. Rather, when the mandible moves to the *right side*, the *right condyle* rotates but remains relatively stationary, while the *left condyle and disc* move forward, downward, and medially within the articular fossa. Table 11-3 on maximum jaw movement reminds us that the mandible can move almost twice as far from side to side as it can directly for-

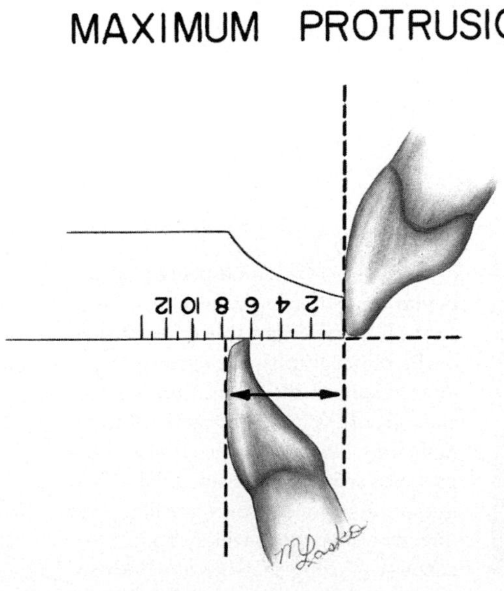

MAXIMUM PROTRUSION

FIGURE 11-23. Maximum protrusive jaw relationship. This is the relationship of mandibular to maxillary central incisors when the mandible is maximally protruded. The mandible has protruded 11 mm because the mandibular central incisor was 3 mm lingual to the maxillary incisor in centric occlusion.

Table 11-3	CAPABILITY OF MANDIBULAR MOVEMENT OF 1114 STUDENTS				
	MAXIMUM JAW OPENING (mm)	MAXIMUM LATERAL JAW MOVEMENT		MAXIMUM JAW PROTRUSION (mm)	ENTIRE LATERAL JAW MOVEMENT (mm)
		Right (mm)	Left (mm)		
DENTAL HYGIENE STUDENTS (796)					
Average	51.01	7.68	7.71	8.44	15.39
Low	27.0	2.5	2.0	3.0	7.0
High	68.5	14.0	15.2	16.0	28.4
DENTAL STUDENTS (318)					
Average	50.99	9.12	9.32	7.95	18.44
Low	35.5	2.0	3.0	2.5	6.0
High	71.0	14.0	15.4	13.5	32.0
Total average (1114 Students)	**50.29**	**8.09**	**8.17**	**8.30**	**16.26**

Research conducted by Dr. Woelfel at the Ohio State University, 1974–1986.

ward. [The maximum average movement to either the right *or* left side was about 8.1 mm. Therefore, the *entire* lateral movement from right to left averaged 16.2 mm compared to an average forward protrusion of only 8.3 mm.]

When the mandible moves to the right or to the left, the side where chewing (or work) occurs is called the working side, while the opposite side is called the nonworking side. In other words, the **working side** is the side toward which the mandible moves during lateral excursion (seen in Fig. 11-24). The **nonworking side** (previously known as the balancing side) is the side opposite the working side, or the side that, during lateral movements, moves toward the median line. These terms are dependent upon which way the mandible is moved. For example, when the mandible moves to the right, the right side is the working side and the left is the nonworking, whereas when the mandible moves to the left, the left side is the working side and the right is the nonworking side.

The working side is the side where the "work" of chewing occurs. As a person with an ideal occlusal relationship moves the mandible laterally, the posterior upper and lower teeth *on the working side* are aligned with the *upper buccal* cusps directly over the *lower buccal* cusps (seen in *Fig. 11-24*) and with the *upper lingual* cusps directly over the *lower lingual* cusps. The condyle on the working side does not move much; it rotates on its vertical axis and moves laterally about 1–2 mm (called **laterotrusion** or Bennett's movement).

On the nonworking side, the *upper lingual* cusps are aligned over the *lower buccal* cusps, but ideally should *not* contact during the opposite side working tooth contacts. **Nonworking side** (or balancing) **interferences** refer to *any* tooth contacts on the nonworking side. The nonworking side mandibular

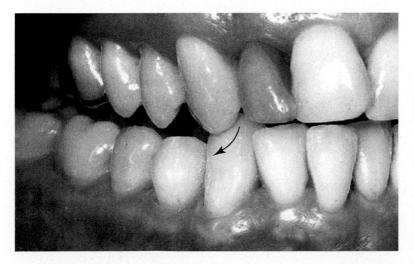

FIGURE 11-24. Canine-protected articulation. When the mandible moves to the patient's right side (the left side of the photograph), the overlap of canines results in the separation (disocclusion) of his posterior teeth on the right side. Notice that this is also the patient's **working side** since the mandibular buccal cusps are lining up directly under the maxillary buccal cusps (as during chewing or working).

Table 11-4	ECCENTRIC OCCLUSAL CONTACTS OF 342 HYGIENE STUDENTS			
	CONDITION	RIGHT QUADRANT	LEFT QUADRANT	TOTAL	PERCENT
WORKING SIDE TOOTH RELATIONSHIPS	Canine-protected articulation	207	205	412	**60.2%**
	Group function	135	137	272	**39.8%**
NONWORKING SIDE TOOTH RELATIONSHIPS	No contact	250	251	501	**73.2%**
	Interference	92	91	183	**26.8%**

CONDITION	STUDENTS	PERCENT
Bilateral canine-protected articulation without nonworking side interference*	129	37.7%
Bilateral canine-protected articulation with nonworking side interference	29	8.5%
Bilateral croup function without nonworking side interference	58	17.0%
Bilateral group function articulation with nonworking side interference	34	9.9%
Different relationships on each side	92	26.9%

* Considered to be the best type of relationship.
Survey conducted by Dr. Woelfel and his carefully trained staff. Doubtful recordings were personally reexamined by him for their validity (1980–1986). More than 30% of these 342 dental hygiene students had undergone orthodontic treatment.

condyle moves medially (**mediotrusion**), downward, and forward perhaps 5–12 mm. If the nonworking side interferences are heavy and frequent, they may actually be destructive to the supportive structures of the involved teeth, and can possibly cause temporomandibular joint pain on the opposite side because of the pivoting of the mandible and the stretching of opposite side ligaments and muscles. Poor occlusal relationships of any type can produce a variety of joint problems.[15-20] Occlusion with considerable vertical overlap of the canines results in canine-protected dentitions and generally does not have balancing side interferences. [As seen in *Table 11-4*, of 342 dental hygiene students examined, 26.8% had nonworking side interferences in at least one side.]

Anterior or **canine-protected occlusion** is an occlusal relationship in which the vertical overlap of the maxillary and mandibular anterior teeth or canines, respectively, produce a disocclusion (separation) of all the posterior teeth when the mandible moves to either side. **Disocclusion** refers to the separation of opposing teeth during eccentric movements of the mandible.[11,12] For example, in Figure 11-31 seen later in this chapter, when the person moves the mandible to the left (working) side, the visible right (nonworking) posterior teeth do not occlude due to the steep canine guidance on the left (working) side. In other words, there are no nonworking or balancing tooth contacts. Also, in Figure 11-24, when the person moves the mandible to the right (working) side, there are no posterior tooth contacts evident on the working side. Many dentists consider canine-protected occlusion to be a desirable or healthy relationship to have. One study of 500 persons indicated that there was a lesser tendency toward bruxism (grinding the teeth together) with canine-protected occlusion.[13] Another study found posterior tooth mobility to be higher in dentitions with canine protection than those with group function.[14] **Group function** (or unilateral balanced occlusion) is an occlusal relationship in which *all* posterior teeth on a working side contact evenly as the jaw is moved toward that side. This is much different from disocclusion, because multiple posterior teeth contact along with the canines on the working side.[7,15] As seen in the chart in Figure 11-21, the average **canine guidance angle** was a little steeper (at 56° and 57°) than the anterior guidance (at 50°). To have a canine-protected articulation where the overlap of the canine teeth disengages the posterior teeth during excursive movements of the mandible, it is usually necessary to have a canine angle of over 60°. [Dr. Woelfel found canine-protected articulation with posterior disocclusion in 60.2% of the natural dentitions of dental hygiene students (Table 11-4).] When not present, it may be achieved through orthodontic treatment or by adding length or lingual thickness to the maxillary canines (by placing restorations).

The desirable type of relationship in a patient who has no teeth and must wear a set of complete dentures is **bilateral balanced occlusion**. This occurs when all of the posterior teeth contact on the working side *and* one or more teeth on the balancing side contact simultaneously. With complete dentures, the bilateral balancing contacts help to prevent the dentures from tipping and coming loose. It is considered undesirable for a patient with natural teeth, however, to have any tooth contact on the nonworking side.

LEARNING EXERCISE

Place a finger just in front of your ears or in your ear openings while you move the mandible to the <u>right</u> side. Do you feel more movement of the condyle on the right side or on the left side? How do you account for this difference? Repeat while moving the jaw to the left side. (See reference 21 for interesting information on this subject.)

SECTION III.	NORMAL MOVEMENTS WITHIN THE TEMPOROMANDIBULAR JOINT

The articular disc divides the articular space into two joint spaces (**synovial spaces**): an upper and a lower compartment[22] (*Fig. 11-25*). [In a healthy joint, with no clinical manifestations of joint disorder, the actual space (determined from radiographs) from the top of the mandibular condyles to the top of the temporal fossae measured 2.5 mm; to the anterior inferior surface of the eminence was 1.5 mm; and to the center of the

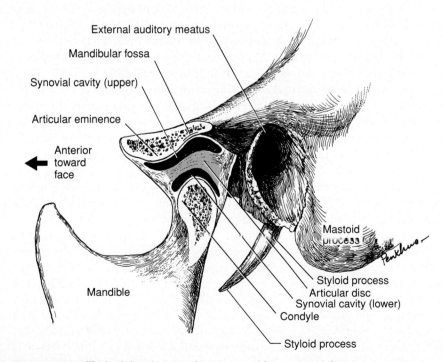

FIGURE 11-25. **Temporomandibular joint** showing the upper and lower synovial spaces.

external auditory meatus was 7.5 mm. This is based on averages from 50 subjects with teeth in centric occlusion, or 100 joints.[23]]

The human temporomandibular joint is unique to mammals in that movement of this joint includes a combination of both hinge and sliding movement. This unique, complex type of joint may be called **ginglymoarthrodial** [JIN gli mo ar THRO de al], where ginglymus refers to a joint that allows movement in only one plane, **rotating** like a door hinge, whereas arthrodia refers to a type of synovial joint that allows **bodily** moving (or **translational movement** where the entire mandible moves bodily in a **gliding** motion). Even in the highest order of apes (chimpanzee), the mandible can only drop open in a simple hinge movement. The *rotational* movement of the condyles (and attached body of the mandible) during limited movements in centric relation occurs beneath the discs in the *lower* joint spaces, whereas the *gliding* (translational) movement of the condyles and the entire mandible *and* discs moving together over the articular eminence occurs in the *upper* joint spaces.

A. MOVEMENTS WITHIN THE LOWER JOINT SPACE

In the lower joint space, only a **hinge-type** or **rotary** motion can occur around a single terminal **hinge axis**. That is, the body of the mandible rotates around a transverse horizontal axis that connects the condyles. This purely rotational (hinge-type) movement of the two rami around a horizontal axis connecting the two condyles can be compared to a playground swing with two supporting chains (similar to the supporting rami) that rotate front to back around a supporting pole (the swing's transverse horizontal bar or axis). The swing itself, like the body of the mandible, moves quite a bit, whereas the highest chain links that attach to the horizontal support bar move little since they attach at the axis of rotation. This purely rotational movement is only possible during the first part of mandibular opening while the jaws maintain a centric relation. [The maximum separation of the incisors for this pure hinge opening (maximum hinge opening in *Fig. 11-26*) averages only 22.4 mm or 44% of maximum opening on 352 subjects (*Table 11-5*).] Further, the rotation of the mandible around a terminal hinge axis is possible only when the mandible is retruded in a centric jaw relation, and only with a conscious effort or by the dentist's guidance.

B. MOVEMENTS WITHIN THE UPPER JOINT SPACE

Translation is the *bodily movement* of the entire mandible downward *and* forward, and occurs within the upper joint spaces. When opening and closing the mouth *wide* (beyond the limit of the purely rotational movement), the discs *and* mandibular condyles together translate forward (upon opening) and backwards (retruding upon closing). During translation, the horizontal axis between the condyles actually moves forward as the condyles *and* discs slide around within the articular fossa and adjacent eminence. Think of this translatory movement as taking the entire playground swing set with its horizontal bar (rotational axis) in the previous example and moving it forward, which moves the swing (condyles and body of the mandible) bodily forward. If the swing is still swinging, a hinge movement is now combined with translation, similar to most movements within the jaw.

When the condyles and discs do not move forward simultaneously, the result may be crepitation. **Crepitation** (**crepitus**) is the crackling or snapping sound or noise emitted from the temporomandibular joints because of a disharmonious movement of the articular disc and the mandibular condyle, sometimes erroneously thought to be caused by the rubbing together of the dry synovial surfaces of joints. When the crackling noise is heard, the articular disc is snapping in or out of position too quickly or it becomes locked in the wrong position.[7,15,16,19,20,26] The frequency of crepitation among 1099 dental hygiene and dental students was presented in Chapter 1 in Table 1-2. Over one-third of these students had some crepitus while opening widely; it was slightly more prevalent on the right side than on the left side, and was more common in women than in men. As you can see, crepitation is *not* a rare occurrence.

Usually, unless crepitation is accompanied by pain, limited jaw opening, or **trismus** [TRIZ mus] (a spasm of masticatory muscles associated with difficulty opening or locking of the jaw), treatment is not indicated.[19,27] The noise may disappear with time, or it may persist for many years being no more than a noisy annoyance. With practice, a person who has crepitus on one or both sides can learn to open the

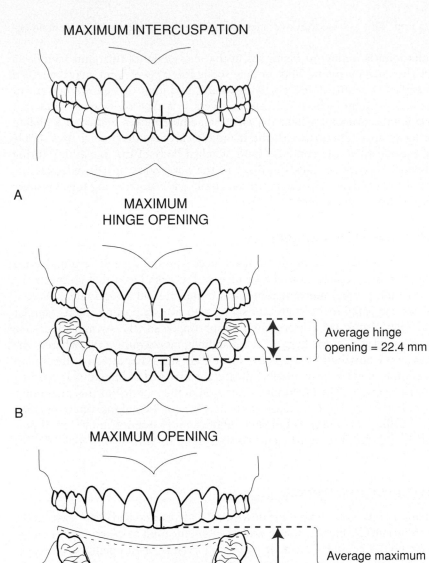

MAXIMUM INTERCUSPATION

A

MAXIMUM
HINGE OPENING

Average hinge
opening = 22.4 mm

B

MAXIMUM OPENING

Average maximum
opening = 51 mm

C

FIGURE 11-26. Range of opening for hinge and translation movements. A. Maximal intercuspal position. **B.** Maximum opening for **hinge movement. C.** Maximum normal **total opening**. Note: Movement from **B** to **C** would include both hinge *and* translatory movement. The curved horizontal line in **C** denotes the **mediolateral curve** (of Wilson) of the occlusal surface from side to side.

Table 11-5	TERMINAL HINGE (ROTARY) OPENING CAPABILITY OF 352 DENTAL HYGIENE STUDENTS†				
TYPE OF JAW OPENING	AVERAGE	RANGE	CONDYLAR ROTATION (AVERAGE IN DEGREES)	RANGE OF CONDYLAR ROTATION (IN DEGREES)
Maximum opening at incisors	51.0 ± 6.3 mm	27.0–68.5 mm	NA*	NA*
Hinge opening at incisors	22.4 ± 5.7 mm	9.5–40.5 mm	12.7	4.4–24.2
Percentage of maximum incisor opening	44.0%	18.9–50.6%	—	—

* Unknown because translation has taken place in upper compartment.
† Results obtained by Dr. Woelfel (1980–1986).

jaw like a hinge in a retruded position without any clicking noise because the discs remain in position as the retruded condyles rotate beneath them.

Both translatory and rotational opening movement occur when a person continues opening beyond about halfway, beginning at the maximum hinge opening limit (Fig. 11-26B) continuing through the maximum possible opening (Fig. 11-26C).

LEARNING EXERCISE

Place your fingers in front of your ears and open and close your jaw to palpate the lateral heads of the mandibular condyles. When you open widely (as in yawning), you will now be rotating *and* translating your mandible. You may feel a bump, or hear a click or popping sound, or hear a grating noise (called crepitation) as the condyles move (translate) forward and slide down under the articular eminences. These sounds may be signs of pathology within the joint such as a disc that does not follow the movements of the condyle. How far are you able to open in the incisor region before you feel the condyles slide or slip forward (translation in the upper part of the joints)? Compare this limited amount of opening with your maximum opening in the incisor region and compare with Dr. Woelfel's measurements shown in Table 11-5.

C. TOTAL JOINT MOVEMENT

During the normal day-to-day activities and functioning of the masticatory complex, a *pure* hinge-type rotation of the mandible does *not* occur since all functional mandibular movements involve some translation with rotation, but not around a stationary, single axis as described earlier. Normal **functional** mandibular movement, such as eating, swallowing, yawning, relaxing the jaw, and talking, occurs simultaneously in both the upper and lower spaces of the temporomandibular joints, resulting in combined translatory and rotary movement.

The combined hinge and translatory motion follows a curved path primarily dictated by the movement of the condyle against the posterior inferior slope of the articular eminence, which is located on the anterior portion of the articular (glenoid) fossa. Most functional movements of the mandible involve translatory motions with curved components because of the shape of the articular fossae and eminences, and because no conscious effort is made to open in a retruded manner.[24,25]

A helpful method for analyzing a patient's mandibular movement is to attach a marking device (stylus) to the mandibular teeth that can trace (on paper) the movements of the mandible as viewed from the front (a frontal view) or from the side (a sagittal view). Figure 11-27 shows examples of these two tracings, both reproducing the outer *maximum* border movements of the mandible, each called an **envelope of motion**. The *frontal* envelope can be visualized, when facing a person, as the outline formed (traced) by a dot located between the mandibular central incisors while the mandible begins at its most intercuspal position (MIP), next with teeth lightly together moves as far to the right as possible, while then, in its most right position, depresses to its most open position, and from there closes in its most left position until teeth lightly touch, and finally returns (with teeth lightly touching) to the MIP.

Now, analyze an actual tracing of a *frontal* envelope in *Figure 11-27A* in order to appreciate what it reveals. Begin in the MIP at the top and following clockwise. The mandible with the teeth in light contact first slides laterally to the patient's left (our right) as far as possible. The outline reveals the amount of canine overlap resulting in the mandible initially moving down as it moves to the side until the canines are end to end, and then moves upward as the canines passing laterally beyond their end-to-end alignment. Next, the jaw opens downward in its most left lateral position until open about 30 mm, then begins veering toward the center to a maximum opening of 51 mm. From this point, the jaw moves to the patient's right (our left) as far as possible as it begins to close. Finally, from the closed maximum right side position, the teeth slide into maximal intercuspal position as the jaw slowly moves back and upward (due to the canine overlap) into the starting point (MIP).

The *saggital* envelope can be visualized, when viewing a person from the side, as an outline formed (traced) by a dot located between the mandibular central incisors while the mandible begins in its most retruded, centric relation (CR) position, just before the teeth move forward into the MIP. Next, with

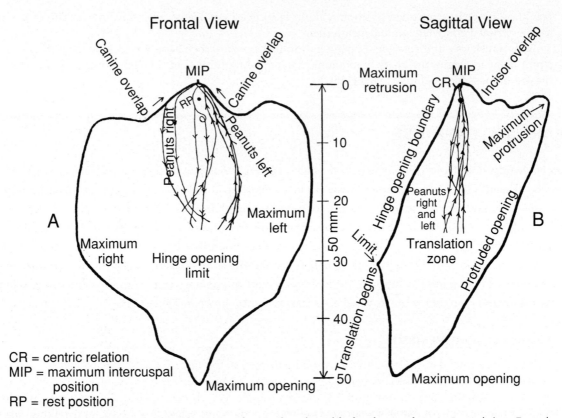

FIGURE 11-27. Frontal and sagittal maximum envelopes of motion with chewing strokes. A. Frontal view: Four chewing strokes are shown within the large envelope of motion as the patient chewed on 3-g portions of peanuts, first on the left and then on the right sides (arrows denote direction of chewing strokes). **B.** Sagittal view of same patient during chewing.

teeth lightly together, the mandible moves into its most anterior position, then to its most open position, and from there the mandible closes in its most posterior position into CR until teeth lightly touch. Finally, the mandible returns (with teeth lightly touching) to the MIP. To analyze the tracing of a *sagittal* envelope of motion in Figure 11-27B, begin at the most retruded posterior position of the mandible (centric relation or CR). Due to a slight deflective (premature) contact, the mandible is directed forward and slightly upward into the MIP. With the teeth held together lightly as the mandible continues to protrude maximally, the initial downward movement of the mandible is due to incisal overlap (normal overbite) where the lingual surfaces of maxillary incisors guide the mandible downward as it goes forward, followed by an upward and forward movement as mandibular incisors move beyond the edge-to-edge position into the most protruded position. With the mandible protruded, it moves down to the maximum opening of 51 mm. From this point, the jaw closes while firmly retruded, which develops the curved *translation* portion of closure, followed by the straighter hinge opening boundary (with rotary motion only), and finally back to the starting point (MIP). We can tell from this envelope of motion that upon opening, this man can *rotate* his retruded mandible open 30 mm at the incisors with a hinge movement before it begins to translate forward.

Now, study *Figure 11-28* to compare the uppermost portions of the frontal envelopes of motion of three subjects in order to visualize differences in the superior portion related to the amount of canine guidance (overlap). Subject A has the smallest and narrowest range of movement for his mandible (32 mm vertically, 21 mm sideways). No lowering of the mandible on either side of the MIP indicates that he did not have canine protection (that is, there are no deeply overlapping canines) to lower the mandible and disocclude the posterior teeth. Subject B can open his mandible 53 mm and move it laterally 31 mm. He has a canine-protected occlusion as indicated by the steep portion where the mandible drops on either side of the MIP. Subject C has a medium-sized envelope of motion with ca-

Frontal envelopes of motion for three young men

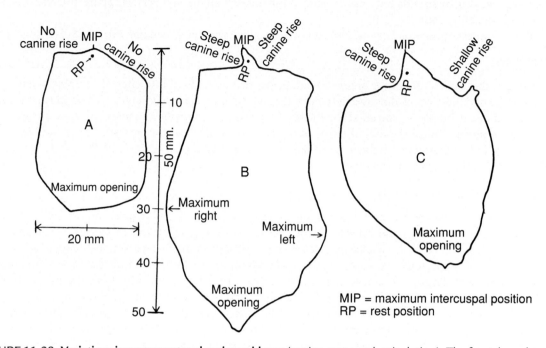

FIGURE 11-28. Variations in movement and canine guidance (canine-protected articulation): The frontal envelopes of motion of three men, demonstrating the wide range of variability between the movement capabilities and their canine guidances.

nine protection on his right side and group function occlusion with shallow canine rise on his left. This patient preferred to chew mostly on his left side where his envelope is lopsided.

An exhaustive study on the temporomandibular joint by Turell includes color pictures of many human temporomandibular joints—some healthy, some with displaced discs, and others diseased with osteoarthritis.[20] This project involved dissection and analysis of joints from 100 cadavers (dead for less than 12 hours). Joint conditions were found to be directly related to existing occlusal relationships. Older people with their teeth and natural occlusion had normal joints. Internal joint changes were determined to be more common in the elderly only because of occlusal interferences, loss of teeth, heavy attrition, and uncorrected malpositions of teeth. It was concluded that many of the alterations seen in osteoarthritic temporomandibular joints had been caused by abnormal, heavy forces within the joints from poor occlusion.[20]

Try to find a copy of reference 27 in your library. It has a glossary, a review of significant research on the temporomandibular joint, and 488 references, and contains original research on the joints of 318 oral rehabilitation patients compared to those of 61 other patients. It is a fascinating treatise.

SECTION IV. FUNCTIONAL MOVEMENTS: CHEWING AND SWALLOWING

Normal **functional movements** of the mandible involve tooth contacts only during eating and swallowing. Eating involves the intake of food by placing it in the mouth, **incising** (bringing incisors together) to bite off a manageable size morsel (small bit of food), chewing (also called **mastication** [mas ti KA shun]), and swallowing (also called **deglutition** [deg loo TISH un]). While you are at rest, the mandibular teeth should not normally occlude with maxillary teeth: there is a space between opposing teeth when the muscles of mastication are relaxed and the mandible is in its **physiologic rest position**. However, this space between the teeth may not be present when a person rests his or her head on the hands to keep awake during a boring lecture. Further, you may think that your teeth must touch when talking but go through the alphabet to see if teeth must touch for any sound. You will find that, for most persons, teeth do not actually touch, although they must come close during sounds like "sss." (Since if the incisors are moved very far apart, the result is more of an "sh" or whistling sound.)

The following descriptions of incising, chewing, and swallowing apply to persons with ideal class I occlusion.

A. INCISING

Incising is the articulation of the anterior teeth performed to cut food into chewable morsels. Eating begins as the mandible drops downward to open the mouth, food is placed between the opposing anterior teeth, and the mandible is protruded (by the lateral pterygoid muscles). The mandible then closes in this protrusive position until the incisal edges of the anterior teeth meet the morsel. The mandible is then moved up and posteriorly with the mandibular incisors against lingual surfaces of the maxillary incisors, thus cutting off a portion of the food.

B. MASTICATING (CHEWING)

Next, food is transferred by the tongue to the posterior teeth; it is held in position on the teeth of the working side by the buccinator muscles in the cheeks (innervated by cranial nerve VII, the facial nerve) and the action of the tongue (whose muscles are controlled by cranial nerve XII, the hypoglossal nerve). The teeth are brought together, engaging the food with the mandible in a slightly lateral position toward the working side. The upper buccal cusps are directly over the lower buccal cusps with the mandible in this lateral position. The closing motion slows as the mandible is forcibly closed[28] (by the masseter, medial pterygoid, and vertical fibers of the temporalis muscles) while the canine overlap and inclines of posterior tooth cusps guide the mandible into maximum intercuspation of the posterior teeth. As this happens, the crushed food is squeezed out through grooves into the buccal and lingual embrasures, and down over the tooth curvatures toward the cheek and onto the tongue where it can be tasted, mixed with saliva, placed back over the teeth, and chewed some more. Once the posterior teeth contact in maximal intercuspal position, there is a pause of about 0.16 second (**silent period**). Next, the mandible opens and moves laterally to commence the next chewing stroke. The duration of each chewing stroke varies from 0.7 to 1.2 seconds in most people.[28] We usually chew like this on one side for several strokes and then switch the food over to the opposite side where a similar chewing cycle occurs.

Tooth cusp slopes and triangular ridges act as cutting blades, whereas major and supplemental grooves serve as escape pathways (**spillways or sluiceways**) for crushed food to squeeze out buccally and lingually. This mechanism significantly reduces lateral forces applied to the teeth that could be damaging to the teeth and their supporting bone.

To appreciate the amount of mandibular movement during chewing relative to the entire envelope of motion, analyze Figure 11-27A. Focus on the smaller pattern of lines with arrows (enclosed within the larger *frontal* envelope of motion) of that person chewing peanuts on the right and left sides. The lines traced during the *opening* stroke (denoted by opening arrows pointing downward) are somewhat straight, whereas the *closing* stroke lines are considerably convex (or bulge) as the mandible moves toward the working side to obtain working side tooth contacts. The chewing cycles occupy only 25 mm of the maximum 51-mm opening range for this man. The chewing strokes on peanuts in a lateral direction utilize only 12 mm of the total side-to-side range of mandibular movement.

On the *sagittal* view (Fig. 11-27B), note that the chewing stroke begins at the MIP and the opening stroke is more posterior than the closing stroke. [The opening stroke is only 7 mm anterior to the hinge opening boundary, whereas the closing stroke is 10 mm anterior to that boundary.] However, as the jaws are closed to crush the food bolus, the mandible is slightly more retruded than the maximal intercuspal position. Crushing of the food bolus (a rounded mass of food) occurs at this maximal intercuspal position.

LEARNING EXERCISE

Look in a mirror and move your jaw as far as possible in all directions (wide open, and from right to left) to discover exactly how wide and long your total envelope (range) of motion is. Then chew some sugarless gum and notice that you use perhaps only half of this overall range of motion. Observe the pattern of movement of your mandible from the facial view during chewing to see if you move your mandible in a tear drop or circle shape similar to the pattern of chewing seen on the frontal view in Figure 11-27. Your side or sagittal view could also be viewed using a second mirror placed at 45°.

C. SWALLOWING (DEGLUTITION)

Swallowing begins as a voluntary muscular act (when we decide to) but is completed involuntarily by reflex action. The mechanics are as follows:

- The anterior part of the mouth is sealed (lips closed).
- The teeth are closed into their maximal intercuspal position.
- The soft palate is raised.
- The hyoid bone is raised as we close off the trachea (windpipe). This prevents food from passing into the lungs.
- The posterior part of the tongue is engaged in a piston-like thrust causing the small mass of chewed food (**bolus**) to be pushed into the oral **pharynx** [FAR inks] (throat).
- The act of swallowing takes place.
- Once the bolus is in the pharynx, the superior portion of the posterior wall presses forward to seal the pharynx, and then the esophageal phase of swallowing commences. This is accomplished by involuntary **peristalsis** (waves of contraction), which moves the food bolus through the entire length of the digestive tract.
- Then the mandible usually drops open, assuming its **physiologic resting posture** where relaxed muscles permit a slight space between upper and lower teeth. Several swallows are necessary to empty the mouth of a given food mass. However, even without food or drink, we swallow a number of times every hour without thinking about it.

LEARNING EXERCISE

Bite off a piece of firm food and analyze your jaw movements by looking in a mirror as you prepare the food for swallowing. This process is called mastication, to be followed by deglutition (swallowing). Observe and feel the hyoid bone above the voicebox move as you swallow. During swallowing, feel the bulge of the suprahyoid muscles located inferior to the mandible (near the midline) but superior to the hyoid bone. Also notice how difficult it is to swallow with your lips and teeth apart. Dental professionals must remember this fact as they keep patients' mouths open for extended periods of time without providing an opportunity for them to close their teeth together and swallow.

SECTION V. PARAFUNCTIONAL MOVEMENT AND TOOTH CONTACTS, SIGNS AND SYMPTOMS

Functional tooth contacts occur during the normal day-to-day processes of mastication and deglutition. Some forces between teeth are actually necessary for maintaining a healthy periodontium. **Parafunctional** contacts, on the other hand, are those which occur outside of these normal functions. Parafunctional movements include oral habits that can result in contacts between teeth, contacts between teeth and hard objects, and contacts between teeth and soft tissue. For example, parafunctional tooth-to-tooth contacts include **clenching** (squeezing the teeth together without jaw movement), **bruxing** (grinding the teeth together in movements other than chewing), and playing a violin (which affects jaw alignment and tooth contacts due to the tilting of the head). Tooth–to–hard object contacts include smoking a pipe (which involves chewing on the pipe stem) and playing a reed instrument such as an oboe. Tooth–to–soft tissue contacts include cheek biting (seen as raw or keratinized mucosa in the area of the linea alba) and lip biting.

Tooth contacts during parafunctional movements may be nothing more than an annoyance, but if these contacts involve considerable force and frequency (beyond that which the tooth and muscles are able to withstand), they can be potentially damaging to teeth, to tooth supportive structures, and to the temporomandibular joint. Unfortunately, when a person develops a bruxing habit, these heavy, potentially damaging tooth contacts may be exercised almost constantly under stressful situations. In a healthy person without occlusal problems, functional tooth contacts over a 24-hour period, including eating three meals, will total only 7–8 minutes. Parafunctional tooth contacts, in contrast, may amount to several hours per day.

Symptoms (that can be felt subjectively by a patient) related to malocclusion and parafunctional contacts include ringing in the ears, sinus pain, dizziness, migraine-type headaches, and joint pain.[10] Parafunctional contacts can result in tired muscles, **trismus** (a disturbance of the trigeminal nerve resulting in spasms of the masticatory muscles and limited jaw opening), a sore tooth or teeth, joint pain, a loose tooth (called **fremitus** [FREM i tus], detectable as a vibration of the tooth upon tapping), tooth **facets** (flattened areas of the tooth due to rubbing away of tooth structure, especially due to heavy or premature tooth contacts), and pain of the face, head, and even the neck. The pain can sometimes be severe.[15–18, 29,30] It is not surprising therefore that parafunctional habits and contacts are undesirable and should be avoided. Teeth that are in heavy occlusion (have premature contacts) may become sensitive to pressure (like forceful chewing) or tapping with an instrument (known as sensitive to **percussion**). **Myofascial** [my o FASH i el] **pain disorder** (MPD) is a common disorder that may result from malocclusion, and it originates in the jaw muscles.[16,17] (Muscle **fascia** is the thin connective tissue covering that connects muscles.) Pain can also be felt as neck aches and back aches. Malocclusion and parafunctional contacts can also result in joint pain.[10] Joint pain may also be due to disease, such as arthritis, or injury. **Temporomandibular disorders** (TMDs) from abnormal functions of the temporomandibular joints can result from loss of vertical dimension from tooth wear or tooth loss, loss of posterior tooth support, and/or other malocclusions. Symptoms of TMD can include headaches, ringing of the ears (**tinnitus** [ti NI tis]), ear pain, and impaired hearing.

Symptoms can be made worse when the force and/or frequency of clenching and grinding increase, as might occur in persons under psychological stress or in persons with poor posture (for example, those who frequently rest one side of their jaw on their arm).

Bruxism

Some people brux their teeth unconsciously during the day and often while sleeping. The signs and symptoms of bruxism include audible tooth grinding (heard by others), worn or chipped teeth, exposed dentin on chewing surfaces, increased tooth sensitivity, jaw pain and muscle tightness, earache, and cheek chewing. It may be worse if a person has malocclusions, anxiety, or suppressed anger, or is hyperactive. Caffeine, tobacco, cocaine, and amphetamines are risk factors. (Refer to the Web site MayoClinic.com; original article address is http://mayoclinic.com/invoke.cfm?id=DS00337.) Clenching and grinding are made worse when the person is under stress. Biting strength in bruxers or clenchers can be as much as six times higher than in the nonbruxers, so it takes little imagination to understand why bruxing can be a dangerous and damaging habit.[24] [Natural dentition chewing forces are well below maximum bite force on average foods, ranging from 0.5 to 33 pounds, seldom exceeding 100 pounds.[25] The human jaw muscles are very powerful, however. The largest maximum bite strength ever recorded was that of a 37-year-old man who maintained a force of 975 pounds for 2 seconds.[24] The average maximum biting force for 20 subjects was 192 pounds (range: 55–280 pounds).]

Signs (objective changes that can be seen) associated with malocclusion include tooth mobility and loose teeth, possibly felt as **fremitus** (when tooth vibrations are felt upon teeth tapping together) and seen as tooth wear (facets). **Radiographic signs** associated with teeth in hyperocclusion include a widened periodontal ligament, angular bone loss, furcation involvement, thickened lamina dura (a defensive mechanism), and **root resorption** (that is, the shortening of a root caused sometimes when teeth are moved too quickly during orthodontic treatment). Open proximal contacts associated with malocclusions can contribute to food impaction and gingivitis and periodontitis if not kept clean.

Signs and symptoms associated with malocclusion may be made worse when only one or two teeth occlude during parafunctional contacts, especially when the patient is a bruxer or clencher. Some tooth contacts are less capable of withstanding forces and more likely to result in muscle or tooth pain. During lateral excursions, any contacts on the nonworking (balancing) side or contacts between only two *posterior* teeth on the working side (in patients with inadequate canine overlap) are not tolerated well. During protrusive contacts, heavy forces on just two or four most posterior teeth (in patients without adequate anterior guidance of overlapping incisors) are not tolerated as well as when ideally overlapped anterior teeth touch and, during protrusive movements, disocclude posterior teeth. Also, heavy forces that are *not* along the vertical axis of the tooth are more likely to be destructive.

Fortunately, we have a natural mechanism that protects teeth from heavy (or deflective) tooth contacts. Our fifth cranial nerve (trigeminal nerve) provides nerve branches to the periodontal ligaments of each tooth, and these nerve fibers send messages to the brain from sensory end organs (called **proprioceptors** [PRO pree o SEP ters]). These stimuli direct movements of the muscles that move the mandible in order for us to *avoid* heavy traumatic or deflective contacts. Several animal studies using cats have found that canines are more richly represented by neuron units (mechanoreceptors in the periodontal ligament) than any other teeth.[31–33] Another study reported that the periodontal ligament proprioceptors were directionally sensitive to forces of a just few grams.[34] Such evidence lends credence to the canine protection theory.[7,11,12] By virtue of this complex protective mechanism, traumatic or deflective tooth contacts are most often avoided during normal function (chewing, talking, and swallowing).[1–3,6,7]

SECTION VI. TREATMENT MODALITIES RELATED TO MALOCCLUSION

Treatment modalities for patients symptomatic due to heavy bruxing, myofascial pain, and/or TMDs may involve or include (a) conscious effort by the patient to avoid clenching, (b) patient education, (c) biofeedback, (d) jaw muscle exercise, (e) nutritional guidance, (f) tranquilizers (medication), (g) muscle relaxants (medication), (h) psychological counseling, (i) an occlusal bite guard (occlusal device) therapy, and (j) occlusal corrections including orthodontics and tooth equilibration (selective recontouring of enamel).[29,30,35] It is appropriate to begin with therapies that are reversible or diagnostic (that is, used to confirm the relationship of malocclusion with the symptoms) before irreversibly moving or reshaping teeth or jaw bones.

Patient Education and Behavior Therapy

It is important to educate a patient on self-treatments that help alleviate muscle pain or tooth pain related to undesireable or premature occlusion. To begin with, teach patients about the association between their pain and their tooth grinding. Just knowing that clenching and bruxing may cause their pain can help the patient to stop bruxing, at least during the day when they notice it. Advise them to try to keep their teeth apart while resting. They need to know that resting the muscles for a while may help, so they need to eat foods that are easy to chew (like casseroles and soups), to avoid foods that require considerable force to chew (like candy-coated peanuts or taco chips), and to avoid foods that increase the frequency of tooth contacts, like chewing gum. Also, limit alcohol, tobacco, and caffeine, all of which may worsen the problem. They should be made aware that bad posture may contribute to muscle pain in the neck and jaws. **Biofeedback** may also be helpful to provide patients with printouts that confirm when they are tightening their muscles so they can learn how to avoid these actions.

Stress Management and Muscle Relaxation

Since persons under psychological stress are more likely to clench and brux more frequently or with more force, therapies that can reduce stress may help. Self-therapies include yoga, meditation, deep breathing, and visualization of a peaceful scene. Referral for psychological counseling may also be necessary. The dentist may prescribe pain medications initially to reduce the pain, tranquilizers to help the patient relax, or muscle relaxants to help reduce muscle tension, but side effects like drowsiness or dry mouth may be undesirable. Botulinum toxin (Botox) has been shown to be helpful for some persons with severe bruxism who have not responded to other therapies.[46] New research has actually shown that taking some antidepressant medications (like seratonin specific reuptake inhibitors) may produce the side effect of bruxing.[47] Therapies that help relieve muscle pain elsewhere in the body could also be used to reduce pain in the muscles of mastication, and these include applying ice for several minutes followed by moist heat to relax muscles.

Dental Approaches

To succeed and to correct a patient's unfortunate parafunctional bruxing habit is not an easy task and takes time, skill, and patience at best. A basic principle of treating occlusal dysfunction is to get the teeth to come together evenly (without premature or undesirable contacts) while the jaw is in the most comfortable position. This can be accomplished through a combination of therapies that includes anterior deprogramming, use of an occlusal device, occlusal equilibration, orthodontics, a full mouth rehabilitation, and/or surgery to improve abnormal jaw alignment.

Anterior deprogramming[8,36–45] is the process of getting the temporomandibular joints into a relaxed or comfortable neuromuscular position (centric relation) by interrupting or negating the proprioceptors surrounding the teeth in the periodontal ligaments. These proprioceptors would otherwise automatically or subconsciously direct the mandible into the habitual or acquired intercuspal position. Anterior deprogramming is usually accomplished in 10 to 15 minutes by interposing something between the anterior teeth[3,37–39,42,43] (such as a leaf gauge, Lucia jig, or sliding guide) while the patient retrudes the mandible and squeezes slightly on the centered anterior fulcrum (see *Figs. 11-29C and 11-30B and C*). The posterior teeth must remain separated several minutes for deprogramming to occur.[3,41] Once it has occurred, the patient will feel as if the posterior teeth occlude (contact) improperly or in a strange way (with deflective contacts). In some instances, the deprogramming will not occur until the patient has worn an occlusal device for several weeks and has maintained a stable and comfortable mandibular position for at least 1 week.[41]

An **occlusal device** (sometimes called a bite plane, bite guard, or night guard) is a removable artificial occlusal surface that can be used to stabilize occlusion, treat temporomandibular disorders, or prevent tooth wear. A detailed description of the method for constructing a maxillary occlusal device is presented in *Figure 11-31*. The occlusal device is constructed of a thin, horseshoe-shaped layer of transparent plastic, and is relatively easy to construct and use. It fits over the upper teeth to provide a smooth, flat surface for the mandibular teeth to contact (without deflective prematurities). A properly constructed occlusal device negates input to proprioceptive sensors in the teeth,[1–3,6,7,15,31] providing a noninvasive, reversible therapy. Its use permits the mandible to seek its centric jaw relation, which is the most neuromuscularly comfortable and stable position.

Patients are advised to wear the occlusal device 24 hours each day except when eating, and the device should be periodically evaluated and adjusted as needed. After a few days, the patient may experience tremendous relief from severe facial muscle pain, headaches, or even some backaches that are related to an imbalance of the temporomandibular joint and tooth occlusion. For example, the patient in Figure 11-16 exhibited trismus and limited jaw opening over a 4-year period. He was only able to open 35 mm at the incisors, but after he wore a maxillary occlusal device for 18 months, his mandible stabilized into a comfortable centric relation position and he was able to open at the incisors 55 mm.

Definitive dental work (restorations, bridges, equilibration, orthodontics, etc.) should be postponed until the patient has remained comfortable for several weeks, and upon return visits requires little if any adjustment of the device.

Occlusal equilibration is the process by which a dentist modifies the occlusal or incisal form of the teeth by using revolving stones or burs in a dental handpiece to remove very small amounts of enamel at the sites of the tooth prematurities.[6] An occlusal equilibration should never be attempted without first having the patient wear a maxillary occlusal device for 1–6 weeks, which ensures natural and comfortable repositioning of the mandible and

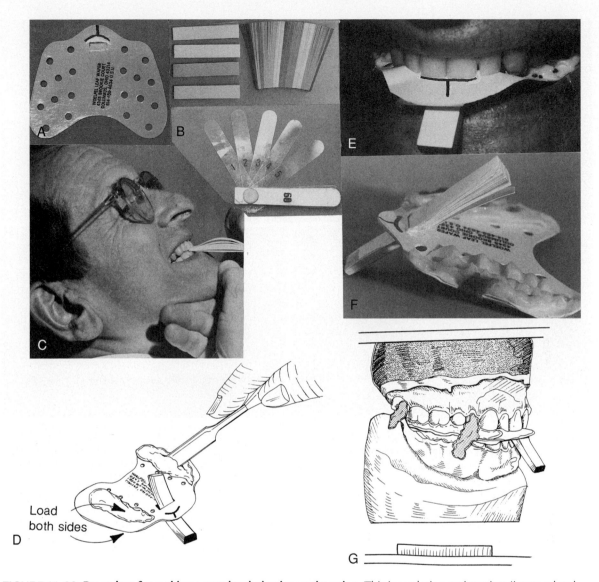

FIGURE 11-29. Procedure for making a centric relation jaw registration. This jaw relation registration (interocclusal record) is used for mounting casts in centric jaw relation on an articulator for analysis and possible tooth alteration or orthodontic movement. **A.** A Woelfel leaf wafer used to carry a leaf gauge (in **B**) of predetermined thickness and the registration medium into the mouth. **B.** Paper leaf gauges above (color-coded for thickness) and below, a numbered plastic leaf gauge. **C.** Patient, with head tipped back, is arcing his mandible in the hinge position and closing on the leaf gauge of minimal but sufficient thickness to separate all teeth to negate any learned habitual closure. **D.** The recording material, polyether rubber, was applied to tooth indentations on the wafer. **E.** The patient closes firmly onto the leaf gauge as the recording material sets. **F.** The centric relation registration with leaf gauge. **G.** The leaf wafer registration is used to orient the lower to upper cast for assembly on an articulator. A brittle, strong sticky wax (shaded areas on drawing) is used to maintain the relationship of the maxillary and mandibular casts until the mounting plaster attaching the casts to the articulator sets.

its temporomandibular joints. Thus, the equilibrated teeth will be in harmony with physiologically relaxed joints. The occlusal equilibration should be reevaluated at appropriate intervals to confirm the need for follow-up treatment.

Long centric articulation or the **intercuspal contact area** is actually a range of mandibular movement where a person can smoothly (without interferences) move the mandible from centric relation directly forward in a horizontal plane to the position of maximum intercuspation. There is no upward or lateral component. This range of movement is often the goal during an equilibration to provide the patient with a long centric relationship by

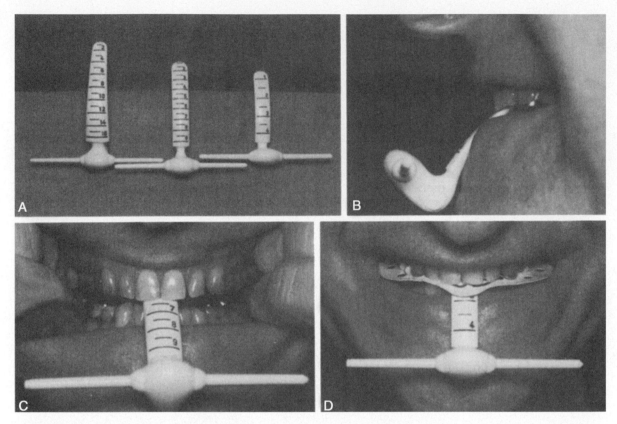

FIGURE 11-30. A. Three sliding guiding inclined gauges. The millimeter scales denote the amount of incisal separation between overlapping incisors (left sliding guide 16 mm, center one 9 mm, right one 4 mm). **B.** A 4-mm sliding guide is held between the incisors at a steep angle to the occlusal plane separating them by 2.5 mm, just enough to keep all of the posterior teeth from touching. **C.** A 9-mm sliding guide is placed in the mouth so the incisors are separated by 6.5 mm during the muscular deprogramming period. **D.** A centric relation jaw registration made with a 4-mm sliding guide inserted into a previously constructed custom "bite deformed Woelfel leaf wafer." The minimal amount of incisal separation (2.5 mm) was determined prior to the centric relation registration that was used to mount diagnostic casts of the patient on an articulator in centric jaw relation.

relieving all deflective or premature tooth contacts that had previously caused the mandible to deviate either sideways or upward from centric relation to the maximal intercuspal position. The patient with a long centric articulation will have a small anteroposterior range (0.5–2.0 mm) of uniform posterior tooth contact occurring at the same vertical dimension of occlusion.

When teeth are so poorly aligned that too much tooth structure would have to be removed during an equilibration (and sensitive dentin or even pulpal tissue would be exposed), the dentist needs to consider other treatment options. **Orthodontic** treatment can be used to bodily move the teeth into an improved alignment. The results of a severe unilateral molar prematurity in the centric relation position was presented in Figure 11-16. This patient underwent 2½ years of orthodontic therapy to correct the enormous discrepancy between centric jaw relation and maximal intercuspal position. Other alternatives would have been surgery (intrusion of molars) or possibly root canal therapy on the molars followed by eight cast crowns (reducing molar cusp height). Ordinarily, centric relation prematurities are not as severe as this and often can be corrected when necessary with minimal occlusal equilibrations or minor orthodontic tooth movement.

Another technique that can be used to perfect the contours and occlusion of teeth that are not too badly out of alignment is to reconstruct the occluding surfaces of all or most teeth by constructing crowns or fixed partial dentures (bridges), or using large, stress-bear-

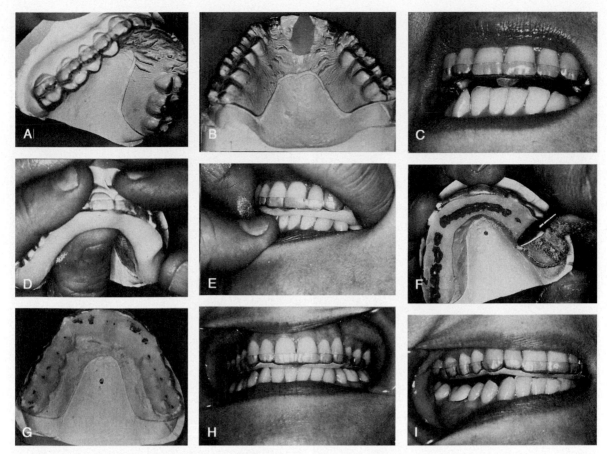

FIGURE 11-31. Stages of construction and adjustment of a maxillary occlusal device (previously called a night guard).
A. A *template* from a thin plastic sheet (1.5–2.0 mm thick) has been heated and vacuum-molded (sucked down) onto a clean, dry, accurate cast of the maxillary teeth. The center palatal portion and excess on the sides and posteriorly has been removed, leaving only a 3-mm overlap on the facial surfaces of the teeth. The occlusal surfaces are roughened with a carbide bur so additional acrylic resin will adhere securely. **B.** A triangular-shaped *anterior ramp* of cold-curing acrylic resin has been added lingually between the central incisors to maintain vertical dimension and to guide the mandible posteriorly (like a leaf gauge or sliding guide). **C.** Contact with the anterior ramp shows an excessive increase of the vertical dimension, so this is *adjusted* leaving only a point of contact with the mandibular incisors, so they will contact at an incline of about 45° upward and posteriorly. **D.** The softened dough roll of orthodontic cold-curing clear acrylic resin is adapted over the roughened occlusal and incisal portion of the template with the anterior portion slightly longer and thinner than the posterior part. **E.** The template with the molded softened acrylic resin dough is *placed in the mouth* and the patient closes gently two or three times in the terminal hinge position and just far enough upward, so that the mandibular incisors are stopped, and the mandible is guided posteriorly by the previously adjusted narrow anterior hard resin ramp. The resin dough is permitted to harden. **F.** With the acrylic resin hardened, return the occlusal device or bite plane to the cast, mark the *cusp indentations* with a bright red felt marker, and then *grind off all excess* acrylic except the imprints of only the tips of the cusps resulting in a flat plane. **G.** *Relieve the anterior portion* of all tooth imprints and slope it sharply upward toward the lingual to provide a ramp for disocclusion during lateral jaw movement. The posterior imprints are correct for initial placement of the device. While on the cast, the roughened acrylic resin is lightly buffed with a rag wheel and polishing compound. **H.** Place the maxillary occlusal device with the patient initially closing in centric relation. The mandibular posterior teeth contact *uniformly* (without deflections) on a flat smooth plane. The mandibular anterior teeth are just barely out of contact until the jaw moves forward or to either side. **I.** The patient slides the mandible to the left, and all teeth on the right side disocclude as the lower left canine slides up the lingual ramp. (Courtesy of Dr. Richard W. Huffman, Professor Emeritus, Ohio State University.)

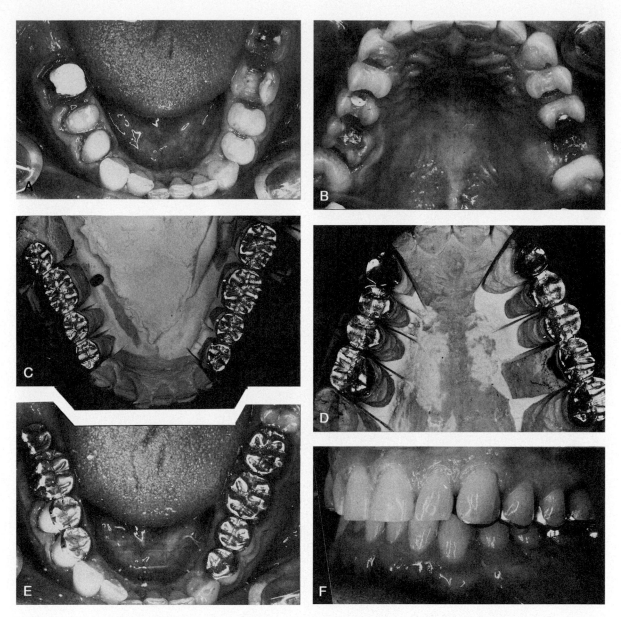

FIGURE 11-32. Stages of a full mouth of rehabilitation. A and B. Preparations of 15 teeth are ready for impressions.
C and D. Completed castings (crowns and inlays or onlays) are constructed on casts of the prepared teeth mounted on
an articulator in centric jaw relation such that the maximal intercuspal position of the newly formed occlusal surfaces is
now simultaneous with the patient's centric jaw relation. The preparations and gold castings were as follows: one DO
inlay-onlay (21), three 3\4 crowns (6, 11, 15), three full cast crowns (28, 29, 30), eight MOD inlay-onlays (3, 4, 5, 12,
13, 18, 19, 20), and two pontics (14, 31). The pontic for tooth 31 is very small for a molar pontic because it has no
posterior support, only the three splinted or soldered units anterior to it (28, 29, 30). Notice the ideal embrasure design
and the multiple small ridges (cutting blades) and grooves or escapeways (gnathologic design) that provide for the
highest possible masticatory effectiveness while directing all forces parallel to the long axes of the teeth. **E.** Mandibular
gold castings in the mouth including the pontic replacing tooth 31. **F.** The patient in maximal intercuspal position,
which is now simultaneous with centric jaw relation. The canines have been lengthened and thickened lingually to provide canine protection. (Courtesy of Dr. John Regenos, Cincinnati, Ohio.)

ing restorations. This technique is a **full mouth rehabilitation**. An example of the stages of
a full mouth rehabilitation performed during the 1980s is presented in *Figure 11-32*. Prior
to having this extensive treatment, the patient in this figure wore a maxillary occlusal
device for 4 months to ensure comfort, stability, and compatibility between his temporomandibular joints and the new occluding surfaces. Upon completion of treatment, his

mandible could move freely to the right or left with all of the teeth disoccluding except the canines, which had been reshaped (lengthened and thickened lingually) to provide this canine protection or steeper guidance angle.

A more contemporary full mouth rehabilitation is presented in Color Plate 21. This patient presented to the dentist with a history of severe gastric (acid) reflux, which contributed to erosion of lingual enamel and much dentin on the lingual surfaces of the anterior teeth. He complained of tooth pain (due to exposed dentinal tubules), muscle pain, and temporomandibular joint pain. He exhibited a deviation between centric relation and maximal intercuspal position of about 2 mm. After preliminary diagnostic procedures were completed, the decision was made to restore all posterior teeth with crowns to correct the deviation, and place all-ceramic crowns or lingual indirect composite veneers to improve contours and cover exposed dentin on all anterior teeth. This Color Plate 21 shows the teeth before, during, and after the full mouth rehabilitation. After therapy, the patient reported no symptoms, and esthetics was improved.

Treatment of class II and class III malocclusions using orthodontics (including braces) usually require much longer correction time and often involves surgical intervention compared to treatment of class I malocclusions. This is due to the greater disparity from an ideal relationship of the corresponding teeth in the maxillae and mandible. When the jaws are so poorly aligned or so different in size that it is impossible to perfect tooth contour using only restorations or orthodontics, **surgical techniques** can be used to reshape and realign jaw bones, usually followed by orthodontic treatment to perfect tooth alignment. A sliding **osteotomy** [ahs te OT o me], where the jaw bones are cut and reshaped, may be used in conjunction with orthodontics to correct severe class II and class III skeletal

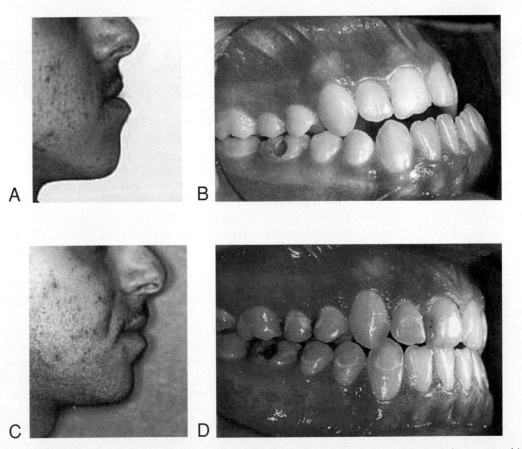

FIGURE 11-33. Changes in jaw alignment before and after orthognathic surgery. A. Pretreatment patient prognathic profile. **B.** Pretreatment class III molar alignment. **C.** Posttreatment orthognathic profile. **D.** Posttreatment class I (almost) molar alignment. (Slide courtesy of Dr. Gluillermo E. Chacon, D.D.S., Ohio State University.)

malocclusions. This technique can dramatically and quickly improve appearance, provide better tooth relationships, and, eventually, better function as well. The change in profile and occlusion from this surgery can clearly be seen in *Figure 11-33*.

SECTION VII. DISLOCATION OF THE MANDIBLE (LUXATION OR CONDYLAR SUBLUXATION)

During an extreme opening of the mandible, the disc and head of the condyle may move forward so far that they slip out of the articular fossa and forward beyond the articular eminence. Thus, the mandible will be partially dislocated or **subluxed**. This dislocation occurs in the upper joint compartment where translation occurs. (The mandibular condyle can also come off of the disc, causing the jaw to lock open.) If the closing muscles suddenly contract, the mandible could become painfully locked open. A person's jaw-opening muscles are not nearly as powerful as the closing muscles and therefore we may not be able to unlock a mandibular dislocation in our own mouth without help. [Perhaps you have seen an alligator trainer hold the alligator's jaws closed with only one hand since their opening muscles are so weak.]

A subluxed position may be released when another person depresses the mandible with heavy force downward and backward to slip the mandibular condyles and discs over the articular emminences and back into the articular fossae. In order to avoid having the person bite down on the fingers of the rescuer as the muscles are released from their state of contraction, the rescuer's thumbs should be placed *not* on the mandibular teeth, but bilaterally on the buccal shelf of the mandible next to the molars. Recall that the disc is loosely attached to the condyle and normally travels with it. The loose capsular tissue surrounding the joint does not usually tear when dislocation occurs, but there would be a lot of pain until the contracted muscles relax after the mandible is depressed and repositioned by the thumbs of the rescuer.

SECTION VIII. ACCURATE RECORDING OF THE CENTRIC RELATION JAW POSITION

The process of obtaining an accurate **centric relation jaw registration** or occlusal record is seen in Figure 11-29. First, a **leaf wafer**[2,8,39] is selected and deformed in the mouth as the patient bites into it. Then a **leaf gauge** or sliding guide (also known as an anterior deprogrammer)[1,6,8,36–39,41] is inserted at an upward angle between the incisors as the patient arcs the mandible open and then closes (hinge type or rotational opening) until the incisors engage the leaf gauge of sufficient thickness so all other teeth separate slightly (Fig. 11-29C). In this manner, the mandible is "tripodized" (stabilized by two condyles and the leaf gauge) by the patient's neuromusculature, and the patient is momentarily unable to aim the jaw into the acquired or habitual occlusion because no signals can be sent to the brain from the proprioceptors in the separated teeth.[31] Otherwise, the teeth could contact deflectively, causing the mandible to move forward from the retruded position. Next, the leaf gauge is inserted in the wafer, and a recording medium (such as the impression material polyether or polyvinylsiloxane) is thinly spread over tooth indentations in the leaf wafer (Fig. 11-29D). Next, the entire assembly is carried to the mouth (Fig. 11-29E), and the patient retrudes and closes firmly, as previously, onto the leaf gauge until the recording medium sets.

This centric relation registration (Fig. 11-29F) is used to relate models (casts) of each arch mounted on the articulator (Fig. 11-29G). This **diagnostic mounting** procedure should always be accomplished prior to attempting any type of tooth equilibration in the mouth.[1,2,6] These dental *stone* models, mounted in their neuromuscularly relaxed centric relation position, can be used to evaluate the extent of tooth malalignment in order to decide the best treatment. The dental stone teeth with interfering or premature contacts can be reshaped (reduced) in order to predict the amount of tooth reduction that will be required during the equilibration. If the amount of tooth structure that must be removed during the equilibration would likely expose dentin or pulp, then orthodontics or surgical procedures must be considered.

Another device used for anterior deprogramming of the mandible and for recording centric jaw relation is the *sliding guiding inclined gauge* or *sliding guide*[36–38,41,45] (Figs. 11-30 and *11-34*). It comes in three maximum thicknesses, and the thickness used is dependent on the severity of the malocclusion (Fig. 11-30A). The thick-

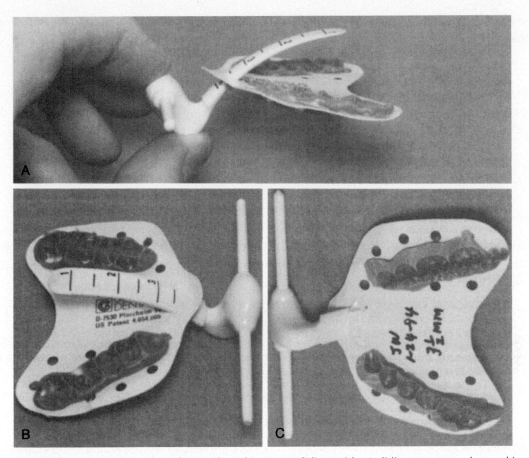

FIGURE 11-34. Three views of a registration made with a 4-mm sliding guide. A sliding gauge may be used in conjunction with the previously bite-deformed leaf wafer and a semi-rigid impression material (polyvinylsiloxane) to obtain the centric relation (retruded) jaw registrations. **A.** The curvature of the sliding guide and its proper angle above the occlusal plane are seen. **B.** Maxillary side of the registration showing the tooth indentations and the 3.5-mm incisal separation. **C.** Inferior view with mandibular tooth imprints in the registration media and pertinent patient information written with a Sharpie fine point marker. This centric jaw relation registration is seen in the mouth in Figure 11-30D.

ness gradually increases from tip to handle, and the curvature of the sliding guide is critical, so that it can be placed in the mouth between overlapping incisors at a relatively steep angle relative to the plane of occlusal without injuring the rugae or hard palate (Fig. 11-30B). The exact thickness between the incisors is read on the millimeter scale (Fig. 11-30C). Minimal incisal separation is the goal for deprogramming and jaw position registration, just so long as no posterior teeth touch, thus avoiding proprioceptive impulses. This is particularly important for the centric jaw relation registration to minimize errors between the articulator and the patient. The sliding guide is made of a nonbrittle autoclavable plastic and works well with a custom bite deformed Woelfel leaf wafer for centric relation jaw registrations (Figs. 11-30D and 11-34).[36-38,41]

LEARNING EXERCISE

Learning Exercise on Your Own Jaw Mobility or Mandibular Movement Capability

It should be an educational and interesting experience for you to complete this simple exercise in order to increase your awareness of your own jaw movements. During this exercise, as you move in each direction as indicated, think about which muscles bring about these jaw movements and which ligaments limit the amount of jaw movement. It will take about 20 minutes to do this exercise.

Obtain a clean, plastic millimeter ruler cut off even with the zero mark. Make the following measurements as described while observing your tooth relationship in a mirror.

1. Horizontal overlap (H) of incisors and canines

Using a mirror, measure the horizontal overlap (**H** in *Fig. 11-35*) in the following three locations while holding your teeth together in maximal intercuspal position (or on handheld tooth models with teeth tightly closed).

     1a. ___ mm = horizontal overlap between the labial surfaces of central incisors at the *midline*

     1b. ___ mm = horizontal overlap between labial surfaces of *left* canines

     1c. ___ mm = horizontal overlap between labial surfaces of *right* canines

2. Protrusive overlap (P) = ___ mm

Measure the protrusive overlap (**P** in Fig. 11-35) with your lower jaw moved forward as far as possible (like a bulldog), between the labial surface of the maxillary central incisors and the labial surface of the mandibular incisors. (This movement requires contraction of both lateral pterygoid muscles simultaneously.)

3. Horizontal overlap of *canines* during lateral excursions (right and left sides)

Measure the horizontal distance between the facial surfaces of the upper and lower canines during maximum movements in lateral excursions, first with the lower jaw moved to the **left** as far as possible as seen in *Figure 11-36A*. This is just like the measurement P in Figure 11-35, only between the facial surfaces of the maxillary and mandibular left canines. This movement requires contraction of the *right* lateral pterygoid muscle.

     3a. ___ mm = **left** horizontal overlap of canines

Next, measure the horizontal distance between the facial surfaces of the upper and lower canines during a maximum lateral movement of the jaw to the **right** side as far as possible, as seen in Figure 11-36B. This movement requires contraction of the *left* lateral pterygoid muscle.

     3b. ___ mm = **right** horizontal overlap of canines

4. Vertical overlap of central incisors (V) = ___ mm

Measure the vertical overlap (**V** in *Fig. 11-37*) at the midline between the incisal edges of your central incisors while holding your back teeth tightly closed, or on your tooth models in maximal intercuspal position.

5. Opening movements (hinge opening and total opening)

The hinge opening is the distance between incisal edges at the maximum hinge-only opening. Practice opening your jaw slowly as far as possible while firmly retruding it in centric relation. Hinge opening is usually

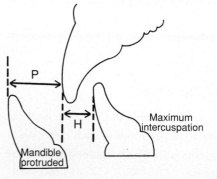

FIGURE 11-35. H is the horizontal overlap of central incisors with the teeth in maximum intercuspation, and **P** is the horizontal overlap with the mandible protruded as far as possible.

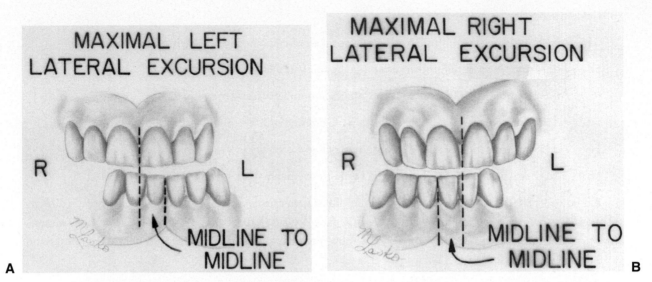

FIGURE 11-36. Lateral jaw movements of the mandibular moved as far as possible to the left **(A)** and to the right **(B)**.

only half or less than half of the maximal opening (first portion of **O** in Fig. 11-37, and represented in Fig. 11-26B as the limit of the hinge opening). If you open properly, there should not be any crepitation because the articular discs and condyles are fixed posteriorly.

5a. ___ mm = hinge opening

Now open as widely as you can and measure the maximum opening (**O** in Fig. 11-37) between the incisal edges (usually you can fit four fingers between your incisors). If you noticed a noise near one or both ears when you opened widely, it is probably caused by a disharmony between the movement of the jaw and the movement of the disc that fits between the jaw condyle and the skull on either side. It is usually not a serious problem, and many people experience crepitation for a while during their lifetime.

5b. ___ mm = maximum opening (**O** in Fig. 11-37)

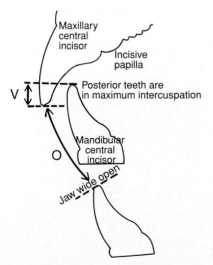

FIGURE 11-37. V is the vertical overlap of central incisors in maximum intercuspation. **O** denotes the maximum opening distance between incisors.

6. Calculate maximum movements

    6a.   Add measurements 4 plus 5b to obtain total incisor opening = ___ mm

    6b.   Add 4 and 5a to obtain maximum hinge opening at incisors = ___ mm

    6c.   Add measurements 1b and 3a to obtain maximum left lateral movement = ___ mm

    6d.   Add measurements 1c and 3b to obtain maximum right lateral movement = ___ mm

    6e.   Add measurements 1a and 2 to obtain maximum protrusion = ___ mm

    6f.   Add totals 6c and 6d to obtain total lateral movement (from right to left) = ___ mm

Are you surprised that you can move your mandible farther from side to side than you can move it directly forward? Usually your jaw can move about twice as far sideways (laterally) as it can protrude or move directly forward. Compare the results of your own jaw movement capability with that of 796 dental hygienists and 318 dental students in Tables 11-2 and 11-3.

LEARNING EXERCISE

Sketch, by memory, the teeth on the right side of the mouth in ideal class I relationship. (Third molars do not need to be included.)

To appreciate the alignment of maxillary and mandibular teeth in ideal class I occlusion, use the following directions to sketch all teeth on the right side of the mouth several times until you can repeat the sketch by memory. Perfection of anatomic form is not as critical as developing the correct proportions and shape of each tooth (incisal edges versus one, two, or three facial cusps), and correct alignment between arches.

1. Use a model of maxillary and mandibular teeth, or a typodont, with teeth in ideal alignment as a guide. First, hold the teeth together in maximum intercuspation but then separate them only enough, so that from the facial view, you can see all maxillary and mandibular facial cusp tips and incisal edges.

2. To make your job easier, do not attempt to reproduce the anterior-posterior curve of Spee. On your paper, place two horizontal, slightly separated, parallel lines that can be used to align the chewing edges of all teeth. Also, place vertical lines to denote the midline of both arches (Fig. A)

3. **Sketch (<u>very lightly</u>) the right maxillary and mandibular central incisors.** View the anterior teeth from the facial view with the midlines lined up. The mesial surfaces of each tooth should touch the midline, the incisal edge should touch the parallel horizontal parallel lines, and the maxillary central should be wider than the mandibular incisor.

        FIGURE A

MIDLINE

4. **Next, sketch (very lightly) the relative shape and width of each incisal edge or cusp in the <u>maxillary</u> arch**, using the top horizontal line as a guide. Note that the models or typodonts must be rotated when viewing more posterior teeth so that each tooth is viewed directly from the facial. Recall that the maxillary lateral incisor is narrower than the central, but the canine and two premolar cusps are about equal in width (except the canine is often slightly longer [beyond the horizontal line]). The first and second molars each have two facial cusps of approximately the same width, neither of which is as wide as the premolars or canine (Fig. B).

FIGURE B

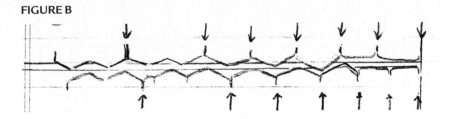

5. **Now sketch the incisal edge or cusp of each tooth in the mandibular arch.** Be sure to reproduce the correct alignment of mandibular cusp tips. For example, the cusp tip of the mandibular canine is aligned with the contact between the maxillary lateral incisor and canine, the cusp tip of the mandibular first premolar is aligned over the proximal contact between the maxillary canine and first premolar, and so forth. Recall that the mandibular first molar most often has three buccal cusps; keep the distal cusp quite small in order to maintain the proper alignment between arches. Begin to form the occlusal/incisal embrasure spaces by rounding the mesial and distal "corners" of each tooth (more so for posterior teeth).

6. **Sketch (very lightly) the proximal and cervical contours of each tooth.** Remember to form the rounded incisal/occlusal embrasures that contour to form proximal contacts with the adjacent tooth, and then taper narrower toward the convex cervical line (which, in health, parallels the free gingival margin). See Figure C.

FIGURE C

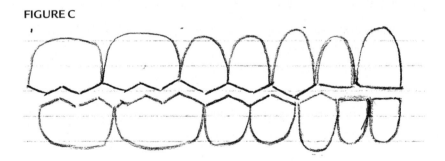

7. Evaluate the overall shape and proportion of each tooth to see if changes are required. If you sketched lightly up to this point, it should be easy to erase and make corrections. Self-evaluate your light sketches using the following criteria:

- **Crown shapes** are recognizable as facial views of each type of tooth.
- **Proportions** for each tooth are reproduced (that is, approximate width versus height).
- **Relative sizes** of teeth are correct.
- **Proximal contacts** are in the incisal or middle thirds but never in the cervical half of the tooth.
- **Embrasure spaces** are reproduced.
- **Cervical line contours** approximate the junction of gingiva and tooth.
- **Correct class I occlusion** is reproduced. (That is, mesiobuccal cusp tip of the maxillary first molar aligns with the mesiobuccal groove of the mandibular first molar, and the cusp tip of the maxillary canine aligns with the embrasure between the mandibular canine and first premolar.)

8. Then, finally, neatly trace and perfect each contour with a darker line in order to perfect the final, distinct shapes for each tooth. Two drawings sketched <u>from memory</u> by two dental students during a final dental anatomy examination are presented in Figure D.

FIGURE D

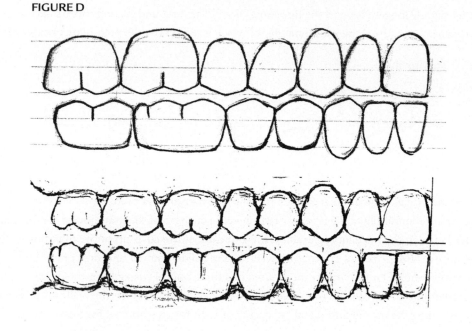

LEARNING QUESTIONS

Answer the following questions with the one best answer based on this sketch of teeth in class I occlusion.

1. In the maximum intercuspal position (MIP), which two teeth occlude with the maxillary first premolar?
   a. mandibular canine and first premolar
   b. mandibular first premolar and second premolar
   c. mandibular second premolar and first molar

2. In MIP, which two teeth occlude with the mandibular second molar?
   a. maxillary first premolar and second premolar
   b. maxillary second premolar and first molar
   c. maxillary first molar and second molar

3. Which two teeth would occlude with the incisal edge of the right mandibular lateral incisor during protrusion of the mandible?
   a. maxillary right central incisor and left central incisor
   b. maxillary right central incisor and right lateral incisor
   c. maxillary right lateral incisor and canine
   d. maxillary right canine and first premolar

4. In MIP, with what landmark would the lingual cusp of the maxillary second premolar occlude?
   a. the mesial marginal ridge of the mandibular second premolar
   b. the mesial fossa of the mandibular second premolar
   c. the distal marginal ridge of the mandibular second premolar
   d. the mesial fossa of the mandibular first molar

5. If this person did not have class I occlusion but had class II occlusion (where the mandible was positioned one full tooth distal to its class I position), which tooth or teeth would contact the maxillary second premolar?
   a. mandibular canine and first premolar
   b. mandibular first premolar and second premolar
   c. mandibular second premolar only
   d. mandibular second premolar and first molar
   e. mandibular first molar only

6. If this person did not have class I occlusion but had class III occlusion (where the mandible was positioned one full tooth mesial to its class I position), which tooth or teeth would contact the maxillary second premolar?
   a. mandibular canine and first premolar
   b. mandibular first premolar and second premolar
   c. mandibular second premolar only
   d. mandibular second premolar and first molar
   e. mandibular first molar only

ANSWERS: 1-b; 2-c; 3-b; 4-c (recall that the lingual cusps of the maxillary premolars are slightly mesial to the crown midline); 5-b; 6-e

REFERENCES

1. Williamson EH, Steinke RM, Morse PK, et al. Centric relation: a comparison of muscle determined position and operator guidance. Am J Orthod 1980;77:133–145.
2. Woelfel JB. New device for accurately recording centric relation. J Prosthet Dent 1986;56:716–727.
3. Carroll WJ, Woelfel JB, Huffman RW. Simple application of anterior jig or leaf gauge in routine clinical practice. J Prosthet Dent 1988;59:611–617.
4. Posselt U. The physiology of occlusion and rehabilitation. Philadelphia: F.A. Davis, 1962.
5. Rosner D, Goldberg G. Condylar retruded contact position correlation in dentulous patients. Part I: three-dimensional analysis of condylar registrations. J Prosthet Dent 1986;56:230–237.
6. Huffman RW. A cusp-fossa equilibration technique using a numbered leaf gauge. J Gnathology 1987;6:23–36.
7. Williamson EH. Occlusion: understanding or misunderstanding. Angle Orthod 1976;46:86–93.
8. Fenlon MR, Woelfel JB. Condylar position recorded using leaf gauges and specific closure forces. Intern J Prost 1993;6(4):402–408.
9. Williamson EH, Woelfel JB, Williams BH. A longitudinal study of rest position and centric occlusion. Angle Orthod 1975;45:130–136.
10. Winter CM, Woelfel JB, Igarashi T. Five-year changes in the edentulous mandible as determined on oblique cephalometric radiographs. J Dent Res 1974;53(6):1455–1467.
11. Brose MO, Tanquist RA. The influence of anterior coupling on mandibular movement. J Prosthet Dent 1987;57:345–353.
12. Kohno S, Nakano M. The measurement and development of anterior guidance. J Prosthet Dent 1987;57:620–630.
13. Barghi N. Clinical evaluation of occlusion. Tex Dent J 1978;96(Mar):12–14.
14. O'Leary J, Shanley D, Drake R. Tooth mobility in cuspid-protected and group function occlusions. J Prosthet Dent 1972;27(Jan):21–25.
15. Ramjford SP, Ash MM Jr. Occlusion. Philadelphia: W.B. Saunders, 1966:142–159.
16. American Dental Association. Temporomandibular disorders. JADA Guide to Dental Health Special Issue 1988;45–46.
17. Locker D, Grushka M. The impact of dental and facial pain. J Dent Res 1987;66:1414–1417.
18. Gross A, Gale EN. A prevalence study of the clinical signs associated with mandibular dysfunction. JADA 1983;107:932–936.
19. Seligman DA, Pullinger AG, Solberg WD. The prevalence of dental attrition and its association with factors of age, gender, occlusion, and TMJ symptomatology. J Dent Res 1988;67:1323–1333.
20. Turell J, Gutierrez Ruiz H. Normal and abnormal findings in temporomandibular joints in autopsy specimens. J Craniomandibular Disord Facial Oral Pain 1987;1:257–275.
21. Sicher H, DuBrul EL. Oral anatomy. 7th ed. St. Louis: C.V. Mosby, 1975:174–209.

22. Montgomery RL. Head and neck anatomy with clinical correlations. New York: McGraw-Hill, 1981:202–214.
23. Ricketts RM. Abnormal functions of the temporomandibular joint. Am J Orthod 1955;41:425, 435–441.
24. Gibbs CH, Mahan PE, Mauderli A, et al. Limits of human bite strength. J Prosthet Dent 1986;56:226–240.
25. Guernsey LH. Biting force measurement. Dent Clin North Am 1966;10:286–289.
26. Renner RP. An introduction to dental anatomy and esthetics. Chicago: Quintessence Publishing, 1985:162.
27. Lindblom G. On the anatomy and function of the temporomandibular joint. Acta Odontol Scand 1960;17(Supp 28):1–287.
28. Woelfel J, Hickey JC, Allison ML. Effect of posterior tooth form on jaw and denture movement. J Prosthet Dent 1962;12:922–939.
29. Green CS. A critique of nonconventional treatment concepts and procedures for TMJ disorders. Comp Cont Educ 1984;5:848–851.
30. Pierce CJ, Gale EN. A comparison of different treatments for nocturnal bruxism. J Dent Res 1988;67:597–601.
31. Crum RJ, Loiselle RJ. Oral perception and proprioception. A review of the literature and its significance to prosthodontics. J Prosthet Dent 1972;28:215–230.
32. Kruger L, Michel F. A single neuron analysis of buccal cavity representation in the sensory trigeminal complex of the cat. Arch Oral Biol 1962;7:491–503.
33. Kawamura Y, Nishiyama T. Projection of dental afferent impulses to the trigeminal nuclei of the cat. Jpn J Physiol 1966;16:584–597.
34. Jerge CR. Comments on the innervation of the teeth. Dent Clin North Am 1965;117–127.
35. Young JL. Successful restorative dentistry for the internal derangement patient. Mo Dent J 1987;67:21–26.
36. Woelfel JB. New device for deprogramming and recording centric jaw relation: the sliding guiding inclined gauge. Advanced Prosthodontics Worldwide, Proceedings of the World Congress on Prosthodontics, Hiroshima, Japan, Sept. 21–23, 1991:218–219.
37. Woelfel JB. A new device for mandibular deprogramming and recording centric relation: the sliding guiding inclined gauge. Protesi occlusionone ATM a cura di Giorgio Vogel FDI 1991. Milan, Italy: Monduzzi Editore III, 1991:35–40.
38. Woelfel JB. Sliding and guiding the mandible into the retruded arc without pushing. The Compendium of Continuing Education in Dentistry 1991(Sept);12(9):614–624.
39. Paltaleao JF, Silva-Netto CR, Nunes LJ, et al. Determination of the centric relation. A comparison between the wax prepared method and the Leaf Gauge-Leaf Wafer System. RGO 1992;40(5):356–360.
40. Tsolka P, Woelfel JB, Man WK, et al. A laboratory assessment of recording reliability and analysis of the K6 diagnostic system. J Craniomandibular Disord Facial Oral Pain 1992;6:273–280.
41. Woelfel JB. An easy practical method for centric registration. Jpn J Gnathology 1994;15(3):125–131.
42. Donegan SJ, Carr AB, Christensen LV, et al. An electromyographic study of aspects of "deprogramming" of human jaw muscles. J Oral Rehabil 1990;17:509–518.
43. Carr AB, Donegan SJ, Christensen LV, et al. An electrognathographic study of aspects of "deprogramming" human jaw muscles. J Oral Rehabil 1991;18:143–148.
44. Christensen LV, Carr AB, Donegan SJ, Ziebert GJ. Observation on the motor control of brief teeth clenching in man. J Oral Rehabil 1991. Jan;18(1):15–29.
45. Yaegashi Y, Tanaka H. An electromyographic study of the effect on masticatory muscle activity applying the leaf gauge. J Prosthet Dent 1994.
46. Tan EK, Jankovik J. Treating severe bruxism with botulinum toxin. J Am Dent Assoc 2000;131(2):211–216
47. Gerber PE, Lynd LD. Selective serotonin reuptake inhibitot induced movement disorders. Ann Pharmocother 1998;32:692–698.

GENERAL REFERENCE

The glossary of prosthodontic terms. J Prosthet Dent 2005;94(1):10–88.

Dental Anomalies

12

I. Anodontia: absence of teeth
    A. Total anodontia
    B. Partial anodontia
II. Extra or supernumerary teeth
    A. Maxillary incisor area
    B. Third molar area
    C. Mandibular premolar area
III. Abnormal tooth morphology
    A. Abnormal crown morphology
    B. Abnormal root morphology

C. Anomalies in tooth position
D. Additional tooth developmental malformations (and discoloration)
E. Reactions to injury after tooth eruption
F. Unusual dentitions

ACKNOWLEDGMENTS

This chapter was originally contributed by Connie Sylvester, R.D.H., B.A., M.S., former faculty of the Ohio State University and the University of Texas Schools of Dental Hygiene. Special thanks to Drs. C.C. Dollens, Rudy Melfi, and Donald Bowers for their gracious assistance in obtaining several of the photographs and radiographs used in this chapter. Also, special thanks to the first-year dental hygiene students at Ohio State University, who brought in numerous anomalies and casts depicting such unusual teeth.

OBJECTIVES

This chapter is designed to help the learner perform the following:

- Identify variations from the normal (anomalies) for the number of teeth in an arch.
- Identify anomalies in **crown** morphology and, when applicable, identify the anomaly by name and give a possible cause (etiology).
- Identify anomalies in **root** morphology and, when applicable, identify the anomaly by name and give a possible cause (etiology).
- Identify anomalies in the alignment of teeth within an arch.

An **anomaly** [ah NOM ah lee] is a deviation from normal, usually related to embryonic development that may result in the absence, excess, or deformity of body parts.[1] Dental anomalies are abnormalities of teeth that range from such "common" occurrences as malformed permanent maxillary lateral incisors that are peg shaped to such rare occurrences as complete anodontia (no teeth at all). Dental anomalies are most often caused by hereditary factors (gene related) or by developmental or metabolic disturbances. While more anomalies occur in the permanent than primary dentition and in the maxilla than the mandible, it is important to remember that their occurrence is rare. For example, only 1–2% of the population have some form of anodontia (one or more missing teeth), while another 1–2% have supernumerary (extra) teeth.[2–4] When specific deformities or abnormal formations of teeth occur with greater frequency, it is difficult to determine whether the deviation is a "true" anomaly or simply an extreme variation in tooth morphology.

Familiarity with dental anomalies is essential to the clinical practice of dentistry and dental hygiene. Recognition and correct labeling of anomalies is important when communicating with other dental team members, especially in the case of referral to or from another dental office. Additionally, your communication with the patient (or, in the case of a child, the parent) should reflect knowledge of abnormal oral conditions. Your assurance that the fused front tooth of a 4-year-old child occurs with 0.5% frequency and rarely affects the number of teeth in the permanent dentition will go a long way to promote the patient's confidence in you and the office. Likewise, the informed patient who understands why the accessory cusp on the buccal of his maxillary or mandibular molar is more prone to decay than normal will likely be more receptive to home care instructions that are specific to his mouth and his needs. Finally, understanding the etiology (cause) of the anomaly is important in determining the course of treatment, if any. Additional information related to the etiology of the following anomalies is found in the study of both oral histology/embryology and oral pathology.

SECTION I   ANODONTIA: ABSENCE OF TEETH

A. TOTAL ANODONTIA

True **anodontia** [an o DON she ah] is the total *congenital* absence of a set of teeth. **Total anodontia** is characterized by the absence of the entire primary and secondary dentitions and is extremely rare. It is most often associated with a generalized congenital deformation (a sex-linked genetic trait) such as the abnormal development of the ectoderm or outer embryonic cell layer. Faulty ectodermal development further affects such structures as hair, nails, sebaceous and sweat glands, and salivary glands.

B. PARTIAL ANODONTIA

Partial anodontia, also referred to as congenitally missing teeth, involves one or more missing teeth from a dentition. Though not proven to be a hereditary trait, tendencies toward missing the same tooth do run in families.

1. MOST COMMONLY MISSING PERMANENT TEETH

The *most commonly missing* permanent teeth are third molars, with the maxillary thirds absent from the dentition more often than the mandibular thirds.

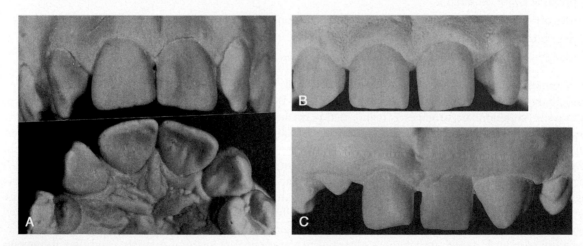

FIGURE 12-1. Partial anodontia. Mouths with congenitally missing maxillary lateral incisors. Notice that canines have moved into the spaces normally reserved for the lateral incisors.

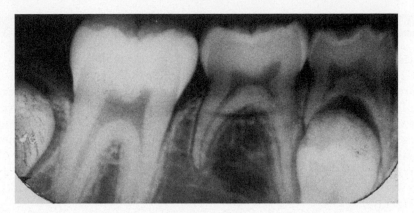

FIGURE 12-2. Partial anodontia. A radiograph revealing a missing second premolar. Routine radiographic examination of a 10-year-old female revealed both mandibular right and left second premolars to be missing. The first premolar can be seen situated under the deciduous first molar crown between its roots. The deciduous second molar is functional and its roots have not begun to resorb. (Notice the fully erupted secondary first molar and the unerupted second molar at the extreme left.)

2.   SECOND MOST COMMONLY MISSING TEETH

The permanent maxillary lateral incisors are the next most commonly missing teeth (*Fig. 12-1*). Approximately 1–2% of the population are missing one or both of these maxillary incisors.[4,5]

3.   THIRD MOST COMMONLY MISSING TEETH

The mandibular second premolars are the third most frequently missing permanent teeth (seen on a radiograph in *Fig. 12-2*), with 1% of the population missing one or both.[4] [Some studies indicate the order of most commonly missing teeth to be third molars, maxillary and mandibular premolars, and maxillary lateral incisors.[6]]

Some observers state that missing teeth follow evolutionary trends in that the teeth most commonly missing from the dentition (third molars) are those that are most expendable in terms of their role in oral function.[4] Conversely, the most stable teeth in the permanent dentition, the canines, are the least likely to be absent from the dentition.[6]

Other congenitally missing permanent and deciduous teeth are evident in *Figure 12-3*.

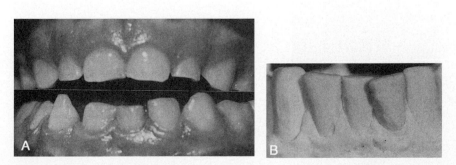

FIGURE 12-3. Partial anodontia. A. Congenitally missing deciduous mandibular central incisor. **B.** Congenitally missing secondary mandibular central incisor.

SECTION II   EXTRA OR SUPERNUMERARY TEETH

Supernumerary **teeth** are teeth that form in excess of the normal dental formulas for each quadrant (deciduous quadrant: I-2, C-1, M-2; permanent quadrant: I-2, C-1, P-2, M-3). They occur in 0.3–3.8% of the population.[22] They are found in both permanent and deciduous dentitions, with 90% of all occurrences in the maxilla.[7] Specifically, the most frequent supernumerary specimens are found in one of two locations: maxillary incisor area (*Fig. 12-4*) or maxillary third molar region. One report states that supernumerary teeth occurred eight times more often in the maxillary than mandibular regions, and twice as frequently in men than in women.[29] Another study of 50 patients from 16 months to 17 years of age found 20% of the supernumerary teeth to be inverted.[23] Fourteen percent of these patients had multiple supernumerary teeth, and 80% of the extra teeth were in a lingual position relative to the dental arch. These teeth can vary considerably in size and shape (*Fig. 12-5*).

A. MAXILLARY INCISOR AREA

A **mesiodens** is a small supernumerary tooth that forms between central incisors. It has a cone-shaped crown and short root (*Fig. 12-6*). It may be visible in the oral cavity or remain unerupted. If unerupted, a diastema (space) may be present.[8] One study of 375 children with mesiodens reports that they are often in an inverted position and rarely erupt into the oral cavity.[29] The prevalence of mesiodens in the permanent dentition in the Caucasian populations is 0.15–1.9%.[9]

Less frequently, supernumerary teeth may be positioned between central and lateral incisors or between lateral incisors and canines. The occurrence of supernumerary teeth in the deciduous dentition is low (approximately 0.5%).[9] The most common supernumerary teeth in the secondary dentition, however, are either midline mesiodens or supplemental lateral incisors.

B. THIRD MOLAR AREA

The presence of supernumerary teeth distal to the third molars is more common in the maxillary arch but does occur in the mandible. These supernumerary teeth are often called **distomolars**, **paramolars, or fourth molars**. These extra teeth rarely erupt into the oral cavity and thus are usually discovered through radiographs (*Fig. 12-7*).

C. MANDIBULAR PREMOLAR AREA

The most common location for supernumerary teeth in the *mandible* is the second premolar region (*Fig. 12-8*). Supernumerary teeth appearing in this area generally resemble normal premolars in size and shape.[10]

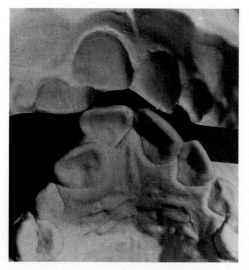

FIGURE 12-4. Supernumerary tooth. Maxillary dentition with three incisors shaped like central incisors (and only one shaped like a lateral incisor).

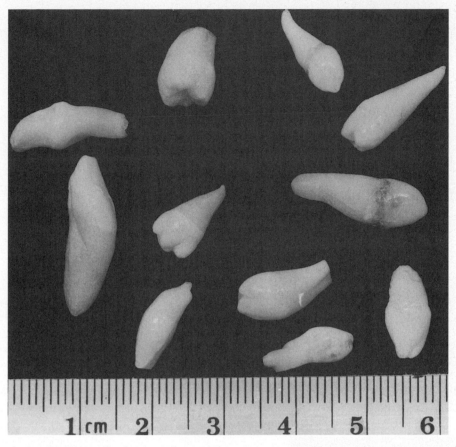

FIGURE 12-5. Supernumerary teeth of various sizes and shapes. Some resemble premolars, some appear like peg-shaped incisors, and others look like very small third molars.

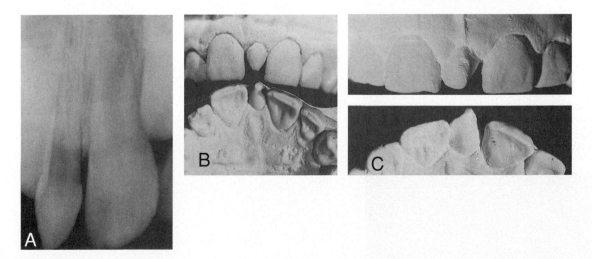

FIGURE 12-6. Supernumerary mesiodens. A. Radiograph: notice the mesiodens next to the fully erupted permanent maxillary central incisor. **B.** An example of a fully erupted mesiodens (facial and incisal views) that has a peg shape. **C.** An example of a fully erupted mesiodens (facial and incisal views) that is shaped more like a small lateral incisor.

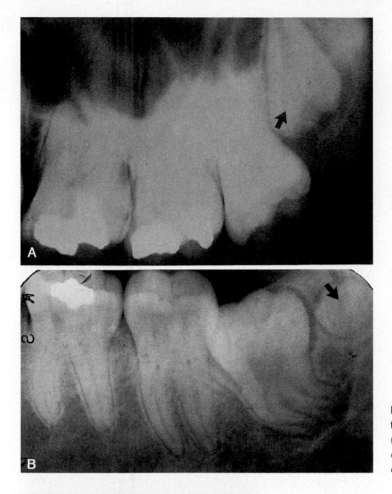

FIGURE 12-7. Paramolars, distomolars, or fourth (supernumerary) molars. A. Maxillary (fourth) distomolar. B. Mandibular (fourth) distomolar. The extra molars (*arrows*) are just distal to the secondary third molars.

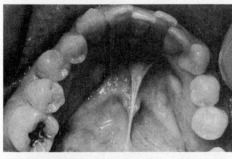

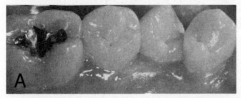

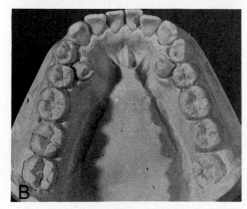

FIGURE 12-8. Supernumerary teeth in mandibular premolar region. A. Two views of an extra mandibular first premolar fully emerged but crowded. (Courtesy of Dr. L. Claman.) B. Extra mandibular first premolars on each side of the mandibular arch are positioned lingually.

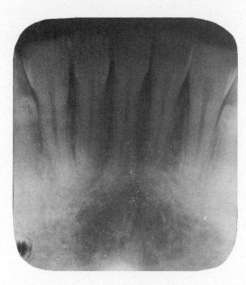

FIGURE 12-9. **Supernumerary mandibular central incisor.** Radiograph of the mandibular incisor region depicting three central incisors and two lateral incisors, all nonfused and with normal pulp cavities.

Extra teeth may also form in other locations in the mouth. For example, a most unusual instance of three mandibular central incisors is seen in the radiograph in *Figure 12-9*.

SECTION III ABNORMAL TOOTH MORPHOLOGY

A. ABNORMAL CROWN MORPHOLOGY

Crown malformations may be seen clinically upon visual inspection of the oral cavity.

1. THIRD MOLAR MALFORMATIONS

Maxillary third molars have the *most variable* crown shape of all permanent teeth followed by mandibular thirds. These anomalies can range in shape from a small peg-shaped crown to a multi-cusped, malformed version of either the first or second molar.

2. PEG-SHAPED LATERAL INCISORS

The most common anomaly in tooth shape in the anterior region of the secondary dentition is the **peg-shaped** (or cone-shaped) **lateral incisor** *(Fig. 12-10)*, occurring in 1–2% of the population.[4] The tooth is generally conical in shape and broadest cervically, and tapers toward the incisal to a blunt point. Several studies of identical twins seem to indicate that missing and peg-shaped lateral incisor teeth may be varied expressions of the same genetic trait.[11,12] A most unusual occurrence is that of peg-shaped maxillary central incisors *(Fig. 12-11)*. Peg-shaped teeth develop from one facial lobe (instead of the three facial lobes normally present on anterior teeth).

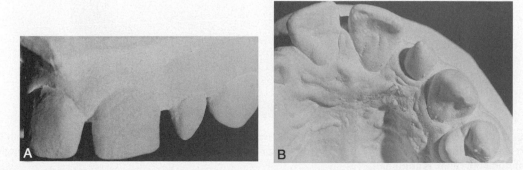

FIGURE 12-10. **Peg-shaped maxillary lateral incisors: A.** Viewed from the facial. **B.** Viewed from the incisal.

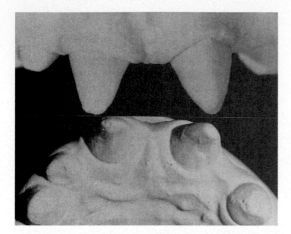

FIGURE 12-11. Peg-shaped maxillary central incisors, a very rare occurrence. **Above:** Facial view. **Below:** Incisal view showing both canines and one lateral incisor.

3. GEMINATION OR TWINNING

Gemination or **twinning** results from the splitting or twinning of a single forming tooth (germ). Since the tooth division is incomplete, the twinned crown appears doubled in width compared to a single tooth and possibly notched *(Fig. 12-12A)*. The single root is not split and has a common pulp canal. Most commonly seen in the anterior area in the region of the maxillary incisors and canines,[3] this condition occurs in less than 1% of the population. It occurs more frequently in the primary dentition than in the permanent dentition. If the doubled tooth is counted as *two* teeth, the dental arch containing the geminated tooth will generally have an *extra* tooth beyond the normal number of teeth. Note in Figure 12-12B that the wide crowns of the anterior teeth of Native Americans may exhibit deep labial grooves that resemble gemination.

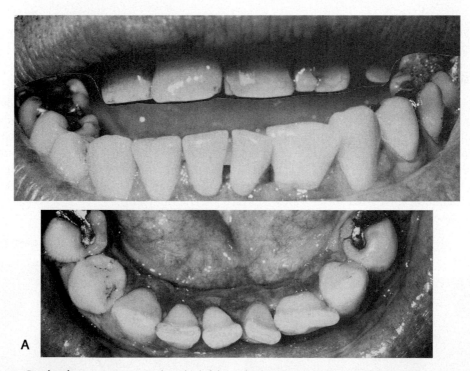

FIGURE 12-12. Gemination. A. It appears that the left lateral incisor germ split or divided into two since, if that tooth is counted as two, there are five incisors, one more than expected. The geminated tooth will generally have a single root and common pulp canal. (continued)

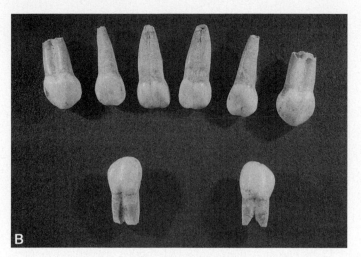

FIGURE 12-12. *(continued)* **B. Deep labial grooves** on all four maxillary central incisors and four canines (maxillary and mandibular) of a Native American. Notice the similarity in crown morphology of these wide, grooved teeth with geminated crowns.

4. FUSION

Fusion is the union of two adjacent tooth germs, always involving the dentin. Upon clinical examination, this condition appears similar to gemination since the fused teeth have one crown that appears doubled in width. However, unlike gemination, radiographs usually reveal two separate but fused roots with separate pulp chambers (*Fig. 12-13*). Another way to differentiate fusion from gemination is to count the teeth in the arch. If the fused teeth are counted as *two*, the total number of teeth will reflect the normal number of teeth in that arch (*Fig. 12-14*).

Like geminated teeth, fused teeth occur more commonly in the anterior portion of the mouth (in less than 1% of the population), and more often in the deciduous dentition than in the permanent dentition. The mandibular incisor area is affected more often than the maxilla.[2,3]

Fusion is thought to be caused by pressure or force during development of adjacent roots. Many of the reports of fusion involve a supernumerary tooth joining with an adjacent tooth, such as the fusion of a mandibular third and fourth molar seen in *Figure 12-15*, and the fusion of a maxillary lateral incisor and anterior supernumerary tooth seen in *Figure 12-16*.[13–15]

5. HUTCHINSON'S TEETH

Unusual incisor and molar shapes may occur in both dentitions as the result of prenatal syphilis. Maxillary and mandibular incisors may be screwdriver shaped, broad cervically, and narrowing incisally, with a notched incisal edge. These teeth are often referred to as **Hutchinson's incisors**. Note in *Figure 12-17* that the crowns of Hutchinson's incisors resemble somewhat the notched crowns of fused teeth seen in Figure 12-14. Also, first molars in these dentitions may have occlusal anatomy made up of multiple tiny tubercles with poorly developed indistinguishable cusps. Because of the berry-like shape on the occlusal, these molars are called **mulberry molars**.

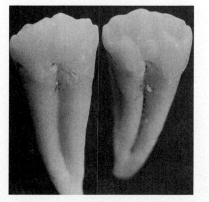

FIGURE 12-13. **Fusion.** Two teeth appearing similar to mandibular first premolars fused together. Buccal aspect (**left**) and lingual aspect (**right**). Some separation between the roots is visible. There would be two pulp canals.

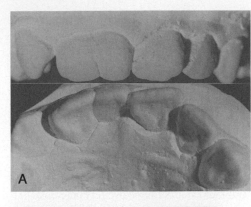

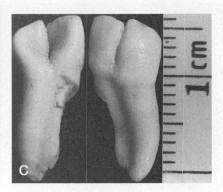

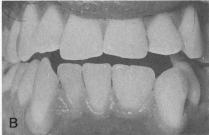

FIGURE 12-14. Fusion. A. If the double wide tooth is counted as two, the number of incisors is four—the expected number. Therefore, we suspect that the maxillary right lateral and central incisor have fused. Another possibility is the fusion of the central incisor and a supernumerary mesiodens, and the lateral incisor is congenitally absent. **B and C.** Fused mandibular central and lateral incisors from different individuals. In **C,** the fused teeth are seen from both lingual and facial aspects.

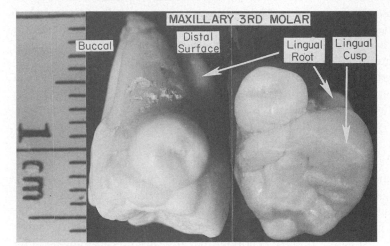

MAXILLARY 3RD MOLAR

Buccal   Distal Surface   Lingual Root   Lingual Cusp

FIGURE 12-15. Fusion. Unusual maxillary third molar with a supernumerary paramolar fused to its distal surface.

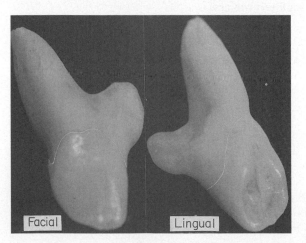

Facial   Lingual

FIGURE 12-16. Fusion. Extracted maxillary central incisor with a fused mesiodens (facial and lingual views).

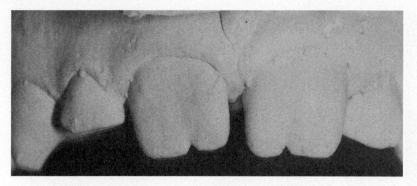

FIGURE 12-17. Hutchinson's (notched) **maxillary incisors** of a 9-year-old female. (Model courtesy of Dmitri J. Harampopoulos, D.D.S.)

6. VARIATIONS IN THE NUMBER OF LINGUAL CUSPS ON MANDIBULAR SECOND PREMOLARS

Mandibular second premolars vary in the number of lingual cusps, ranging from one to three (recall Table 6-4). Occlusal morphology can vary greatly in terms of groove and fossa patterns established by the number of lingual cusps.[16]

7. ACCESSORY CUSPS, TUBERCLES, OR RIDGES

Any tooth may exhibit extra small enamel projections called **tubercles** *(Fig. 12-18)*, or extra accessory cusps. These enamel projections may result from developmental localized hyperplasia (increase in volume of tissue caused by growth of new cells), or crowded conditions prior to eruption may result in fusion of a supernumerary tooth, which may be appear similar to an extra cusp *(Fig. 12-19)*. A third lingual cusp may develop on mandibular molars on the lingual surface, and is called a **tuberculum** [too BER ku lum] **intermedium** *(Fig. 12-20)*. If this extra cusp were located on the distal marginal ridge, it would be called a **tuberculum sextum**. Finally, an unusual prominent ridge is seen on the facial surface of a maxillary central incisor in *Figure 12-21*.

a. Enamel Pearls

Enamel pearls are small, round nodules of enamel with a tiny core of dentin. They are found most frequently on the distal of third molars and the buccal root furcation of molars[17] *(Fig. 12-22)*.

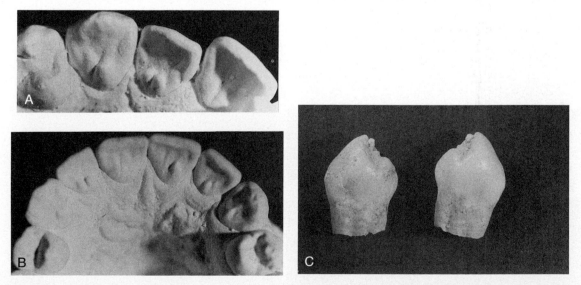

FIGURE 12-18. Tubercles. A. Two elevations or tubercles (or cusplets) on the canine and three on the lateral incisor. **B.** Pronounced tubercles on the cingula of maxillary anterior teeth, most noticeable (due to lighting) on the patient's *left* central and lateral incisor and canine. **C.** Proximal views of contralateral first premolars from a young Native American showing tubercles emanating from the buccal triangular ridges just lingual to the buccal cusps.

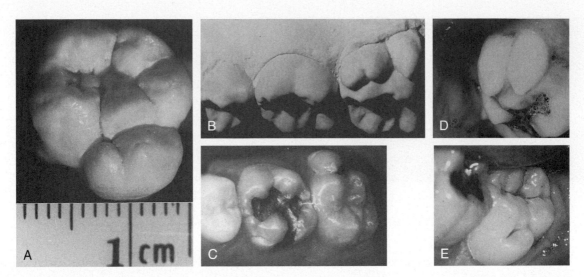

FIGURE 12-19. Extra cusp, cusps, or paramolar fused to mandibular third molar in **A**, and to the buccal surfaces of maxillary second molars in **B**, **C**, and **D**, and **E**.

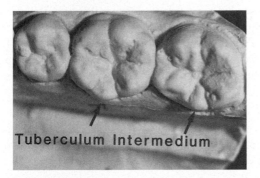

FIGURE 12-20. Tuberculum intermedium. Mandibular first and second molars with extra, midlingual cusps called tuberculum intermedium.

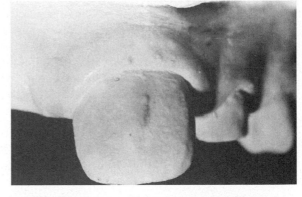

FIGURE 12-21. Unusually prominent labial ridge on a secondary maxillary central incisor.

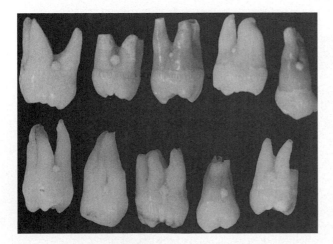

FIGURE 12-22. Enamel pearls of various sizes on maxillary third molars.

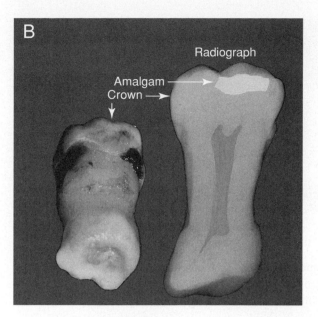

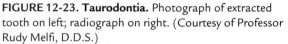

FIGURE 12-23. **Taurodontia.** Photograph of extracted tooth on left; radiograph on right. (Courtesy of Professor Rudy Melfi, D.D.S.)

Radiographically, enamel pearls appear as small round radiopacities (that is, areas appearing light or white on the exposed film). Being covered with enamel, they prevent the normal connective tissue attachment and consequently may channel disease (periodontal problems) into this region.

b. Taurodontia

In **taurodontia**, or so-called bull or prism teeth, the pulp chamber is very long, without a constriction near the cementoenamel junction *(Fig. 12-23)*. This occurs only in permanent teeth, with a frequency of less than 1 in 1000 among American Indians and Eskimos.[24] Taurodontia is caused by a disorganization of the calcified tissues and possibly occurs in dentitions subjected to heavy use.

c. Talon Cusp

A small enamel projection in the cingulum area of maxillary or mandibular anterior permanent teeth is a **talon** ("claw of an animal") **cusp** *(Fig. 12-24A)*. Frequently, the cusp has a pulp horn so that radiographically it may be mistaken for a supernumerary tooth superimposed over an anterior tooth or dens in dente (described later in this chapter). Removal of this cusp is often neces-

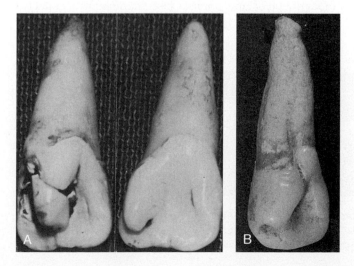

FIGURE 12-24. **Talon cusps. A.** Lingual view of two maxillary central incisors with talon cusps. **B.** Lingual view of a maxillary left lateral incisor shows a deep lingual groove at the junction of the unusually prominent mesial and distal ridges, which might, at first glance, be confused with a talon cusp.

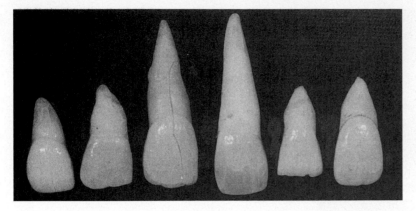

FIGURE 12-25. Variation in tooth size from **microdontia** (very small) to **macrodontia** (very large). Microdontia of four very short central incisors with dwarfed roots (one tooth only 16 mm long) and macrodontia of two very long incisors (one 34 mm long).

sary because of its interference in jaw closure in the maximum intercuspal position. Since the pulp horn is present, endodontic treatment is usually required when this cusp is removed.[2,18] Notice that the deep lingual grooves found on some anterior teeth may somewhat resemble the grooves of a talon cusp *(Fig. 12-24B)*.

8. VARIATIONS IN TOOTH SIZE

Microdontia (very small, but normally shaped teeth) and **macrodontia** (very large, but normally shaped teeth) may occur as a single tooth, several teeth, or an entire dentition.[36] Macrodontia most frequently involves incisors and canines, whereas microdontia affects maxillary lateral incisors and third molars.[8,19,20] Some examples of variation in size of teeth are shown in *Figure 12-25*. One report shows a maxillary canine 39 mm long and a maxillary first molar 31 mm long (compared to average lengths of 26.3 mm and 20.1 mm, respectively), both removed from a pituitary giant.[36]

9. SHOVEL-SHAPED MAXILLARY INCISORS

Possibly not a true anomaly, **shovel-shaped incisors** are a frequently occurring trait that reflect biologic differences between races.[4] The lingual anatomy includes a pronounced cingulum and marginal ridges, thus the scoop or "shovel" appearance *(Fig. 12-26A)*. These teeth are observed most frequently in the Asian, Mongoloid, Eskimo, and American Indian races. Double shoveling refers to the pronounced *lingual* marginal ridges, as well as prominent ridges on the mesial and distal portions of the *labial* surface as seen in *Figure 12-26B*.

B. ABNORMAL ROOT MORPHOLOGY

Root malformations are not usually obvious without the aid of radiographs. Close examination of extracted specimens reveals wide variations.

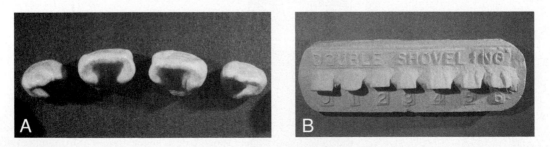

FIGURE 12-26. A. Shovel-shaped permanent incisors from a young Native American dentition (incisal view). Note the prominent marginal ridges on the lingual surface. **B.** The range of prominent labial ridges on **double-shovel–shaped incisors** varies from barely discernible labial ridges on the left to prominent labial ridges on the right.

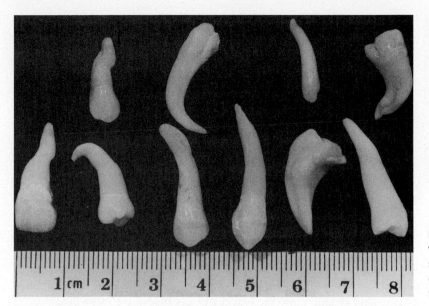

FIGURE 12-27. Dilaceration, where the root and/or crown are severely twisted. Maxillary teeth crowns are down; mandibular teeth crowns are above the roots.

1. DILACERATION OR FLEXION

Dilaceration [di las er A shun] is a severe bend or distortion of a tooth root and/or crown, often approximating an angle from 45° to more than 90° (*Fig. 12-27*).[25] This unusual occurrence may be the result of a traumatic injury or of insufficient space for development, as is often the case with third molars (*Fig. 12-28*). **Flexion** is another term used to describe a sharp curvature or bend (less than 90°) on a tooth root. Dilaceration and flexion are often observed in teeth with accessory roots.

2. DENS IN DENTE

Dens in dente (literally "tooth within a tooth") is a developmental anomaly resulting from the invagination of the enamel organ within the crown of a tooth. Clinically, it appears as a deep crevice primarily in the cingulum region of incisors. Most commonly found in maxillary lateral incisors, it can appear in upper central incisors and in mandibular incisors. Radiographically, dens in dente appears as a mass of elongated enamel within the dentin of a normal-sized tooth (*Fig. 12-29A and B*). Usually, it appears in the coronal third of the tooth, but may extend the entire root length. Often peg-shaped lateral incisors, with failure of mesial and distal lobes to develop, are found to have dens in dente upon radiographic examination. Their occurrence is from 1 to 5% of the population.[2]

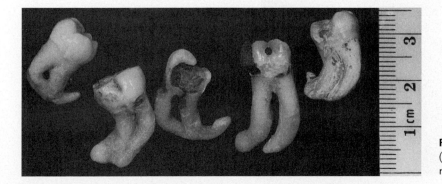

FIGURE 12-28. Dilaceration (severe) of the roots of mandibular molars.

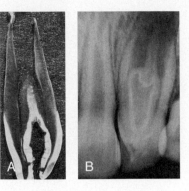

FIGURE 12-29. Dens in dente ("tooth within a tooth"). **A.** Faciolingual cross section of a maxillary lateral incisor with a dens in dente (tooth within a tooth). This tooth section is only 50 micrometers thick. **B.** Radiograph of dens in dente on maxillary right central incisor. It connects with the lingual pit as clearly seen in **A.** It is caused by an invagination of the epithelium of the enamel organ before the formation of hard tissue. (Courtesy of Professor Rudy Melfi, D.D.S.)

3. CONCRESCENCE

Concrescence [kon KRES ens] is a type of superficial fusion or growing together of two adjacent teeth at the root through the *cementum only (Fig. 12-30)*. Unlike fusion, the teeth involved are originally separate but become joined, usually after eruption into the oral cavity, because of the close proximity of the roots and excessive cementum deposition.[6] This anomaly occurs most frequently in the maxillary molar region.

4. DWARFED ROOTS

Maxillary teeth often exhibit normal-sized crowns with abnormally short (**dwarfed**) roots (seen in Fig. 12-25). The incisal edge is usually displaced lingually as in the mandibular incisors. This condition is often hereditary; however, isolated or generalized dwarfing of roots may also result from orthodontic movement of the teeth (with braces) when the movement has occurred too rapidly.

5. HYPERCEMENTOSIS

Hypercementosis is the excessive formation of cementum around the root of a tooth after the tooth has erupted *(Fig. 12-31)*. It may be caused by trauma, metabolic dysfunction, or periapical inflammation. The excess amount of cementum may cause webbing of the roots.

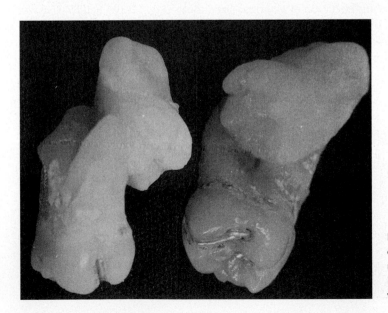

FIGURE 12-30. Concrescence. The junction or joining of cementum between adjacent maxillary first and second molars. **Left:** Lingual view. **Right:** Disto-occlusal aspect with the buccal toward the right.

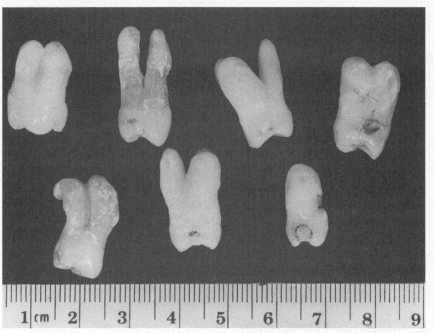

FIGURE 12-31.
Hypercementosis or excess cementum thickness. **Top row:** Maxillary third molar, first premolar, and two first molars. **Lower row:** Mandibular first molar, maxillary first molar, and second premolar.

6. ACCESSORY (EXTRA) ROOTS

Usually occurring in teeth whose roots form after birth, accessory roots are probably caused by trauma, metabolic dysfunction, or pressure. Third molars are the multirooted teeth most likely to exhibit accessory roots (*Fig. 12-32A*).[2] Other molars may also develop extra roots, as seen on a mandibular second molar in *Figure 12-32B*. The single-rooted teeth most frequently affected are

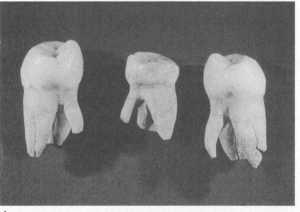

A

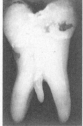

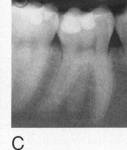

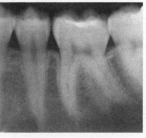

B   C

FIGURE 12-32. A. Three examples of distolingual **extra (accessory) roots** in a young Native American: two permanent contralateral first mandibular molars and a deciduous second molar. **B.** Secondary mandibular left second molar with extra root-like appendage in the furcation area. **C.** Two radiographs showing a right and left mandibular first molar, each with three (instead of two) roots.

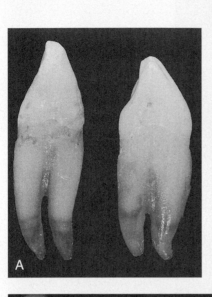

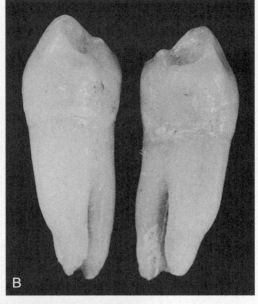

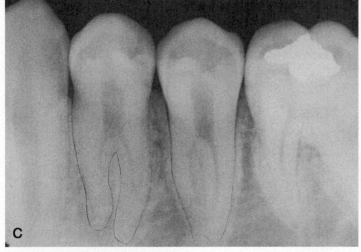

FIGURE 12-33. Unusual bifurcated roots.
A. Two mandibular canines with an uncommon furcated root (one facial and one lingual). **B.** Two mandibular right first premolars with bifurcated roots, a condition that is less common for this tooth than on mandibular canines. **C.** Radiograph showing both first and second mandibular premolars with mesial and distal roots. This mesiodistal split is quite rare. A more common occurrence is for mandibular first premolars to have their root divided buccolingually (as in **B**). (Root and pulp cavity images have been enhanced.)

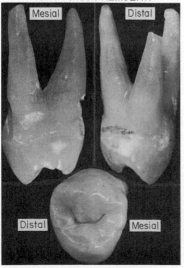

MAXILLARY
RIGHT FIRST PREMOLAR

Mesial   Distal

Distal   Mesial

FIGURE 12-34. Unusual trifurcation of a maxillary premolar. Three views of a maxillary right first premolar with a normal-looking crown, but with three roots: two buccal and one lingual root (mesiobuccal, distobuccal, and lingual). Except for a lesser spread, these roots resemble those found on maxillary molars.

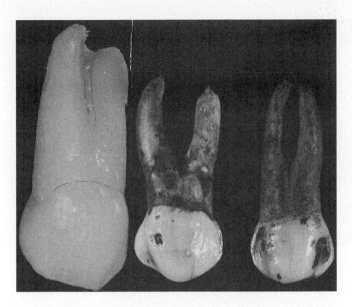

FIGURE 12-35. Unusual bifurcation seen on buccal views of primary maxillary canines.[41] The left tooth was extracted from a 9-year-old African American child (mesial surface is to the right.) The middle and right teeth came from a 5-year-old Native American child in Woods County, Ohio, believed to be 2580 years old. Mesial sides face each other. (Courtesy of Dr. Ruth B. Paulson.)

the mandibular canines and premolars. Two roots (one facial and one lingual) are found rarely enough on mandibular canines to be interesting, but frequently enough not to be amazing (*Fig. 12-33A*). Mandibular first premolars may also exhibit a bifurcated root, one buccal and one lingual (*Fig. 12-33B*), a condition less common for this tooth than for mandibular canines. A Japanese study of 500 mandibular first premolars found that this type of bifurcation occurred in 1.6% of their teeth. These researchers also found one very rare specimen with three roots, two buccal and one lingual.[40] A somewhat rare occurrence of two roots on mandibular premolars (one mesial and one distal) is evident in the radiographs in *Figure 12-33C*.

Another unusual root formation includes maxillary first premolars with three roots (two buccal and one lingual) similar to the roots of a maxillary molar (*Fig. 12-34*). The somewhat rare occurrence of the *primary* maxillary canines with their root divided mesiodistally is shown in *Figure 12-35*.[30–36] There have been six reported cases of contralaterally bifurcated roots on primary maxillary canines: five discovered from routine radiographic examination, the sixth on a routine dental recall examination.[30–35]

C. ANOMALIES IN TOOTH POSITION

1. UNERUPTED (IMPACTED) TEETH

Unerupted teeth are embedded teeth that fail to erupt into the oral cavity because of a lack of eruptive force. **Impacted** teeth, on the other hand, fail to erupt due to mechanical obstruction, often related to the evolutionary decreasing size of modern man's jaw. At least 10% of the population have impacted teeth, which most often include maxillary and mandibular third molars (*Fig. 12-36*) and maxillary canines.[2,4,21]

2. MISPLACED TEETH (TRANSPOSITION)

Occasionally, tooth buds seem to get out of place, causing teeth to emerge in peculiar locations. The most common tooth involved is the maxillary canine seen in *Fig. 12-37* (20 of 25 cases reported),[26] followed by the mandibular canine (*Fig. 12-38*). Maxillary canines can even be transposed to the central incisor region.[37,38]

3. TOOTH ROTATION

Rotation is a rare anomaly, most common for the maxillary second premolar, sometimes the maxillary incisor, first premolar, or mandibular second premolar.[27] A tooth may be rotated on its axis by as much as 180° (see rotated maxillary second premolar in *Fig. 12-39*).

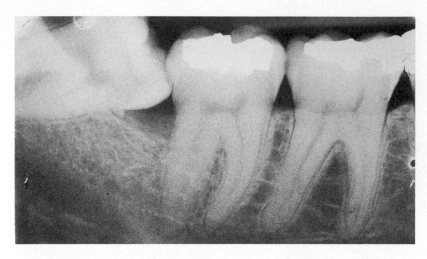

FIGURE 12-36. Impacted mandibular third molar. Because of its horizontal position, it is mechanically locked beneath the distal bulge on the second molar.

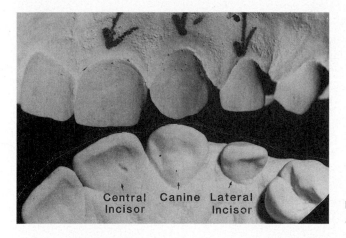

FIGURE 12-37. Switched positions for the secondary left maxillary lateral incisor and canine.

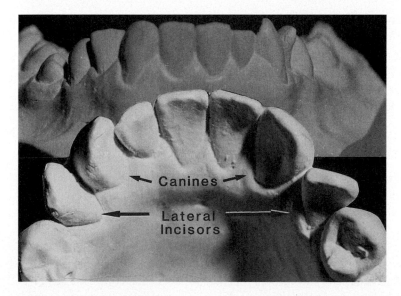

FIGURE 12-38. Bilaterally **misplaced** mandibular canines and lateral incisors, a rare occurrence. Also note the small retained left deciduous lateral incisor.

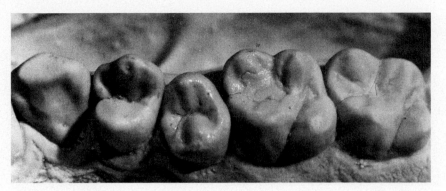

FIGURE 12-39. Rotation of a secondary maxillary second premolar with its buccal surface rotated 180° so that it is now facing to the lingual.

4. ANKYLOSIS

Teeth that erupt into the oral cavity but fail to reach occlusion with the opposing arch appear submerged or ankylosed. **Ankylosis** [ang ki LO sis] may be initiated by an infection or trauma to the periodontal ligament. The ankylosed tooth has lost its periodontal ligament space and is truly fused to the alveolar process or bone. Deciduous mandibular second molars most often fail to continue erupting as the jaw grows. Many times, the ankylosis occurs when the permanent successor is missing. Consequently, the ankylosed tooth will be 2–4 mm short of occluding with an opposing tooth.

D. ADDITIONAL TOOTH MALFORMATIONS AND DISCOLORATIONS

Additional tooth malformations, including those that tend to affect the entire dentition rather than one or two specific teeth and those related to heredity and injury during formation, should be recognized.

1. ENAMEL DYSPLASIA

Enamel dysplasia is a broad term used to describe abnormal enamel development. Specifically, it is any disturbance in the ameloblasts during the enamel matrix formation. Enamel hypocalcification, on the other hand, is a disturbance in the maturation of the enamel matrix. Enamel dysplasia may be hereditary (amelogenesis imperfecta), or could result from systemic causes (such as drugs, infection, and nutritional deficiencies) or local disturbances (such as trauma and periapical infection). Generally, variations in color (from white to yellow and brown) or morphology (pitted and roughened enamel) can result. Relatively common occurrences include the following:

a. Amelogenesis Imperfecta

Amelogenesis imperfecta [ah mel o JEN e sis im per FEC ta] is a hereditary disorder that affects the enamel formation of both dentitions (*Fig. 12-40* and Color Plate 22). The partial or complete lack of enamel results in rough yellow to brown crowns that are highly susceptible to decay. This condition is extremely rare, with an incidence in the United States of 1 in 15,000.[2]

b. Fluorosis

Fluorosis is a condition caused during enamel formation by the ingestion of a high concentration of fluorine in drinking water that *greatly exceeds* the concentration recommended for controlling decay. The fluorine content of some naturally occurring mineral water that causes this condition is *many times greater* than the one part per million that is added to drinking water in many cities to effectively reduce the prevalence of decay. If during enamel formation unerupted teeth are exposed to high concentrations of ingested fluoride, the tooth can exhibit

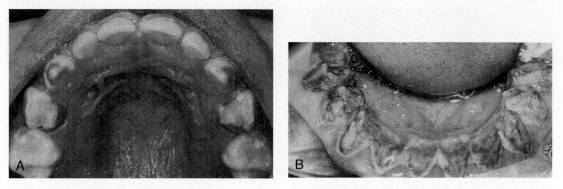

FIGURE 12-40. Amelogenesis imperfecta. A. Deciduous maxillary dentition. **B.** Severe amelogenesis imperfecta on the permanent mandibular dentition. (Courtesy of Professors Donald Bowers and Rudy Melfi.)

a color change from white to yellow/brown spots called mottled enamel, and if severe, the tooth enamel can undergo a morphologic change resulting in the formation of pits within the enamel (**pitted enamel**) (seen in *Fig 12-41* and on erupting secondary maxillary incisors in Color Plate 23). Clinically, all *permanent* teeth may be involved. These teeth are generally very resistant to decay.

c. Enamel Damage Due to High Fever

Pitted enamel on permanent teeth is often the result of early childhood fever from such diseases as measles.[4] Usually, the specific crowns that are developing at the time of the fever are affected (*Fig. 12-42*). Thus, there are identifiable patterns, such as the pitting of enamel in all permanent first molars as well as the permanent incisors.

d. Focal Hypomaturation

Focal hypomaturation or hypoplasia is seen as a localized chalky white spot on a tooth. During enamel formation, this condition may result from trauma, a local infection of an adjacent abscessed primary tooth, or some other interference in enamel matrix maturation, most likely to occur in succedaneous teeth (called **Turner's tooth**, or Turner's hypoplasia seen in *Fig. 12-43*). Unlike decalcification (early decay), which usually forms around the cervical thirds of teeth or occlusal surfaces of posterior teeth, hypomaturation generally appears in the middle third of the smooth crown surfaces (facial and lingual surfaces). The underlying enamel is usually soft, and thus, the area is susceptible to decay (Color Plate 24).

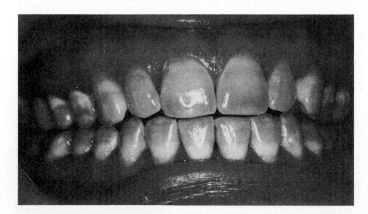

FIGURE 12-41. Fluorosis. This example of mottled enamel is generalized in a 25-year-old female. It is seen as a chalky white coloration in the cervical and/or middle third of all of these permanent teeth. Some pitting of the enamel surface is also visible.

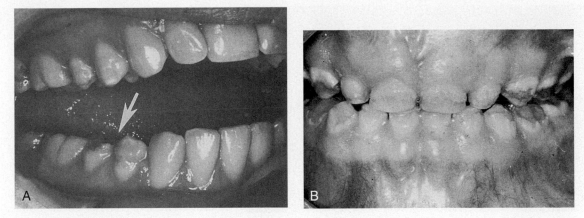

FIGURE 12-42. Dysplasia of the enamel due to **high fever. A.** Permanent dentition. Patient reported a history of high fever between the ages of 2 and 3 years. Notice that the teeth whose enamel matrix was forming at the time of the fever are affected: mandibular first and second premolars and second molar, and maxillary second premolar and second molar. **B.** Deciduous dentition. Patient had a high fever during the first 6 weeks after birth. (Courtesy of Professor Donald Bowers.)

2. DENTIN DYSPLASIA

Dentin dysplasias occur twice as often as those in enamel (1 in 8000).[28] Anomalies of the dentin include those with hereditary and systemic causes as follows.

a. Dentinogenesis Imperfecta

Dentinogenesis [den ti no JEN e sis] **imperfecta** is a hereditary disorder that affects the dentin formation of both dentitions. Clinically, all teeth have a light blue-gray to yellow, somewhat opalescent appearance (*Fig. 12-44* and Color Plate 25A), hence the term opalescent dentin. Radiographically, there is partial or total absence of pulp chambers and root canals (Color Plate 25B). These teeth are weak because of a lack of support in the dentin and, as with amelogenesis imperfecta, are esthetically displeasing.

b. Tetracycline Stain

When antibiotic tetracyclines are taken either by a pregnant woman, an infant, or a child during the time of tooth formation and calcification, it can be incorporated in developing dentin. Clinically, the resultant staining is generalized in the deciduous dentition, ranging in color, depending on the dose of the drug, from yellow to gray-brown (*Fig. 12-45* and Color Plate 26). Some permanent teeth may also be affected, depending on the age at which tetracycline was prescribed. Since only the teeth that are calcifying during the tetracycline therapy are stained, it is

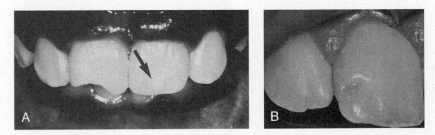

FIGURE 12-43. Enamel hypoplasia (focal hypomaturation) caused by a disturbance during the formative stage of the enamel matrix. **A.** Focal hypomaturation (*arrow*). **B.** A defect on the labial surface of the maxillary central incisor (a so-called **Turner's tooth**) caused by an infection (abscess) on the deciduous central incisor that preceded it. (Courtesy of Professor Donald Bowers.)

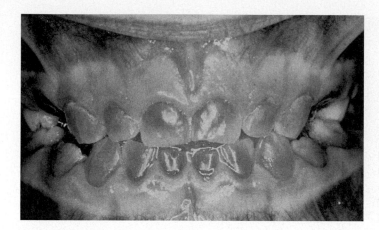

FIGURE 12-44. Dentinogenesis imperfecta (opalescent dentin), a hereditary disorder that affects the dentin and external appearance of all teeth. This condition occurs only once in 8000 people. (Courtesy of Professor Donald Bowers.)

possible to confirm this condition by noting the age when tetracycline was given and comparing this to the teeth that were calcifying at that age (see Table 10-1). Staining from **tetracycline** antibiotic therapy during tooth formation has often been erroneously blamed by some on community fluoridated drinking water, which is beneficial for both teeth and general health.

E. REACTIONS TO INJURY AFTER TOOTH ERUPTION

Reactions to injury are not really anomalies but are unique changes in tooth morphology associated with a specific cause. It is important to recognize these conditions so that their etiology (causes) can be identified and modified, when possible, to avoid the causative factor(s) that could worsen the condition.

1. ATTRITION

Attrition is the wearing away of enamel and dentin from the movement of mandibular teeth against maxillary teeth during normal function and is made worse by excessive grinding or gritting together of teeth known as **bruxism**. Two examples of severe attrition are shown in *Figure 12-46*. Stress greatly increases bruxism. This condition must be recognized and distinguished from other forms of tooth wear such as abrasion and erosion.

2. ABRASION

The wearing away of tooth structure by *mechanical* means is called **abrasion**. Abrasion from improper tooth brushing most often results in worn enamel on the facial surfaces of premolars and canines at the cementoenamel junction *(Fig. 12-47)*. It is caused by use of a hard toothbrush and/or a horizontal brushing stroke and/or a gritty dentifrice. Occlusal abrasion results from chewing or biting hard foods or objects, or from chewing tobacco, and results in flattened cusps on all posterior teeth and worn

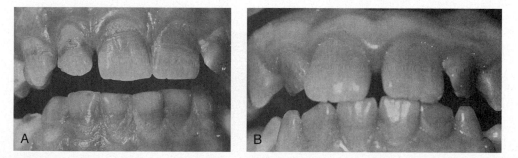

FIGURE 12-45. Tetracycline staining in permanent dentitions resulting from the administration of this antibiotic during the time that these crowns were forming. **A.** The horizontal bands in the enamel are a result of a high fever that required antibiotic therapy. **B.** The staining is again evidenced but the antibiotic controlled the fever sufficiently to prevent the deeply grooved bands seen in **A.** (Courtesy of Professor Donald Bowers.)

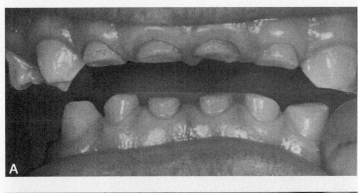

FIGURE 12-46. Attrition from prolonged bruxism or grinding of the teeth. **A.** The anterior teeth have been worn down almost to the gingival sulcus. **B.** The secondary mandibular incisors are worn down to a level where the pulp chamber had been at one time many years previously. (Note the darker circular and oval areas of exposed secondary or reparative dentin visible on the incisal ridges.)

incisal edges (appearing similar to attrition). An unusual type of abrasion, caused by the use for many years of a toothpick between the maxillary central incisors, has been reported by Melfi.[39] The same type of proximal abrasion has been reported from the use of a straight pin for the same purpose over many years. A similar-looking condition resulting from tooth bending (flexure) of the tooth caused by heavy occlusal forces is called **abfraction** [ab FRAC shun]. Although not yet supported by research, this condition is thought to result in loss of tooth structure due to separation of enamel rods near the cervical line.

3. EROSION

Erosion is the loss of tooth structure from *chemical* (nonmechanical) means and affects smooth and occlusal surfaces. Erosion can be the result of excessive intake or use of citric acid (lemons),

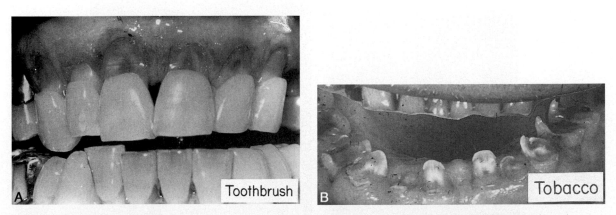

FIGURE 12-47. Abrasion. A. Abrasion (sometimes called toothbrush abrasion) due to incorrect horizontal tooth brushing over areas of cementum that are now exposed due to the recession of the gingiva. Flexing of the teeth during heavy occlusal forces and subsequent enamel loss (called **abfraction**) contributes to and appears similar to abrasion. **B.** Abrasion from chewing tobacco over a 30-year span. Notice that it is the patient history of chewing tobacco that confirms abrasion since the condition appears similar to attrition, which is caused by tooth-to-tooth contact. (Courtesy of Professor Rudy Melfi.)

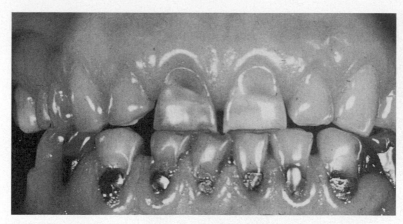

FIGURE 12-48. Erosion from an unknown cause (idiopathic). Restorations have been placed in the cervical regions of the mandibular teeth, but the erosion process continues beyond the amalgam margins and is most obvious in the cervical half of the maxillary central incisors. This *facial* erosion is similar to that caused by holding pieces of acidic fruit like lemons next to the teeth and sucking on them for an extended period of time, a habit practiced by some persons in southeast Asia. *Lingual* surface erosion is often associated with acid reflux or repeated regurgitation in bulimic persons.

A MOST UNUSUAL MANDIBULAR DENTITION

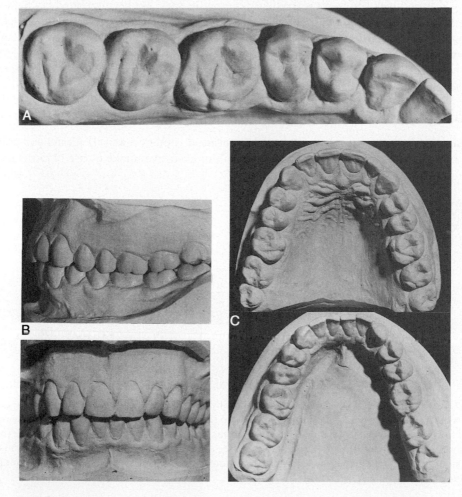

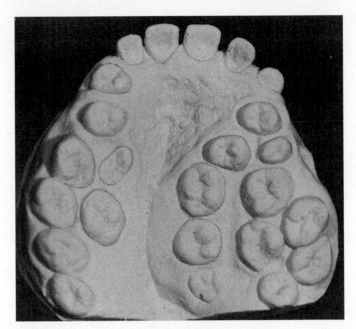

FIGURE 12-50. Very unusual permanent maxillary dentition with 24 teeth, including 13 molars. This cast was furnished courtesy of J. Andrew Stevenson (D.T.L.) and Dr. Robert Stevenson, Columbus, Ohio.

carbonated beverages, or industrial acids, or the result of regurgitated stomach acids (seen in bulimic individuals who habitually induce vomiting, as in the "binge and purge" syndrome).[2] Erosion can also occur from an unknown cause (idiopathic) *(Fig. 12-48)*. Severe erosion of the lingual enamel of all maxillary anterior teeth is evident in Color Plate 27. Careful inspection reveals that at least one pulp horn has been exposed on the maxillary left lateral incisor.

F. UNUSUAL DENTITIONS

During a routine check of a dental hygiene student's completed oral prophylaxis on a 23-year-old man, the instructor noticed what appeared to be an oblique ridge and cusp of Carabelli on the left mandibular first molar. Alginate impressions were made and casts poured *(Fig. 12-49)*. Careful examination of the casts by both the instructor and Dr. Woelfel revealed not only that the mandibular left first molar closely resembled a maxillary first molar, but also that first and second mandibular premolars and first, second, and third mandibular molars on both sides were remarkably similar morphologically to maxillary posterior teeth. The mandibular six anterior teeth unquestionably belonged to the mandibular dentition. The occlusion of the young man's teeth was remarkably good considering the fact that maxillary posterior teeth were occluding against practically identical maxillary teeth on both sides!

A most unusual maxillary dentition with a total of 24 erupted or partially erupted teeth is seen in *Figure 12-50*. This was the maxillary dentition of a foreign exchange student from Africa. There are 4 incisors, 1 canine, 6 premolars, and 13 molars (5 of which somewhat resemble mandibular molars).

FIGURE 12-49. A most unusual mandibular dentition. **A.** A close-up of the ***mandibular*** dentition of a 23-year-old man who has premolars and molars with crown morphology more similar to *maxillary* premolars and molars, particularly on the left side. **B.** The teeth as they fit together well into the maximum intercuspal position. **C.** Both dentitions are seen from the occlusal aspect, maxillary in the top photo and mandibular in the bottom photo. Lower premolar crowns do not resemble mandibular premolars in any fashion but are more similar to maxillary premolars. The six mandibular anterior teeth appear truly mandibular, however. The mandibular right first molar has three buccal cusps, but otherwise seems to be a mixture of both maxillary and mandibular first molars: oblong mesiodistally like a lower, but with a much larger mesiolingual cusp and a Carabelli-like cusp similar to upper first molars. The mandibular left three molars seem to have only morphologic characteristics of maxillary molars. This man's maxillary dentition seems entirely normal. It is most interesting to note that the lower left posterior teeth (particularly the premolars) have the morphology of maxillary right-side teeth. Likewise, the lower right teeth appear similar to those found in an upper left quadrant.

LEARNING QUESTIONS

Circle the correct answer(s).

1. What may result when a forming succedaneous tooth is located next to an abscess on an adjacent deciduous tooth?
   a. Turner's tooth
   b. fluorosis
   c. tetracycline staining
   d. dentinogenesis imperfecta
   e. amelogenesis imperfecta

2. When you observe that only three maxillary incisors but one crown is doubled in width and notched, what do you suspect?
   a. fusion
   b. twinning
   c. gemination
   d. concrescence
   e. cementosis

3. Which condition may be caused by habitually sucking on lemons (which are quite acidic)?
   a. attrition
   b. erosion
   c. abrasion
   d. amelogenesis imperfecta
   e. hypoplasia

4. Which *three* of the following locations are most likely to have supernumerary teeth form?
   a. mandibular premolar area
   b. maxillary premolar area
   c. maxillary incisor area
   d. mandibular incisor area
   e. third molar area

5. Which *one* of the following teeth that are normally single rooted are most likely to have a bifurcated root?
   a. maxillary central incisors
   b. maxillary lateral incisors
   c. mandibular canines
   d. mandibular first premolars
   e. mandibular second premolars

6. Which *two* of the following are most likely to exhibit unusually formed crown morphology?
   a. maxillary central incisors
   b. maxillary lateral incisors
   c. mandibular canines
   d. maxillary third molars
   e. maxillary first molars

ANSWERS: 1-a; 2-a; 3-b; 4-a, c, e; 5-c; 6-b, d.

REFERENCES

1. Dorland's pocket medical dictionary. Philadelphia: W.B. Saunders, 1965.
2. Smith RM, Turner JE, Robbins ML. Atlas of oral pathology. St. Louis: C.V. Mosby, 1981
3. Croll TP, Rains JR, Chen E. Fusion and gemination in one dental arch: report of case. ASDC J Dent Child 1981;48:297.
4. Rowe AHR, Johns RB, eds. A companion to dental studies: dental anatomy and embryology. Vol. 1, Book 2. Boston: Blackwell Scientific Publications, 1981.
5. McDonald TP. An American Board of Orthodontics case report. Am J Orthod 1981;80:437–442.
6. Fuller JL, Denehy GE. Concise dental anatomy and morphology. Chicago: Year Book Publishers, Inc, 1984: 264–265.
7. Jones AW. Supernumerary mandibular premolars. Report of a case in a patient of mongoloid origins. Br J Oral Surg 1981;19:305–306.
8. Robinson HB, Miller AS. Colby, Kerr and Robinson's color atlas of oral pathology. Philadelphia: J.B. Lippincott, 1983:38.
9. Primosch RE. Anterior supernumerary teeth—assessment and surgical intervention in children. Pediatr Dentistry 1981;3:204–215.
10. Ranta R, Ylipaavalniemi P. Developmental course of supernumerary premolars in childhood: report of two cases. ASDC J Dent Child 1981;48:385–388.
11. Rubin MM, Nevins A, Berg M, et al. A comparison of identical twins in relation to three dental anomalies. Multiple supernumerary teeth, juvenile periodontosis, and zero caries incidence. Oral Surg 1981;52:391–394.
12. Zvolanek JW. Maxillary lateral incisor anomalies in identical twins. Dent Radiogr Photog 1981;54:17–18.
13. Hemmig SB. Third and fourth molar fusion. Oral Surg 1979;48:572.
14. Good DL, Berson RB. A supernumerary tooth fused to a maxillary permanent central incisor. Pediatr Dentistry 1980;2:294–296.
15. Powell RE. Fusion of maxillary lateral incisor and supernumerary tooth. Oral Surg 1981;51(3):331.
16. Speiser AM, Bikofsky VM. Premolars with double occlusal surfaces. JADA 1981;103:600–601.
17. Melfi RC, Alley KE. Permar's oral embryology and microscopic anatomy: a textbook for students in dental hygiene. Philadelphia; Lippincott Williams and Wilkins, 2000.
18. Myers CL. Treatment of a talon-cusp incisor: report of case. ASDC J Dent Child 1980;47:119–121.
19. Hayward JR. Cuspid gigantism. Oral Surg 1980;49:500–501.
20. Ruprecht A, Singer DL. Macrodontia of the mandibular left first premolar. Oral Surg 1979;48:573.
21. Becker A, Smith P, Behar, R. The incidence of anomalous maxillary lateral incisors in relation to palatally-displaced cuspids. Angle Orthod 1981;51:24–29.
22. McKibben DR, Brearley LJ. Radiographic determination of the prevalence of selected dental anomalies in children. J Dent Child 1971;28:390–398.
23. Nazif MM, Ruffalo RC, Zullo T. Impacted supernumerary teeth: a survey of fifty cases. JADA 1983;106:201–204.
24. Hamner JE, Witkop CJ, Metro PS. Taurodontism. Oral Surg 1964;18:409–418.
25. Pindborg JJ. Pathology of the dental hard tissues. Philadelphia: W.B. Saunders, 1970:15–73.
26. Schachter H. A treated case of transposed upper canine. Dent Rec 1951;71:105–108.
27. DeJong TE. Rotatio dentis. Gegenbaurs Morphologisches Jahrbuch 1965;108:67–70.
28. Schulze C. Developmental abnormalities of the teeth and jaws. In: Gorlin RJ, Goldman HM, eds. Thoma's oral pathology. 6th ed. St. Louis: C.V. Mosby, 1970:138–40.
29. Rothberg J, Kopel M. Early versus late removal of mesiodens: a clinical study of 375 children. Comp Cont Educ Pract 1984;5:115–120.
30. Paulson RB, Gottlieb LJ, Sciulli PW, et al. Double-rooted maxillary primary canines. ASDC J Dent Child 1985;52: 195–198.
31. Bimstein E, Bystrom E. Birooted bilateral maxillary primary canines. ASDC J Dent Child 1982;49:217–28.
32. Kelly JR. Birooted primary canines. Oral Surg 1978;46:872.
33. Brown CK. Bilateral bifurcation of the maxillary deciduous cuspids. Oral Surg 1975;40:817.
34. Kroll SO. Double rooted maxillary primary canines. Oral Surg 1980;49:379.
35. Bryant RH Jr, Bowers DF. Four birooted primary canines: report of a case. ASDC J Dent Child 1982;49:441–442.
36. Goldman HM. Anomalies of teeth (part 1). Comp Cont Educ Pract 1981;2:358–367.
37. Jackson M, Leeds, LD. Upper canine in position of upper central. Br Dent J 1951;90:243.
38. Curran JD, Baker CG. Roentgeno-oddities. Oral Surg 1973;41:906–907.
39. Dr. Rudy Melfi, Columbus, Ohio, personal communication.
40. Takeda Y. A rare occurrence of a three-rooted mandibular premolar. Ann Dent 1988;44:43–44.
41. Paulson RB, Gottlieb LJ, Sciulli PW, et al. Double rooted maxillary primary canines. ASDC J Dent Child 1985; 52:195–198.

13 Operative Dentistry

CONTRIBUTED BY ROBERT G. RASHID, DDS, M.A.S. PROFESSOR, THE OHIO STATE UNIVERSITY

OBJECTIVES

After studying this chapter, readers should be able to:

- Define operative dentistry, dental caries, dental plaque, intra- and extracoronal restorations, and restorative dentistry.
- Classify dental caries according to pit and fissure versus smooth surface and describe the pattern of spread of each within enamel and dentin.
- Define and identify root caries.
- Describe and identify each G.V. Black class of dental caries clinically and radiographically.
- List and describe the principles of cavity preparation.
- Describe the indications for restoring a tooth for each class of caries.
- List and describe characteristics of commonly used restorative materials.
- For each class of caries, describe the unique application of the principles of cavity preparation dependent upon the material used.
- For each class of caries, define terms used to describe cavity walls, cavosurfaces, line angles, and point angles.
- Define and identify the types of restorations used to restore large tooth defects.
- Define and identify the restorations used to replace lost teeth.

SECTION I

OPERATIVE AND RESTORATIVE DENTISTRY: DEFINITIONS

Tooth destruction can occur from dental caries (decay), attrition or abrasion, erosion, fracture, and the breakdown of old restorations. **Dental caries** [CARE eez] (always plural, never a carie), known more commonly as tooth decay, is the most common cause of tooth destruction. Caries (which literally means "rotten") results from the **demineralization** of mineralized tooth structures (that is, the loss of minerals or inorganic content from enamel, dentin, and cementum). This demineralization process occurs when specific bacteria firmly adhere to teeth (in a layer called **dental plaque** or biofilm) *and* are exposed to certain carbohydrates over extended periods of *time* to form acids (such as lactic acid), which react with the hard tooth structure, causing mineral loss. *Streptococcus mutans* and lactobacilli are bacteria known to contribute to the caries process. Sugar-containing food items, such as candy, honey, pastries, and especially non-diet soft drinks, contribute to acid formation that can destroy mineralized tooth structure.[1]

Demineralization can be reversed if plaque is removed frequently enough through good oral hygiene measures, if sweets in the diet are limited, and if minerals (especially calcium in healthy saliva and fluoride) are available for uptake (remineralization) into the porous demineralized tooth. This tug-of-war between demineralization and remineralization is constant and is the basis for prevention methods that are applied and taught by dental professionals.

Patient education and **preventive treatment** are important aspects of dental patient care. Prevention and treatment should be based on personalized risk-based assessment of each patient's caries history, which includes their history of fluoride use, their salivary flow rate, and the frequency of sugar uptake (especially snacks).[2,3] **Fluoride** applied to teeth in appropriate concentrations has been shown to reduce dental caries incidence because it increases the tooth's resistance to breakdown by caries-forming acids. Therefore, caries prevention includes daily use of fluoride-containing paste and fluoride-containing mouthwashes (either prescription or over the counter), as well as office-applied fluorides that contain higher concentrations. Further, when saliva flow is reduced (from damage to the salivary glands due to radiation therapy or as a side effect to many medications), the teeth are more susceptible to tooth decay. Artificial saliva or sugarless chewing gum (which stimulates saliva flow) could be used to alleviate this problem. Finally, snacks provide the ingredients that, with certain bacteria found in dental plaque, form acids that contribute to demineralization. (Most soft drinks are quite acidic themselves, as well as containing sugars that can produce even more acid during the caries-forming process.) Therefore, frequent snacking must be curtailed.

In a 1979–1980 survey representing 45.3 million U.S. school children between the ages of 5 and 17 years, the estimated prevalence of breakdown in permanent dentition was 4.77 decayed, missing, or filled surfaces per child.[4] Comparing data from two studies conducted for the Centers for Disease Control and Prevention, the number of carious permanent teeth (both treated and untreated) in children from 6 to 18 years old decreased by 57% from 1971–1974 through 1988–1994 [decreasing from 4.44 to 1.9 carious teeth].[5] These studies also showed a 40% decline in the number of carious primary teeth in 2- to 10 year olds [from 2.29 to 1.38].

These and other reports have shown a worldwide decrease in the incidence of coronal caries, especially in children and adolescents, ranging from 10 to 60% depending on the article cited. However, the number of adults older than 65 is expected to double by 2025, and people are keeping their teeth longer (53% of persons older than 65 still have at least 20 natural teeth).[6] Further, the prevalence of root caries in the elderly is increasing,[7] with one study reporting 75% of elderly women with clinically detectable root caries.[8] Therefore, the restoration of damaged teeth (from caries and other reasons) will continue to be a part of the practice of general dentistry for some time to come. Additionally, with improvements in the properties of contemporary esthetic restorative materials, the decline in caries rate is being offset by the increased number of patients who ask for dental procedures that improve esthetics.

Operative dentistry is the phase of dentistry involving the art and science of the diagnosis, treatment, and prognosis of defects in teeth that do *not* require restorations that cover the entire tooth (full coverage). Restoring *conservative* tooth defects, such as those resulting from small carious lesions that are confined to enamel or have progressed just beyond the dentinoenamel junction (DEJ), usually requires placement of **intracoronal** restorations whose preparations are cut *within* the tooth and, if located occlusally, are small (narrower buccolingually than the distance between the cusps).

As tooth destruction increases in size, **extracoronal** restorations may be a more appropriate restoration of choice. These larger extracoronal restorations surround and cover all or part of the exposed tooth, and include crowns (also known by many as "caps") or onlays (which have an intracoronal component but also include coverage of cusp tips). Treatment with extracoronal and intracoronal restorations should result in the restoration of proper tooth form, function, and esthetics while maintaining the physiologic integrity of the teeth in harmonious relationship with the adjacent hard and soft tissues, all of which enhances the general health and welfare of the patient.[9] **Restorative dentistry** is the phase of clinical dentistry that includes not only the prevention and treatment of defects of individual teeth, but also the replacement of teeth that were lost or never formed. Lost teeth can be replaced using a fixed partial denture (also known as a bridge or **fixed dental prosthesis**), a removable partial denture (**removable dental prosthesis**), an **implant** (surgical insertion or placement of an artificial root over which a crown may be constructed), or complete dentures (also known as false teeth or a **complete removable dental prosthesis**). Thus, restorative dentistry involves the restoration of lost tooth structure *and/or lost teeth* with the ultimate goal of reestablishing a healthy, functioning, and comfortable dentition.

SECTION II CLASSIFICATION OF CARIOUS LESIONS

There are two *broad* classifications of tooth decay based on the anatomy of the tooth surface involved: *pit and fissure*, and *smooth surface*. The pattern by which the spread of dental caries occurs as it enlarges and deepens differs in these two types.

Pit and fissure carious lesions begin in the depth of pits and fissures, which form from incomplete fusion of enamel lobes during tooth development and are nearly impossible to keep clean. Note the deep occlusal fissure in cross section of a tooth in Figure 13-1B. Fissures and pits are most often located on the occlusal surfaces of posterior teeth (molars and premolars), as well as on the lingual surface of maxillary molars, on the buccal surface of mandibular molars, and in the lingual fossae of maxillary incisors, especially lateral incisors.

A small pit and fissure lesion can be almost undetectable externally (Color Plate 28), but as it progresses deeper, the caries widens within the fissure as it approaches the DEJ, and then, once within dentin, spreads out at the DEJ (occlusal surface in *Fig. 13-1A and B*). This widening in dentin occurs because decay can spread more quickly in dentin that is less mineralized than enamel, especially at the DEJ.

In contrast to pit and fissure caries, **smooth surface** carious lesions occur on the smooth surfaces of the anatomic crown of a tooth in the areas that are least accessible to the natural cleansing action of the lips, cheeks, and tongue. These areas include the proximal surfaces of teeth just *cervical* to the proximal contact (Color Plate 29) and the facial and lingual surfaces just *cervical* to the crest of curvature of the crown (in the gingival one-third of the crown) as seen in Color Plate 30. The pattern of spread within enamel for smooth surface caries is different than for pit and fissure caries since it begins as a relatively broad area of destruction just beneath the outer layer of enamel, but it *narrows* as it progresses more deeply toward the dentinoenamel junction. Once it reaches dentin, however, it spreads out wider at the dentinoenamel junction, just like pit and fissure caries. (The sectioned tooth in Color Plate 31 shows the spread of decay through enamel and into dentin through a pit occlusally, and on a smooth surface mesially.)

Root surface caries is another type of smooth surface caries that occurs on cementum, most frequently in patients with disease of the periodontium, in patients with decreased saliva flow, or in older patients who have had gingival recession, which increases the potential for accumulation of caries-forming plaque on the cementum of root surfaces. This type of caries is a softening, destructive process that may not require a restoration if there is only minimal involvement.[10] Treatment in these cases can include polishing the root, applying fluoride (topical or fluoride-containing varnishes), and keeping the roots clean through good oral hygiene.

In 1908, Dr. G.V. Black developed a comprehensive method of classifying carious lesions that has been useful when describing specific principles of cavity preparation.[11] The original classifications were G.V. Black classes I, II, III, IV, and V. All pit and fissure type lesions are class I, whereas class II, III, IV, and V caries are all smooth surface–type lesions.

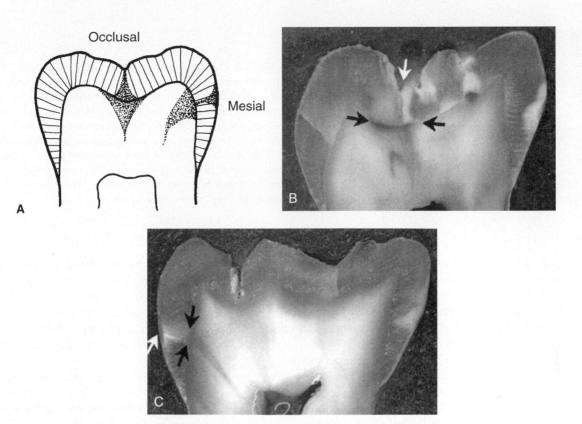

FIGURE 13-1. Pattern and location of pit and fissure and smooth surface caries. A. Drawing of a cross section of a mandibular molar showing the usual pattern of spreading decay. The occlusal lesion (class I, pit and fissure) is small externally, widening toward the depth of the fissure as it approaches the dentinoenamel junction. Once within dentin, the caries spreads out laterally, as well as progressing toward the pulp. The mesial lesion (class II, smooth surface) is broad externally, narrowing toward the dentinoenamel junction (DEJ). Once within dentin, this lesion spreads out laterally (like the class I) as well as progressing toward the pulp. **B.** Cut section of a mandibular molar. Notice the very deep fissure beneath the central groove (*top arrow*) and the lateral spread of decay at the dentinoenamel junction (*arrows*). **C.** Cut section of a smooth surface class II lesion. Note the width of the lesion near the surface of enamel, the narrowing as it progresses toward the DEJ, and then the spread of the decay once it reaches dentin.

A. IDENTIFICATION OF CLASS I CARIES

Class I lesions *(Fig. 13-2)* form in enamel pits and fissures, and may form wherever deep inaccessible pits and fissures occur. In a 1979–1980 survey of U.S. schoolchildren aged 5–17 years, 54% of all carious lesions were found on the occlusal surfaces,[4] which constitute one-fifth of the surfaces of any premolar or molar. More recently, studies of teeth at risk show that the occlusal surfaces of the first molars are at greatest risk for *initial* caries, followed by the occlusal surfaces of lower, then upper second molars.[12]

Detecting class I lesions clinically requires visual inspection and tactile evaluation. Careful visual analysis of a clean, dry, well-lighted occlusal surface will reveal this type of caries as a fissure or pit surrounded by enamel that is chalky or more opaque (less translucent) than the adjacent enamel (Color Plate 28). Some dentists prefer to confirm caries within these suspicious defects by probing with a very sharp explorer. After pressing the explorer into the defect with moderate to firm pressure, sensing a resistance to removing the explorer (known as **tugback**) helps to confirm the presence of softness and therefore caries within the defect or fissure wall. However, the firm use of the explorer for the detection of occlusal caries should be used with caution. One study suggests that the sensitivity and specificity of this technique is poor, and excessive force could actually damage fragile enamel rods on the tooth.[13] Even in the absence of obvious tugback, loss of translucency of enamel around a pit or fissure may be considered to be reliable evidence of attack. It is especially important to avoid undue pressure with the explorer point in larger, frank lesions (as seen in Fig. 13-2, right tooth) because injudicious probing may cause pain or additional enamel rod destruction.

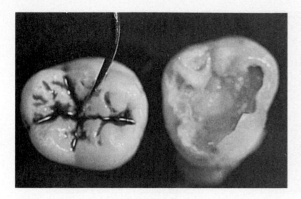

FIGURE 13-2. Class I carious lesions. On the left is a small lesion in the central pit on tooth #18 at the depth of stained grooves, which must be evaluated for color changes that indicate demineralization or be detected with a sharp explorer by feeling for tugback. On the right is an enormous, clinically obvious lesion on tooth #2 that has resulted in the collapse of most of the occlusal enamel by the undermining spread of the decay in dentin. Both teeth appear to be restorable, but the one with extensive decay would probably require endodontic therapy (root canal) and an inlay-onlay or crown.

A class I lesion is usually not detectable on a radiograph until it is quite deep into dentin because the lesion is superimposed between the thick buccal and lingual surfaces of enamel, which show up whiter (radiopaque), thereby masking the darker caries. By the time the cavity is visible on the radiograph (*Fig. 13-3*), the size of the preparation required to remove all of the decay would be considerably deeper (toward the pulp) than if the decay had been detected during a good clinical examination when the lesion was smaller. Thus, early class I decay can be best diagnosed during a thorough, systematic *clinical* examination of clean, dry teeth using good lighting and a sharp exploring point.

A class I lesion in cross section in *enamel* is somewhat triangular in shape with the point of the triangle barely visible on the enamel surface and its wide base located along the DEJ. Once into *dentin*, the spread at the DEJ is like a second triangle with its base along the DEJ and its point following the dentinal tubules toward the pulp (as seen in Fig. 13-1A). That is, the shape of the spread of class I caries through enamel and into dentin is like two triangles with their bases touching at the DEJ.

B. IDENTIFICATION OF CLASS II CARIES

A **class II** lesion is one that forms on the smooth proximal surface of *posterior teeth* just cervical to proximal contact (*Fig. 13-4A* and Color Plate 29). It results from inadequate plaque removal in these hard to reach interproximal surfaces. Judicious use of dental floss is one method for preventing (or reversing) class II (and class III) caries.

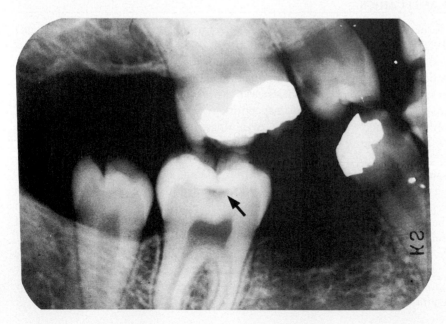

FIGURE 13-3. Radiograph of a class I lesion on tooth #31. By the time the lesion appears this deep on the radiograph, the caries has destroyed dentin to such a depth that a thermal-insulating base of some type of dental cement will possibly be needed to protect the pulp from thermal conductivity through the metal filling. This pit and fissure caries should have been detected earlier with a good clinical examination. [There is also a large distal class II lesion on tooth #4, which appears to be rotated (top right)].

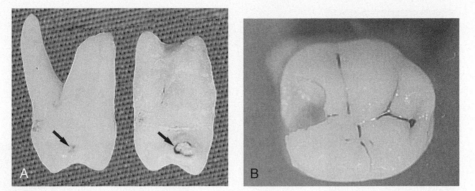

FIGURE 13-4. Class II lesions. A. Left: An incipient (beginning) lesion without cavitation on the mesial surface of tooth #14, probably visible only on a radiograph if an adjacent tooth were present. **Right:** A larger class II lesion with cavitation on the mesial surface of tooth # 15, with color changes to the enamel that would be evident beyond the proximal contact area in the mouth. **B.** A class II lesion on the mesial surface of tooth #30, which resulted in the collapse of the entire mesial marginal ridge of enamel.

Clinical detection of small class II lesions in the mouth without the aid of radiographs is often difficult due to the inability to visualize or probe the areas where they form. A loss of translucency of the enamel seen when examining the overlying marginal ridge may be the first clinical evidence of class II caries (Color Plate 32). As the carious lesion increases in size, it may appear as a dark, cavitated area (hole) that can be detected by a thin probe (explorer) in the buccal or lingual embrasure. A very large class II lesion may actually undermine the entire marginal ridge, permitting the entire ridge of enamel to break off during mastication *(Fig. 13-4B)*.

Radiographic detection of an incipient (beginning, small) class II lesion is most predictably accomplished using bitewing radiographs because the class II lesion is normally visible on the radiograph before it can be detected clinically *(Fig. 13-5)*. A class II lesion is seen as a narrow triangular shadow within the enamel *just cervical to the proximal contact* (Fig. 13-5A, arrow). Unlike the spread pattern of class I caries, the wide base of the triangle is located at the enamel surface, and it tapers to a point toward the DEJ. When the lesion gets large enough to reach dentin, the spread pattern is the same as for class I caries: It is like a triangle with its base spread out along the DEJ, and its point follows the dentinal tubules toward the pulp (seen in two large lesions in Fig. 13-5B and in the diagram and crown cross section in Fig. 13-1A and C).

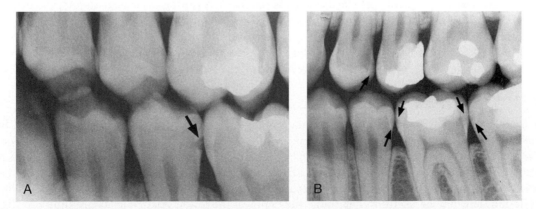

FIGURE 13-5. Radiographs of class II lesions. A. Radiographic evidence of a class II lesion that has barely spread into dentin on the distal surface of tooth #20 *(arrow)*. Note the location of the lesion just cervical to the proximal contacts, and that the lesion is wider at the surface of enamel than at the dentinoenamel junction. **B.** Several class II lesions *(arrows)*, some of which are confined to enamel and two (# 12 and # 13, distal) that have spread out in dentin. [Note the existing class II amalgam on tooth #13 with a deep base and large undesirable overhang (that is, excess bulk of amalgam beyond the gingival cavosurface margin).]

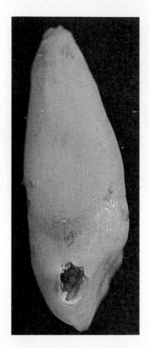

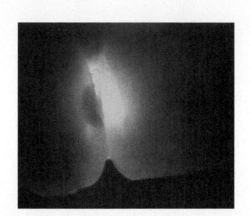

FIGURE 13-6. Class III lesion on the mesial of tooth #6 with an area of obvious cavitation or hole in the enamel surface. If this lesion involved any more of the mesial incisal angle, it would become a class IV, rather than a class III, lesion.

FIGURE 13-7. Transillumination. A light source is directed through the proximal surfaces of these anterior teeth to reveal a change in translucency just cervical to the proximal contact area, indicating the presence of class III caries.

C. IDENTIFICATION OF CLASS III CARIES

Class III lesions are smooth surface lesions located on the proximal surfaces of *anterior teeth*, just cervical to the proximal contact, but *not* involving the incisal angle (or corner) of the tooth (*Fig. 13-6*).

An incipient (small or beginning) class III lesion can usually be detected clinically by carefully examining the enamel facially or lingually for changes in translucency *just cervical to the proximal contact* (Color Plate 33). The underlying lesion causes overlying enamel to appear slightly darker or more opaque than surrounding, sound enamel. These changes are most evident when a source of light (such as fiber optics) is placed lingually against the proximal enamel of the tooth, revealing the change in translucency facially (*Fig. 13-7*). This method of clinical detection is called **transillumination**.

Periapical radiographs of the anterior teeth (and the bitewing radiographs for the distal of canines) may also be used to confirm a class III lesion (*Fig. 13-8*, arrow). The location (just cervical to the proximal contact) and pattern of spread is typical of smooth surface lesions as described earlier for a class II lesion.

D. IDENTIFICATION OF CLASS IV CARIES

A **class IV** lesion involves the proximal surface of an anterior tooth (as does a class III lesion), but, *in addition*, it involves the incisal angle (or corner) of the tooth (*Fig. 13-9*). The class IV lesion is frequently the result of a class III lesion that became so large that the undermined tooth angle broke off. A similar-shaped defect occurs when the tooth corner fractures off due to a blow to the mouth. The loss of an incisal angle is plainly visible upon clinical examination. Radiographs are not needed to detect the class IV lesion, but may be useful to determine the depth of the lesion relative to its proximity to the pulp chamber (*Fig. 13-10*).

E. IDENTIFICATION OF CLASS V CARIES

The **class V** lesion is located in the cervical one-third of the facial or lingual surface of any (anterior or posterior) tooth crown (*Fig. 13-11* and Color Plate 30). It is a smooth surface lesion that results from

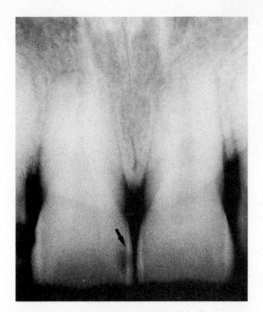

FIGURE 13-8. Radiograph of a class III lesion on the mesial of tooth #8. Note the location of this decay just cervical to the proximal contact and the characteristic spread or widening of the decay at the dentinoenamel junction.

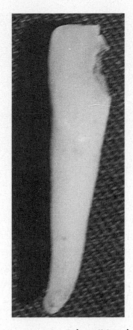

FIGURE 13-9. An enormous **class IV carious lesion** involving the mesioincisal angle of tooth #26.

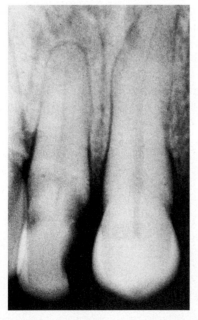

FIGURE 13-10. Radiograph of a class IV lesion involving the distoincisal angle of tooth #10.

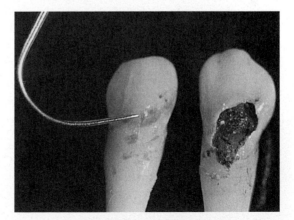

FIGURE 13-11. Class V lesions. Left: Incipient (beginning) facial lesion that is seen as chalky and discolored and is flaking away. **Right:** An obvious cavitated class V facial lesion that has destroyed much of the enamel on the buccal surface of the crown and adjacent cementum and dentin of the root.

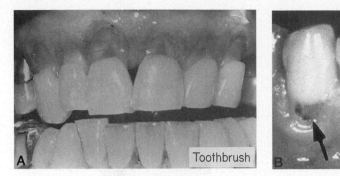

FIGURE 13-12. Types of root cavitation.
A. Maxillary anterior teeth showing cervical **abrasion**, possibly due to poor tooth brushing technique and abrasive pastes. These areaa are prone to caries and often become sensitive. Each tooth should be evaluated carefully to determine if application of a desensitizing solution or a restoration is indicated. **B. Root caries** on an area of exposed cementum after gingival recession.

poor hygiene in the area of the tooth just cervical to the buccal or lingual crest of curvature, adjacent to the gingiva, where the natural cleansing action of the lips, tongue, and cheeks is ineffective. This area of the tooth is susceptible to plaque accumulation and resultant caries. Over the lifetime of a tooth, the gingiva and supporting bone may recede apically, exposing greater amounts of the root surface. With decreased salivary flow and/or poor oral hygiene, the incidence and severity of caries increases in this area (Fig. 13-11, right tooth).

The **class V** lesion is best detected by careful visual examination of the smooth gingival portion of the tooth crown with good lighting to determine a chalky white or stained appearance, often with a break (**cavitation** or hole) in the enamel surface (Color Plate 30). *Care should be taken with the explorer* not *to break through an area of beginning demineralization that has not yet cavitated*, since excellent oral hygiene and fluoride has been shown to reverse the caries process. These lesions may extend slightly apical to the level of inflamed gingiva, so that the use of the tactile sense obtained through the explorer is critical for detection of cavitation,[10] and to distinguish these lesions (which are cavitated) from a calcified buildup of calculus (which is felt as a bump attached to the surface of the tooth).

Other areas of cavitation (or depressions) located in the cervical of the crown and the adjacent root surface include defects formed from erosion by acids, or from **abrasion** (most commonly caused by abrasive toothpastes and improper tooth brushing), and a process known as **abfraction** (the loss of hard tooth structure, which appears similar to abrasion but is caused by flexure or bending of the tooth caused by heavy occlusal forces). Caries may develop at the depth of these defects. Also, as the root becomes exposed to the oral environment due to gingival recession, the cementum, which is much less mineralized than enamel, is more susceptible to caries compared to enamel. The result is **root caries**, a condition that is occurring more frequently in our aging population (*Fig. 13-12*).

As with a radiograph of a class I lesion, the class V lesion is superimposed over buccal or lingual surfaces of enamel that show up whiter (radiopaque), thereby masking the darker (radiolucent) caries (*Fig. 13-13*). By the time a class V lesion is evident on radiographs, it has progressed far beyond the incipient

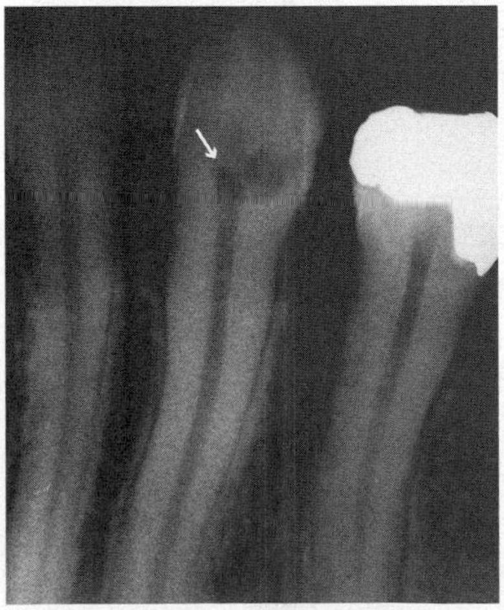

FIGURE 13-13. Radiograph of a class V lesion on tooth #22. It is impossible to tell from the radiograph whether it is on the buccal or lingual surface or whether it is decay or a radiolucent (dark looking on the radiograph) composite restoration.

stage, and will require a much larger restoration than would have been required if it were *clinically* diagnosed at its earliest stages. Therefore, the examiner should not depend on radiographs for detection of these lesions. However, when discovering a cervically located radiolucency on a radiograph, the dentist should carefully evaluate the tooth to clinically prove or disprove the presence of class V caries. Darker (radiolucent) areas of cervical abrasion, as well as older types of radiolucent restorative materials, can appear like class V or root surface caries on radiographs.

F. CLASS VI TYPE OF DENTAL CARIES

A **class VI** type of dental caries or restoration is not one of Black's original classifications. In Baum's text, it is defined as the cavity or defect found on the tips of cusps or along the biting edges of incisors.[10] In Sturdevant's text, class VI caries includes lesions on the cusp tips of posterior teeth.[9]

SECTION III | INDICATIONS FOR RESTORING A TOOTH

A. CLASS I CARIES: WHEN TO RESTORE

Some class I lesions are difficult to differentiate from noncarious deep enamel defects. If tugback occurs with a sharp explorer in a deep pit or fissure and the surrounding enamel is chalky or less translucent, a restoration is indicated (recall Fig. 13-2). Certainly, by the time caries is obvious on the radiograph, it would be evident clinically and should be restored. However, if tugback is minimal and without the accompanying evidence, the dentist might consider periodically reevaluating the area during recall appointments, especially if the patient is older and has a low caries rate. Beware, however, that tugback can occur when probing in deep fissures even if caries is not present. Generally, multiple signs should be present to make a clinical diagnosis of caries, and then consider the need for a restoration. Finally, it is important to know that pit and fissure decay on adult teeth can be prevented or delayed by applying **sealants** shortly after tooth eruption. For permanent first molars, this would be age 6, and for second molars, age 12.

B. CLASS II CARIES: WHEN TO RESTORE

Clinically obvious class II lesions, when cavitated (with a break or hole in the surface), should be restored (Fig. 13-14A, tooth on the right). The radiographic indication for restoring a small lesion is when the lesion has penetrated to the DEJ and begins to spread out into dentin (recall Fig. 13-5B). If the lesion is small enough to be confined to enamel on the radiograph, the dentist must consider the patient's previous history of carious activity, oral hygiene, and age in order to decide whether to restore now or to reevaluate at subsequent recall intervals. The use of fluoride and fluoride varnishes has improved the potential to arrest early lesions. However, a young patient with a small carious lesion only two-thirds of the way through

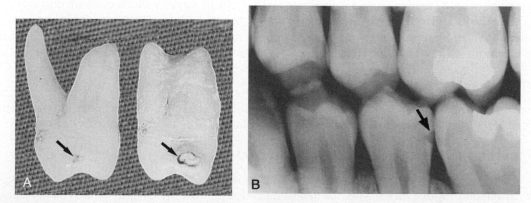

FIGURE 13-14. A. Class II lesions. B. Radiographs of class II lesions.

enamel, but with many deeper lesions and poor oral hygiene that is not improving, should probably have the tooth restored, especially since a *lesion extends deeper in the tooth than it appears on the radiograph.*[10]

C. CLASS III CARIES: WHEN TO RESTORE

The indications for restoring a class III lesion are the same as for a class II lesion: That is, if the surface is cavitated or decay has reached the dentin as seen on the radiograph or through transillumination, a restoration is indicated (recall Figs. 13-6 and 13-8).

D. CLASS IV CARIES: WHEN TO RESTORE

The class IV restoration is indicated when active caries is detected (recall Fig. 13-9). Many class IV restorations are indicated, however, not because of caries but because the corner of the tooth has fractured off in an accident. In these instances, the extent of the fracture, the proximity of the exposed tooth structure to the pulp chamber, hypersensitivity to temperature changes, and, most often, the patient's concern for esthetics are important in determining when to restore the tooth. If the fracture is not into the dentin and the patient is not concerned about the appearance of the tooth, smoothing the rough edges of the tooth may suffice. If, however, dentin is involved or if there is evidence of decay, a restoration is indicated to prevent discomfort from the exposed dentin and to stop the spread of decay.

E. CLASS V CARIES: WHEN TO RESTORE

Not all areas at the cervical of the tooth that are cavitated and white or darkly stained require a class V restoration (as in Color Plate 30), since these areas of beginning (incipient) decay could respond to fluoride and improved oral hygiene, and actually remineralize so no restoration is required. Also, these defects could be areas of arrested (old, inactive) decay, or noncarious cavitated defects due to abrasion, erosion, or abfraction. Class V lesions require restorations when tooth structure is *soft* or cavitated (recall Fig. 13-11). Restorations should also be considered for noncarious defects (like abrasion defects) that occur in this part of the tooth if the tooth is sensitive and does not respond to desensitizing agents, if the lesion is very deep and cannot be kept clean, or if it appears that it will continue to get worse due to poor oral hygiene or parafunctional habits.

There are times when caries extends beyond the previously defined classification categories. For instance, a class V lesion may initially start at the gingival third of the facial surface of a tooth and progress around the proximal line angle into the interproximal area, possibly connecting with a class II lesion. Restoring this tooth may require two separate preparations that abut one another (one to remove the class II caries and one to remove the class V caries).

SECTION IV   PRINCIPLES OF CAVITY PREPARATION

Basic principles of cavity preparation were developed by Dr. Black in the early 1900s and were uniquely applied to each class of caries and type of restorative material. Today, the application of his principles has been modified due to the introduction of new dental restorative materials that were not available in his day. Each principle that the dentist must consider when preparing a tooth for a restoration is described here.

A. ESTABLISH AN OUTLINE FORM

The outline form of a preparation is the external shape of the preparation on the tooth. It is developed by *removing the least amount of tooth structure* possible, yet adhering to the following principles:

1. EXTEND THE PREPARATION TO SOUND ENAMEL

The dentist enlarges the preparation outline, so it extends to solid enamel that has no signs of cavitation or active caries. Also, the dentist must determine if the integrity of the enamel margins is adequate to support function. In many cases, this involves extending the preparation to enamel that is supported by, or resting on, sound dentin (that is, enamel that is not undermined by the spread of caries within the dentin). Since enamel is brittle, if it is not sufficiently supported by sound dentin and/or bonding techniques, the unsupported enamel rods will fracture off, leaving a gap between the tooth and restorative material.

2. EXTEND THE PREPARATION FOR PREVENTION

The dentist evaluates the need to enlarge the preparation within enamel beyond the specific area of decay in order to include adjacent tooth structure felt to be prone to the development of future decay. This may involve enlarging a preparation for a pit and fissure lesion to include adjacent deep pits and fissures thought to be caries prone, even though they have not yet become carious. Similarly, when developing the cavity preparation for smooth surface carious lesions, the outline of the preparation may be extended to include adjacent smooth surface areas likely to become carious. For example, if one small area of tooth next to the gingiva has decay, the preparation might be enlarged to include more of the tooth adjacent to that caries-prone area (particularly if the adjacent area shows signs of early decay such as white decalcified areas).

Over the past 30 years, there has been a tremendous increase in the use of fluoride (in community water, toothpaste, rinses, and topical applications applied periodically by the dentist), as well as improved efforts by dental professionals to educate the population in prevention techniques. Therefore, the need for preventive extension on smooth surface lesions must be weighed against the possibility that excellent hygiene and fluoride could stop or even reverse the decay process, especially if it has not progressed too far. The degree of extension should be based on such factors as the age of the patient (younger enamel is more susceptible to caries than mature enamel), his or her rate of caries activity, personal oral hygiene, and dietary habits. For example, extension for prevention for a tooth preparation on a younger patient with multiple areas of active decay, poor oral hygiene, and frequent intake of high-sugar snacks and sugar-containing carbonated beverages who is unwilling to change is more appropriate than it would be on an older patient with a lower caries rate, better eating habits, and good or improving oral hygiene.

3. PROVIDE ADEQUATE ACCESS

A restoration outline must be large enough for the dentist to ensure that all carious tooth structure has been removed, and that instruments required to place the filling material will fit. A small, narrow initial cut through the enamel might not permit the dentist to confirm the removal of all caries that may have spread laterally at the dentinoenamel junction. Further, even when the removal of all caries can be verified visually or by probing, a very small initial preparation might be too small for the instruments required to place the restorative material to be placed into the preparation without voids.

4. PROVIDE RESISTANCE FORM

The dentist must design a preparation to ensure room for an adequate thickness of restorative material for strength, and sufficient remaining solid tooth structure to withstand occlusal forces. If preparation depth is inadequate for the material of choice to withstand occlusal forces, the restoration could break. If the remaining tooth is too thin or undermined, it could fracture. One solution to protect thin remaining tooth structure is to cover it with cast metal onlays or crowns, as discussed in Section VI of this chapter. Another solution is to bond on a layer of composite material to increase the strength of the thin remaining enamel.

B. PROVIDE RETENTION FORM

Retention form is the design of a preparation (traditionally provided by internal retentive grooves or pits) that will prevent the restoration from falling out or becoming dislodged. The methods for providing retention differ depending on the restorative material and on the location of the carious lesion. The appropriate methods for establishing retention form with different restorative materials are described later in Section V of this chapter.

C. REMOVE CARIES AND TREAT THE PULP

All principles of the cavity preparation described up to this point assume that caries has spread minimally into dentin, not more than 0.5 mm deeper than the dentinoenamel junction. The dentist usually prepares the outline form and retention for cavity preparations with a high-speed dental handpiece using carbide or diamond burs that cut quickly, minimizing the potentially damaging heat by use of an effective water coolant spray. When removing carious lesions that have progressed deeper than 0.5 mm into dentin, the dentist selects slowly rotating round burs (in slow-speed handpieces) or hand instruments. The slow-speed handpiece permits the dentist to differentiate between the *softer* carious dentin and the harder, sound dentin.

When caries extends close to the pulp, it may be advisable to protect the vital tissues of the tooth (odontoblasts, blood vessels, and nerves within the pulp) with dental liners and cement bases prior to placing the final restoration. Various dental materials have been developed for this purpose. When used in the appropriate combination and in the correct order, they can prevent bacterial penetration, provide thermal insulation, sedate the pulp, and stimulate the production of secondary dentin.

D. FINISH THE PREPARATION WALLS

This step entails using a handpiece with appropriate burs, discs, and hand instruments (chisel type) designed to smoothly plane the walls while removing unsound enamel (i.e., enamel that is crazed or cracked or not supported by sound dentin).

E. CLEAN THE PREPARATION

Prior to the restoration of any cavity preparation, the operator must remove excess cement base that is too close to the preparation margins, along with tooth debris, hemorrhage, and saliva from the walls of the preparation. In this way, the restorative material will contact only sound clean tooth structure.

F. FINAL EVALUATION OF THE PREPARATION

Finally, a most important last step is to evaluate the finished preparation to ensure that all of the principles of cavity preparation have been addressed.

SECTION V — PRINCIPLES OF CAVITY PREPARATION BASED ON RESTORATIVE MATERIAL, CLASS, AND SIZE OF LESION

A. RESTORATIVE (FILLING) MATERIALS

The success of decay prevention techniques taught in dental practices and presented in the media are important factors in the reduction of the number and size of restorations being placed in the adult population. Also, the early protection of susceptible pits and fissures with sealants before the caries process has begun reduces the number of invasive (surgical or cutting) procedures. Finally, susceptible smooth surfaces can be protected by the application of fluoride and fluoride varnish, which strengthens the enamel and can even reverse early bacterial damage in smooth surface lesions (classes II, III, and V).

When prevention methods have not been successful and it is deemed necessary to use surgical techniques, materials of choice for restoring small conservative defects requiring intracoronal restorations include amalgam, composite, glass ionomer, resin ionomer, and porcelain or cast metal inlays that are placed into intracoronal preparations within the tooth. The materials of choice for restoring larger defects that require protection (extracoronal coverage) of thin remaining tooth structure include gold, semi- or nonprecious metal, or porcelain, which surround or cover the entire tooth in a relatively thin outer shell.

1. AMALGAM

Amalgam has been a widely used restorative material owing to its ease of placement and relatively low cost. It is silver in color and is packed into a preparation in successive small increments that, within

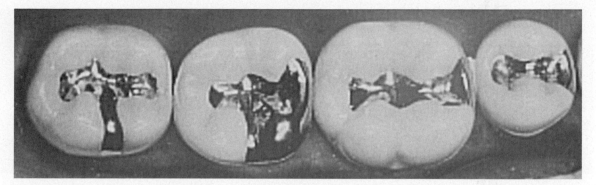

FIGURE 13-15. Class I and II amalgam restorations, mandibular arch. **Left:** Class I OB-A (occlusobuccal amalgam) on tooth #32. **Left-center:** Class II MOB-A (mesio-occlusobuccal amalgam) with a mesiobuccal cusp buildup or replacement on tooth #31. **Right-center:** Class II MO-A (mesio-occlusal amalgam) on tooth #30. **Right:** Class II MO-A on tooth #29.

several hours, cohere and become hard enough to withstand chewing forces. Therefore, it is used for restorations on the chewing (or occlusal) surfaces of posterior teeth and other restorations when maintenance of proximal and occlusal contacts is important but when esthetics is not a factor (*Figs. 13-15* and *13-16*).

2. ESTHETIC RESTORATIVE MATERIALS

Esthetic restorative materials, such as composite resin and glass ionomer, are being increasingly used due to patients' demands for esthetic restorations. **Composite resin** is a tooth-colored restorative material that is applied as a plastic-like mass into a preparation. It can be hardened quickly with a light source. Due to initial concerns about the strength and abrasion resistance of composite resins,[14,15] it was historically used primarily for restoring the proximal surfaces of anterior teeth and the facial surfaces of teeth on which esthetics is a chief concern. An example of composite restoration used to close a diastema is shown in *Figure 13-17* and to restore class III lesions in *Figure 13-18*. Note that the shade of the composite restorations in Figure 13-18 is dark in order to visualize the size, outline, and location of these restorations.

With newer generations of esthetic restorative materials showing better performance in posterior areas, composite is replacing amalgam as the restoration of choice for small class I and II lesions. One

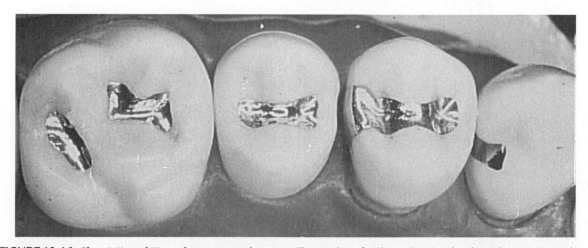

FIGURE 13-16. Class I, II, and III amalgam restorations, maxillary arch. **Left:** Class I O-A (occlusal amalgams) on tooth #3 with two parts separated by a strong intact oblique ridge. **Left-center:** Class I O-A (occlusal amalgam) on tooth #4. **Right-center:** Class II DO-A (disto-occlusal amalgam) on tooth #5. **Right:** Class III DL-A (distolingual amalgam) on tooth #6. These are all very conservative restorations, extended only as wide as necessary for access and prevention.

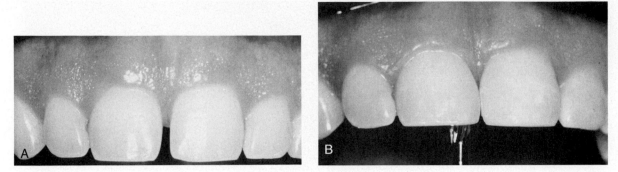

FIGURE 13-17. A. Teeth #8 and 9 with diastema. **B.** Same teeth during final finishing stages after placement of **composite veneers** used to close the diastema. No tooth preparation was necessary. (Courtesy of Dr. Roland Pagniano, D.D.S.)

longitudinal study rated composite restorations after 10 years (using a U.S. Public Health system of evaluation) to be over 90% satisfactory for color stability, surface smoothness, anatomic form, lack of recurrent caries, and pulp response.[16] Only marginal adaptation was scored below 90%, with a score of 81%. With recent physical property improvements,[17] a new generation of dentin bonding agents that can etch enamel and dentin simultaneously,[18] and a new generation of packable composite-based resins, they will be used even more widely in the future.

When esthetics is a factor, tooth-colored materials can be used as inlays or onlays, using either a direct technique (constructed within the mouth) or an indirect technique (constructed outside the mouth and then cemented in place). Also, when there are large cavities, an adhesive (bonded) indirect composite restoration that has adequate wear resistance can be used to strengthen the remaining tooth.[9]

Glass ionomer and related materials such as resin-modified glass ionomer are recommended for the treatment of root surface caries and erosion lesions.[19] These materials bond to dentin chemically, are reasonably esthetic, and contain fluoride, which reduces the possibility of recurrent caries.

3. CAST METAL RESTORATIONS

Cast gold or semiprecious alloys, when used for inlays and onlays (and full crowns as discussed later), are constructed from an accurate model (or die) of the patient's teeth (*Fig. 13-19*). These cast metal restorations require considerably more time to construct than composite resin or amalgam restorations because of the laboratory procedures. Consequently, they are more expensive for the patient.

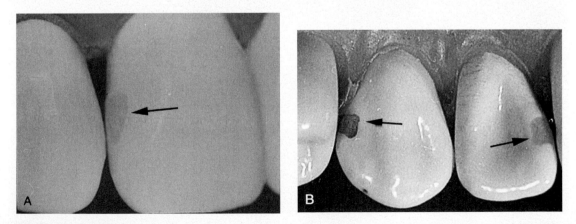

FIGURE 13-18. Class III restorations. A. A DF-C: distal composite with labial approach on tooth #8. **B. Left:** A DL-A: distal amalgam with lingual approach on tooth #11; metal is used here to maintain the distal contact. **Right:** A ML-C (mesial composite) with lingual approach on tooth #10. (The dark shade of the composite was used to make the restoration visible in this photograph.)

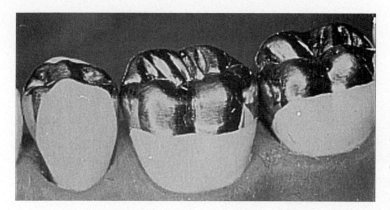

FIGURE 13-19. Class II cast metal inlay and onlay restorations. Left: An MOD-I (mesio-occlusodistal **inlay**) on tooth #20. **Center and right:** A MOD-On (extensive mesio-occlusodistal **onlays**) on teeth #19 and 18.

An **inlay** is a cast restoration that fits within the prepared tooth cavity but does not overlay the cusps, in contrast to an **onlay**, which overlays or replaces cusps (Fig. 13-19). Onlays and full crowns are recommended when the tooth structure remaining after tooth preparation is frail and needs to be protected from occlusal forces. The greater strength of the cast metal in thin layers compared to amalgam permits optimum protection and strength with less bulk of metal, resulting in less occlusal reduction of tooth structure. Further, cast metal restorations can be contoured more perfectly on a **die** (which is a precise dental stone reproduction of the individual prepared tooth) than in the mouth. Finally, cast restorations are more inert (less likely to change) in the mouth compared to amalgam (that is, cast restorations have better marginal stability over time). For these reasons, a cast inlay may be selected over amalgam for patients who desire and can afford the cast restoration, even when the restoration will be quite conservative and not require onlaying.

4. PORCELAIN: INLAYS, ONLAYS, AND VENEERS

Indirect (i.e., constructed outside of the mouth and cemented) **ceramic inlays and onlays** are becoming esthetic alternatives to cast metal inlays and onlays due to advanced processing methods and bonding techniques that improve fit.[20,21] Advances are also occurring in the generation of these restorations by computer.[22] Conservative techniques for veneering the labial surfaces of anterior teeth to improve esthetics include porcelain (or direct composite) veneers that require minimal or no tooth reduction and fees that are generally less than for a crown with a porcelain veneer. A mouth with many porcelain crowns and indirect composite restorations can be seen in Color Plate 21. Porcelain veneers used to improve the esthetics of anterior teeth with old, unesthetic composite restorations are shown in *Figure 13-20*.

B. PRINCIPLES OF CAVITY PREPARATION AND NOMENCLATURE FOR EACH G.V. BLACK CLASS OF CARIES BASED ON MATERIAL USED

The discussion of tooth restoration that follows assumes that the tooth to be prepared is periodontally sound (that is, has a stable alveolus and healthy gingiva) and that the maintenance of the tooth is an integral part of the overall treatment for that patient. The five classifications of decay devised and published by Dr. G.V. Black in 1908 are still appropriate to consider, although the principles of cavity preparation are now applied uniquely for each class of decay and each new restorative material. Successful cavity preparations for restorative materials such as dental amalgam, composite, resin, or cast metal are designed to allow placement and maintenance of each restorative material and, at the same time, to ensure the preservation of remaining tooth structure.

1. CLASS I CARIES: PRINCIPLES OF CAVITY PREPARATION AND TERMINOLOGY

Pit and fissure sealants can be used as a preventive measure to prevent class I caries in deep caries-prone pits and fissures, especially for the young patient. A sealant is a "flowable" resin that is applied over noncarious but caries-prone, unprepared pits and fissures of recently erupted teeth. These sealants have been shown to be an effective means of preventing caries in pits and fissures.[23–25] An initial sealant

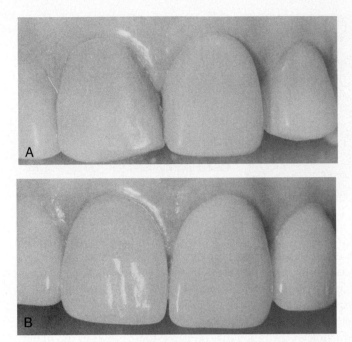

FIGURE 13-20. Porcelain veneers used to replace old unesthetic composite veneers. **A.** Teeth #8, 9, and 10 with old composite resin veneers that have chipped and exhibit a loss of translucency. **B.** These same teeth after placement of esthetic porcelain veneers that cover the entire facial surfaces. (Courtesy of Dr. Roland Pagniano, D.D.S.)

application for all permanent molars and premolars requires only 15–20 minutes per child.[26] A transitional restoration involving composite resin in a very conservative preparation confined within enamel, plus a sealant over adjacent pits and fissures, is called a **conservative resin restoration** (previously called preventive resin restorations). Conservative preparations can also be formed using an **air-abrasion system** where abrasive particles are blown forcefully toward the tooth to actually remove tooth structure. This technique permits removal of only the most conservative amounts of tooth structure, but the principles of cavity preparation for this new technology (such as retention, access, extension to sound enamel, etc.) must still be considered. **Bonding agents**, similar to sealants, can be used for retention when placing composite restorations over the abraded (roughened) tooth.[27]

Amalgam is frequently chosen for stress-bearing class I restorations on occlusal surfaces. For small class I pits or fissures on posterior teeth where esthetics are important, composite resins may be used, possibly in conjunction with sealants to protect, rather than cut into, adjacent susceptible pits and fissures. Cast gold or porcelain onlays would only be considered for class I restorations if there were few restorations in the mouth with a low evidence of new decay or the size of the restoration necessitated onlaying cusps.

Certain of G.V. Black's principles of cavity preparation are uniquely applied when restoring the class I cavity with amalgam as described here. Differences in preparation requirements will be noted for resin materials.

a. Extension for Prevention (Class I)

Extension for prevention, to include those pits and fissures adjoining the defects with active decay, should be considered when the patient is young, has a high caries rate, and/or exhibits poor oral hygiene, but sealants may also be used to protect adjacent pits and fissures. Examples of amalgam preparations including all major grooves can be seen in *Figures 13-21* and *13-22*.

b. Resistance Form (Class I)

When amalgam is used on a stress-bearing surface, a minimum depth of 1.5–2 mm is recommended due to the brittleness of amalgam in thinner layers, whereas if cast metal is used, a thickness of 1 mm may be sufficient to withstand occlusal forces. Ideally, amalgam meets the unprepared tooth surface at right angles to provide resistance form, whereas gold ends in an overlapping bevel *(Fig. 13-23)*.

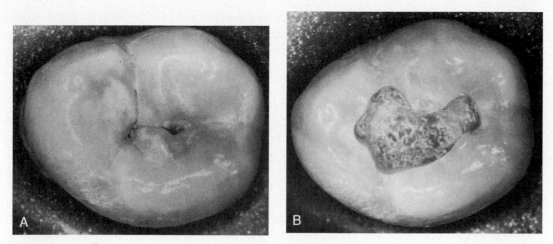

FIGURE 13-21. Extending a class I preparation for access and extending to sound enamel. A. Class I lesion seen as small pits on the occlusal surface. **B.** The same tooth after preparation showing the extension necessary to obtain access (convenience form) to remove decay, which spread out laterally beneath the dentinoenamel junction. This outline form is also necessary to end the preparation on sound enamel walls, which are supported by sound dentin (not softer caries).

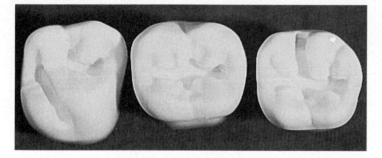

FIGURE 13-22. Class I amalgam preparations showing various degrees of extension for prevention. Left: Tooth #3 with an occlusal and an occlusal-lingual preparation. The preparations are separate since in this case, there was no need to cross the oblique ridge. **Center:** An occlusal amalgam preparation of tooth #31. **Right:** An occlusobuccal amalgam preparation on tooth #30.

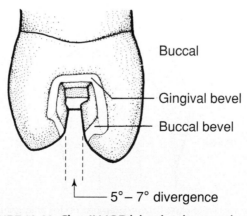

FIGURE 13-23. Class II MOD inlay showing retentive form provided by opposing walls diverging very slightly (only 5–7°) so the inlay fits snuggly like a stopper in a wine decanter bottle. Also, note the preparation design, which includes **bevels** that permit thin metal to be burnished or adapted more closely to the enamel with a blunt instrument.

Resin restorations can be thin in low-stress areas (as when used as a sealant or preventive resin restorations) or as thick as amalgam in high-stress areas. Because the resin mechanically bonds to the tooth structure, it can meet the prepared tooth surface at right angles or be beveled.

c. Retention (Class I)

For amalgam, retention is provided in an occlusal preparation by a slight *convergence* of the buccal and lingual preparation walls toward the occlusal surface, which, due to the slope of the triangular ridges, is coincidentally accomplished by ending the buccal and lingual cavity walls at right angles to the unprepared triangular ridges (*Fig. 13-24C*).

For composite preparations, additional retention is provided by acid etching the enamel to produce *microscopic* irregularities (minute undercuts) on the surface. Then, flowable resin **bonding agents** can flow into the irregularities to form retentive resin tags that *mechanically* lock into the *microscopic* retentive features of the etched enamel (*Fig. 13-25*). Layers of the stronger composite resin can subsequently be *chemically* bonded to the flowable resin layer. When using newer adhesive agents, additional retention is gained by chemical bonds formed between tooth and resin.

For inlays or onlays (cast gold or porcelain), retention is provided by preparing the opposing *internal* walls of the preparation with a slight (5–7°) *divergence* toward the occlusal surface (as seen within the class II inlay preparation in Fig. 13-23), thus allowing the solid casting to be seated snugly within the tooth, somewhat like a glass stopper fitting into the opening of a decanter. The

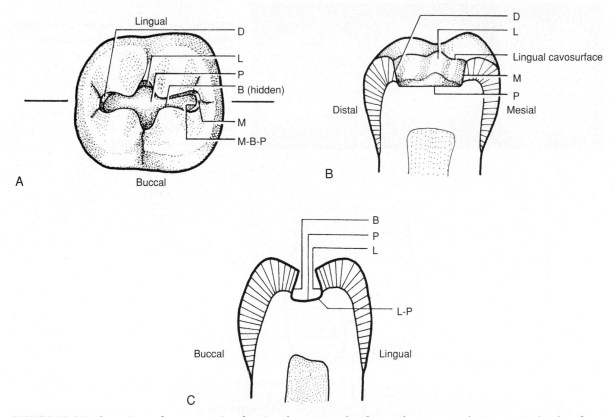

FIGURE 13-24. Three views of a conservative **class I cavity preparation for amalgam** on tooth #31. **A.** Occlusal surface showing extension for prevention into the major grooves. **B.** Mesiodistal cross section of the same tooth showing the ideal depth of the pulpal floor, just into dentin (about 0.5 mm). The lingual cavosurface is also identified where the lingual wall of the preparation joins the unprepared surface of the tooth. **C.** Buccolingual cross section of the same tooth showing the convergence of the vertical buccal and lingual walls toward the occlusal for retention and resistance form. **Key for nomenclature: B** = buccal wall; **L** = lingual wall; **M** = mesial wall; **D** = distal wall; **P** = pulpal wall or floor. Example of a line angle: **L-P** is the linguopulpal line angle. Example of a point angle: **M-B-P** is the mesiobuccopulpal point angle in **A.**

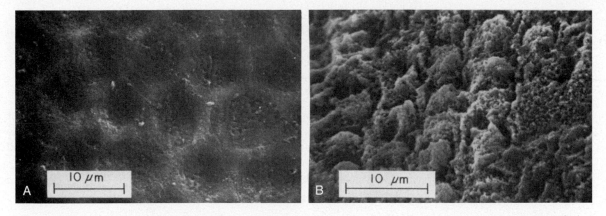

FIGURE 13-25. The effect of etching enamel. A. Magnified view of a nonetched enamel surface (×3260). **B.** Magnified view of an etched enamel surface (×3600) after application of 50% phosphoric acid. This etched surface allows the resin bonding agent of the composite systems to flow into the irregular microscopic undercuts, thus affording mechanical retention for the material. (Courtesy of Dr. Ruth Paulson, Ohio State University.)

dental cement used between the inlay and tooth provides retention by sealing the margins and by setting to hardness at the interface between the slight irregularities of the enamel walls of the preparation and those of the inlay/onlay. Some dental cements chemically bond to the calcium of the tooth and can be mechanically attached to the etched surface of metal castings (resin cements, glass ionomer, and polycarboxylate cements).

d. Cavity Nomenclature (Class I)

The traditional occlusal preparation can be compared to a room (with no ceiling) that has four vertical walls and a horizontal floor or wall. The four vertical walls are named after the most closely related tooth surfaces, namely, buccal, mesial, lingual, and distal; the horizontal floor is called the **pulpal floor (or wall)** because it is over the pulp (abbreviated as B, M, L, D, and P in Fig. 13-24A). A **line angle** in the preparation is the line formed when two walls join. There are eight internal line angles in a conservative class I preparation (if it is confined to the occlusal surface and is not extended into a buccal or lingual groove). These are named by combining the terms for the two walls that join to make up each line angle, changing the suffix of the first word from "al" to "o." It makes no difference which wall is named first. For example, the junction of the pulpal floor and distal wall is the distopulpal *or* pulpodistal line angle. All possible line angles in a class I occlusal preparation include four horizontal ones—distopulpal, mesiopulpal, buccopulpal, and linguopulpal—and four vertical ones—mesiobuccal, distobuccal, mesiolingual, and distolingual.

The term that describes the junction of any wall of the preparation with the unprepared tooth structure is called the **cavosurface**. The cavosurface therefore is the *outline* that encircles the preparation and restoration. An occlusal restoration where the buccal wall of a preparation meets the uncut surface is the buccal cavosurface, where the lingual wall ends is known as the lingual cavosurface, and so on (Fig. 13-24B).

Finally, there are four **point angles** in a class I preparation, each formed by the junction of three walls (as in the corner of a room where two walls meet the floor). Point angles are named after the three walls that form them: mesiobuccopulpal (abbreviated M-B-P in Fig. 13-24A), mesiolinguopulpal, distolinguopulpal, and distobuccopulpal. Since the junction of walls in a preparation is often rounded, line angles and point angles may be small, general areas rather than distinct, sharp angles or points.

A class I *restoration* is properly described and identified by naming the surfaces involved and material used. For example, an amalgam on tooth #14 involving the occlusal surface with a lingual extension would be abbreviated OL-A, #14. The letter O represents the occlusal portion of the preparation, the L represents the lingual extension, and the letter A represents the restorative material, amalgam. (Test yourself by referring to Figs. 13-15 and 13-16 where the legends give the correct abbreviations for several types of amalgam restorations.) If composite had been used, the representation would have been OL-C, #14. A lower right third molar with an occlusal amalgam and buccal extension would be an OB-A, #32. A buccal or lingual pit restored with composite would be a B-C or L-C, followed or preceded by the tooth number.

2. CLASS II CARIES: PRINCIPLES OF CAVITY PREPARATION AND TERMINOLOGY

The preparation for a class II carious lesion can be restored with amalgam, direct composite, inlays, or onlays (cast metal or tooth colored). The larger the preparation (and therefore the thinner the remaining tooth structure), the more appropriate an onlay restoration might be to cover the cusps and protect the remaining thin tooth and provide adequate resistance form (recall Fig. 13-19). Improvements in composite restorative materials and techniques have resulted in the increased use of this tooth-colored material for class II restorations, especially when esthetics is an important factor.

a. Extension for Prevention (Class II)

To reach class II lesions, the dentist must, in most cases, prepare a **proximal box** that extends apically through the marginal ridge in order to reach the decay, which forms just cervical to the proximal contact. The class II preparation often extends over some of the occlusal surface to include adjacent defective or carious occlusal pits and fissures as in a class I preparation, whereas the proximal box might be compared to a stair step descending gingivally off of the occlusal portion (*Fig. 13-26*). When proximal decay is present but there is no decay or deep fissures on the occlusal surface, the dentist may prepare a **slot preparation**. This conservative preparation is just the proximal box of the traditional class II amalgam preparation with no extension into the occlusal grooves (Fig. 13-26C). Notice that in Figure 13-26A, the maxillary molar prepara-

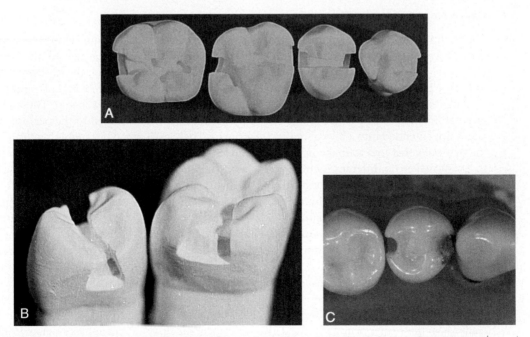

FIGURE 13-26. Models of conservative **class II amalgam preparations. A. Occlusal views: Left:** MO-A (mesio-occlusal amalgam) preparation on tooth #30. **Left-center:** MO-A, DO-A (mesio-occlusal and disto-occlusal amalgam) preparation on tooth #3 with the oblique ridge intact. **Right-center:** MOD-A (mesio-occlusodistal amalgam) preparation on tooth #5. **Right:** DO-A (disto-occlusal amalgam) preparation on tooth #28 with the transverse ridge intact. **B. Proximal views** of class II amalgam preparations. **Left:** MOD-A preparation on tooth #4. **Right:** MO-A preparation on tooth #30. Note the convergence of the buccal and lingual walls toward the occlusal for retention and resistance form. When the decay process has progressed deeper and wider, the prepared walls by necessity will be farther apart than these.
C. Conservative **slot preparation** involving the distal and occlusal surfaces of typodont tooth #28; note the amalgam restoration (MO-A) in a similar slot preparation on the mesial and occlusal surfaces. This conservative preparation may be preferred to reach interproximal caries when there is proximal caries without any occlusal involvement.

tion does not extend over the oblique ridge since there is seldom a susceptible groove in this area. Also, the DO-A preparation on the mandibular first premolar does not cross the transverse ridge (which seldom has a deep groove) nor does it include the mesial pit if it is not deeply fissured or carious.

The class I portion follows the principles for restoring a class I lesion already discussed, but the proximal extension (box) adds new features. For example, the buccal and lingual walls of the proximal box of class II preparations are extended beyond the proximal contact areas just into the buccal and lingual embrasures. In this way, the margins of the restoration can be better evaluated by the dentist and kept clean by the patient.

b. Retention Form (Class II)

For class II *amalgam* cavity preparations, the buccal and lingual walls of the occlusal portion and the proximal boxes are prepared so that they *converge slightly toward the occlusal* to prevent the restoration from dislodging occlusally as in the class I preparation. **Retentive grooves** may be prepared buccally and lingually in a proximal box as extensions of the internal vertical wall of the box that is aligned along the long axis of the tooth, and is therefore called the **axial wall.** These retentive grooves are designed to prevent the amalgam restoration from dislodging in a proximal direction. They are located at the axiobuccal (A-B) and axiolingual (A-L) line angles seen later in Figure 13-29. Resin restorations are generally prepared in a similar fashion to amalgam. However, with additional retention gained from the enamel etching and bonding, there is less need for internal retention grooves.

For *cast metal* inlays, opposing buccal and lingual walls must *diverge slightly toward the occlusal.* The two axial walls in a mesio-occlusodistal inlay preparation must *converge slightly toward the occlusal* so that an accurate wax model (pattern) and subsequent casting can be seated within the preparation and then removed while constructing and refining the casting prior to cementation (*Figs. 13-27* and *13-28*). **Bevels** are angular enamel reductions placed at the cavosurface in order for the margins (or outer edges) of the casting to be thin enough, so the dentist can perfect the adaptation and minimize the cavosurface gap between tooth and metal. The goal is to minimize the gap between the casting and tooth since this gap is to be filled with a dental cement, which is not as strong nor as durable as the metal.

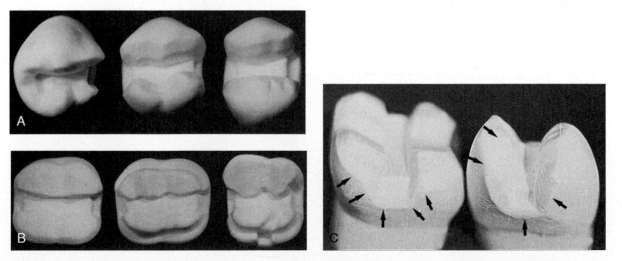

FIGURE 13-27. Models of **class II inlay and onlay preparations. A.** Three inlay preparations. **Left:** An MO-I (mesio-occlusal **inlay**) preparation on tooth #21. **Center and Right:** MOD-I (mesio-occlusodistal inlay) preparations on tooth #20 and 13, respectively. **B.** Three **onlay** preparations. **Left:** A conventional MOD-O (mesio-occlusodistal onlay) preparation on tooth #18. **Center:** An MOD-O preparation (for ledge-type onlays) on tooth #19. **Right:** An MODL-O (mesio-occlusodistolingual onlay) with conventional onlayed buccal cusps on tooth #14. **C.** Proximal views of an onlay preparation (left) and of an inlay preparation (right) showing the continuous **bevel** surrounding the preparation and the divergence of the buccal and lingual walls toward the occlusal. The **cavosurface,** or outline of the preparation (marked with arrows), is at the outer end of the prepared bevels.

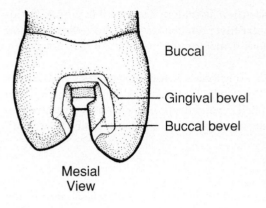

Buccal

Gingival bevel

Buccal bevel

Mesial
View

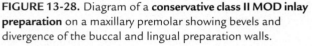

FIGURE 13-28. Diagram of a **conservative class II MOD inlay preparation** on a maxillary premolar showing bevels and divergence of the buccal and lingual preparation walls.

c. Cavity Nomenclature (Class II)

Class II lesions can involve just one or both proximal surfaces of a posterior tooth, but since obtaining access into the proximal lesion normally requires breaking through the occlusal marginal ridge, these restorations involve a minimum of two (occlusal and mesial *or* occlusal and distal) or three (mesial, occlusal, and distal) surfaces. A proximal box has vertical buccal, lingual, and axial walls (the axial wall is along the long axis of the tooth) and a horizontal **gingival wall** (or floor) (all labeled with abbreviations in *Fig. 13-29*).

The line angles that are present in a mesial or distal proximal box are axiopulpal, axiogingival, buccogingival, linguogingival, axiobuccal, and axiolingual. The axiobuccal and axiolingual line angles (labeled A-B and A-L in Fig. 13-29) are where the **retentive grooves** for an amalgam preparation are placed. In a mesio-occlusodistal preparation, each line angle is differentiated by

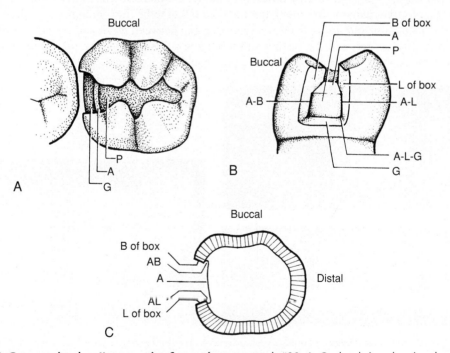

FIGURE 13-29. Conservative class II preparation for amalgam on tooth #30. **A.** Occlusal view showing the proximal box extending just through the proximal contact buccally and lingually. **B.** The mesial view showing the slight convergence toward the occlusal of the buccal and lingual walls of the box and axiobuccal (A-B) and axiolingual (A-L) line angles where retentive grooves are placed. An example of a point angle: A-L-G for axiolinguogingival is seen. **C.** A cross section of this prepared tooth in the middle third of the crown showing the placement of the retentive grooves entirely within dentin at the axiobuccal and axiolingual line angles. Key for nomenclature: Walls, **B** = buccal; **P** = pulpal; **L** = lingual; **A** = axial; **G** = gingival. Example of line angles: **A-B** = axiobuccal; **A-L** = axiolingual (location of retentive grooves).

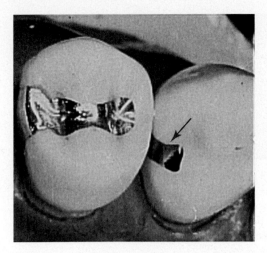

FIGURE 13-30. **A class III amalgam preparation on the distal of a canine** (#6). This area would most likely be restored with composite today.

stating whether it is in the mesial or distal box. For example, there are two axiopulpal line angles in the mesio-occlusodistal amalgam preparation: One is the axiopulpal line angle of the mesial box and the other is the axiopulpal line angle of the distal box. The point angles in each box include axiolinguogingival (A-L-G in Fig. 13-29B), axiobuccogingival, axiobuccopulpal, and axiolinguopulpal.

Class II preparations for amalgam involving only two surfaces, such as mesio-occlusal or disto-occlusal, are traditionally abbreviated MO-A or DO-A (not OM-A or OD-A). A mesio-occlusodistal amalgam preparation is abbreviated MOD-A (not DOM-A). A class II preparation for composite material involving only two surfaces would be abbreviated similarly, with the abbreviation of "C" such as MO-C or DO-C. For inlays (I) or onlays (O), the abbreviation would be MO-I and DO-I, MOD-I and MO-O, and DO-O and MOD-O, respectively.

3. CLASS III CARIES: PRINCIPLES OF CAVITY PREPARATION AND TERMINOLOGY

Since the class III lesion occurs in a non–stress-bearing area that is often of esthetic concern to the patient, a tooth-colored composite resin is usually the restoration of choice. The distal proximal surface of the canine is less visible so it could be restored with a conservative class III amalgam *(Fig. 13-30)*. However, composite materials are used most often in this class III area.

a. Extension for Prevention: Class III

Extension for prevention is minimal in the class III composite preparation since the dentist wants to preserve as much enamel as possible for esthetic reasons and because the anterior teeth may be easier to keep clean. For all class III lesions, the approach to the decay, whenever possible, is from the lingual of the tooth, so the facial enamel is preserved for maximum esthetic effect *(Fig. 13-31A and C)*, but when the decay has already destroyed the facial plate of enamel, a facial approach can be used *(Fig. 13-31B)*.

b. Retention: Class III

When restoring teeth with larger carious lesions, retention form may be obtained by simply removing the decay that has spread out at the dentinoenamel junction, resulting in a preparation that is wider internally than externally. Historically, retentive pits or grooves have been used as extensions of the axial wall in order to improve retention for either a composite or amalgam class III preparation (seen in *Fig. 13-32*). However, the more conservative method of affording retention and reducing leakage at the cavosurface margin of a composite restoration is by bonding the composite resin to an acid-etched, beveled enamel surface (recall Fig. 13-25B). The first layer of flowable resin (bonding agent) can form resin tags that fill the microscopic etched irregularities and harden, thus locking the restoration in place. The preparation shape therefore can be more conservative, without the need for internal retentive grooves or pits.

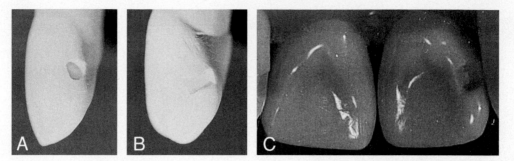

FIGURE 13-31. Class III cavity preparations. A. Model of a DL-A: distal amalgam preparation with lingual approach on tooth #6. Note the box-like shape and axioincisal retentive groove in the shadow (the axiogingival retentive groove is hidden). The preparation for composite would be similar but would not require retentive grooves. **B.** Model of the DF-C: distal composite preparation with facial approach on tooth #10. Note the generally triangular form. **C.** DL-C: distal composite preparation with lingual approach on tooth #8. Note the axioincisal retentive feature. (The axiogingival retentive feature is less visible here.)

c. Cavity Nomenclature: Class III

As previously stated, because the class III resin restoration gains retention from bonding of resin to enamel and dentin, the final shape of a resin class III preparation may be somewhat amorphous, removing only carious tooth structure while conserving as much healthy tooth structure as possible. Sometimes, however, a more defined, traditional preparation may be desirable. The traditional preparation for the *lingual approach* for a class III composite has the same terminology as the lingual approach for a class III amalgam and is represented in Figure 13-32A and B. This lingual approach preparation can be compared to the four-walled proximal box portion of a class II preparation, which is also cut through the marginal ridge. However, due to the more horizontal alignment of the box of a class III preparation, the names assigned to the walls differ. Here, the four walls are called gingival, facial, incisal, and axial (as abbreviated in Fig. 13-32A and B). There are only five internal line angles: gingivofacial, incisofacial, gingivoaxial, facioaxial, and incisoaxial. There are only two internal point angles: gingivofacioaxial and incisofacioaxial.

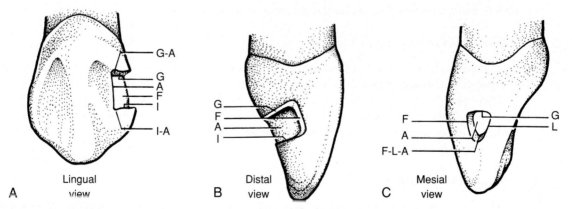

FIGURE 13-32. Class III preparations. A. The lingual view of the class III amalgam preparation, lingual approach, on the distal of tooth #6. Retentive grooves are evident at the cavosurface of the gingivoaxial and incisoaxial line angles. **B.** The distal view of a class III composite preparation, lingual approach. Note the slight convergence of the incisal and gingival wall toward the lingual for retention. This preparation also has retentive grooves (or pits) at the incisoaxial and gingivoaxial line angles, but they do not extend to the cavosurface. The gingivoaxial groove is in the shadow between G and A. **C.** The mesial view of a class III composite preparation, labial approach. Note the triangular shape. Retentive features are found internally at the axiogingival line angle and the faciolinguoaxial point angle. **Key for nomenclature: for lingual approach (A and B): G** = gingival; **A** = axial; **F** = facial; **I** = incisal. Examples of the angles are the retentive features **G-A** and **I-A** for the gingivoaxial and incisoaxial line angles, respectively. **Key for the facial approach (C): F** = facial; **A** = axial; **G** = gingival; **L** = lingual.

The traditional preparation for a composite with a *facial approach* may be more triangular in shape with three walls and a floor (Fig. 13-32C). The three walls are the facial, lingual, and gingival walls, and the fourth wall (or floor) is the axial. Subsequently, this preparation has six internal line angles: facioaxial, linguoaxial, gingivoaxial, faciolingual, linguogingival, and gingivofacial. There are only three internal point angles: faciolinguoaxial (abbreviated F-L-A in Fig. 13-32C), linguogingivoaxial, and faciogingivoaxial.

Class III composite or amalgam restorations may be abbreviated by identifying the proximal surface, as well as the surface through which access was gained, and the material used. For example, a composite on the mesial surface of tooth #7 with access to the decay through the lingual enamel would be identified as M-C, #7, lingual approach, or more precisely, ML-C, #7. A distal composite restoration on tooth #24 approached from the facial would be identified as D-C, #24, facial approach, or DF-C, #24. Note that instead of using "L" to denote the labial (or facial) surface, "F" is used to denote the facial surface in order to avoid confusion with "L," which is used to denote the lingual surface.

4. CLASS IV CARIES: PRINCIPLES OF CAVITY PREPARATION AND TERMINOLOGY

If a class IV preparation is conservative, a composite, particularly one that utilizes an acid-etching technique, is the restoration of choice. An alternative treatment is a veneer of porcelain bonded to the facial surface of the tooth, replacing the fractured incisal area *(Fig. 13-33)*. If the preparation is extensive or if the whole incisal edge of the tooth and both proximal surfaces are involved, but there is sufficient remaining tooth structure, it may be better to recommend a full cast crown with facial porcelain, or a full porcelain crown for the best esthetics and longevity (Fig. 13-40).

Caries removal and smoothing extremely rough or unsupported enamel may be all that is needed to prepare the tooth for a class IV composite. The occlusion, as always, must be analyzed to be sure that there is room for the restoration when the patient chews and incises, especially in a protrusive direction. Retention is most commonly achieved by acid-etch techniques that permit resin tags to bond the composite to the tooth. A thin sleeve or skirt of excess composite material can cover beveled enamel that has been acid etched to maximize retention (Fig. 13-33B) and to improve esthetics by blending the color differential between composite and enamel.

Depending on the degree of involvement, this preparation may have only one flat wall (as in a fracture; similar to the shape seen in Fig. 13-33) or may be made up of two main surfaces: a gingival surface and a more axial surface. These two portions may join at an angle called the axiogingival line angle. There are no point angles.

A composite restoration that restores one incisal angle actually restores parts of four surfaces, so it may be abbreviated as either an MIFL-C or DIFL-C, to denote the involvement of all surfaces of either the mesioincisal or the distoincisal angle of the tooth. If both proximal surfaces are involved, the restoration would be designated as MIDFL-C. As usual, the tooth number can be added either before or after the abbreviation, for example, #9, MIDFL-C, or MIDFL-C, #9.

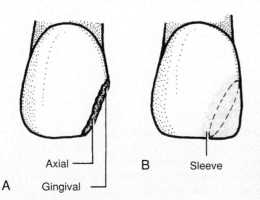

A   Axial ⎤
     Gingival ⎦

B   Sleeve

FIGURE 13-33. **Class IV carious lesion or fracture** on tooth #8 and the resultant restoration. **A.** View of the lesion or fracture showing the gingival and axial portions of the defect. **B.** After smoothing the preparation and acid etching the enamel, the restored tooth with a sleeve or skirt (thin film of bonded resin that extends beyond the original cavosurface margin) of composite overlaps the etched enamel surface, **thus establishing maximum retention and enhancing (blending) the color match.**

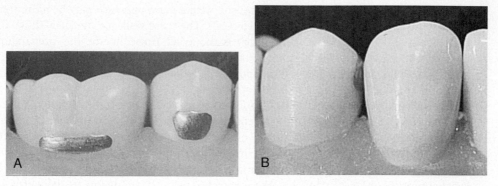

FIGURE 13-34. Class V restorations. A. Two B-As (buccal amalgams) on teeth #29 and 30. The extent of these amalgams is usually dictated by the extent of the caries. **B.** Class V B-C (buccal composite) on tooth #27. If the shade of the material is good, these restorations are difficult to detect, and their surface grittiness felt by an explorer or scaler might be confused for incipient calculus formation. (Restorations by Gregory Blackstone, second-year dental student.)

5. CLASS V CARIES: PRINCIPLES OF CAVITY PREPARATION AND TERMINOLOGY

Since a class V lesion occurs in non–stress-bearing areas, when esthetics is a factor a composite may be used, even though it may be less resistant to abrasion than amalgam (*Fig. 13-34B*). In gingival abrasion lesions and areas of root caries, the dentist may restore the tooth with a glass ionomer or resin-modified glass ionomer because they both bond to dentin and contain fluoride. Amalgam may be used when the esthetics are *not* of prime concern (*Fig. 13-34A*). In rare cases, primarily at the patient's request, a cast metal inlay (or porcelain inlay) could be used to replace lost tooth contour.

The preparation for a class V composite restoration is usually kept as conservative as possible, with an equally deep, convex axial wall (*Fig. 13-36C*) and little or no extension for prevention (*Fig. 13-35*). Prevention of future caries occurs through patient education in oral hygiene techniques and from periodic application of topical fluoride. The retention of amalgam restorations is obtained by preparing retentive **grooves** that are extensions of the axial wall in an occlusal and gingival direction (A-O and A-G in *Fig. 13-36B*). When using composite, similar retentive grooves could be used, but more often, retention is dependent on beveled enamel surfaces that have been acid etched (recall the discussion under class III preparations). A glass ionomer restoration in an area of deep cervical abrasion (V-shaped or notched) may require no preparation, only a treatment with a dentin conditioner or primer that aids in the chemical bond between dentin and a glass ionomer restoration. A class V inlay must have walls *slightly divergent toward the tooth surface* to allow the wax model (pattern) removal from the tooth model (die), and as for all gold castings, there should be short bevels prepared at the cavosurface margins.

The class V preparation is somewhat box shaped and consists of five walls: distal, occlusal, mesial, gingival, and axial. There are eight line angles: axiomesial, axiogingival, axiodistal, axio-occlusal, mesiogingival, distogingival, mesio-occlusal, and disto-occlusal. The axio-occlusal and axiogingival line angles are prepared with retentive grooves labeled as A-O and A-G in Figure 13-36B. There are

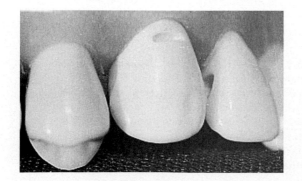

FIGURE 13-35. Class V preparation. Class V labial composite preparation on tooth #6. [A class III D-C (distal composite) preparation with labial approach can also be seen in the facial embrasure on tooth number 7.] (Preparations by Gregory Blackstone, second-year dental student.)

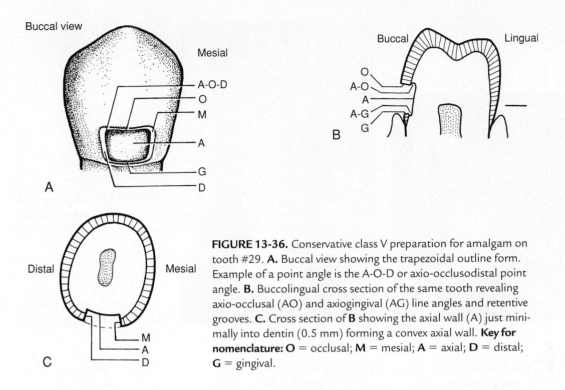

FIGURE 13-36. Conservative class V preparation for amalgam on tooth #29. **A.** Buccal view showing the trapezoidal outline form. Example of a point angle is the A-O-D or axio-occlusodistal point angle. **B.** Buccolingual cross section of the same tooth revealing axio-occlusal (AO) and axiogingival (AG) line angles and retentive grooves. **C.** Cross section of **B** showing the axial wall (A) just minimally into dentin (0.5 mm) forming a convex axial wall. **Key for nomenclature: O** = occlusal; **M** = mesial; **A** = axial; **D** = distal; **G** = gingival.

four point angles: axio-occlusodistal (A-O-D in Fig. 13-36A), axio-occlusomesial, axiodistogingival, and axiomesiogingival.

The restoration is identified by surface and material. For example, a buccal amalgam on tooth #19 is B-A, #19, a facial composite on tooth #7 is F-C, #7, and a glass ionomer on the facial surface of tooth #11 would be F-GI, #11. Typically, the term facial (F) is applied to anterior teeth, whereas buccal (B) is applied to posterior teeth.

6. CLASS VI: TYPE OF DENTAL CARIES OR RESTORATION

The resultant preparation for a class VI lesion conservatively follows Black's principles of cavity preparation, and the restoration of choice depends on size and location of the lesion and the need for strength and esthetics.

SECTION VI	RESTORING LARGE TOOTH DEFECTS AND TOOTH REPLACEMENT

When a tooth is too badly broken down to be restored with an intracoronal restoration because only a thin shell of enamel remains, it may be necessary to remove decay and replace some or all of the lost tooth structure with amalgam or composite to develop a "core" of tooth and filling around and over which an extracoronal crown can be constructed. The core restoration that replaces tooth structure prior to preparing a tooth for a crown may be called a restoration under crown (RUC) or amalgam under crown (AUC). When the remaining tooth crown is almost completely gone, a cast metal *core* (resembling a tooth prepared to receive a crown) must be designed with a metal *post,* which fits snugly into one of the previously endodontically treated and prepared root canals. The post is necessary to provide retention. This restoration is called a cast **post and core** (*Fig. 13-37*).

On posterior teeth, a crown will sometimes be constructed entirely of cast metal, and can be called a **complete crown** or a **complete veneer crown** (CVC) (*Fig. 13-38B*). To prepare a tooth for a complete crown, the previously restored anatomic tooth crown (or prepared core) is externally reduced with diamond burs to make room for the required thickness of the metal cast crown. The preparation usually extends gingivally beyond the

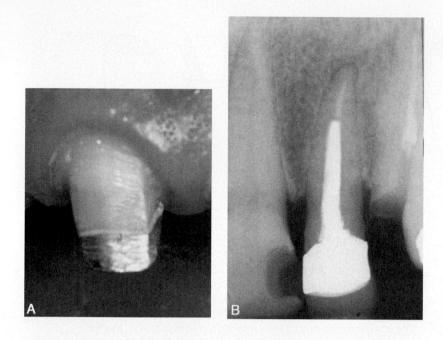

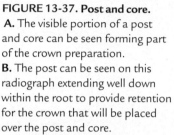

FIGURE 13-37. Post and core.
A. The visible portion of a post and core can be seen forming part of the crown preparation.
B. The post can be seen on this radiograph extending well down within the root to provide retention for the crown that will be placed over the post and core.

core filling material, so that the crown margins end on sound tooth structure. Full metal crown preparations end at the gingival cavosurface with a rounded shape called a **chamfer** (*Figs. 13-38A* and *13-39A*).

When esthetics are a factor, especially on anterior teeth and maxillary premolars, further reduction of tooth structure is necessary on the facial surface to make room not only for the thin cast metal, but also for an additional thickness of tooth-colored porcelain veneer over the metal. This restoration is called a **metal ceramic restoration** (also called a **metal ceramic crown** [MCC] or **porcelain veneer crown** [PVC]). The preparation for

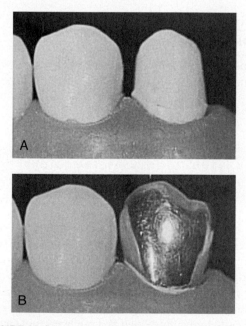

FIGURE 13-38. A. Crown preparation on tooth #20 for a full cast metal crown that will eventually support the framework of a removable partial denture with clasps. **B.** The resultant solid metal **cast metal crown** in place. The facial surface of a crown like this can be veneered with porcelain if visible when speaking or laughing.

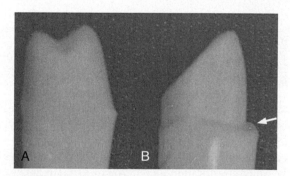

FIGURE 13-39. Proximal views: **Crown preparations** with their facial surface toward the right. **A. Full metal crown** (no veneer) preparation on a mandibular premolar with **chamfer** finish lines. **B.** Preparation on a maxillary canine that will have baked-on **porcelain veneer** covering the facial surface for esthetics. The finish line on the lingual is a **chamfer**, but on the facial, to make room for porcelain, a **ledge with bevel** (*arrow*) is necessary.

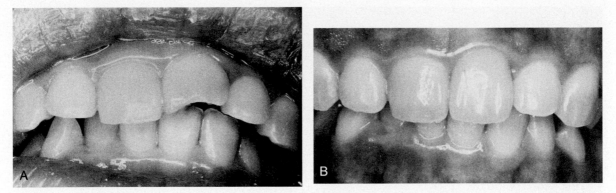

FIGURE 13-40. A. Tooth #9 with a fracture that includes the entire incisal edge. A large class IV composite could be used to restore this defect but would be more susceptible to fracture and discoloration than a crown with a porcelain facing. **B.** The same patient with an **esthetic cast metal crown and porcelain facing** on tooth #9. (Photographs courtesy of Dr. Steven Rosenstiel, Section Head of Restorative and Prosthetic Dentistry, Ohio State University.)

this type of crown ends at the gingival margins with a ledge that may have a bevel (*Fig. 13-39B*). Photographs of a crown with a porcelain facing used to improve the esthetics of a severely fractured tooth #9 is shown in *Figure 13-40B*. Crowns gain retention from the encompassing shape, nearly parallel walls that slightly converge toward the occlusal, accurate fit, and the cement. Retention of large onlays and crowns may be enhanced through mechanical bonding by etching the tooth or crown and chemical bonding utilizing a glass ionomer, polycarboxylate, or resin cement.

Another esthetic solution for a full coverage restoration is an **all ceramic restoration** or all ceramic crown. Teeth are prepared with a wide chamfer completely around the tooth. There is no internal metal support under the porcelain, permitting increased translucency that more closely resembles a natural tooth (seen on all maxillary anterior teeth in Color Plate 21).

Even when little or no caries or breakdown is evident, a crown may be recommended if the tooth is cracked or when needed to support an adjacent false tooth (pontic) that replaces a missing tooth. The crowned teeth and the replaced tooth or teeth together are called a **fixed dental prosthesis** (also called a fixed partial denture [FPD] or a fixed bridge) (*Fig. 13-41*). The false tooth is called a **pontic**, and the teeth that are crowned on either side that are attached to and support the pontic are called the **abutment teeth**, which are covered by their crowns called **retainers**. An FPD replacing tooth #4 with an abutment metal ceramic crown on tooth #5 and a complete veneer crown (CVC) on tooth #3 is shown in Figure 13-41. The metal pontic replacing #4 is veneered with porcelain.

In the 1980s and 1990s, techniques for replacing lost teeth with **dental implants** (titanium alloy roots surgically embedded into the bone) were perfected and are now widely used (*Fig. 13-42*). A dental implant

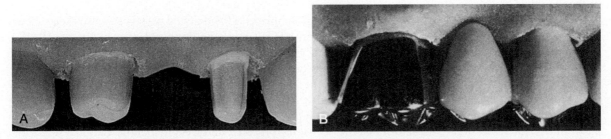

FIGURE 13-41. Fixed dental prosthesis (fixed partial denture or bridge). **A.** Buccal view of full crown preparation on tooth #3 (on left) and a crown veneer preparation on tooth #5 for the attachment of a bridge to replace tooth #4. **B.** The completed three-tooth fixed partial denture (bridge) for replacing tooth #4. The premolar **retainer** (abutment tooth crown) and **pontic** (replacement tooth) in the photograph are porcelain veneered to metal.

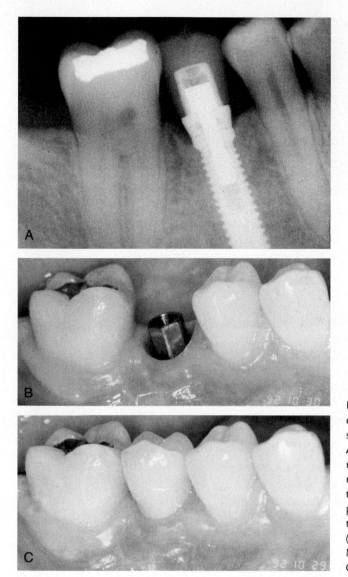

FIGURE 13-42. An implant. Tooth #29 has been extracted and replaced with a dental implant. It supports a crown veneered with porcelain. **A.** A radiograph of the implant with the screw-retained component and crown. **B.** The screw-retained component (crown support) attached to the implant and extending above the tissue prior to placement of the crown. **C.** The crown cemented on the screw-retained component of the implant. (Photographs courtesy of Ed McGlumphy, D.D.S., M.S., Associate Professor, Ohio State University, College of Dentistry.)

involves embedding an artificial root (titanium alloy) into the bone. Three to six months after surgical placement, the embedded implant can be used to provide retention for a crown or a screw-retained fixed dental prosthesis, or to provide support for a removable partial denture. Ten-year success rates of 91% for dental implants in the mandible have been reported.[28]

Groups of lost teeth can also be replaced with multiple implants, a fixed dental prosthesis (also called a fixed partial denture or bridge), or a **removable dental prosthesis** (also called a removable partial denture [RPD]). One type of removable dental prosthesis is made of an acrylic saddle over the edentulous area that contains the artificial replacement tooth crowns, and a **framework** (usually metal) that provides stability and retention (*Fig. 13-43A*). The part of the framework that connects the left and right sides of the prosthesis is called a **major connector**. The framework also contains **clasps**, which surround abutment teeth and adapt to these teeth just cervical to the height of contour facially or lingually to provide retention. It also has **rests** that are designed to adapt into small depressions (**rest seats**) that the dentist has prepared in the enamel of the marginal ridges and adjacent tooth structure in order to keep the partial denture from seating too firmly against the mucosa. When all teeth have been lost, a **complete removable dental prosthesis** (also called a complete denture [CD] or false teeth) can be constructed (*Fig. 13-43B*).

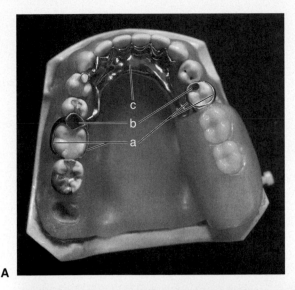

FIGURE 13-43. A. **Removable dental prosthesis** on a typodont replacing teeth #30 and 31, and attached to abutment teeth #19 and 29 using **clasps** (a) and **rests** (b) that retain and position the prosthesis in the mouth. The **major connector** (c) of the metal framework that connects the left and right sides of the prosthesis has a **linguoplate** that adapts to the lingual surfaces of all of the mandibular anterior teeth, providing additional stability. **B. Complete removable dental prosthesis.** The upper denture on the left is designed to cover the palate, while the lower denture on the right is designed to maintain room for the tongue.

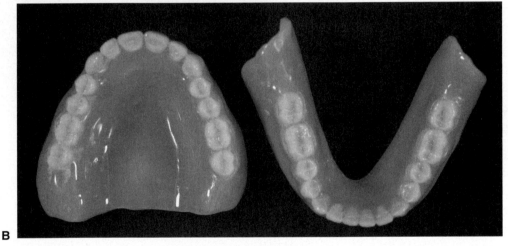

LEARNING EXERCISE

Without looking at the key to each photograph of restorations in this chapter, identify the material used, the surfaces involved, and the abbreviation that could be used to denote the restoration. Do the same with extracted teeth that have existing restorations. Looking in your mouth using a mirror or in a friend's mouth, identify the classification of the existing restorations (according to Dr. G.V. Black). Note that some restorations are extended over more of the tooth than others. Could this be because the dentist extended the preparations, or was it due to the spread of caries? Do you suspect any areas of decay? (If so, check with a dentist.)

LEARNING QUESTIONS

Answer each of the following test items by selecting the correct answer, or answers, for each item.

1. What is the class of decay found in the buccal pit of tooth #19?
    a. class I
    b. class II

    c. class III

    d. class IV

    e. class V

2. Which material is more likely to be used for a *conservative* class III restoration (mesial and facial surfaces) on tooth #8?

    a. amalgam

    b. cast gold crown

    c. composite resin

    d. cast porcelain inlay

    e. cast gold onlay

3. Caries in the cingulum area of tooth #7 is an example of which class of caries?

    a. class I

    b. class II

    c. class III

    d. class IV

    e. class V

4. Throughout the end of the 20th century, has dental caries occurrence in children increased, decreased, or stayed about the same?

    a. increased

    b. decreased

    c. stayed about the same

5. Which class(es) of caries occur(s) in posterior teeth, but not in anterior teeth?

    a. class I

    b. class II

    c. class III

    d. class IV

    e. class V

6. Which class(es) of caries occur(s) in anterior teeth, but not in posterior teeth?

    a. class I

    b. class II

    c. class III

    d. class IV

    e. class V

7. A point angle is the junction of how many cavity preparation walls?

    a. one

    b. two

    c. three

    d. four

    e. five

8. Which of the following are point angles in a conservative class I preparation (if it has not extended onto the buccal or lingual surfaces to include buccal or lingual grooves)?

    a. gingivobuccoaxial

    b. occlusobuccoaxial

   c. mesiobuccopulpal

   d. distolinguopulpal

   e. buccolinguopulpal

9. Which of the following are line angles *within* a DO-A preparation?

   a. axiobuccal

   b. axiopulpal

   c. distopulpal

   d. distoaxial

   e. mesiopulpal

ANSWERS: 1-a; 2-c; 3-a; 4-b; 5-b; 6-c, d; 7-c; 8-c, d; 9-a, b, e

REFERENCES

1. DiOrio LP. Clinical preventive dentistry. East Norwalk, CT: Appleton-Century-Crofts, 1983.
2. Newbrun E. Problems in caries diagnosis. Int Dent J 1993;43:133–142.
3. Powell LV. Caries risk assessment: relevance to the practitioner. JADA 1998;129:349–353.
4. National Caries Program. The prevalence of caries in U.S. children, 1979–80. NIH Publication No. 82–2245, December 1981.
5. Brown JL, Wall TP, Lazar V. Trends in total caries experience: permanent and primary teeth. JADA 2000;131:223–231.
6. American Dietetic Association. Position of the American Dietetic Association: oral health and nutrition. Available at www.eatright.org/aoral.html.
7. Hicks MJ, Flaitz CM. Epidemiology of dental caries in the pediatric and adolescent population: a review of past and current trends. J Clin Pediatr Dent 1993;18:43–49.
8. Heinrich R, Heinrich J, Kunzel W. Prevalence of root caries in women. Z Stomatol 1989;86:241–247.
9. Robertson T. Sturdevant's art and science of operative dentistry. 4th ed. St. Louis: C.V. Mosby, 2002.
10. Baum L, Phillips RW, Lund MR. Textbook of operative dentistry. Philadelphia: Saunders, 1995.
11. Black GV. A work on operative dentistry. Vol. 1. Chicago: Medico-Dental Publishing Company, 1908;203–234.
12. Hannigan, A, O'Mullane DM, Barry D. Caries susceptibility classification of tooth surfaces by survival time. Caries Res 2000;34:103–108.
13. Radike AW. Criteria for diagnosis of dental caries. In: Proceedings of the Conference on the Clinical Testing of Cariostatic Agents. Chicago: American Dental Association, 1972.
14. Leinfelder KF. Posterior composite resins. JADA 1988;11(Special Issue):21E–26E.
15. Roulet JF. The problems associated with substituting composite resins for amalgam: a status report on posterior composites. J Dent 1988;16:101–113.
16. Ishikawa A. 10-year clinical evaluation of a posterior composite resin [Abstract 2178]. J Dent Res 1996;75:290.
17. Leinfelder KF. Posterior composite resins: the materials and their clinical performance. JADA 1995;126(May): 663–676.
18. Kugel G, Ferrari M. The science of bonding: from first to sixth generation. JADA 2000;131:20S–25S.
19. Shaw K. Root caries in the older patient. Dent Clin North Am 1997;41(4):763–793.
20. Nathanson D, Riis D. Advances and current research on ceramic restorative materials. Curr Opin Cosmetic Dent 1993;34–40.
21. Leinfelder KF. Porcelain esthetics for the 21st century. JADA 2000;131:47S–51S.
22. Leinfelder KF. Advances in biorestorable materials. JADA 2000;131:35–41.
23. Simonsen RJ. The clinical effectiveness of a colored sealant at 36 months. J Dent Res 1980;59:406.
24. Simonson RJ. Preventive resin restorations: three-year results. JADA 1980;100:535.
25. Craig RG, O'Brien WJ, Powers JM. Dental materials properties and manipulation. 3rd ed. St. Louis: C.V. Mosby; 1983:33–44.
26. Harris NO, Cristen G. Primary preventive dentistry. Reston, VA: Reston Publishing, 1982.
27. Guirguis R, Lee J, Conry J. Microleakage evaluation of restorations prepared with air abrasion. Pediatric Dent 1999;21,6:311–315.
28. Rosenstiel S, Land M, Fujimoto J. Contemporary fixed prosthodontics. 3rd ed. St. Louis: Mosby, Inc., 2001.

14 Guidelines for Drawing, Sketching, and Carving Teeth

I. Drawing teeth
   A. Materials needed
   B. How to accurately reproduce a tooth outline
   C. Example: accurately reproduce the shape of a mandibular canine (copying an actual tooth or tooth model)

II. Sketch teeth recognizably from memory

III. Carving teeth
   A. Materials needed
   B. How to carve a tooth
   C. Example: how to carve a maxillary central incisor
   D. Notes

OBJECTIVES

This chapter is designed to prepare the learner to perform the following:
- Carefully draw a tooth to reproduce its contours precisely from various views.
- From memory, sketch (quickly) teeth from various views, so the sketch is recognizable as the tooth being sketched.
- Reproduce the contours of a tooth in wax.

SECTION I   DRAWING TEETH

A. MATERIALS NEEDED

- Graph paper ruled eight squares to the inch
- Drawing pencil, sharpened to a fine point
- Eraser
- Ruler with millimeter scale
- Boley gauge
- Teeth or tooth model
- Chart with dimensions of tooth to be drawn (such as Table 3-2)

B. HOW TO ACCURATELY REPRODUCE A TOOTH OUTLINE

To accurately reproduce the outline of any object, not only must you must look at the object, but you must also see or visualize it. Rarely is there a person, however lacking in artistic skill, who cannot make a reasonably good drawing of a human tooth. Those who are not skilled in accurate drawing (extensive art training does not necessarily result in accuracy of outline) may find a solution in using graph paper ruled eight squares to the inch. The tooth specimen is measured in millimeters with a Boley gauge, and the measurements are transferred to the graph paper, allowing one square to equal 1 mm. Drawings may be made to scale of each type of tooth: maxillary and mandibular incisors, canines, premolars, and molars. All drawings should depict maxillary teeth with crowns down and mandibular teeth with crowns up, the same orientation they have in the mouth.

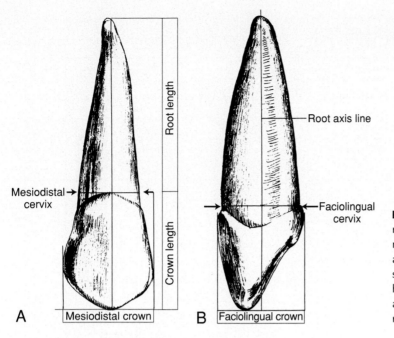

FIGURE 14-1. A. Facial side of a maxillary right canine tooth model showing how measurements of a tooth may be made to assist in drawing and carving. **B.** Mesial side of the same maxillary canine showing how tooth measurements can be made and how the incisal portion is positioned relative to the root axis line.

Using an undamaged extracted tooth or tooth model for a specimen, make the following six measurements with the Boley gauge *(Fig. 14-1A and B)*:

- Crown length
- Mesiodistal crown
- Faciolingual crown
- Root length
- Mesiodistal cervix
- Faciolingual cervix

Using a consistent method of measurement avoids confusion. On anterior teeth, measure the crown length on the facial side from the cervical line to the incisal edge. On premolars, measure the crown length on the facial side from the cervical line to the tip of the buccal cusp. On molars, which have more than one buccal cusp, crown length is always to the mesiobuccal cusp tip. Make the other cusps their proper length relative to the measured cusp, that is, either longer or shorter. With more than one root, the overall tooth length will be from the mesial or mesiobuccal root apex to the mesiobuccal cusp (refer to Table 3-2).

Plan how you want to place your drawings on the graph paper. One convenient arrangement is facial aspect, upper left corner; lingual aspect, upper right; mesial aspect, lower left; distal aspect, lower right; and incisal aspect, center *(Figs. 14-2 and 14-3)*. These views will be centered nicely if you allow a four-square border on all sides as shown in the same illustrations.

C. EXAMPLE: ACCURATELY REPRODUCE THE SHAPE OF A MANDIBULAR CANINE (COPYING AN ACTUAL TOOTH OR TOOTH MODEL)

1. FACIAL VIEWS

Use the measurements you have made of the tooth specimen you intend to draw. In the upper left corner of the page, count down from the upper four-square border the number of squares and fraction thereof equal to the crown length in millimeters and draw a horizontal line. From this line, count down the number of squares equal to the root length in millimeters and draw a second horizontal line. From the inside of the left four-square border, count to the right the number of squares equal to the mesiodistal crown measurement and draw a vertical line. You will

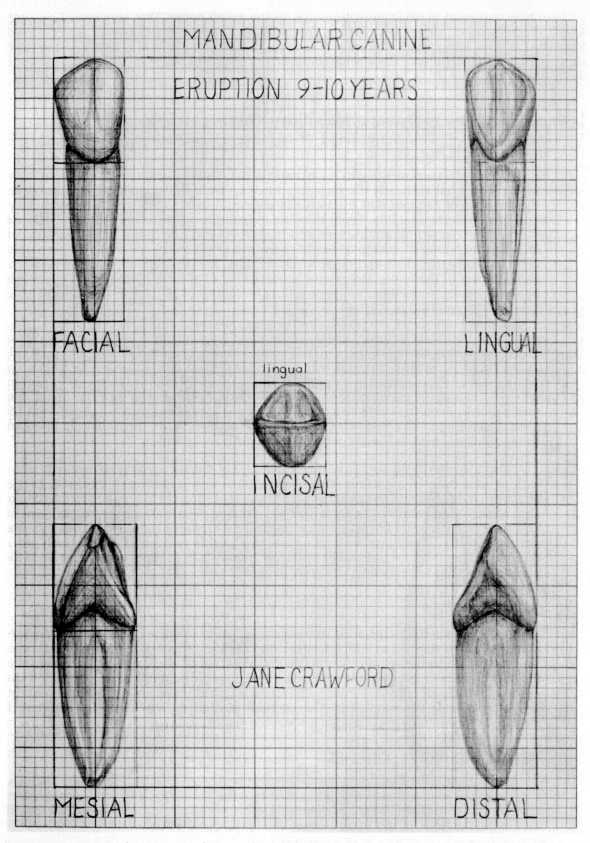

FIGURE 14-2. A precise drawing on graph paper of a model of a mandibular right canine by a first-year dental hygiene student.

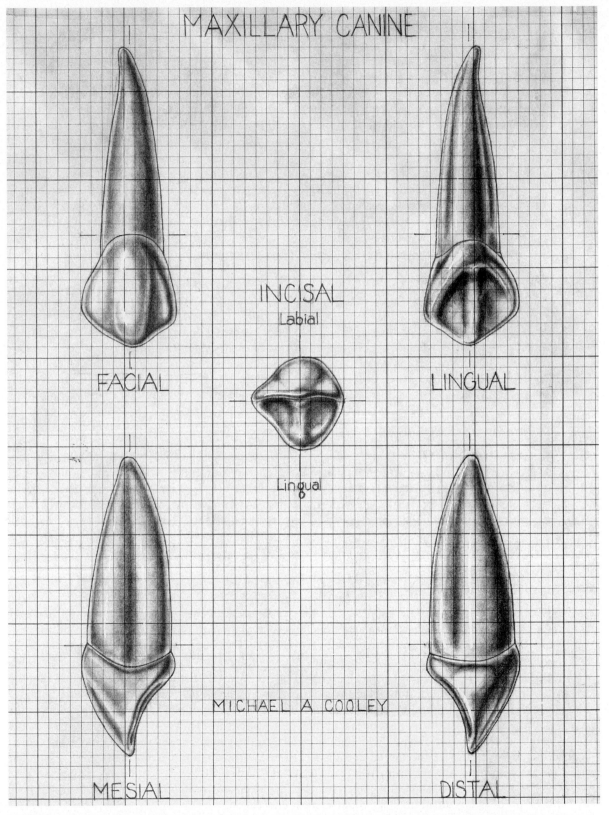

FIGURE 14-3. Professional drawing (by medical artist) of a model of a maxillary canine based on dimensions given in Table 3-2.

draw the facial aspect of the tooth inside the box. Make your lines *very light at first*, so that corrections can be made easily. Remember to begin from the four-square margin (top and side) as seen in Figure 14-2.

Before you start to draw, make a light mark at the locations of the mesial and distal contact areas of the crown. (A pencil or straight edge held against the side of the tooth parallel to the root axis line will help you determine where to put the small marks.) Also, mark the location of the apex of the root. Estimate the location mesiodistally of the cervix of the tooth. When you fit the crown into the box, if you remember to keep the root vertical, the axis will not always be an equal distance from the mesial and distal sides because the crowns of some teeth are tilted distally. Mark off the mesiodistal cervical measurement very lightly.

Now draw in the curvature of the crown at the contact areas (you marked the location) and draw in a portion of the cervical line and the incisal cusp ridges. Draw the root apex and the cervical part of the root. Correct any errors in location or shape, and then connect the lines you have drawn. You have a drawing of a tooth. You may be pleasantly surprised how natural and morphologically correct this first sketch appears. Many professional artists are unable to depict natural teeth accurately because they are unfamiliar with tooth morphology, and they do not have the proportions that were dictated by your measurements.

2. LINGUAL VIEWS

In the upper right corner of the page (Fig. 14-2) use the same set of measurements to make the box in which to draw the lingual aspect of the tooth. Remember that almost all teeth taper toward the narrower lingual surface, but the overall outline from the lingual is the same width as from the facial view. The cingulum is narrower than the cervical portion on the labial sketch, and it should be drawn centered or a little toward the distal.

3. MESIAL AND DISTAL VIEWS

Draw these two boxes in the lower left and right corner of the page (Fig. 14-2) using the same root and crown lengths. However, use the faciolingual crown measurement instead of the mesiodistal measurement. Before you start to draw the tooth, lightly mark the locations of the incisal edge, the labial crest of curvature (that is, where the curve or greatest convexity of the labial surface will touch the line of the box), and the crest of curvature on the cingulum (Fig. 14-1B) and the root tip. Mark the faciolingual width of the cervix. Then draw the tooth. Remember to leave the four-square border at each side and below these views.

4. INCISAL VIEW

Near the center of the page draw a box with the distance between the upper and lower horizontal lines the exact number of squares for the faciolingual measurement of the crown in millimeters. The distance between right and left vertical lines of this box should equal the number of the squares of the mesiodistal crown measurement in millimeters. Hold the tooth facial side down and in such a position that you are looking exactly in line with the root axis line. Be sure that the tooth is not tilted up or down. On the sides of the box, mark the places where you are going to put the mesioincisal and distoincisal angles. The incisal edge of the tooth will normally have a slight lingual twist of the distoincisal corner (not evident in Fig. 14-2) and will lie either in the center of the box faciolingually or slightly lingual to the center (in the same position it is shown on your drawings of the mesial and distal aspects). The cingulum is normally centered on, or slightly distal to, the root axis line.

Do you find any straight lines (ruler-straight, that is) on any tooth other than those lines that have been produced by attrition? This would be most unusual.

Using the same approach, you will be able to draw other types of teeth. Labeling the grooves, the fossae, and the ridges on the occlusal surfaces of the posterior teeth will help to fix the morphology in your mind.

SECTION II   SKETCH TEETH RECOGNIZABLY FROM MEMORY

The extremely precise and accurate drawings described in Section I of this chapter have the value of developing skills to accurately visualize and reproduce the subtle outlines and exact grooves of a specific tooth from various views. However, this time-consuming method of copying teeth may have limited value in helping the student to quickly *sketch* a tooth from memory for a specified view as might be expected during a conversation with an instructor or a patient. Therefore, the authors are including guidelines that can be useful for dental and dental hygiene students when learning how to *quickly* sketch a specific tooth and view from memory.

In order to sketch a recognizable tooth from memory, the drawer must have knowledge of the following characteristics related to the tooth being drawn: (a) approximate crown-to-root ratio (that is, how much longer is the root compared to the crown); (b) approximate crown proportions (width compared to length); (c) location of the crown heights of contour (crests of curvature); (d) crown shape (taper, incisal edge shape or number and relative size of cusps, and cementoenamel junction shape); and when drawing the entire tooth, (e) root shape (taper and number of roots). If one considers each of these tooth characteristics in the appropriate order, sketching a tooth becomes a relatively easy task, and is an excellent exercise to apply all of the knowledge of dental morphology that has been presented throughout this text.

As an example, consider a sketch of *a right maxillary central incisor from the facial view*. Follow along with Figure 14-4 as you read about each step.

Step A: Consider the **root-to-crown ratio**. It is not expected that a student will remember the exact ratio of this tooth (1.16 to 1), but rather the student should recall that all roots are normally longer than the crown. On maxillary central incisors, the root is only *slightly* longer than the crown. Based on this fact, three parallel horizontal lines can be drawn to denote the distance of the *crown length* from incisal edge to the cervical line *relative to* the *root length* from cervical line to root apex (only slightly longer). Position the smaller *crown length* on top for the mandibular teeth and on the bottom for maxillary teeth. For this maxillary central incisor, the crown length is on the bottom.

Step B: Consider the **proportions of the crown**, that is, the crown height (incisocervically) compared to its width (mesiodistally). Again, you do not need to memorize that the average crown width for this tooth is 8.6 mm and its average length is 11.2 mm, but you should recall that the maxillary central incisor crown is slightly longer than it is wide. Using this knowledge, two parallel *vertical* lines can be placed perpendicular to the horizontal lines to establish the proportion for the tooth crown. Extending these vertical lines along the entire tooth length results in the formation of two boxes: a *crown box* that will surround the crown and a *root box* that will enclose the root. At this time, label the mesial (M) and distal (D) surfaces of the crown box that is dependent on whether you are viewing a right or left incisor. For this right incisor, the mesial surface is on the right side and the distal is on the left side, as if you were facing the patient.

Step C: Consider the **heights of contour** (crests of curvature) on the mesial and distal surfaces. Since these two points are the widest parts of the tooth crown where the mesial and distal surfaces bulge out the most, they are therefore the points where the crown outline touches the *crown box* established in the previous step. When the teeth are in ideal alignment, they are the location of the proximal contacts. On all incisors, the proximal heights of contour on incisors occur in the incisal one-third and are

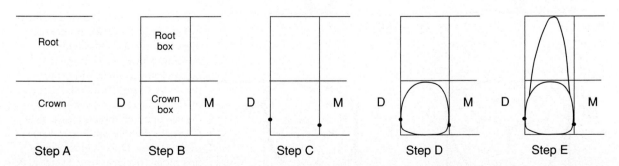

FIGURE 14-4. Five steps involved in **sketching** the facial view of a tooth (in this case, a right maxillary central incisor).

located more incisally on the mesial surface than on the distal surface (EXCEPT on the symmetrical mandibular central incisor). With this knowledge, a dot can be placed on the mesial and distal crown box outline at the appropriate levels. It is not until this step is complete that you actually begin sketching the tooth crown shape (outline).

Step D: Begin sketching the **crown outline**. Use as many of the criteria presented in the Appendix as you can recall to make your sketch recognizable. For example, on a maxillary central incisor, we know that the areas immediately surrounding all contact areas are convex; mesial and distal crown walls taper *slightly* toward the root; and the incisal edge is almost flat or slightly convex and is a little shorter toward the distal. We also know that the cervical line from the facial view is broad and curves toward the apex. Based on this knowledge, begin sketching the crown outline by placing subtle convexities that touch the crown box at the heights of contact points (dots). These convexities blend apically to become the mesial and distal crown walls, and these walls converge (just slightly) toward the cervical line. The proximal convexities also curve incisally to blend with the relatively straight incisal edge that touches the incisal line of the crown box in the mesial half and tapers shorter (farther from the box outline) toward the distal. Finally, the cervical line appears as a continuation of the mesial and distal walls and curves toward the apex, just touching the cervical line of the crown box. If a sketch of the crown is all that you required, you would be finished. If, however, you wish to add the root, proceed to the final step.

Step E: Sketch the **root**. We know that the apex of the root is near or just distal to the center of the tooth root axis (a vertical line in the center of the root at the cervix). We also know that roots are broadest in the cervical third (but not very much narrower than the width of the crown), may be nearly parallel in the cervical third, and taper toward the rounded apex. Based on this knowledge, you can finish the sketch. Be aware that part of the root outline where it joins the crown is actually visible within the *crown box,* and the rounded apex just touches the apical line of the *root box.*

When sketching other teeth from the **facial views**, use steps A through C as described earlier for developing the "boxes" and crests of curvature, and refer to the Appendix pages for tooth traits when sketching the actual tooth outlines. With practice, teeth can be sketched without the boxes in less than a minute while still maintaining the approximate proportions and heights of contour. See the student sketch of a recognizable mandibular second molar from the buccal view in *Figure 14-5A.*

The steps used to sketch the **lingual view** of all teeth are the same as for the facial view EXCEPT the *outline* is a mirror image of the facial view. Also, on this surface of anterior teeth, there is normally evidence of a

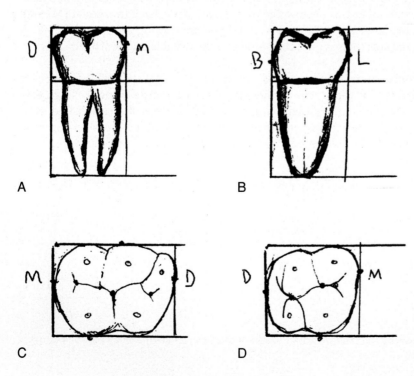

FIGURE 14-5. Four sketches of teeth by first-quarter dental and dental hygiene students. Although not perfectly drawn, each sketch is recognizable as the tooth being drawn. **A.** Right mandibular second molar, facial (buccal) view. **B.** Right mandibular first molar, mesial view. **C.** A right mandibular first molar, occlusal view. **D.** A right maxillary first molar, occlusal view. Sketches **A** and **B** would look nicer if the lines were not so wide and dark.

narrower crown cingulum, marginal ridges, a lingual fossa, and a cervical line that often includes a partial view of the proximal cementoenamel junction due to the taper of teeth toward the lingual. On maxillary molars, the lingual root is now in the foreground.

When sketching the **proximal view** of teeth, the first two steps are similar to steps A and B above except the crown outline box is developed for this view by using the faciolingual and mesiodistal *crown proportions*. The *facial crest of curvature* is similar for **all teeth**: in the cervical third. *Lingually*, the crest of curvature is in the cervical third on the cingulum for anterior teeth, but in the middle third for posterior teeth. Develop a *crown and root shape* according to guidelines in the Appendix. See the student sketch of a mandibular second molar from the mesial view in Figure 14-5B.

Posterior teeth from the **occlusal view** are viewed looking directly down along the axis of the root. Crown-to-root ratios do not apply from this view. The crown outline box is developed for this view by using the mesiodistal and faciolingual *crown proportions*. On **mandibular premolars**, the crown proportions are slightly longer buccolingually than mesiodistally, but close to square. **Maxillary premolars** from the occlusal view are similar to mandibular premolars except crown proportions are less square, more rectangular: proportionally wider buccolingually than mesiodistally. **Mandibular molars** from the occlusal view are wider mesiodistally than buccolingually, whereas **maxillary molars** are slightly wider buccolingually than mesiodistally.

The *crests of curvature* on molars and premolars on the mesial and distal surfaces are located in the center or slightly to the buccal of the buccolingual midline. The buccal and lingual crests of curvature for molars are located mesial to the middle, except on the buccal of the mandibular first molar where it is close to the middle. After the outline "box" is sketched and crests of curvature have been noted, sketch the crown outlines using descriptions from the Appendix pages. An additional challenge on these views involves reproducing the location of the *cusp tips, grooves,* and *pits* (as must be accomplished by dental personnel every time a restoration is placed on an occlusal surface, finished and polished, or constructed or carved in wax in the laboratory).

Cusp tips can be identified by placing small dots or circles on the sketches at these locations. It may be helpful to remember these basic guidelines regarding *pits and grooves*. Most premolars have a mesial and distal pit connected by a groove running mesiodistally between buccal and lingual cusps. Molars (and three-cusped mandibular second premolars) have three pits (mesial, central, and distal) that are also connected by a groove passing mesiodistally between buccal and lingual cusps. Molars also have one or two buccal grooves that separate the two or three buccal cusps, respectively. On mandibular molars, the lingual groove comes off near the central pit, but on maxillary molars, a lingual (distolingual) groove comes off of the distal pit and parallels the oblique ridge. Developmental triangular or fossa grooves or supplemental grooves may angle off from the mesial and distal pits of most posterior teeth, directed toward the "corners" of the tooth. See the student sketches of the occlusal views of two recognizable molars in Figure 14-5C and D.

SECTION III   CARVING TEETH

A.   MATERIALS NEEDED

- Blocks of carving wax (34 × 17 × 17 mm for molars or 32 × 12 × 12 for other teeth)
- Boley gauge (Vernier caliper)
- Millimeter ruler
- Office knife and sharpening stone
- Roach carver, No. 7 wax spatula, and PKT-1 (for melting and adding wax)
- No. 3, No. 5-6, 6C, and PKT-4 carvers
- Sharpened drawing pencil
- Large or small tooth model and its measurements

B.   HOW TO CARVE A TOOTH

Carving a tooth helps you to see the tooth in three dimensions and also to develop considerable manual skill and dexterity. Examples of carvings by dental hygiene students are shown in *Figure 14-6*. While eventually you may be able to carve a tooth from a block of wax without preliminary measurement, the

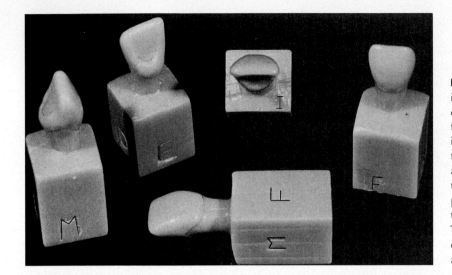

FIGURE 14-6. Maxillary central incisor wax carvings by first-year dental hygiene students as seen from the mesial (M), lingual (L), incisal (I), facial (F), and mesial-facial (M, F) aspects. The crown and half of the root were carved to specific dimensions that were proportional to the tooth model they viewed during the carving. These excellent carvings were each done in less than 3 hours as a required skill test.

beginner can only do well by approaching the carving systematically in the same way you approached the drawings: first, by outlining a box on the wax block; second, by sketching an outline of the tooth in the box; and third, by carving around the sketch or outline, one view or aspect at a time (sequence is shown in Fig. 14-7).

When approaching the task of carving a tooth, consider Michelangelo, who conceived of his task of producing a marble statue by "liberating the figure from the marble that imprisons it." And remember that he, too, sometimes made mistakes and had to discard a half-finished statue [like that of St. Matthew, which appears to the casual observer to be all right from the front, but from the side, the leg, bent at the knee, is seen to be hopelessly out of position]. The same can happen to your tooth carving. To minimize this, as you cut away wax, repeatedly examine your carving from all sides; turn it around and around and compare it with your specimen from each view. Where it is too bulbous, the fault is easily correctable by further reductions. Where too much wax has been removed, you have one of three choices: add molten wax to the deficient region, make the entire carving proportionally smaller, or start with a new block of wax.

C. EXAMPLE: HOW TO CARVE A MAXILLARY CENTRAL INCISOR

Refer to *Figure 14-7* as you follow the following guidelines:

1. Use the measurements you used for drawing. (Again, use the measurement of the buccal cusp on premolars and of the mesiobuccal cusp and mesiobuccal or mesial root on molars.) This consistency of method prevents confusion. Allowance is made for the greater length of some lingual cusps, which are longer than the measured buccal cusp.
2. Shave the sides of the block flat and make all angles right angles.
3. Measure 2 mm from one end of the block and draw a line at this level, encircling the block (on all four sides). (This end of the block will be the incisal or occlusal end of the tooth and the 2-mm allowance here is to provide for the extra length of the lingual cups on molars that are longer than the mesiobuccal cusp that established crown length. Although it is convenient to allow the 2 mm on all carvings, it is essential only for molars.)
4. From the 2-mm line, measure the crown length and draw a second line around the block at this level. This line is the location of the cervical line on the facial, mesial, distal, and lingual sides of the tooth (Fig. 14-7A).
5. From this cervical line, measure one-half of the length of the root and draw a third line around the block. (The end of the block beyond this line will be referred to now as the base.)
6. On the base of the block, carve, on appropriate sides, F (facial), L (lingual), M (mesial), and D (distal). Be sure to put M and D in the proper relation to F and L, so that you will carve a right or a left tooth, whichever you intend.

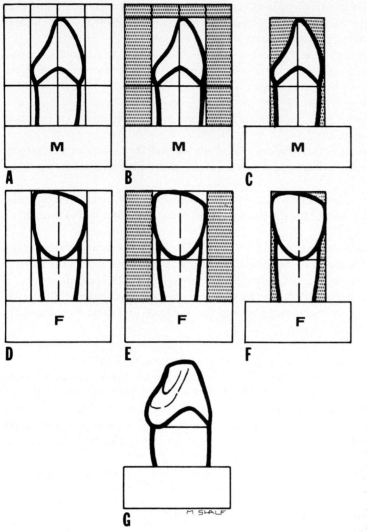

FIGURE 14-7. The sequential method described in this chapter for carving a tooth from a block of wax. The final product should look like those shown in Figure 14-6. The large letter M denotes the mesial aspect of the carving. Likewise, F indicates the facial side of the block.

7. Using a very sharp pencil, draw a shallow line lengthwise on the block in the center of the mesial surface. Do the same on the distal surface and **be sure that these lines are exactly opposite**.

8. Add 0.5 mm to the faciolingual measurement of the crown. Divide this number by 2. Using this measurement, draw a line this distance on either side of the center line on the mesial and distal sides of the block (Fig. 14-7A). These two outer lines should be parallel to the center line and extend from the top of the block to the base. These two lines form a box whose dimension faciolingually is equal to the crown dimension plus 0.5 mm. The extra 0.5 mm is an allowance for safety in carving. Do not make trouble for yourself by allowing more than this extra 0.5 mm.

9. On the *mesial* side of the block marked M, draw, within the box, an outline of the mesial side of the tooth as you drew it on the graph paper. Be careful to place the incisal edge and the labial and lingual crests of curvature accurately. Your carving will probably be no better than this drawing.

10. Draw a similar outline on the *distal* side of the block. Be sure that on both sides, the drawings are oriented so the facial surface of the tooth is toward the side of the block you have marked F. (It is easy to make a mistake here.) These drawings of the crown may appear slightly fat due to the extra 0.5 mm width allowance confining the crown size faciolingually.

11. Carve away the shaded portions of wax in Figure 14-7B from the facial, lingual, and incisal sides of the block so it is now shaped like Figure 14-7C. At this time, do not carve around the outline of the tooth, but rather carve up to the straight vertical lines that form the box in which the tooth picture is drawn.

12. Check the distance between the two parallel carved surfaces carefully with your Boley gauge. Be sure they are perfectly flat and smooth. Be sure the thickness of the column of wax between these parallel surfaces exactly equals the given faciolingual crown dimension plus 0.5 mm.

13. Now carve away the shaded regions seen in Figure 14-7C around and down to the facial and lingual outlines of the tooth. Follow the drawing carefully, making the tooth shape the same all the way through the block. Keep the carving surface smooth; if it becomes chopped up, it will be impossible to smooth it without losing both the shape and the size of the carving.

14. With a sharp pencil, very lightly draw center lines on the curved facial and lingual sides of the carving as in Figure 14-7D. Be sure they are exactly opposite.

15. Add 0.5 mm to the mesiodistal crown measurement and draw two lines one-half this distance on either side of the center line. This makes a box on the curved surface as wide as the greatest mesiodistal crown measurement plus 0.5 mm (Fig. 14-7D).

16. Redraw a horizontal line the exact crown length distance from the incisal edge on the facial and lingual sides (since the original line was carved away). Then draw the facial outline of the crown and half of the root on the curved facial side of the block (Fig. 14-7D).

17. On the lingual surface of the block, draw an outline the same shape as the one on the facial surface except, of course, that it is a mirror image; the distal side of the tooth must be toward the same side of the block in each case. Check the crown length on the lingual surface too, so the crown will not be too long.

18. Carve away all the wax outside the drawing box, removing all the shaded portions as shown in Figure 14-7E. On some first molars their spreading roots may extend beyond the box lines, and these roots should be carved accordingly. Check your measurements again.

19. Shape the tooth by carefully carving the mesial and distal contours by removing the shaded portions of Figure 14-7F, so that it resembles your tooth specimen outline from the facial and lingual sides.

20. Now it is time to round off the corners, narrow the lingual surface, shape the cingulum (it is distal to the center line, and the mesial marginal ridge is longer than the distal), and carve out the lingual fossa. Be sure to look at all aspects of the tooth as you are finishing the carving. Include, of course, the incisal (occlusal) aspect (seen in Fig. 14-6). Four nice carvings of maxillary canines, made by dental hygiene students at Ohio State University, are shown in *Figure 14-8*. Five aspects of another very fine carving by a dental student are seen in *Figure 14-9*.

21. Carve your initials on the bottom of the base of the block. Be an honest critic of your work, constantly looking for regions where the carving could be improved.

You can work toward becoming proficient in drawing teeth by sketching outlines (lightly at first) in the blank boxes that are proportionally the correct size for the view and tooth listed in *Figures 14-10, 14-11*, and *14-13*. You should have a tooth model or extracted tooth specimen to view as you make these sketches. One example of how to sketch teeth into the blank boxes of Figure 14-11 is shown in *Figure 14-12*.

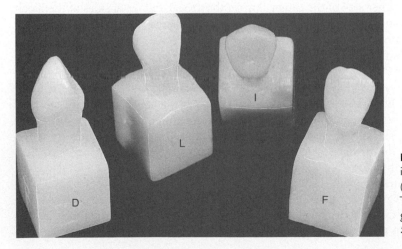

FIGURE 14-8. Maxillary canine wax carvings viewed from the distal (D), lingual (L), incisal (I), and facial (F) aspects. These were done by first-year dental hygiene students during a skill test (2 hours, 50 minutes time limit).

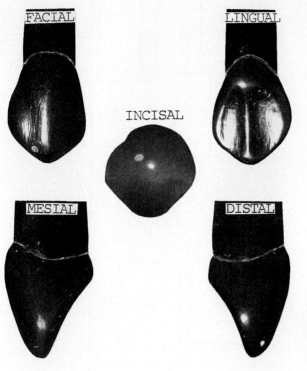

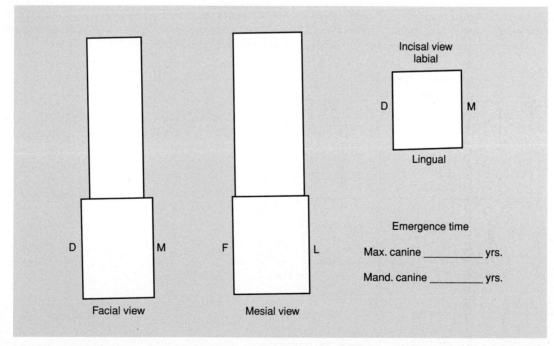

FIGURE 14-9. Maxillary right canine carving done by senior dental student Keith Schmidt. Observe the nearly perfect contours from all aspects and that the root is not becoming narrower as it joins the crown (a very common carving error in attempting to refine the cervical line).

FIGURE 14-10. Outlines within which you may draw three views of a maxillary canine. The boxes are proportional to the natural tooth average measurements in Table 3-2. The widest portions of the crown (mesial and distal contacts) should touch the sides of the wider lower box. Only the widest part of the root should touch the sides of the narrower box above with the root apex touching the top of this box. On the incisal view, be sure to position the incisal ridge just labial to the faciolingual middle of this box. Drawing these three views will be helpful to you when you outline similar contours on a block of wax for carving a maxillary canine.

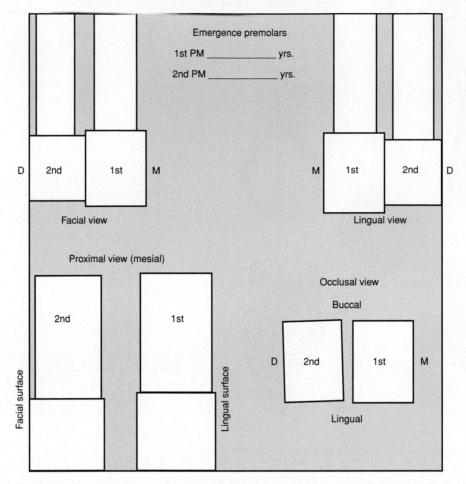

Emergence premolars

1st PM _____ yrs.

2nd PM _____ yrs.

FIGURE 14-11. Outlined proportional boxes for drawing several views of the maxillary first and second premolars in their usual relationship to each other. Use the same guidelines given in the legend for Figure 14-10. A dental hygiene student's drawing of these two teeth within the outlined boxes is seen in Figure 14-12.

Maxillary premolars

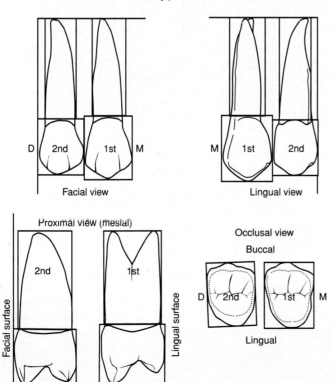

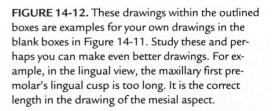

FIGURE 14-12. These drawings within the outlined boxes are examples for your own drawings in the blank boxes in Figure 14-11. Study these and perhaps you can make even better drawings. For example, in the lingual view, the maxillary first premolar's lingual cusp is too long. It is the correct length in the drawing of the mesial aspect.

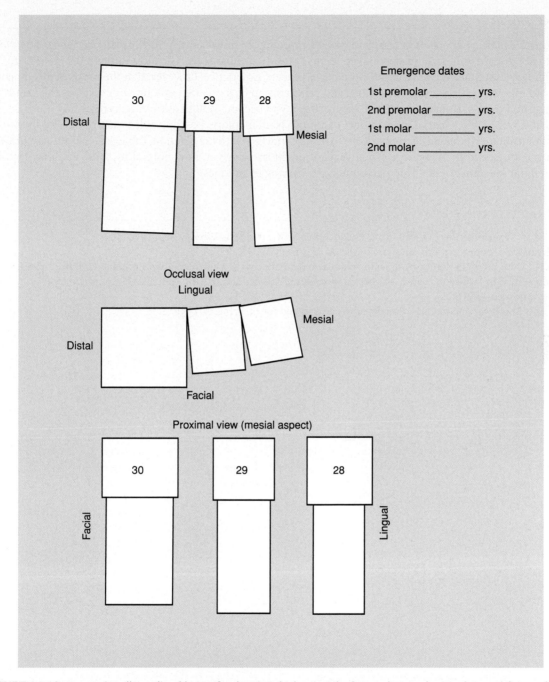

FIGURE 14-13. Proportionally outlined boxes for drawing the lower right first and second premolars and first molar in their usual relationship to one another. Select three nice tooth specimens or tooth models and go to work.

D. NOTES

Practice makes perfect, or at least you will see pronounced improvement in your later carvings. Therefore, do not discard your first ones, but keep them for future comparisons. The most difficult task is to begin for the very first time. We have found from many years of experience, however, that the inexperienced people who follow these or similar directions and proceed step by step often end up with some of the best carvings in the class. Do not be afraid to begin. When you become skillful at carving teeth, it may surprise you that it is possible to carve the contours of a tooth from memory, possibly aided only by several important dimensions. Average measurements from 4572 extracted teeth are given in Table 3-2. Should you draw or carve a tooth to these average dimensions, it might surprise you how normal it looks. You may find the General References helpful in perfecting your carving techniques.

GENERAL REFERENCES

Ash MM Jr. Wheeler's atlas of tooth form. Philadelphia: W.B. Saunders, 1984.

Beaudreau DE. Tooth form and contour. J Am Soc Prev Dent 1973;3:36–37.

Burch JG. Coronal tooth contours: didactic, clinical and laboratory. 3rd ed. Worthington: James G. Burch, 1980.

Grundler H. The study of tooth shapes: a systematic procedure. Berlin: Buch-und Zeitschriften-Verlag "Die Quintessenz," 1976.

Linek HA. Tooth carving manual. Pasadena, CA: Wood and Jones, Printers, 1948.

Forensic Dentistry

15

I. Forensic dentistry defined

II. Dentistry and human identification

III. Civil litigation (including abuse and neglect)

IV. Bite marks

V. Mass disasters

VI. Importance of forensic dentistry to practicing dentists

ACKNOWLEDGMENTS

This chapter was contributed by Daniel E. Jolly, D.D.S., D.A.B.S.C.D., Professor of Clinical Dentistry and Director of the General Practice Residency program at Ohio State University College of Dentistry and University Medical Center. He is a diplomate of the American Board of Special Care Dentistry, Chief Forensic Odontologist for the Franklin County Coroner's Office in Columbus, Ohio, Core team member of the Ohio Dental Association's Forensic and Mass Disaster Team, member of the American Society of Forensic Odontology, and associate member of the American Academy of Forensic Sciences.

Most illustrations shown in this chapter are from cases with which the author was directly involved as part of his duties with the Franklin County Coroner's Office and other agencies in Ohio. The final three figures are from Dr. Theodore Berg, the author of this chapter in previous editions, and are used with permission.

OBJECTIVES

This chapter is designed to prepare the reader to perform the following:

- Cite examples of the importance of dentistry in human identification and crime investigation.
- Recognize the role of the dentist in identifying and reporting cases of abuse.

SECTION I   FORENSIC DENTISTRY DEFINED

Forensic dentistry, or **forensic odontology**, is the area of dentistry that encompasses concepts and practices related to the oral and maxillofacial structures in the context of the legal or judicial system. Forensic odontology is a part of the much larger field of forensic sciences, which includes all the areas of practice and activity used in a judicial setting. The forensic sciences are accepted by the legal system, as well as the scientific community as the means of separating truth and untruth.

Forensic dentistry as a science is represented in the United States by numerous forensic dentistry teams on local levels, including the Odontology Section of the American Academy of Forensic Sciences, the American Board of Forensic Odontology, and the American Society of Forensic Odontology. Each year more dentists become involved as law enforcement becomes increasingly aware of dentistry's potential and reliable contribution.

This chapter provides an overview and introduction to forensic dentistry, while illustrating its elemental dependence on dental anatomy. This textbook is cited in the American Society of Forensic Odontology Manual as the prime dental anatomy reference on this subject.

The forensic sciences include many areas of specialization and special interest. The American Academy of Forensic Sciences (AAFS) is the largest forensic professional organization in the world with over 5600 members worldwide (http://www.aafs.org). The AAFS recognizes 10 areas of forensic endeavors as noted below:

1. **Forensic anthropology** is the study of skeletal evidence in a manner similar to the field of archeology. The forensic anthropologist examines evidence such as bones, teeth, hair, clothing, artifacts, and other aspects

of the scene of a legal matter such as the crime of murder. This person addresses considerations such as time of death, age, sex, race, ethnicity, culture, body size and weight, and cause and manner of death.

2. **Forensic pathology and biology** is the field that uses autopsy techniques and the analysis of tissues in the investigation of a crime or suspicious death such as homicide, suicide, and accidental death or if the subject is unidentified. This duty is legally the responsibility of a coroner or medical examiner with specialized training in pathology and forensic sciences. A forensic pathologist attempts to determine such matters as the cause and manner of death (for example, a gunshot wound to the chest resulting in laceration of the left ventricle, which resulted in cardiac arrest as a result of a homicide).

3. **Criminalistics** is the forensic science that analyzes fingerprints; ballistics; tool marks (knife, saw, hammer, etc.); and other physical evidence from the investigated scene to reconstruct the crime (or other event) and to confirm or eliminate the connection between suspects and victims.

4. **Toxicology** uses chemistry, photography, and biology to identify harmful substances in the victim such as medications, poisons, and illegal drugs.

5. **Forensic psychiatry and behavioral sciences** examine and provide legal opinions regarding such matters as sanity, human motivation, and personality profiles that are relevant to the investigation of an event such as a crime.

6. **Forensic engineering** investigates such events as airplane and other vehicular accidents, as well as structural collapse as part of the legal process.

7. **Questioned documents** is a field where technicians study and provide legal testimony about printing, handwriting, typewriting, ink, paper, and other features of documents.

8. **General forensics** involves other specialists who are qualified to analyze specific evidence such as designers, photographers, and technical experts. They might report, for example, in a case of product liability associated with death or injury.

9. **Forensic jurisprudence** involves criminal and civil lawyers using the earlier described specialists, reports, and testimony to pursue their case in our system of justice.

10. **Forensic odontology** is divided into five major areas: (a) human dental identification, (b) mass disaster human dental identification, (c) bite mark analysis, (d) human abuse, and (e) legal issues such as the standard of care considerations in personal injury cases.

SECTION II   DENTISTRY AND HUMAN IDENTIFICATION

Teeth are the most durable parts of the body, and dentitions are as individual as fingerprints. Therefore, individual tooth morphology, as well as the restorations that exist in teeth, are useful for human identification. Situations involving decomposition and skeletal remains may yield no recognizable facial features or fingerprints. **Postmortem** (after death) teeth, jaws, prostheses, and appliances can yield a positive identification, given the existence and accuracy of **antemortem** (before death) records. Even DNA, a popular and valuable identification tool, relies on accurate and complete antemortem (before death) records. Therefore, accurate, comprehensive, and current radiographs and dental charting are critical to the successful confirmation or elimination of an individual as a victim.

Even with the lack of antemortem records, evaluation of the dentition is a worthwhile aid for investigators to provide information regarding the age, sex, and estimated socioeconomic (sometimes called race or cultural heritage) grouping. This information is derived from tooth and dental arch morphology and anatomy, restorative materials, attrition patterns, periodontal status, eruption patterns, skeletal features, and serology (the study of body fluids like blood).

Forensic dental techniques most commonly include collection and preservation of dental and jaw remains, dental radiographs, photographs, impressions and casts, antemortem and postmortem charting, and the comparison of these records. Points of comparison (specific features) include (a) the number, class, and type of teeth, (b) tooth rotation, spacing, and malposition, (c) anomalies and general morphology (*Fig. 15-1*); (d) restorations (*Fig. 15-2*) and prostheses or appliances (*Fig. 15-3*); (e) caries and other pathology (in some situations); (f) endodontic treatment; (g) implants and surgical repairs; (h) bony trabecular patterns; and (i) occlusion, erosion, and attrition.

DNA can be recovered from periodontal and pulpal tissues, as well as the hard tissues, of the teeth. Although DNA analysis has become an important tool in the forensic science armamentaria, its limitations include high

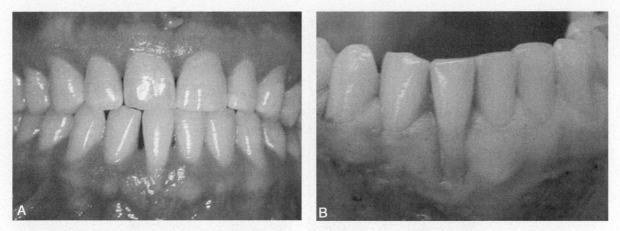

FIGURE 15-1. Comparison of antemortem and postmortem radiographs looking for similarities in general morphology. **A. Antemortem dental photograph** showing gingival clefting. **B. Postmortem photograph** showing similar clefting found in the victim at autopsy. Similar dental arch form is observed as is the overall morphology of the dental coronal structure.

costs and lengthy processing times. And like all methods, the use of DNA requires antemortem information. A DNA collection kit is shown in *Figure 15-4*. Forensic dentistry techniques retain a valuable place in the scope of forensic sciences because of the accuracy, low cost, generally available antemortem records, and speed with which a conclusion can be reached.

The forensic dentist must carefully organize all evidence, so that it is analyzed in a systematic manner using consistent and standardized methods that are easily understood by other professionals and defensible in a legal action. A well-organized and thorough approach results in accurate comparisons and minimizes the chance of error. The examiner should record each feature of the postmortem teeth, jaws, and radiographs on a standardized dental chart (Fig. 15-5B). The same is done for antemortem records, radiographs, casts, and pictures on a

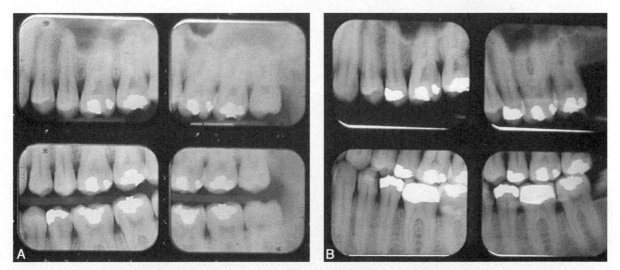

FIGURE 15-2. Comparison of antemortem and postmortem radiographs looking for similarities of restorations and general morphology. **A. Antemortem radiographs** in the same victim shown in Figure 15-1 demonstrate multiple dental restorations, unique root and sinus morphology, pulp chamber shape, interdental bone height, and trabecular patterns. **B. Postmortem radiographs** show consistency in some restorations when compared to the antemortem radiographs, but note that several teeth have had restorations placed after the antemortem radiographs were obtained. For example, an MOA was placed on tooth #13, a crown was placed on tooth #19, an MOA on tooth #20 was replaced with an MODA, and third molars #16 and 17 were extracted. Also noted are identical matching restorations that had not been replaced, as well as the unique root and sinus morphology, pulp chamber shape interdental bone height, and trabecular patterns. This was sufficient to prove positive identification of this individual.

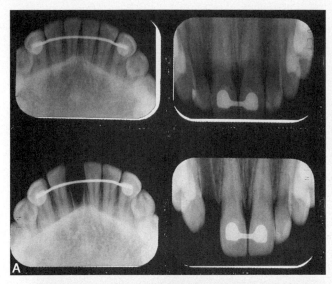

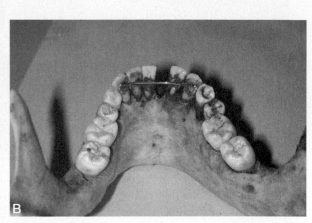

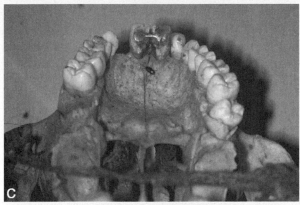

FIGURE 15-3. Comparison of antemortem radiographs with postmortem findings (photographs). A. These radiographs show antemortem (**top**) and postmortem (**bottom**) radiographs of a homicide victim with orthodontic appliances in place, which are identical to actual postmortem findings (seen in **B** and **C**) and served to confirm the identity. Note also the restoration of tooth #10, a peg lateral, that matches as well. **B.** This postmortem photograph shows the orthodontic retainer in the mandibular arch as evident in the antemortem radiographs. **C.** This postmortem photograph shows the orthodontic retainer in the maxillary arch as evident in the antemortem radiographs.

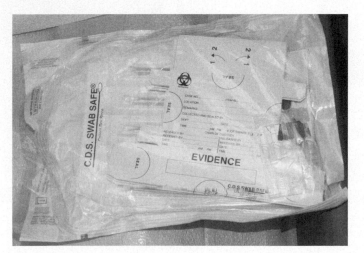

FIGURE 15-4. This is a **DNA collection kit** as used the by the FBI to obtain swabbings of bite marks or other human tissues for comparison to antemortem records.

Antemortem Dental Record ID#: ___05-1111_____

Last: ___Doe_____ First: ___John_____ MI: ___E_____

Date: _3/15/05__ Sex: ___M__ Race: _ C___ Age/DOB : __8/8/1951_____

Height: _____ Weight: ____ Eye: _____ Hair: _____ Blood Type: _____

Team Member: Daniel E. Jolly, DDS

☐ Confirmed by: William Baldwin, DDS

Type, Date, and Number of X-Rays _____

Panorex and 2 bitewings 11/10/04

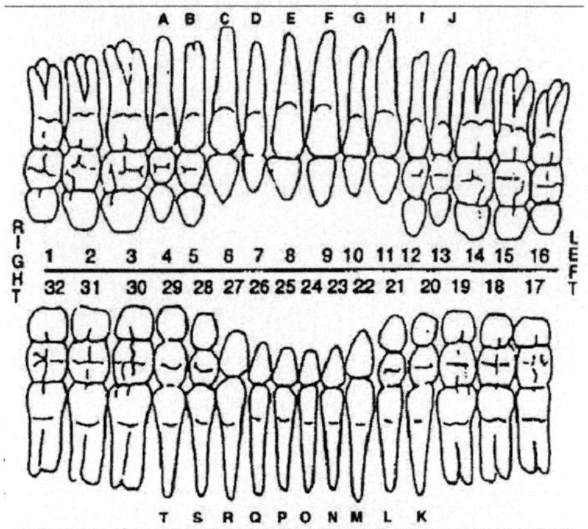

				Description	Code
1	18				OS
2	17				OS
3	16				MODFS
4	15	A	55		V
5	14	B	54	ORTHO EXT	X
6	13	C	53		V
7	12	D	52		V
8	11	E	51		V
9	21	F	61		V
10	22	G	62		V
11	23	H	63		V
12	24	I	64	ORTHO EXT	X
13	25	J	65		V
14	26				OFS
15	27				OFS
16	28				OS
17	38				OS
18	37				OS
19	36				MOS
20	35	K	75		V
21	34	L	74	ORTHO EXT	X
22	33	M	73		V
23	32	N	72		V
24	31	O	71		V
25	41	P	81		V
26	42	Q	82		V
27	43	R	83		V
28	44	S	84	ORTHO EXT	X
29	45	T	85		OS
30	46				OS
31	47				OS
32	48			? OFS	OS

Codes	
Primary Codes	**Secondary Codes**
M - Mesial	A - Annotation
O - Occlusal	B - Decidious
D - Distal	C - Crown
F - Facial	E - Resin
L - Lingual	G - Gold
I - Incisal	H - Porcelain
U - Unerupted	N - Non-precious
V - Virgin	P - Pontic
X - Missing	R - Root Canal
J - Missing Cr	S - Silver Amalgam
/ - NoData	T - Denture Tooth
	Z - Temporary

A: _____

B: _____

C: _____

Comments: _____
____Aircraft crash victim_____
_____
_____

ID As: _____

A

FIGURE 15-5. A. An **antemortem** dental chart using the WinID format and coding. *(continued)*

Postmortem Dental Record   ID#: __05-1111_____

Date: _3/15/05___   Sex: ___M__   Race: __C____   Estimated Age: __53__

Height: _____   Weight: ____   Eye: _____   Hair: _____   Blood Type: _____

Code	Description				
OS				18	1
OS				17	2
MODFS				16	3
V		55	A	15	4
X		54	B	14	5
V		53	C	13	6
V		52	D	12	7
V		51	E	11	8
V		61	F	21	9
V		62	G	22	10
V		63	H	23	11
X		64	I	24	12
V		65	J	25	13
OFLS				26	14
OFS				27	15
OS				28	16
OS				38	17
OFS				37	18
MOFS				36	19
V		75	K	35	20
X		74	L	34	21
DE		73	M	33	22
V		72	N	32	23
V		71	O	31	24
V		81	P	41	25
V		82	Q	42	26
V		83	R	43	27
X		84	S	44	28
OS		85	T	45	29
OFS				46	30
OFS				47	31
OFS				48	32

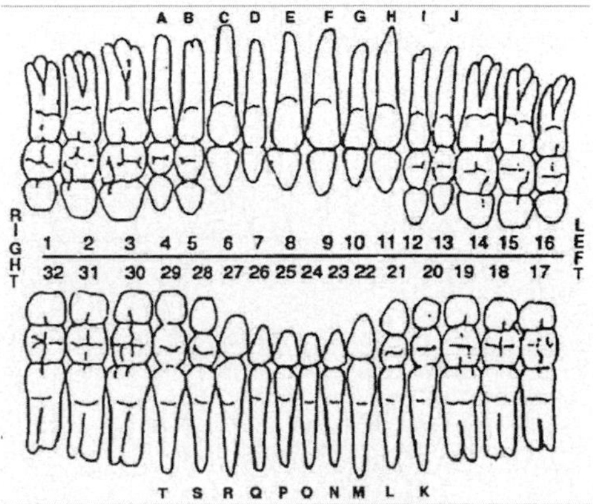

Comments: _____
_____
_____

Copyright © 2001 James McGivney, DMD

Team member: Daniel E. Jolly, DDS

☐ Confirmed by: William Baldwin, DDS

Type and Number of X-Rays _____

_____Full mouth radiographs with bitewings____

WinID Codes	
Primary Codes	**Secondary Codes**
M - Mesial	A - Annotation
O - Occlusal	B - Decidious
D - Distal	C - Crown
F - Facial	E - Resin
L - Lingual	G - Gold
I - Incisal	H - Porcelain
U - Unerupted	N - Non-precious
V - Virgin	P - Pontic
X - Missing	R - Root Canal
J - Missing Cr	S - Silver Amalgam
/ - NoData	T - Denture Tooth
	Z - Temporary

A: _____
B: _____
C: _____

Body ID As: _____

B

FIGURE 15-5. *(continued)*, **B.** A **postmortem** dental chart using the WinID format and coding. Notice how the two forms can be placed side by side for easy comparison.

separate, but identical, chart *(Fig. 15-5A)*. Antemortem records vary widely in quality and completeness. Some dentists mount radiographs as viewed from the front of the patient (with the film bump facing toward the viewer), which is the standard in forensic dentistry, while others still prefer mounting them as viewed from the lingual (film bump facing away from the viewer). Charting tooth identification in dental offices (the antemortem record) is not always done using the Universal system. (See Chapter 3 for other tooth identification systems such as Palmer and the FDI or International systems.)

A real test of the value of dental identification is found in the case of John Wayne Gacy of Chicago, convicted of 33 counts of murder. Only five of the human remains found still had soft tissue, making the identification process a challenge. However, 20 of the 33 known victims were identified through their dental records.

<table>
<tr><td>SECTION III</td><td>CIVIL LITIGATION INCLUDING HUMAN ABUSE AND NEGLECT</td></tr>
</table>

Civil litigation (violations of the standard of care or malpractice) and human abuse and/or neglect are two distinct areas of endeavor for the forensic dentist. Due to the focus of this text (the relevance of dental anatomy), only brief comments will be made about these topics.

In **civil litigation** cases, a person might claim that improper dental care was rendered (malpractice) as illustrated in the radiographs in *Figure 15-6*; damage was sustained at the hands of another person (criminal assault and battery); damage was sustained due to food contaminated with a foreign body (glass, shell, etc.) (product or corporate liability); or a dentist failed to provide specific treatment that had been billed to the patient and/or third-party payor (fraud). Investigators of these situations often require examinations, comparisons, and testimony by expert witnesses including the forensic dentist. This may involve examining a person and studying records and radiographs from prior dentists. All of the techniques and careful comparisons described previously are useful.

Dentists and other health caregivers have a responsibility to report suspected **abuse and neglect** of their patients by others. This includes recognition and differentiation of the signs, symptoms, and body areas involved in accidents compared to the injuries that are sustained by a child, a spouse (male or female), or an elderly or disabled individual. One abuse scenario is described here. A young adult male brought his girlfriend into the dental office for emergency treatment of several broken front teeth and lacerated lips. The woman was silent

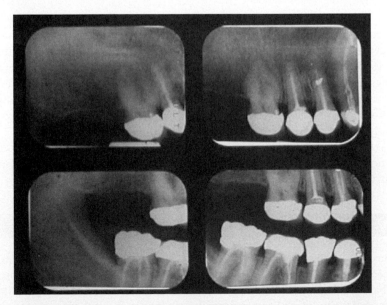

FIGURE 15-6. These bitewing radiographs were used in a **standard-of-care** case. One can see marginal discrepancies between tooth contours and restoration contours (especially on the mesial crown margin on tooth #3) and poor endodontic procedures that are the basis for the malpractice claim.

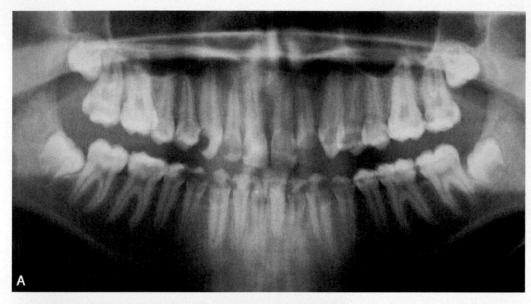

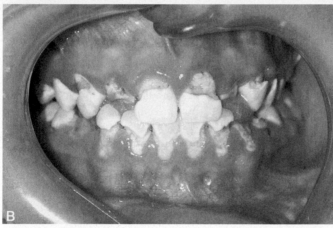

FIGURE 15-7. A. This is a Panorex radiograph of a 14-year-old girl showing rampant caries that progressed over many years resulting in a treatment recommendation to extract all teeth. This evidence of **parental neglect** was reason for the dentist to contact legal authorities for suspected child abuse/neglect. **B.** This is a photograph of this same 14-year-old girl showing rampant dental caries.

while the man related an accident as the cause of the injuries. The man insisted on being present during the treatment and was evasive about answering questions. As required by all state laws, the situation was reported immediately to the appropriate law enforcement agency. The dentist's suspicions had been aroused sufficiently regarding the incongruity of the story and the injuries sustained. Toward the end of treatment, the police arrived, and the man was arrested. Radiographs, the dental record, and the dentist's testimony were critical since the victim was fearful of future revenge from her abuser. Injuries the dentist might observe include fractured bones and teeth, bruises, lacerations, and bite marks.

Neglecting dental pathology is also a reportable and potentially criminal offense. As often seen by this author, children may not be taken to a dentist for treatment of dental caries. This can result in pain and infection and in some cases may result in the loss of all teeth at an early age *(Fig. 15-7)*.

SECTION IV   BITE MARKS

Bite marks are in the category described as pattern injuries. Pattern injuries can result from teeth, belt buckles, and other blunt objects such as a hammer or pipe. Homicides and assault and battery cases have been solved by bite mark identification, analysis, and comparison. Many bites are severe and leave telltale marks long after an assault. One of several techniques of comparison and analysis is shown here, comparing bite mark tracings to the suspect's or defendant's tooth imprint pattern tracings. Dental casts and photographs from the suspect or suspects are made after obtaining a court-ordered search warrant *(Fig. 15-8A and B)*.

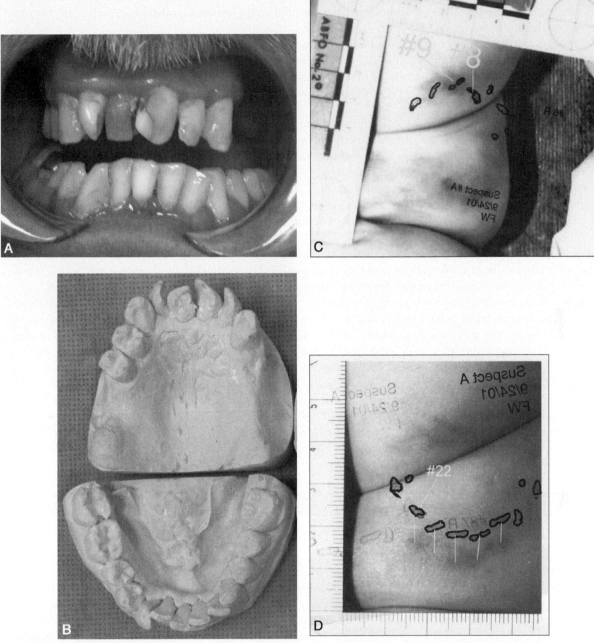

FIGURE 15-8. Bite mark evidence. A. A photograph of the dentition of the perpetrator of child abuse of a 2-year-old girl resulting in her death. **B.** Models of the suspect show a distinct dental pattern that matches well to the injuries depicted in **C. C.** This photograph shows the bite marks on the victim depicting the relationship of the maxillary teeth as shown in **A** and **B. D.** This photograph shows the bite marks on the victim depicting the relationship of the mandibular teeth as shown in **A** and **B.**

In all cases of bite mark analysis, the forensic dentist must have a thorough knowledge and understanding of tooth morphology, occlusion, dental arch characteristics, and the physiology of jaw function. Teeth that are malpositioned, not in occlusion, fractured, or restored may not leave the same mark on a victim as teeth that are in ideal alignment. This aberration from normal (or differences from one suspect to another) could benefit the forensic dentist in analysis and identification.

Although these techniques can be useful in solving some child abuse cases, assaults, and homicide, bite marks cannot generally be used to a level of absolute certainty in suspect identification. A potential suspect is either "ruled out or eliminated" as the perpetrator of the crime or "included" as a suspect. (See Figure 15-8C and D.) Additional evidence is usually required to obtain a firm conviction. However, in this author's experience, suspects often admit their guilt prior to trial when faced with a forensic dentist who would testify in court regarding the bite mark.

Photography can be used to assist bite mark identification. Color and black-and-white film photography is still the standard, but digital photography has become fairly well accepted. The use of infrared photography can be used to identify subcutaneous evidence of damage from a bite mark that is not visible on the surface of the skin. Ultraviolet photography can serve to depict a bite mark in an area with extraneous other marks such as tattoos and skin damage.

The forensic dentist must first establish the mark as a human bite mark, then identify, if possible, the teeth involved in the mark. Aberrations include teeth that are missing, extruded (supererupted), hypoerupted or ankylosed, rotated (torsiversion), tilted, chipped, and anomalous. The chapter in this text on anomalies should be reason enough to remain open-minded and diligent when considering bite marks! The dental forensic examiner must also consider the possibility of animal bites, victim self-bites, and marks from foreign objects that might be mistaken for a bite mark. Separate analysis of those markings may be useful to law enforcement agencies by connecting the victim's injuries to a tool or instrument owned by a suspect.

A bite mark may also provide DNA evidence of the perpetrator of the crime. Techniques are available to obtain this information. Today, when DNA can be collected, amplified, and analyzed with the standard accepted modern methods (for example, polymerase chain reaction [PCR]) of mitochondrial or nuclear DNA), it is possible to quantify the numerical probability of the association between the biter and the bite mark injury.

Law enforcement agencies are becoming increasingly aware of potential identifications from the dental profession. In a landmark bite mark case in California, *State v. Marx*, Dr. G. Vale, a forensic dentist, recognized bite marks on the autopsy photograph of a nose. After alerting investigators, the body was exhumed and studied with the resultant identification and conviction of the murderer based on the victim's nose bite mark and the suspect's dentition! An appeal was made to the Supreme Court on the grounds that the dental techniques were unique, untested, and not scientific. The appeal was denied, making this the first US bite mark case to withstand the appellate process. Thus, the reliability of this method of identification was legally verified [People (of California) versus Marx, 54 Cal. App. 3rd 100, 126 Cal. Reptr. 350, Dec. 29, 1975]. Since the outcome of the decision in this landmark case, it has been cited many times in most state, federal, and military courts.

The notorious mass murderer Ted Bundy (executed January 1989) was positively identified as the perpetrator by his bite marks found on the buttocks of one of his young female victims.

SECTION V   MASS DISASTERS

Mass disasters are relatively common occurrences in our world and are of various forms. Most of us vividly recall the mass disaster that occurred on September 11, 2001, at the World Trade Center in New York City as well as at the Pentagon and in Pennsylvania. However, there are many natural disasters that cause mass fatalities. These include the August and September 2005 hurricanes (Katrina, Rita, and Wilma) affecting the Gulf Coast of the United States, the December 2004 tsunami in Indonesia and the Indian Ocean, and other hurricanes, earthquakes, floods, and tornados. Manmade mass disasters include the various forms of terrorist acts, armed conflicts, building collapses, large freeway motor vehicle accidents, industrial accidents, airplane crashes, and train wrecks. Mass disasters cannot be predicted with any accuracy, but they will certainly continue to happen in our immediate future and beyond.

The role of the forensic dentist in mass disasters is primarily to identify human remains. Knowledge of dental anatomy is crucial to this role. Human fatalities in mass disasters can number from a relative handful of individuals to thousands or hundreds of thousands. Management of small disasters can be relatively easily managed while larger disasters are more complex. The management of any-size disaster will necessarily include considerations for harmful chemicals or other biologic agents (such as in bioterrorism). The dentist must be able to coordinate and function well in these situations from the initial occurrence of the disaster. This requires that the forensic dentist and the dental team be well trained, led by experienced individuals and completely integrated into the operation.

Preparation and Training

A forensic dental team must be trained at the individual level and as a team. The Armed Forces Institute of Pathology (AFIP) course is the premier international training course held annually in Bethesda, Maryland (http://www.afip.org). The Southwest Symposium is offered biannually in June at the University of Texas Health Sciences Center at San Antonio (http://www.uthscsa.edu). Additionally, the American Society of Forensic Odontology (http://www.asfo.org) offers annual training and scientific programs and information on other courses nationally and internationally. All forensic dentists and teams who were initially called to New York City for the World Trade Center attack on 9/11/2001 were required to be AFIP trained and/or board certified by the American Board of Forensic Odontology.

Initial Response

In the event of a mass disaster, local law enforcement agencies and emergency medical teams respond first. Legal authority and jurisdiction is by the legal entity such as city or county in which the disaster occurs. Rescue of injured individuals is the first priority for emergency medical services (EMS) personnel. Site security is the first priority for the law enforcement agency.

The initial response may include the mobilization of federal and statewide assistance. Responding agencies may include the National Transportation and Safety Board (NTSB), the Federal Emergency Management Agency (FEMA), the Disaster Mortuary Operational Response Team (DMORT), the FBI, the National Disaster Medical System (NDMS), the Department of Homeland Security, and related state agencies.

It is critical for a dentist to be available at the disaster site to identify human remains and dental components of human remains that may not be recognizable by a non–dental-trained person. There should be a dentist onsite during the entire operation of search and recovery. Obviously the knowledge of dental anatomy is critical to this aspect. A general recommendation is to have a forensic dentist accompany each body recovery team to ascertain that all relevant dental information necessary for identification is retained in a useful and trackable manner. All body parts are initially flagged on site and in situ, then photographed in place prior to removal. Extreme burn cases may require stabilization of the dentition with a spray lacquer such as polyurethane or even hair spray. This will stabilize the fragile dental evidence from damage during transport.

All body parts are given separate identification numbers, which will often mean that several parts of a single individual's dentition may possess different and unique identifiers that will ultimately be connected to a single identified body. In New York City after the World Trade Center disaster, as many as 200 individually identified and numbered body parts were later associated with a single victim. A single tooth found separated from a portion of a jaw or body would have a different number than the jaw part from which it is later associated. An appropriate tracking method is used to locate within the site grid and diagram the original location of each body and part. Aspects of this process can be used later in the forensic determination of cause and method of progression of the disaster event.

Morgue and Forensic Dental Identification Operations

The dental section of the morgue operation is divided into three major components: antemortem examination, postmortem examination, and a comparison of each. Each of the three major sections has two forensic dentists. There is a minimum of one *experienced* forensic dentist in each of the teams. A team leader generally functions in a supervisory capacity as a shift commander. There are usually additional secretarial support personnel for overall coordination. Figure 15-9 depicts the dental radiographs and actual dissected jaws with dentition used to identify an actual aircraft incident victim for which a dental identification was required.

A critical component for dental identification procedures is the computer-based **WinID program** developed by Dr. James McGivney. An example of the document used for gathering information for this program is seen in Figure 15-9D. It is a database program that utilizes specific codes of antemortem and postmortem dental findings and identifies records that have a possible identification match. The hardcopy records are then examined by the forensic dental team for final verification. This program can be downloaded at no cost from http://www.winid.com.

The personnel in charge of **antemortem records** obtain antemortem dental records from dentists of likely victims. These records must include copies of all dental chart information and notations, as well as *original* dental radiographs that are identified by name, date, and position (left, right, etc.). The antemortem team verifies and inputs this information into the WinID program to create a digital database.

The dental radiographs alone are not adequate to complete antemortem charting. One must also consider the time span between antemortem information and the presumed time of death. Additional dentists may have provided dental care and therefore, additional antemortem records may exist. The dental chart must be reviewed in detail to determine what additional restorations or other treatments (such as extractions) were provided subsequent to the date of the radiographs. For example, even though there is no antemortem radiographic evidence of a new mesio-occlusal amalgam, the postmortem charting can still be considered consistent with the antemortem radiographs if the radiographs were obtained prior to the placement of this more recent restoration, and if all other findings match. A paper record is filed in the antemortem file area. (See Figure 15-2 for a comparison of antemortem and postmortem radiographs to illustrate the changes that can occur between the antemortem and postmortem radiographs.)

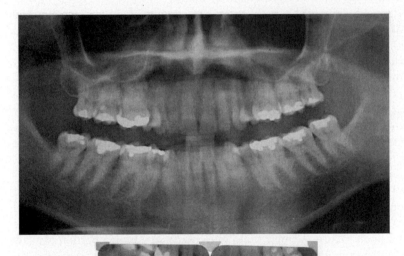

A

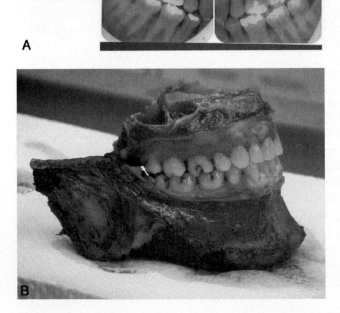

B

FIGURE 15-9. A. Antemortem films from the victim of an aircraft crash and severe burning. Original films must always be provided to the forensic dentist, so that appropriate anatomic orientation can be made. Bitewings are the most helpful images for use in comparison of restoration morphology and pulpal conditions such as recession, pulp stones, etc. The antemortem charting of this individual's dentition can be seen in Figure 15-5A. **B.** For this victim, the jaws had to be resected to permit appropriate detailed clinical and radiographic examination. When properly dissected and cleaned, all tooth surfaces can be directly visualized, examined, photographed, and radiographed. (The forensic dentist must have appropriate permission from the medical examiner or coroner to remove body parts such as the jaws. Only when the victim is not viewable in a funeral home open casket setting can this procedure be permitted.)

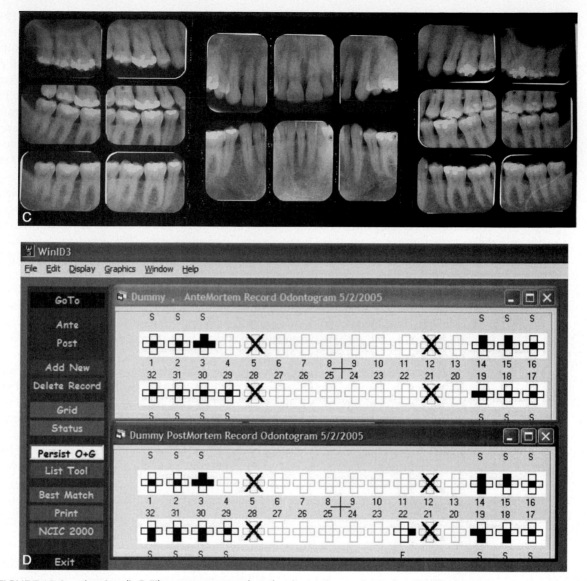

FIGURE 15-9. *(continued)* **C.** The **postmortem** dental radiographs are shown here and can be easily compared to the antemortem records found in **A.** Close attention must be paid to tooth and root morphology, sinuses, trabecular patterns, bone levels, and restorations. **D. Antemortem and postmortem** information is transferred from the paper charts shown in Figure 15-5A and B to the WinID database. The database can then be used to search all unidentified victims for possible matches to antemortem records. The computer will provide a report as shown here in graphic fashion. The forensic dentist is still required to visually compare the dental radiographs and other examination information to ascertain identity, which was "positive" in this case.

Dental records could be provided in a language other than English, so translation may be necessary. When reviewing the antemortem chart, it is important, as noted earlier, to convert any numbering systems used by the dentist of record (Palmer, FDI, etc.) to the Universal numbering system common in the United States (numbered 1–32 for permanent teeth and A–T for primary teeth). One should also be attentive to esthetic treatments (composites, veneers, etc.) that could be missed on postmortem examination of remains that are covered with debris or damaged by fire and trauma. Finally, in reviewing dental records, the quality of the handwriting and/or completeness of the record may pose significant barriers to determining accurate antemortem information.

A thorough **postmortem examination** is performed by a team of two forensic dentists who verify each other to reduce the chance of errors. In severe burn cases, resection of the jaws may be required to accurately observe and take radiographs of the dental conditions (Fig. 15-9B). The victim's condition is recorded photographically, radiographically, and in written notes as received in the morgue area. The process of postmortem dental examination, both clinical and radiographic, must consider numerous factors. On clinical examination, the forensic personnel must prepare the specimens by careful cleaning of debris, with care taken not to destroy fragile tooth fragments or the relation of teeth and tooth fragments to the rest of the dental arch. This is most critical in the burned victim. As noted earlier, the preservation of fragile dentition can be aided with spray lacquer or hair spray. Failure to do so can cause enamel to separate from the dentin, restoration loss, and/or destruction of porcelain restorations. The use of disclosing solution or transillumination can aid in the identification of composite restorations or other esthetic restorations.

The postmortem examination must also take into account the following: (a) identification of existing and missing teeth; (b) developmental and eruption stage; (c) estimated dental age; (d) occlusion and alignment of teeth; (e) structure of tooth crown (basic dental anatomy, anthropologic features, restorations, wear patterns, appliances, etc.); (f) root structure (such as apical development, dilacerations, root numbers, and endodontic therapy); (g) pulpal anatomy (pulp stones, recession of pulp chamber); (h) pathologic changes; (i) retained primary and supernumerary teeth, impactions, and retained root tips; (j) anatomy of sinuses; (k) bony architecture and trabeculation as seen radiographically; (l) bony pathology (exostoses, cysts, tumors, periodontal condition, periapical pathology, fractures, and foreign objects); (m) bone plates, screws and wires, etc.; and (n) evidence of systemic diseases and conditions as well as congenital abnormalities.

At this time, the postmortem record can be completed according to the appropriate coding as shown on the forms. Coding used in the WinID program is slightly different from that used in the average dental practice. Failure to use the appropriate codes will prevent the comparison feature of WinID from functioning properly. As a result, a match may not be found and a victim may not be properly identified.

The final step is **comparison** of the antemortem and postmortem records. In cases of individual identifications or the review of a few charts, this may be done manually. However, in large disasters the use of a comparison program such as WinID is critical. In the management of a disaster on the scale of the World Trade Center disaster in 2001 involving the analysis of several thousand antemortem records and over 1000 postmortem dental examination records, WinID and computerized assistance are mandatory.

In the comparison process, there are three outcomes possible. Ideally a positive identification is obtained. The other possible outcomes are either "consistent with" or "not a match or unidentified." If any of the following conditions exist in the antemortem record *but not in the postmortem record*, there is an immediate **nonmatch**: missing teeth, restored tooth surfaces, unusual root morphology, or chronic pathology. However, it is possible for teeth to be removed, restored, or even orthodontically moved between the date of antemortem information and time of death (recall Fig. 15-2A compared to B). These postmortem findings would not rule out a match between a person and an unknown victim. Pathology present in antemortem information could have been treated, or pathology present in the postmortem condition may not have existed in antemortem information. All of these situations must be readily and reliably explained.

Final "sign-off" of the comparison is legally the responsibility of a licensed dentist with appropriate forensic odontology credentials.

Forensic Anthropology

Another component of forensic identification may involve determining the age, race (cultural heritage), and sex of the victim. Age can be estimated in some cases by the evaluation of the teeth, especially during the time of primary or mixed dentition as described in detail in Chapter 10. Growth and development of the dentition is complete by about 18 years of age. Once all primary teeth are exfoliated and third molars are fully developed, whether impacted or erupted, the ability to gauge age by dental development is no longer reliable. Wear patterns

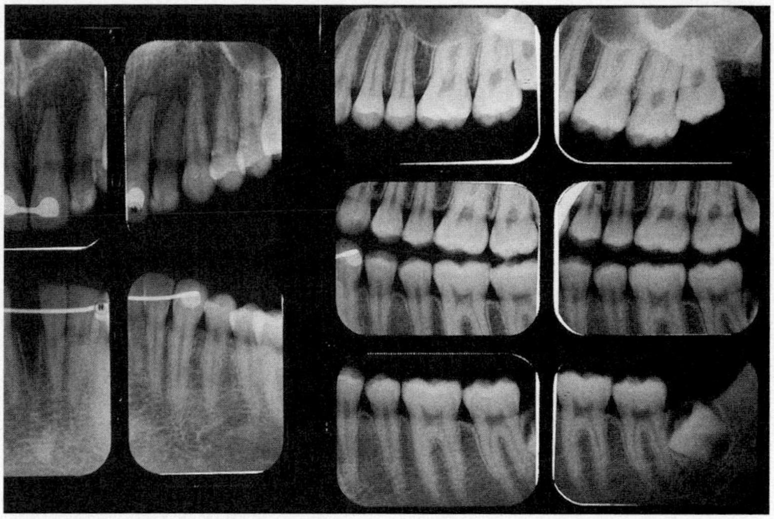

FIGURE 15-10. Dental aging can be variable as shown in this same homicide victim case depicted in Figures 15-3. The development of the root of tooth #17 appears to be of a person around 15 years of age as shown in dental growth and development charts elsewhere in this textbook. However, tooth #16 appears to be of an individual at least 18 years of age. The actual victim's age was 20 years. Although dental growth, eruption patterns, tooth apex development, and closure patterns are well documented, the reality of human variations can still be problematic in accurately assessing an individual's age.

and pulp chamber changes such as pulp stones and pulpal recession are not accurate. This author has worked with forensic cases where dental wear and pulpal recession appeared to indicate a person of 35–50 years of age when in reality the victim was in the early 20s. In another homicide case a known 21-year-old female presented with an impacted tooth #16, which suggested a developmental age of 15 years, and an impacted tooth #17, which suggested a developmental age of at least 18. (See *Figure 15-10*).

Other anthropologic aspects of the dentition can provide indicators of racial or cultural backgrounds. Shovel-shaped incisors may indicate a person of Asian or Mongolian background. Other indicators of this ancestry include prominent zygomatic processes, moderate prognathism, rotation of the incisors, buccal pitting, an elliptical dental arch form, a straight mandibular border, and a wide and vertical ascending ramus. The presence of a cusp of Carabelli is most often an indicator of Caucasian ancestry. Other traits of Caucasian ancestry include a parabolic dental arch form, bilobate (two-lobed) and/or prominent chin, slanted and pinched vertical ramus, canine fossae, retreating zygomatic bones, and lack of prognathic mandible. The African American population may show vertical zygomatic bones, a noticeably prognathic mandible, molar crenelations (scalloped or notched), hyperbolic dental arch form, blunt and vertical chin, and a pinched and slanting ascending ramus. However, one must be cautious when making an ancestral determination due to the increasing number of mixed racial and ethnic backgrounds that can blur these findings.

Anthropologic determinants also include overall skull characteristics for ethnic, as well as sexual determination. The cranial sutures will ossify and obliterate as a person ages and can be used for age determination.

Mass Disaster Case Studies

Several disasters highlight the value of a forensic dental team in the accurate identification of bodies. On the July 17, 1996, off East Moriches, New York, TWA flight 800 (a Boeing 747 aircraft) bound for Paris, France, exploded with 230 passengers aboard. Within the first 12 hours, a team of 30 dentists began the painstaking work of identifying the recovered bodies, which were devoid of clothing. Two and a half weeks later, 208 of the 210 recovered bodies and body parts had been positively identified. Ninety-five bodies were identified by dental records alone, and another 60 by dental records along with medical records (radiographs, magnetic resonance images, etc.), medical anomalies, and fingerprints.

For the first time ever, all relatives were screened for DNA samples to compare with the more than 400 recovered body parts, enabling the return of each to the families for an appropriate resting place. Nuclear DNA samples were extracted from both bone and dental pulps (which was all that remained after the first week). Mitochondrial DNA was also extracted from ground tooth structure, but it is only effective in matching maternal family connections. One victim was identified by examining DNA on toothbrushes in his home (*Columbus Dispatch*, Columbus, Ohio, April 1, 1997) since, during toothbrushing, microscopic bits of tissue from the gums and mucosa are scrubbed off and collect on the brush bristles. In all, seven people were identified by DNA alone because no other method was available.

One month later, Norwegian researchers were able to identify 139 of 141 people who died in a plane crash in Spitsbergen, Norway, in August 1996 (*Journal of Nature Genetics*, April 1997). They proved that 257 recovered body parts belonged to 141 people. They collected DNA samples from close relatives. When relatives were not available, investigators collected DNA from hairbrushes, dirty laundry, and toothbrushes in the victims' homes.

On September 11, 2001, both towers of the World Trade Center in New York City were destroyed by terrorist hijacked aircraft, and 2726 people were killed in the disaster, more than those who died at the attack of Pearl Harbor by the Japanese Navy in 1941. The dental identification team consisted of over 200 dental personnel working for more than 1 year to identify bodies and body parts by dental records. Approximately 50% of all known victims (less than 1500) were identified, about half of those by dental records and half by DNA means. On November 12, 2001, American Airlines flight 587 crashed in Queens on Long Island due to mechanical failures and air turbulence. All 265 victims were processed for dental identification through the same facility serving the victims of the World Trade Center disaster. The identification process was completed in approximately 1 month and attention returned to World Trade Center victims by the Dental Identification Unit of the Office of the Chief Medical Examiner of New York City.

On December 26, 2004, the tsunami struck many communities around the Indian Ocean, causing an estimated death toll in excess of 212,000 people. The challenges for dental iden-

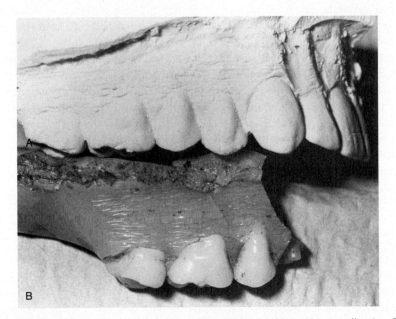

FIGURE 15-11. The dental stone cast of an upper denture (**A**) was obtained in evidence collection for investigation of an airliner crash. A denture fragment (**B**) recovered from the crash site, with teeth #2, 3, and 4 present, matches the antemortem cast. The impact broke off a distal piece of tooth #2. Unique horizontal grooves in the buccal resin of the denture precisely match those seen in the antemortem cast. (Photograph was provided by Dr. Theodore Berg.)

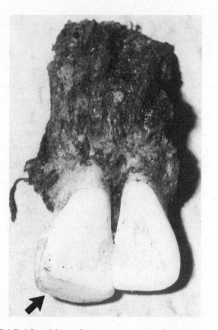

FIGURE 15-12. Although one or two teeth might seem scant evidence for identification, they should be thoroughly examined and radiographed. The labial laminate bonded veneer (*arrow*) made this specimen especially unique since this was in the early period of such technique. Also useful can be crown, root, and pulp shape; tooth positions; other restorations; pin and base buildups; endodontic therapy; posts; and bone trabecular patterns. (Photograph was provided by Dr. Theodore Berg.)

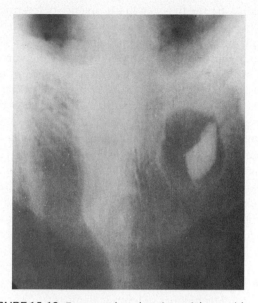

FIGURE 15-13. Even an edentulous jaw might provide a big clue to identification with some unique feature such as the dentigerous cyst shown in the maxillary canine region. Each case challenges the investigator to carefully consider all possibilities and to make no premature assumptions. (Photograph was provided by Dr. Theodore Berg.)

tification in this situation included the loss of dental records from destroyed dental offices and the socioeconomic and cultural situation that precluded many people from visiting a dentist and having antemortem information available for comparison.

On August 29, 2005, Hurricane Katrina, which had slightly weakened from a Category 5 to Category 4 storm, struck the New Orleans, Louisiana, area of the Gulf Coast of the United States. At least 1386 people lost their lives. The primary challenge for the dental identification teams was obtaining antemortem records. Many dental offices had been destroyed in the hurricane, and records were either lost entirely or too damaged by water to be usable. Only a minority of victims have been identified by any of the available techniques.

Figures 15-11 through 15-13 provide three additional examples of dental evidence that was useful for identifying the vicitm of a mass disaster. *Figure 15-11* shows a denture, *Figure 15-12* shows a two-tooth jaw fragment with a unique restoration, and *Figure 15-13* shows a radiograph of a uniquely impacted tooth.

SECTION VI — IMPORTANCE OF FORENSIC DENTISTRY TO PRACTICING DENTISTS

Forensic dentistry is a large area of special interest. This short chapter could only provide a brief overview of the importance of dental anatomy as a foundation for the effective practice of the specialty. All dental professionals must maintain accurate and comprehensive dental records for legal, standard-of-care, and forensic purposes. This includes written records, radiographs, and models that accurately describe or reproduce the oral anatomic and anthropologic form in detail. The weakest link in the dental identification process (subsequent to locating the antemortem dentist of record) is the quality of the dental written and radiographic record. These records are the first step in the practice of forensic dentistry by every dental professional.

Even if the average dentist does not intend to be involved in forensic dentistry, the probability is that eventually he or she will be contacted regarding questions about quality of care or observed injuries (such as suspected child or spousal abuse), or from law enforcement agencies requesting help. A valuable contribution can be made by understanding the role of dentistry in forensic science, by recognizing dental evidence or a bite mark, and by helping to properly preserve crucial evidence for later analysis.

The dental professional must understand how dental anatomy knowledge is valuable in forensic procedures. Other chapters of this text describe in more detail some of these anatomic features. The presence of a cusp of Carabelli on a maxillary first molar will identify a person as Caucasian heritage. Shovel-shaped incisors will identify a person of mongoloid or Asian origin. Tooth root apex development is an age indicator. Cuspal contours of lower premolars assist in the orientation of bites in a bite mark case when one understands cuspal anatomy of lower versus upper premolars. Root dilacerations, pulp stones, pulpal recession in the elderly or bruxing patient, maxillary sinus morphology, and virtually all aspects of dental anatomy are useful in the forensic identification of an individual or for assessing standard-of-care issues. In some cases, as in the World Trade Center disaster, the ability to identify a single tooth as a maxillary versus mandibular premolar was the key to the ability to search the database of antemortem records and confirm an identification.

You will find dental anatomy the foundation or basis for any forensic dentistry investigation. The references offered within this chapter were selected to give the novice a practical and representative introduction to the field and techniques of forensic dentistry.

GENERAL REFERENCES

American Board of Forensic Odontology. Guidelines for bite mark analysis. JADA 1986;(Mar). Available at: http://www.abfo.org.

American Society of Forensic Odontology's information source via the Internet: http://www.asfo.org.

Bowers CM. Forensic dental evidence. Boston: Elsevier Academic Press, 2004

Bowers CM, Bell GL, eds. Manual of forensic odontology. Saratoga Springs, NY: American Society of Forensic Odontology. 3rd revised ed. 1997. This manual can be obtained from the American Society of Forensic Odontology at http://www.asfo.org.

Clark DH, ed. Practical forensic odontology. Boston: Wright (Butterworth-Heinman Ltd.), 1992.

Cottone JA, Standish SM. Outline of forensic dentistry. Chicago: Year Book Medical Publishers, Inc., 1982.

deVilliers CJ, Phillips VM. Person identification by means of a single unique dental feature. J Forensic Odontostomatol 1998;16(1):17–19.

Dorion RB. Bitemark evidence. New York: Marcel Dekker, 2005.

Gill GW, Rhine S. Symposium Ed: skeletal attribution of race—methods for forensic anthropology. Manual available from Maxwell Museum of Anthropology at the University of New Mexico, Albuquerque, NM, 1990.

Guidelines for bite mark analysis by the American Board of Forensic Odontology. JADA 1986;March.

Harvey W. Dental identification and forensic odontology. London: Henry Kimpton Publishing, 1976.

Journal of California Dental Association: May 1996: Vol.24(5): 28-66) (seven concise articles with overview introduction on subjects of bite marks, crime investigation, child abuse, photography, computers, and mass disasters).

Krogman W. The human skeleton in forensic medicine. Springfield, IL: Charles C. Thomas Publishers, 1973.

Lampe H, Roetzcher K. Age determination from adult human teeth. Med Law 1994;13(7–8):623–628.

Luntz L, Luntz P. Handbook for dental identification. Philadelphia: J.B. Lippincott, 1973.

Melia E, Carr M. Forensic odontology and the role of the dental hygienist. Access 2005;19(3);15–23.

Nuckles DB, Herschaft EE, Whatmough LN. Forensic odontology in solving crimes: dental techniques and bite mark evidence. Gen Dent 1994;42(3):210–214.

Rothwell BR. Bitemarks in forensic dentistry: a review of legal, scientific issues. 1995;126(2):223–232.

Sopher M. Forensic dentistry. Springfield, IL: Charles C. Thomas, 1976.

Standish SM, Stimson PG. Symposium on forensic dentistry: legal obligations and methods of identification for the practitioner. Dent Clin North Am 1977: Vol 21(1).

Stimson PG, Mertz CA. Forensic dentistry. Boca Raton, FL: CRC Press, 1997: Vol 21(1).

Wood JD, Gould G. Mass fatality incidents: are California dentists ready to respond. Calif Dental J 2004;32(8):681–688.

Wright FD. Integrating new technologies in bitemark analysis. Am Soc Forensic Odontol News 1999;Winter.

Wright FW. Forensic dentistry: an introduction. Columbus: Ohio Dental Association 2005. Available from the Ohio Dental Association, 1305 Dublin Road, Columbus, Ohio 43215.

Appendix

This Appendix includes numerous drawings of permanent and primary teeth, which are labeled (with letters) to highlight features of each tooth. Traits represented by each letter are described on the back of each page following the same letter used on the drawings.

The pages in this Appendix section are perforated, so they can be torn out to facilitate study for Chapters 4 through 9, thus minimizing page turns. For example, while reading about the morphology of incisors in Section I of Chapter 4, when you see the word "Appendix" followed by a number and letter (e.g., **Appendix 1a**), refer to the appendix page (page 1) and item (letter a). Find that letter on the line drawings, and it will illustrate the concept being described in the text.

General Class Traits of All Incisors
(using the maxillary right lateral incisor #7 as an example)

Class Traits

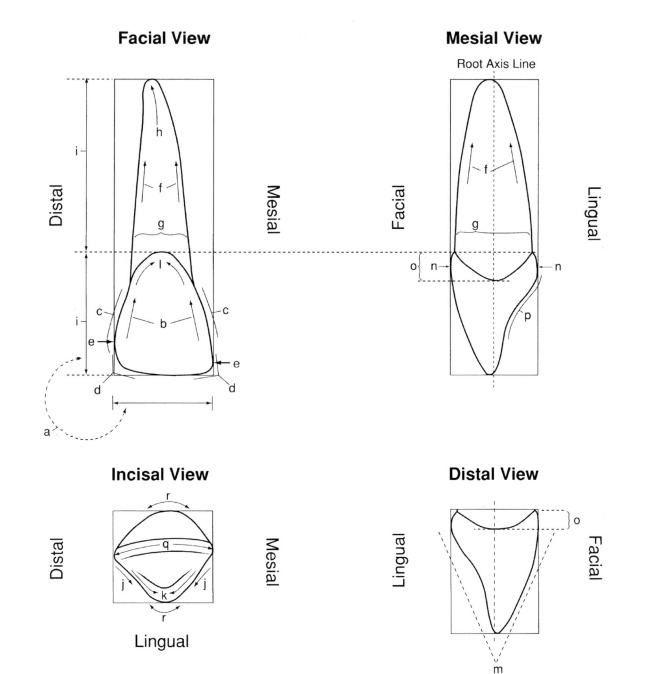

Facial View

Mesial View

Incisal View

Distal View

Refer to letters a–r on back, which describe these features.

GENERAL CLASS TRAITS OF ALL INCISORS

a. Crown shapes are rectangular, longer incisogingivally than mesiodistally (facial views).

b. Crowns taper from the contact areas to cervical lines (facial views).

c. Crown outlines on the distal are more convex than on the mesial (facial views) EXCEPT on mandibular central incisors, which are known for their symmetry.

d. The mesioincisal angles are more square (or acute) than the distoincisal angles, which are more obtuse (facial views) EXCEPT on mandibular central incisors.

e. Mesial contact areas are in the incisal third; distal contact areas are more cervical than the mesial (facial view) EXCEPT on mandibular central incisors, where mesial and distal contacts are at same height (facial views).

f. Roots taper from the cervical line toward the apex (facial and proximal views) and from the facial toward the lingual (best seen on an actual tooth or model).

g. Roots are wider faciolingually than mesiodistally (comparing proximal to facial view) EXCEPT maxillary central incisors, where dimensions are about equal.

h. When bent, roots often bend to the distal in the apical third (facial views).

i. Roots are slightly to be considerably longer than crowns (facial and proximal views).

j. Crowns taper from proximal contact areas toward the lingual (incisal views).

k. The mesial and distal marginal ridges converge toward the lingual cingulum (incisal and lingual views).

l. Cervical lines on the facial (and lingual) surfaces are convex (curve) toward the apex (facial and lingual views).

m. Proximal outlines are wedge shaped (proximal views).

n. Facial and lingual crests of curvature are in the cervical third (proximal views).

o. Proximal cervical lines are convex (curve) toward the incisal AND more so on the mesial than on the distal surfaces (compare mesial to distal views).

p. Lingual outlines are S-shaped with a concave lingual fossa and convex cingulum, and the lingual outlines of the marginal ridges are more vertical than horizontal (proximal views).

q. Incisal edges terminate mesially and distally at the widest portion of the tooth crown (incisal views).

r. Facial outlines are more broadly rounded than lingual outlines due to lingual convergence (incisal views).

Incisors

Maxillary

Lateral (#7) **Central (#8)**

Mandibular

Lateral (#26) **Central (#25)**

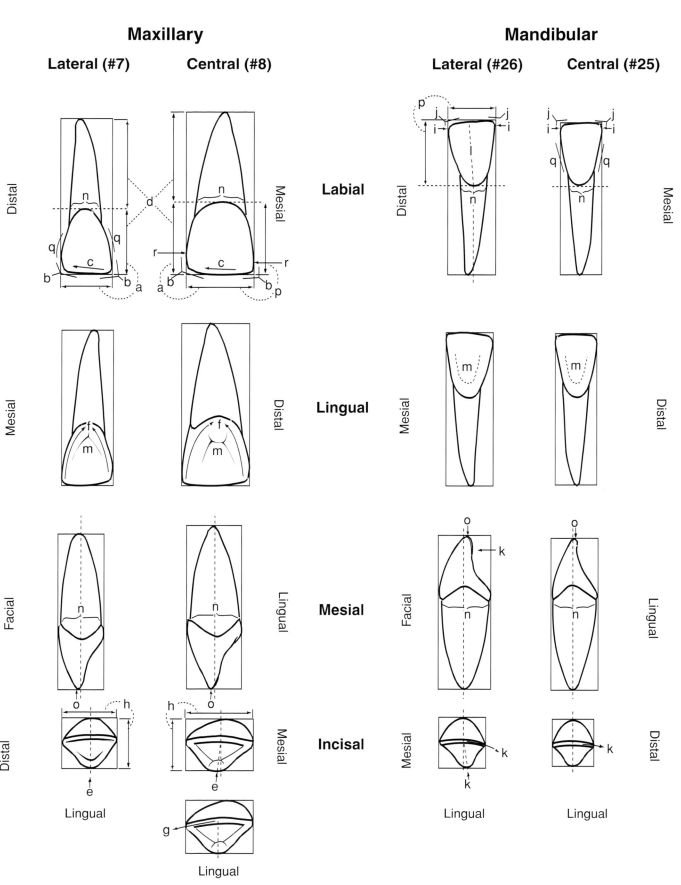

Refer to letters a–r on back, which describe these features.

TYPE TRAITS THAT DISTINGUISH THE <u>MAXILLARY</u> CENTRAL INCISOR FROM THE MAXILLARY LATERAL INCISOR

a. Although the crowns of both types of maxillary incisors have a larger cervicoincisal dimension than mesiodistal, maxillary central incisors are closer to square. Lateral incisors are more oblong cervicoincisally (facial views).

b. On both maxillary incisors, the mesioincisal angles are close to 90°; the distoincisal angles are more rounded (facial views), but both angles are more rounded on the lateral compared to the central incisor (facial views).

c. Incisal edges slope cervically toward the distal (facial views), more so on lateral incisors (facial views).

d. Maxillary central incisors have crowns and roots closer to the same length. Lateral incisors have proportionately longer roots relative to crowns (facial views).

e. When the incisal edges are aligned horizontally, cingula of maxillary central incisors are off-center to the distal versus cingula of lateral incisors, which are centered (incisal views).

f. Mesial marginal ridges are longer than the distal marginal ridges (in central incisors due to the distally displaced cingulum, and in lateral incisors due to the cervical slope of the incisal edge to the distal) (lingual views).

g. From the incisal view, when the crest of curvature of the cingulum is positioned directly downward, the incisal edge of maxillary central incisors has a slight distolingual twist with the distoincisal corner more lingual than the mesioincisal corner. Lateral incisor ridges run mesiodistally with no twist (incisal and mesial views).

h. Mesiodistal dimensions on central incisors are considerably wider than faciolingual dimensions (rectangular shaped). On lateral incisors, these dimensions are more nearly equal (closer to square) (incisal views).

TYPE TRAITS THAT DISTINGUISH THE <u>MANDIBULAR</u> CENTRAL INCISOR FROM THE MANDIBULAR LATERAL INCISOR

Mandibular central incisors are very symmetrical versus lateral incisors, which are not. Examples of the relative lack of symmetry in lateral incisors include the following:

i. Lateral incisors have the distal proximal contacts more apical than the mesial contacts. Central incisor contacts are at the same level (facial views).

j. Lateral incisors have the distoincisal angles more rounded than the mesioincisal angles. On central incisors the mesio- and distoincisal angles are quite similar (facial views).

k. Incisal edges of lateral incisors have a slight distolingual twist (relative to a line bisecting the cingulum). Central incisors have their incisal edges at right angles (with no twist) to this bisecting line (incisal and mesial views).

l. The crown of the mandibular lateral incisor tips slightly to the distal relative to the root (facial views).

ARCH TRAITS THAT DISTINGUISH MAXILLARY FROM MANDIBULAR INCISORS

m. Lingual fossae are more pronounced on maxillary incisors (often with a lingual pit, especially on the maxillary lateral incisor). Mandibular incisors have smoother lingual anatomy without grooves and pits (lingual views).

n. Maxillary incisors have roots that are more round in cross section. Mandibular incisors have roots that are more ribbon-like (that is, are thin mesiodistally and much wider faciolingually). Compare proximal views to facial views.

o. Incisal edges of maxillary incisors are often labial to the root axis line. Mandibular incisal edges are often lingual to the root axis line (proximal views).

p. Mandibular crowns are smaller and narrower mesiodistally relative to the length compared to maxillary incisors, which are wider (facial views).

q. Mandibular crowns have outlines mesially and distally that are flatter than on maxillary incisors (facial views).

r. (r compared to i). Proximal contact points (crests of curvature or heights of contact) are closer to the incisal edge on mandibular incisors (i) than on maxillary incisors (r) (although all incisor mesial proximal contacts are in the incisal third of the crowns, and distal contacts are more cervically positioned) (facial views).

General Class Traits of All Canines
(using the maxillary right canine #6 as an example)

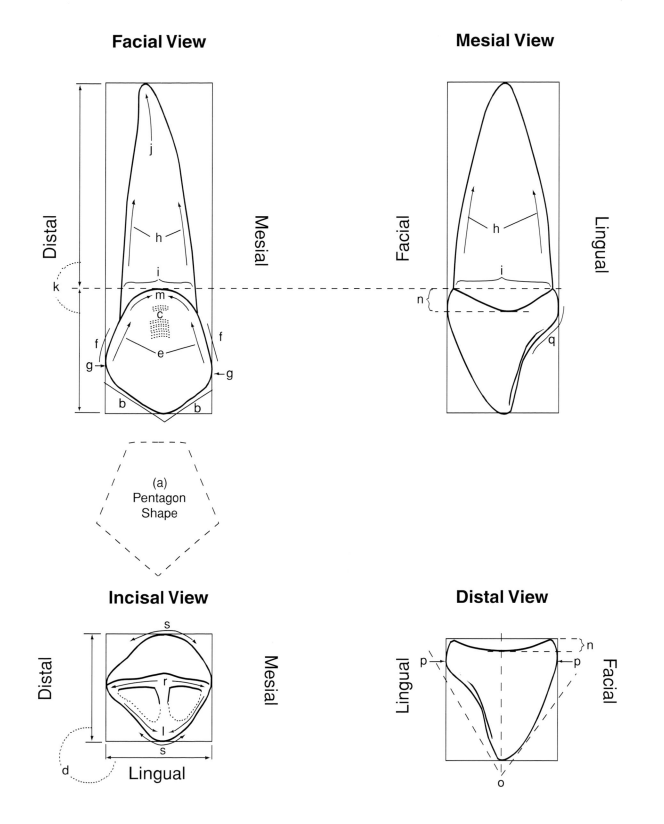

Facial View

Mesial View

Distal

Mesial

Facial

Lingual

j

h

i

k

m
c

f   f

e

g   g

b   b

n

h

i

q

(a)
Pentagon
Shape

Incisal View

Distal View

Distal

Mesial

Lingual

Facial

s

r

l

s

d

Lingual

n

p   p

o

Refer to letters a–s on back, which describe these features.

GENERAL CLASS TRAITS OF ALL CANINES

a. Crowns are pentagon shaped (facial views).
b. Cusps have mesial cusp ridges shorter than distal cusp ridges (facial views).
c. Vertical labial ridges are prominent (more so on maxillary canines) (facial views).
d. Crowns are wider faciolingually than mesiodistally (similar to mandibular incisors) (incisal views).

General Canine Characteristics Similar to Incisors

e. Crowns taper from contact areas toward the cervical line (facial views).
f. Crown outlines are more convex on the distal and less convex (flatter) on the mesial (facial views).
g. Mesial contact areas are located in the incisal third of the crown (or at the junction of the incisal and middle thirds); distal contact areas are more cervically positioned (facial views).
h. Roots taper from the cervical line toward the apex (facial and proximal views), and from facial toward lingual (which is best viewed on an actual tooth or model).
i. Roots are wider faciolingually than mesiodistally (compare proximal to facial views).
j. If roots are bent, they more often bend toward the distal in the apical third on maxillary canines (facial views).
k. Roots are considerably longer than crowns (facial views).
l. Crowns taper from the proximal contacts toward the lingual (incisal views), so the mesial and distal marginal ridges converge toward the cingulum (incisal views).
m. Cervical lines on the facial (and lingual) surfaces curve toward the apex (facial and lingual views).
n. Proximal cervical lines curve toward the incisal, more so on the mesial than on the distal surface (compare proximal views).
o. Canines (like incisors) are wedge shaped when viewed from the proximal.
p. Facial and lingual crests of curvature are in the cervical third (proximal views).
q. Lingual outlines are S-shaped with a concave lingual fossa and convex cingulum; the marginal ridges are oriented more vertically than horizontally (proximal views).
r. Incisal edges run from the mesial to the distal contact areas (incisal views).
s. Facial outlines are more broadly rounded than lingual outlines due to lingual convergence (incisal views).

Canines

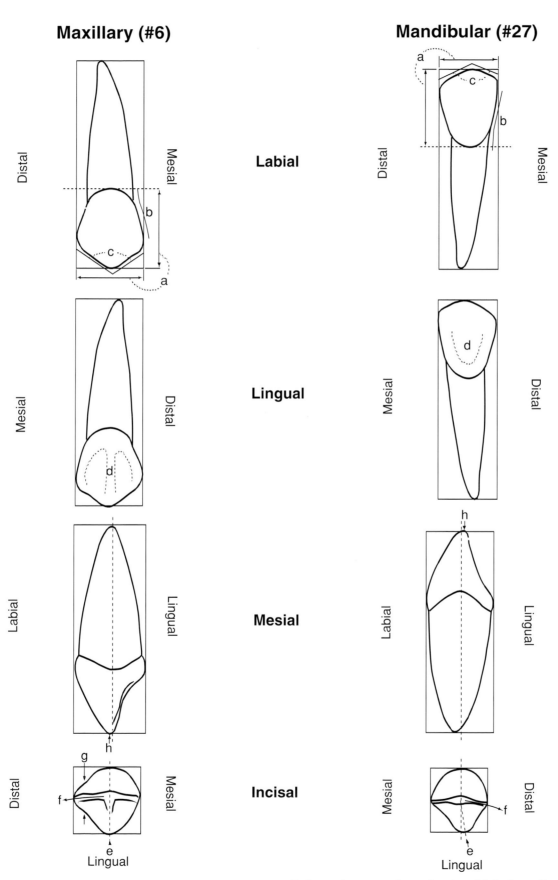

Maxillary (#6)

Mandibular (#27)

Labial

Lingual

Mesial

Incisal

Refer to letters a–h on back, which describe these features.

TYPE (AND ARCH) TRAITS THAT DISTINGUISH THE MAXILLARY CANINE FROM THE MANDIBULAR CANINE

a. Both maxillary and mandibular canine crowns are oblong (rectangular) with the mesiodistal dimension less than the incisocervical dimension, but the mesiodistal dimension is narrower on mandibular canines than on maxillary canines (facial views).

b. Maxillary canines have mesial crown contours convex to flat cervically versus mandibular canines, which have mesial crown contours more in line with the contour of the root (facial views).

c. The angle formed by the cusp slopes of maxillary canines is more pointed or acute (averaging about 105°), resulting in a sharper cusp, compared to the broader (less pointed or obtuse) angle on the mandibular canine, which averages 120° (facial views). The mesial cusp ridge of the mandibular canine is often close to horizontal when the tooth is held with the long axis vertically.

d. Lingual ridges that separate mesial and distal fossae are more prominent on maxillary canines than on mandibular canines (lingual views).

e. Cingula on maxillary canines are large and centered mesiodistally. On mandibular canines, they are often slightly to the distal (incisal views).

f. Incisal ridges on maxillary canines are straighter mesiodistally. On mandibular canines, the distal cusp ridge bends distolingually (incisal views).

g. The distal half of the crown of maxillary canines is compressed (squeezed) faciolingually more than on mandibular canines (incisal views).

h. The cusp tip of the maxillary canine is on or labial to the root axis line, whereas the mandibular cusp tip is lingual to this line (proximal and incisal views).

General Class Traits of All Premolars
(using the maxillary right second premolar #4 as an example)

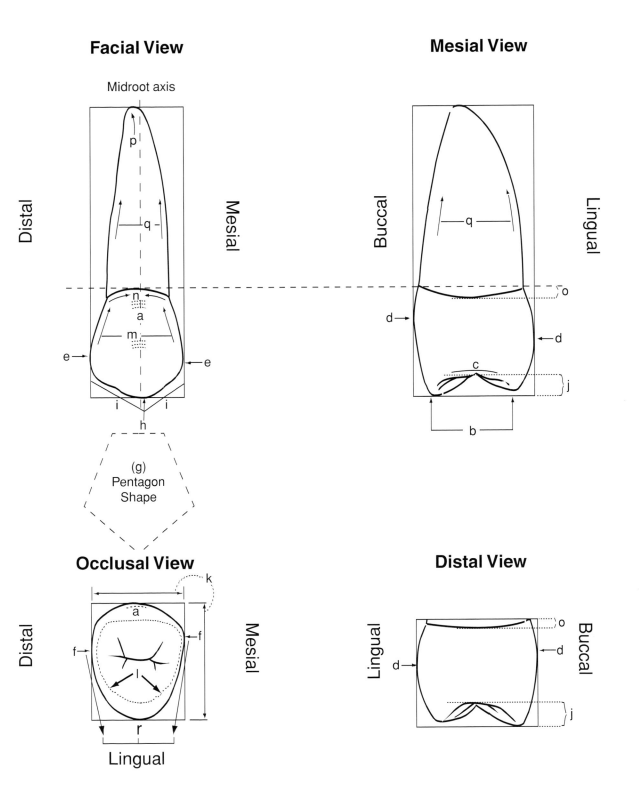

Facial View

Midroot axis

p

q

Distal

Mesial

n
a
m
e ← → e
i i
h

(g)
Pentagon
Shape

Mesial View

Buccal

q

Lingual

d →
← d
o
c
j
b

Occlusal View

Distal

Mesial

k
a
f ← → f
f
l
r

Lingual

Distal View

Lingual

Buccal

o
← d
d →
j

Refer to letters a–r on back, which describe these features.

GENERAL CLASS TRAITS OF ALL PREMOLARS

a. Buccal ridges are present (similar to canine labial ridges) (facial and occlusal views).

b. Usually, premolars have two cusps: one buccal and one lingual cusp (EXCEPTION is the mandibular second premolar, which often has three cusps: one buccal and two lingual) (proximal views).

c. Marginal ridges are aligned relatively horizontally (EXCEPT on mandibular first premolars, where the mesial marginal ridge is closer to a 45° angle from horizontal) (proximal views).

d. Buccal and lingual crests of curvature are more occlusal than on anterior teeth (still in cervical third on the facial, but in the middle third on the lingual) (proximal views).

e. Mesial proximal contacts (heights of contour) are near the junction of the occlusal and middle thirds, and the distal contacts are often slightly more cervical in the middle third (EXCEPT on mandibular first premolars, where mesial contacts are more cervical than the distal contacts) (facial views).

f. Proximal contacts (crests of curvature) from the occlusal view are buccal to the center faciolingually (occlusal views).

g. From the facial, premolars are roughly pentagon shaped (similar to canines) (facial view).

h. The buccal cusp tip is mesial to the midroot axis (EXCEPT on the maxillary first premolar, where the cusp tip is distal to the midroot axis) (facial views).

i. The mesial cusp ridge of the buccal cusp is shorter than the distal cusp ridge (EXCEPT on the maxillary first premolar, where the mesial cusp ridge is longer) (facial views).

j. Mesial marginal ridges are generally more occlusal than distal marginal ridges, which are more cervical (EXCEPT on mandibular first premolars, where distal marginal ridges are in a more occlusal position) (compare the proximal views).

k. Crowns are oblong from the occlusal view, wider faciolingually than mesiodistally relative to anterior teeth (maxillary premolars are decidedly oblong or rectangular, whereas mandibular premolars are closer to square [or round] in shape) (occlusal views).

l. Cusp ridges (or slopes) and marginal ridges form the boundary of the occlusal surface or occlusal table (occlusal views).

m. Crowns taper from proximal contact areas toward the cervical (facial views).

n. Cervical lines curve apically on the facial and lingual surfaces (facial and lingual views).

o. Cervical lines curve occlusally on the proximal surfaces, with the mesial cervical line more convex than the distal (compare mesial to distal proximal views).

p. The apical third of roots bend distally more often than mesially (facial views).

q. Roots taper toward the apex (both proximal and facial views).

r. The crowns taper narrower from the contact areas toward the lingual (occlusal views).

Premolars

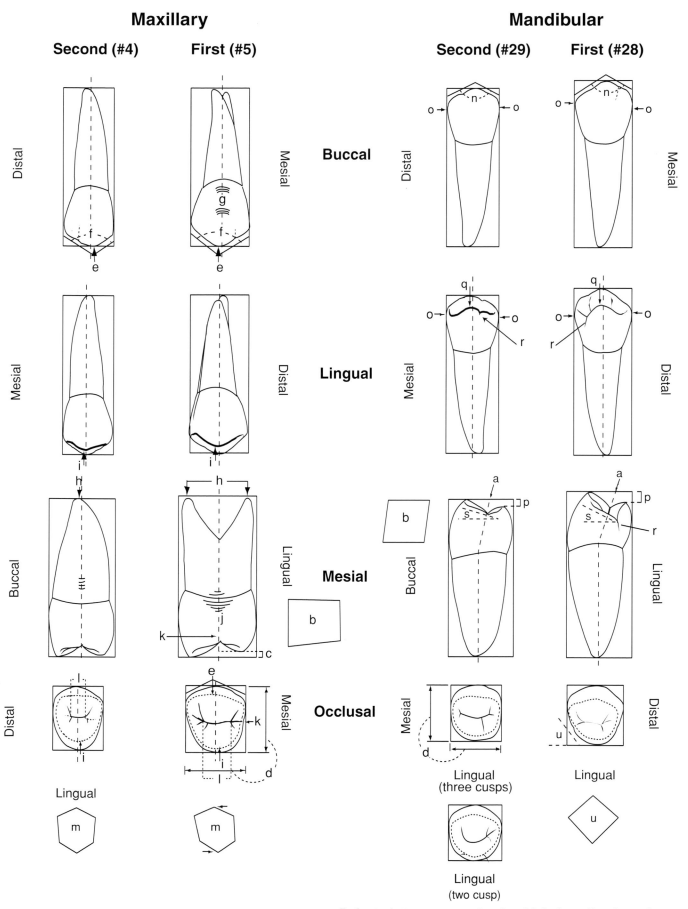

Maxillary

Second (#4)   **First (#5)**

Mandibular

Second (#29)   **First (#28)**

Buccal

Lingual

Mesial

Occlusal

Lingual
(three cusps)

Lingual

Lingual
(two cusp)

Refer to letters a–u on back, which describe these features (t is not shown).

ARCH TRAITS OF PREMOLARS THAT DISTINGUISH MAXILLARY FROM MANDIBULAR PREMOLARS

a. Mandibular premolar crowns tilt to the lingual, so mandibular lingual cusp tips may be lingual to the root (proximal views). Maxillary crowns do not tip noticeably.

b. The outline of the mandibular premolars are rhomboid in shape (four-sided with all opposite sides parallel), and the maxillary premolars are trapezoidal (four-sided with only two opposite walls parallel) (proximal views).

c. (compared to p). Although lingual cusps are shorter than buccal cusps for all premolars, the mandibular lingual cusps are relatively much shorter than buccal cusps (p) compared to maxillary lingual cusps, which are closer to the same length (c) (maxillary second premolar cusps are almost equal in length) (proximal views).

d. Mandibular premolars are more square or round from the occlusal view; maxillary premolars are more rectangular or oblong (relatively wider buccolingually) (occlusal views).

TYPE TRAITS DISTINGUISHING MAXILLARY FIRST FROM MAXILLARY SECOND PREMOLARS

e. Buccal cusps of maxillary first premolars are tipped more to the distal and mesial cusp ridges are longer than distal cusp ridges (THESE ARE THE ONLY PREMOLARS WITH THIS TRAIT) (facial and occlusal views).

f. Buccal cusps of maxillary first premolars are more pointed (average: 105°) than on second premolars, where they are more obtuse (120°) (facial views).

g. Buccal ridges are more prominent on maxillary first premolars (occlusal and facial views).

h. Maxillary first premolars usually have a divided root versus second premolars, which usually have one root (proximal views).

i. Maxillary premolars have their lingual cusps tipped (bent) toward the mesial (lingual and occlusal views).

j. Both maxillary premolars have mesial and distal *root* depressions, but only the maxillary first premolars exhibit a mesial *crown* concavity (mesial views).

k. Mesial marginal ridge grooves are almost always present on maxillary first premolars and are less common on second premolars (occlusal and mesial views).

l. The central developmental grooves on maxillary first premolars are longer (from mesial to distal pit) than those of second premolars, where they are only one-third or less of the mesiodistal dimension (occlusal views).

m. Occlusal outlines of maxillary first premolars are more *a*symmetrical with the lingual cusp tip positioned more to the mesial and the buccal cusp tip more to the distal versus second premolars, which are more symmetrical overall (occlusal views).

TYPE TRAITS DISTINGUISHING MANDIBULAR FIRST FROM SECOND PREMOLARS

n. Mandibular first premolar buccal cusps are more pointed (110°) versus on second premolar, where they are more obtuse or blunt (130°) (facial views).

o. Mesial proximal contacts (and marginal ridges) of mandibular second premolars are more occlusal than distal contacts (following the general rule), whereas the reverse is true on mandibular first premolars (EXCEPTION), where *mesial* contacts (and marginal ridges) are more cervical (facial views).

p. Lingual cusps of mandibular first premolars are very small and nonfunctional. On second premolars the lingual cusps function and are relatively longer (proximal views).

q. Lingual cusps of mandibular second premolars are positioned to the mesial (or, if there are two lingual cusps, the mesiolingual is the more prominent) (lingual views).

r. Mandibular **first** premolars have a **mesiolingual** groove separating the mesial marginal ridge from the lingual cusp. **Second** premolars (three-cusp type) have a **lingual** groove separating the two lingual cusps (lingual and mesial views).

s. Mesial marginal ridges of first premolars slope cervically toward the lingual at about 45° from horizontal. On second premolars they are more horizontal (mesial views).

t. The mesial root surfaces of mandibular second premolars are the only premolar root surface (maxillary and mandibular, mesial and distal) not likely to have a midroot depression (best seen on models or actual teeth, not labeled in drawings).

u. Mandibular first premolars are the only premolars that have the mesiolingual corner, with its mesiolingual groove and low marginal ridge, pinched or squeezed in, forming about a 45° angle with the lingual surface. This makes the occlusal outline somewhat diamond shaped (occlusal views).

General Class Traits of All Molars
(using the second mandibular molar #31 as an example)

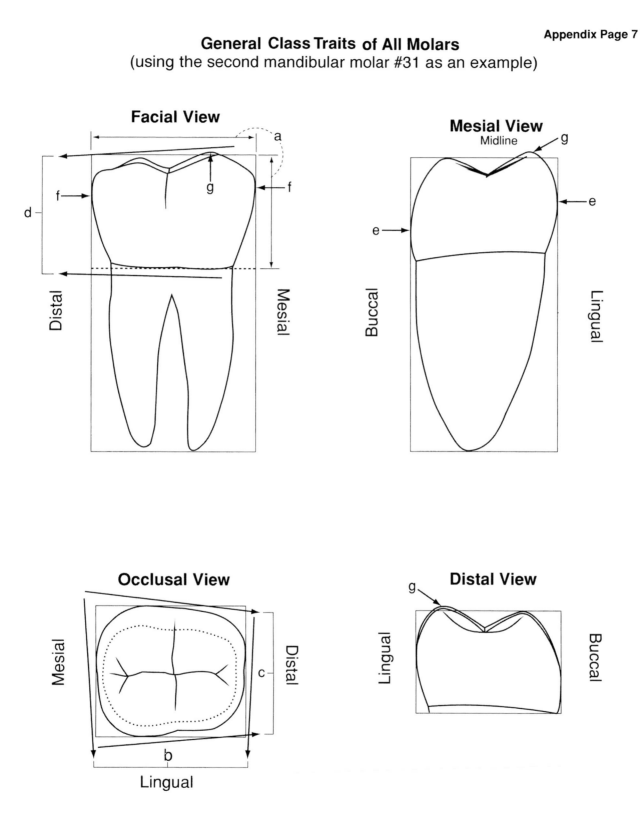

Facial View

Mesial View
Midline

Occlusal View

Distal View

Refer to letters a–g on back, which describe these features.

GENERAL CLASS TRAITS FOR ALL MOLARS

a. Molar crowns are wider mesiodistally than cervico-occlusally (facial views).

b. Crowns taper (get narrower) from the buccal to the lingual; that is, the mesiodistal width on the buccal half is wider than on the lingual half (EXCEPT some maxillary first molars with large distolingual cusps, where crowns taper to the buccal and the mesiodistal dimension on the lingual is greater than on the buccal) (occlusal view).

c. Crowns taper (get narrower) from the mesial to the distal; that is, the buccolingual width is less on the distal half than on the mesial half (occlusal view).

d. Crowns taper (get shorter) from mesial to distal; that is, the crown height on the distal half is less than on the mesial half (facial view).

e. As with premolars, the buccal crests of curvature (heights of contour) of crowns are in the cervical one-third, and the lingual crests of curvature are in the middle third (proximal views).

f. Proximal contacts (heights of contour) on the mesial are at or near the junction of the occlusal and middle thirds, and distal proximal contacts are more cervical in the middle third near the middle of the tooth (facial views).

g. Lingual cusps on mandibular molars (and mesiolingual cusps on maxillary molars) are longer than buccal cusps when molars are oriented on a vertical axis (facial, mesial, and distal views).

Molars

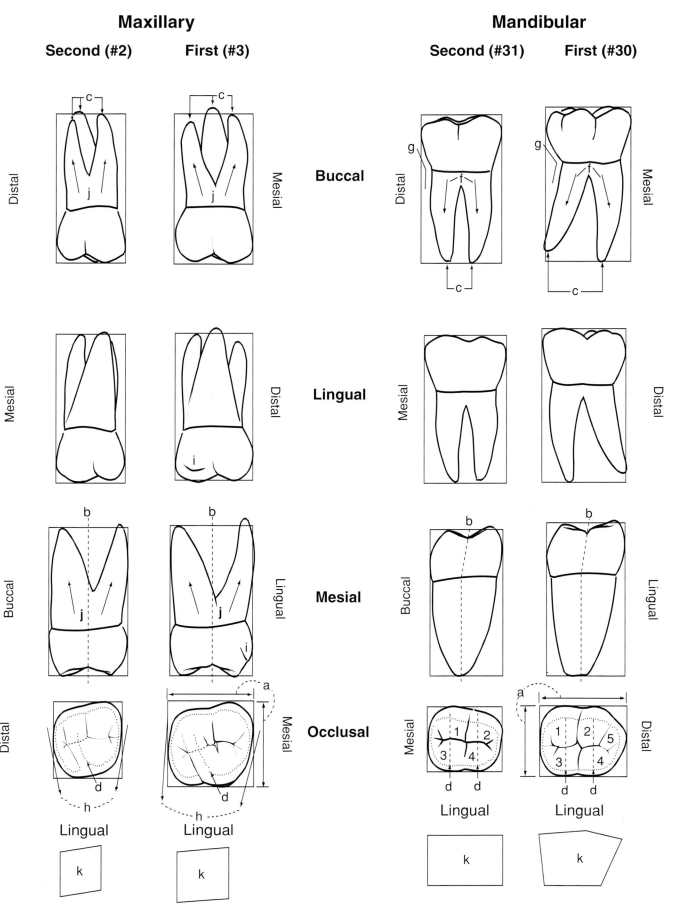

Refer to letters a–k on back. which describe these features.

ARCH TRAITS THAT DISTINGUISH MAXILLARY FROM MANDIBULAR MOLARS

a. Mandibular crowns are wider mesiodistally than faciolingually, resulting in a more rectangular or pentagon outline. Maxillary molar crowns have the faciolingual dimension slightly greater than the mesiodistal dimension, and are more square or rhomboid in outline (k) (occlusal views).

b. Mandibular molar crowns tilt lingually at the cervix (like mandibular premolars), whereas maxillary crowns are aligned directly over the roots (proximal views).

c. Mandibular molars usually have two roots (a larger mesial and a smaller distal root) versus maxillary molars, which have three roots (the longest lingual root, the shorter mesiobuccal, and the shortest distobuccal root) (facial or lingual views).

d. Maxillary molars have oblique ridges that run diagonally across the tooth from the mesiolingual to the distobuccal cusp compared to mandibular molars, which primarily have two transverse ridges that run directly buccolingually (occlusal views).

TYPE TRAITS THAT DISTINGUISH MANDIBULAR FIRST FROM MANDIBULAR SECOND MOLARS

e. Mandibular second molars have four cusps (mesiobuccal = 1, distobuccal = 2, mesiolingual = 3, and distolingual = 4) with a "cross" pattern of occlusal grooves compared to first molars, which most often have five cusps (the same four cusps as on the second molar, plus a smaller distal cusp = 5) with a zigzag central groove pattern (facial or occlusal views; see corresponding numbered cusps, not labeled as "e").

f. First molar roots are more divergent and widely separated compared to second molars roots, which are more parallel and closer together (facial and lingual views).

g. There is more taper (narrowing) from the distal proximal contact to the cervical line on first molars than on second molars due to the presence of the distal cusp on first molars (facial views).

TYPE TRAITS THAT DISTINGUISH MAXILLARY FIRST FROM MAXILLARY SECOND MOLARS

h. There is more taper (narrowing) from the buccal to lingual on second molars due to their smaller distolingual cusp compared to less taper on maxillary first molars with their wider, prominent distolingual cusps (occlusal views).

i. First molars are more likely to have a fifth cusp, the cusp of Carabelli (located on the mesiolingual cusp) compared to second molars, which rarely have the cusp of Carabelli (occlusal, lingual, and mesial views).

j. Roots of first molars are more spread apart than on second molars (similar to mandibular molars) (facial and proximal views).

k. The parallelogram outline shape of maxillary molars (with more acute or sharper mesiobuccal and distolingual angles and more obtuse or less sharp distobuccal and mesiolingual angles) is more twisted on second molars than on first molars (that is, acute angles are more acute and obtuse angles are more obtuse on maxillary second molars) (occlusal views).

Primary Anterior Teeth

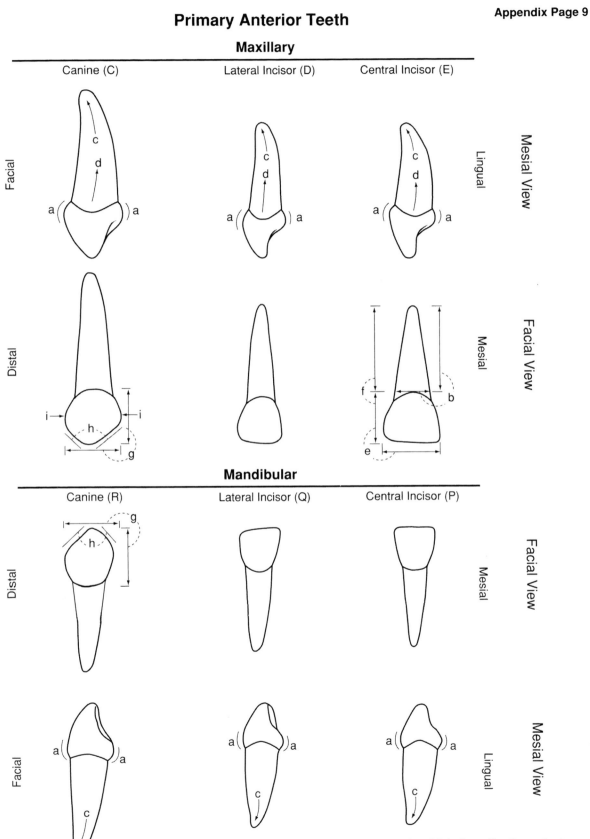

Maxillary

Canine (C) Lateral Incisor (D) Central Incisor (E)

Mandibular

Canine (R) Lateral Incisor (Q) Central Incisor (P)

Refer to letters a–i on back, which describe these features.

UNIQUE PROPERTIES OF ANTERIOR PRIMARY TEETH

a. Primary anterior tooth crowns have bulges in the cervical third of the labial and lingual surfaces. The lingual bulge is seen as a relatively large cingulum that occupies up to one-third of the cervicoincisal crown length, and the labial bulge is seen as a prominent convex cervical ridge (proximal views).

b. Roots are long in proportion to crown length and narrower (thinner) mesiodistally than on secondary anterior teeth (facial view).

c. Roots of maxillary and mandibular primary anterior teeth bend as much as 10° labially in their apical third, less so in mandibular canines (proximal views).

d. Roots of maxillary incisors bend (bow) lingually in the cervical third to half, whereas the mandibular incisors are straight in their cervical third (proximal views).

e. Primary <u>central</u> incisors are the only incisors, primary or permanent, where the crown is wider mesiodistally than incisocervically (facial views).

f. Primary incisor crowns are shorter relative to the root length compared to permanent teeth (facial views).

g. Primary maxillary canines are about as wide mesiodistally as they are long incisogingivally. Mandibular canines are longer incisocervically and narrower mesiodistally (facial views).

h. Primary mandibular canines have their distal cusp slopes longer than on the mesial (as do all secondary canines and premolars EXCEPT secondary maxillary first premolars) (facial views). Primary maxillary canines have their mesial cusp slopes longer than the distal cusp slopes (which is UNIQUE to only this tooth and maxillary first premolars).

i. Primary maxillary canines have mesial proximal contacts more cervical than the distal (which is UNIQUE to this tooth and the permanent mandibular first premolar) (facial views). All other primary and permanent teeth have the distal contact area more cervically located than on the mesial.

Primary Molars

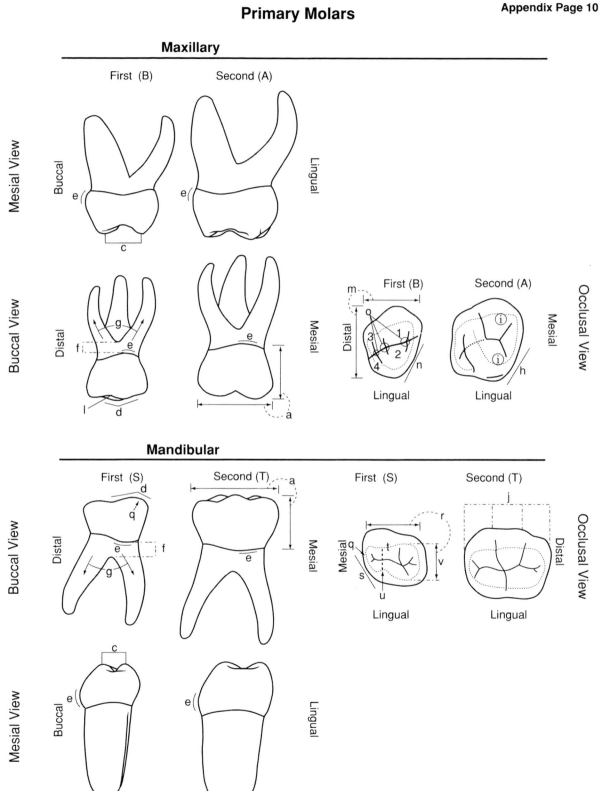

Maxillary

First (B)   Second (A)

Mesial View

Buccal — e — c

Lingual

Buccal View

Distal — g, f, e, l, d

Mesial — e, a

Occlusal View

First (B) — m, o, 3, 1, 2, 4, n

Second (A) — i, i, h

Lingual   Lingual

Mandibular

Buccal View

First (S) — d, q, e, f, g

Second (T) — a, e

Distal

Mesial

First (S) — r, q, t, s, u, v

Second (T) — j

Lingual   Lingual

Occlusal View

Mesial View

First (S) — c, e, Buccal

Second (T) — e

Lingual

Refer to letters a–v on back, which describe these features.

GENERAL CHARACTERISTICS OF ALL PRIMARY MOLARS

a. Primary molars crowns are wider mesiodistally and shorter cervico-occlusally, as on secondary molars (buccal views).

b. Primary first molars are decidedly smaller than primary second molars compared to permanent or secondary molars, where the first molars are larger (compare all views, not labeled as "b").

c. Primary molar crowns have a narrow chewing surface, or occlusal table, buccolingually compared to the entire tooth width buccolingually (proximal views).

d. Buccal cusps are not sharp; cusp ridges meet at a wide (obtuse) angle (buccal views).

e. Mesial cervical ridges are prominent (proximal views) with cervical lines curved more apically on the mesial half of the buccal surface (buccal views).

f. Root furcations are nearer to the crown with little or no root trunk compared to secondary molars (buccal views).

g. Roots are thin, slender, and widely spread (buccal views).

Additional Characteristics Unique to Primary Maxillary Second Molars (which most closely resemble the permanent [secondary] maxillary first molars)

h. Mesiolingual corner of the occlusal surface is compressed toward the distal (occlusal views).

i. Primary mesiobuccal cusp is about equal in size to the mesiolingual cusp compared to permanent or secondary teeth, where the mesiolingual cusp is larger than the mesiobuccal cusp (occlusal views).

Additional Characteristics Unique to Primary Mandibular Second Molars (which most closely resemble the permanent [secondary] mandibular first molars)

j. The three buccal cusps are of nearly equal size versus permanent first molars, where the distal cusp is usually considerably smaller (buccal views).

Additional Characteristics Unique to Primary Maxillary First Molars (which, from the occlusal view, somewhat resemble permanent maxillary premolars)

k. There are often four cusps: two larger cusps (like a maxillary premolar), the mesiobuccal cusp (1) widest and longest and the mesiolingual cusp (2) the smaller but sharpest; and two smaller cusps, the distobuccal (3) and the inconspicuous, sometimes absent, distolingual (4) (occlusal views; see corresponding numbered cusps).

l. A notch (distal to center) divides the large mesiobuccal cusp from the indistinct distobuccal cusp (buccal views).

m. The crown is wider faciolingually than mesiodistally like a maxillary *pre*molar (occlusal views).

n. The mesial marginal ridge is directed distolingually (occlusal views).

o. There are three fossae: a large mesial triangular fossa, a medium central fossa, and a minute distal fossa (occlusal views).

p. The grooves form an "H" pattern (somewhat similar to a maxillary premolar) (not labeled with a letter; seen on occlusal views).

Additional Unique Characteristics of Primary Mandibular First Molars (resembling no other tooth)

q. The mesial marginal ridge is overdeveloped, almost resembling a cusp (buccal and occlusal views).

r. The occlusal table is wider mesiodistally than buccolingually like secondary (permanent) mandibular molars (occlusal views).

s. The mesial surface converges to the lingual with an acute and prominent mesiobuccal angle of the occlusal table (occlusal views).

t. The mesiobuccal cusp is the largest and longest cusp, covering nearly two-thirds of the buccal surface (occlusal views), but is not wide buccolingually (occlusal views).

u. A pronounced transverse ridge runs between the mesiobuccal and mesiolingual cusp (occlusal views).

v. The occlusal table is larger distal to the transverse ridge with a larger distal fossa and a smaller mesial triangular fossa (no central fossa) (occlusal views).

Index

Page numbers in *italics* indicate figure; page numbers followed by t indicate table; those followed by cp indicate color plate.

A

Abducent nerve, 51t
Abfraction, 427, *427*, 440
Abrasion, 426–427, *427*, 440
Abuse and neglect, forensic dentistry in, 487–488, *488*
Abutment teeth, defined, 461
Access openings, for endodontics, 310, *310*, 316
Accessory (extra) root, 419, *419*, 421
Acoustic, defined, 8
Acoustic meatus
  external, *14*, 15
  internal, 15, *15*
Adult dentition (*See also* Permanent teeth)
  defined, 324
Afferent (sensory) nerves, 50
  facial nerve, 60–61
  glossopharyngeal nerve, 61
  to tongue, 62–63
  trigeminal nerve, 50
Air-abrasion system, 448
Alveolar artery
  anterior superior, *67*, 68
  inferior, 65, *67*
  middle superior, *67*, 68
  posterior superior, *67*, 68
Alveolar bone, in periodontal health, 281–282
Alveolar canals, 19, *20*
Alveolar eminences, 17–18, *20*
Alveolar mucosa, *104*, 105
Alveolar nerve
  anterior superior, 54, *55*
    local anesthetic technique for, 83, *85–86*
  inferior, 56, *57*, *58*
    local anesthetic technique for, 95–96, *96–98*
  middle superior, 54, *55*
    local anesthetic technique for, 83, *85–86*
  posterior superior, 53, *55*
    local anesthetic technique for, 83, *84–85*
Alveolar process, *17*, 17–18, *20*
  oral examination of, 103
Alveolar vein, inferior, 68, *68*
Alveolingual sulcus, 100, *101*
Alveolus (alveoli), 6, 17

Amalgam, restoration materials, 444–445, *445*, 450, 453
Ameloclasts, 115
Amelogenesis imperfecta, 22cp, 423, *424*
American Academy of Forensic Sciences (AAFS), 481
Anatomic crown
  defined, *115*, 116
  morphology of, 120–129
Anatomic root
  defined, *115*, 116
  morphology of, 129, *130*
Anesthetic injections
  anterior superior alveolar nerve, 83, *85–86*
  general technique for, 82
  greater palatine nerve, 91–92, *93*
  inferior alveolar nerve, 95–96, *96–98*
  infraorbital nerve, 83, *87*
  long buccal nerve, 88–89, *89–90*
  middle superior alveolar nerve, 83, *85–86*
  nasopalatine nerve, 91, *92–93*
  posterior superior alveolar nerve, 83, *84–85*
Angle, Dr. Edward H., *360*, 360–361
Angular artery, 65, *67*
Angular spine, *12*, 13
Anguli, defined, 38
Ankylosis, 423
  defined, 363
Anodontia
  partial, *404*, 404–405, *405*
  total, 404
Anomalies, 403–429
  anodontia, *404*, 404–405, *405*
  crown, 409–416
    fusion, 411, *411*, *412*
    Hutchinson's teeth, 411, *413*
    lingual cusps, 413
    peg-shaped lateral incisor, 409, *409–410*
    third molar, 409
    tubercles, 413, *413*, *414*, *415*, 415–416
    twinning, 410, *410–411*
  defined, 403
  dentin dysplasia, 425–426
  enamel dysplasia, 24cp, 423–424

root, 416–421
  accessory roots, 419, *419*, 421
  concrescence, 418, *418*
  dens in dente, 417, *418*
  dilaceration, 417, *417*, *418*
  dwarfed, *416*, 418
  hypercementosis, 418, *419*
  supernumerary teeth, 406, *407–409*, 409
  in tooth position, 421–423
    ankylosis, 423
    impacted, 421, *422*
    rotation, 421, *423*
    transposition, 421, *422*
  tooth size, 416, *416*
  unusual dentitions, 428–429, 429
Antemortem, defined, 482
Antemortem records
  for human identification, 482, *483–485*
  in mass disasters, 492–493, *492–493*
Anterior arch, 94
Anterior deprogramming, 388, *389*, *390*, 394–395, *395*
Anterior guidance, 374, *375*
Anterior protected articulation, 374, *375*
Anterior superior alveolar artery, *67*, 68
Anterior superior alveolar nerve, 54, *55*
  local anesthetic technique for, 83, *85–86*
Anterior teeth, 4
Anteroposterior curve, 130, *132*
Anthropology, forensic, 481, 494–495, *495*
Antrum, 19–20, *20*
Aperture, defined, 7
Apex, of root, 129, *130*
Apical foramen, 116, 304
Apical foramina, of root, 129, *130*
Arteries, 65, *67*, 68
  flow of blood to teeth, *66*
  to mandible, 65
  to maxillae, 65, 68
  to muscles, 65
Articular disc, 32, 33–34
Articular eminence, 13, *14*, *30*
Articular fossa, 13, *14*, *30*, 32–33